Handbuch der experimentellen Pharmakologie

Vol. 42 Heffter-Heubner New Series

Handbook of Experimental Pharmacology

Neuromuscular Junction

Contributors

Ruth E. M. Bowden · B. Collier · R. D. Dripps
L. W. Duchen · G. E. Hale Enderby · B. L. Ginsborg
S. Head · F. Hobbiger · D. H. Jenkinson
F. C. MacIntosh · Jennifer Maclagan · S. E. Smith
Eleanor Zaimis

Editor

Eleanor Zaimis

Assistant Editor

Jennifer Maclagan

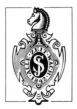

Springer-Verlag Berlin   Heidelberg   New York 1976

ELEANOR ZAIMIS, Prof., MD., F.R.C.P., Royal Free Hospital, School of Medicine, University of London, London/Great Britain

With 194 Figures

ISBN 3-540-07499-6 Springer-Verlag Berlin Heidelberg New York
ISBN 0-387-07499-6 Springer-Verlag New York Heidelberg Berlin

Library of Congress Cataloging in Publication Data. Main entry under title: Neuromuscular junction. (Handbook of experimental pharmacology: New series; v. 42). Includes bibliographies and indexes. 1. Neuromuscular blocking agents. 2. Myoneural junction. 3. Neuromuscular transmission. I. Bowden, Ruth E. M. II. Zaimis, Eleanor. III. Series: Handbuch der experimentellen Pharmakologie: New series; Bd. 42. [DNLM: 1. Neuromuscular junction–Drug effects. 2. Neuromuscular blocking agents–Pharmacodynamics. 3. Cholinesterase inhibitors–Pharmacodynamics.
Library of Congress Cataloging in Publication Data. QV34 H236 v. 42] QP905.H3 Bd. 42 [RM312] 615'.1'08s 76-1957 ISBN 0-387-07499-6 [615'.77]

Foreword

Has the neuromuscular junction been over-exposed or is it perhaps already a closed book? I asked myself this at a recent International Congress when an American colleague complained that the Journal of Physiology had articles on nothing but the neuromuscular junction, while another colleague asked why I was editing a volume on a subject about which everything was already known. It is worrying to think that these views may be shared by other people. I hope that this volume will convince my two colleagues and other readers that the neuromuscular junction is very much alive and continues to attract the interest of many workers from a variety of fields; strange as it may seem, the synapse between a motor nerve ending and muscle fibre, with its relatively simple architecture, is one of the most interesting sites in the body—I do hope we have done it justice.

The various chapters of this volume present a cross section of knowledge as viewed by a group of 13 individuals, actively engaged in research. Multi-author volumes such as this are frequently criticised on the grounds that chapters or sections overlap. I believe that such criticium is only valid where the overlap is repetitious. Where it results in the reader having available discussions of material from differing stand-points, overlap becomes a valuable feature of this type of publication.

My co-authors have taken time from their busy lives to survey their fields of interest; for this I am greatly indebted to each. For them and for myself I wish to thank those colleagues and publishers who have allowed us to reproduce illustrations previously published elsewhere.

I am delighted to record my deep appreciation of the competence and cheerfulness with which my secretary, JAN COLES, has borne the heavy burden of her additional duties. My heartfelt thanks to PETER UPTON for reading the manuscripts and commenting on our English, and to my colleague, RON OWEN, who has helped me in so many ways, especially with the bibliographic references. I also wish to express my gratitude to the Publishers in the persons of their representatives Mr. W. BERGSTEDT, Mrs. I. FISCHER, Mrs. TH. DEIGMÖLLER and last but not least Mr. E. ERFLING, whose patience and skilled work have facilitated the metamorphosis of our manuscripts into a fine handbook.

Unfortunately I have to end on a sad note—the loss of a good friend and colleague, Dr. ROBERT DRIPPS. BOB DRIPPS was a brilliant anaesthetist and in his life was responsible for so much in clinical research, academic administration and the training of young anaesthetists from all over the world. We are honoured to have among the contributions of this volume what I am told is the last article he wrote.

February, 1976   ELEANOR ZAIMIS

Table of Contents

CHAPTER 2

Neurochemistry of Cholinergic Terminals. F. C. MacIntosh and B. Collier
With 12 Figures

CHAPTER 3

Transmission of Impulses from Nerve to Muscle. B. L. GINSBORG and D. H. JENKINSON
With 36 Figures

CHAPTER 4A

Depolarising Neuromuscular Blocking Drugs. ELEANOR ZAIMIS and S. HEAD
With 35 Figures

CHAPTER 4B

Competitive Neuromuscular Blocking Drugs. JENNIFER MACLAGAN
With 14 Figures

CHAPTER 4C

Pharmacology of Anticholinesterase Drugs. F. HOBBIGER
With 25 Figures

CHAPTER 5A

The Clinician Looks at Neuromuscular Blocking Drugs. R. D. DRIPPS

CHAPTER 5B

Neuromuscular Blocking Drugs in Man. S. E. SMITH
With 28 Figures

CHAPTER 5C

Twenty Years' Experience with Decamethonium. G. E. HALE ENDERBY
With 4 Figures

List of Contributors

RUTH E. M. BOWDEN, D.Sc., F.R.C.S.Eng., Professor of Anatomy, University of London, Royal Free Hospital School of Medicine, London, WC1N 1BP

B. COLLIER, Ph.D., Associate Professor, Department of Pharmacology, McGill University, Montreal, P.Q., Canada

R. D. DRIPPS†, M.D., University of Pennsylvania, 110 College Hall, Philadelphia, P A. 19174, USA

L. W. DUCHEN, M.D., Ph.D., D.C.P., F.R.C.Path., Professor of Experimental Neuropathology, University of London, Institute of Psychiatry and Maudsley Hospital, London, SE5

G. E. HALE ENDERBY, M.B., B.Chir., F.F.A.R.C.S.Eng., Senior Consultant Anaesthetist, Queen Victoria Hospital, East Grinstead, Sussex RH19 3DZ

B. L. GINSBORG, Ph.D., Reader in Pharmacology, University of Edinburgh Medical School, Edinburg EH8 9JZ

S. HEAD, Ph. D., Lecturer in Pharmacology, Royal Free Hospital School of Medicine, London, WC1N 1BP

F. HOBBIGER, M.D., Ph.D., D.Sc., Professor of Pharmacology, University of London, Middlesex Hospital Medical School, London W1P 7PN

D. H. JENKINSON, Ph.D., Reader in Pharmacology, University College London, London WC1

F. C. MACINTOSH, F.R.S., M.A., Ph.D., Professor of Physiology, McGill University, Montreal, P.Q., Canada

JENNIFER MACLAGAN, Ph.D., Senior Lecturer in Pharmacology, Royal Free Hospital School of Medicine, London WC1N 1BP

S. E. SMITH, D.M., Ph.D., Reader in Applied Pharmacology and Therapeutics, St. Thomas's Hospital Medical School, London SE1

ELEANOR ZAIMIS, M.D., F.R.C.P., Professor of Pharmacology, University of London, Royal Free Hospital School of Medicine, London, WC1N 1BP

The Neuromuscular Junction: Areas of Uncertainty

ELEANOR ZAIMIS

During a Symposium in Philadelphia in 1954, Sir HENRY DALE discussed the beginnings of chemical transmission and told us that before Otto Loewi's discovery in 1921 the general climate of physiological opinion still remained hesitant and sceptical. "Transmission by chemical mediators" Sir HENRY DALE said "was like a lady with whom the neurophysiologist was willing to live and to consort in private, but with whom he was reluctant to be seen in public". Progress since then has been more than spectacular, and today nobody doubts that the transmission from motor nerve to skeletal muscle is chemical and that the transmitter substance is acetylcholine. After its release the acetylcholine diffuses across the synaptic gap and acts on a component of the post-synaptic membrane, the so-called acetylcholine receptor. The molecular properties of these receptors at the neuromuscular junction have been intensively studied during the last three years and the evidence that they exist as actual chemical substances is now quite strong[1].

In a survey of the literature belonging to the field of neuromuscular junction, one comes across a degree of disagreement between the results of various investigators, and especially between results obtained in man and those reported from animal experiments. Having edited a volume containing results obtained from both animals and man and from both isolated muscle preparations and experiments *in vivo*, it seems almost an obligation to indicate some aspects which may be of special significance for work in man, and also to consider certain variations in results and conclusions which may be the product of experimental conditions.

Neuromuscular Block by Prolonged Depolarisation

There is strong evidence that in the cat and man decamethonium and suxamethonium produce a neuromuscular block by prolonged depolarisation. This comes from analyses of the pharmacological characteristics[2] of the blockade *in vivo* and from

---

[1] Some of this work has been discussed in Chapters 2 and 3, but no attempt has been made to include a special section in the present volume. Fortunately, H.P.RANG has just published (1975) a most excellent and comprehensive review on "Acetylcholine receptors".

[2] You may wonder why in 1975 I still discuss "characteristics" based on pharmacological data. The reason is, that if various results are put together, one cannot help reaching the conclusion that for an analysis of drug action, pharmacological reactions *still* provide very fine tools. Drug reactions in the intact animal or man are, undoubtedly, a good indication of differences which determine the properties of various excitable membranes, properties which must be at the molecular level. Morphological studies or electrophysiological techniques alone have often proved unable to differentiate structures which differ profoundly in their functional properties. It is well known, for example, that many pharmacologically distinct varieties of membranes can all generate similar types of electrical responses.

electrophysiological analyses either *in vivo*, based on measurements of end-plate depolarisation by means of external electrodes, or *in vitro* by studying the effects of depolarising drugs on the electrical properties of single muscle cells (see Chapter 4 A).

Depolarising neuromuscular blocking drugs were first described in 1948. Twenty-eight years later investigations of their actions still produce contradictory results and controversial interpretations of those results. These drugs mimic acetylcholine in their action. Acetylcholine, however, under physiological conditions makes contact with the post-synaptic membrane for an extremely short period of time and therefore at the end of its action the motor end-plate and the surrounding membrane return to their normal state. With acetylcholine in the presence of an anticholinesterase drug the process is far from being a short one any more. STEPHEN KUFFLER[3] gave recently a very elegant description of the action of acetylcholine on the post-synaptic membrane in the presence or absence of an anticholinesterase drug: "A nerve impulse", he said "releases approximately 300 quanta. These act independently of each other and the post-synpatic currents generated by each quantum sum in a linear manner. This functional isolation of quanta is brought about by AChE which hydrolyses ACh molecules immediately after they have interacted with receptors. On the average, ionic gates are opened only once for about 1 msec, and the diffusion of ACh within the synaptic cleft is severely limited, to an area less than $2\,\mu m^2$. In contrast, when AChE is inhibited, quanta are free to diffuse within the clefts, so that they cover overlapping areas and react repeatedly on the receptors. This leads to a prolongation of synpatic currents; under such conditions quanta interact and potentiate each other's synaptic effect. This post-synaptic potentiation is a result of the non-linear properties of receptors whose responses vary with the concentration of ACh."

Drugs such as decamethonium and suxamethonium persist at the neuromuscular junction for a longer time and produce a long-lasting interruption of neuromuscular transmission. A neuromuscular block by prolonged depolarisation of the end-plate, however, presents a complex picture, for a sequence of excitation followed by depression of transmission is always detectable. The depolarisation, although limited to the end-plate region, spreads slightly beyond the area in which end-plate potentials can normally be recorded, the extent of this spread of depolarisation increasing with time (BURNS and PATON, 1951). The manifestations of this sequence vary with different species and with different muscles in the same species so that the same process may give rise to a situation in which either repetitive firing, or contracture or block of transmission predominates.

During a prolonged depolarisation of the end-plate region the muscle may lose significant amounts of potassium and gain significant amounts of sodium, calcium and chloride. The ionic concentrations, therefore, on either side of the muscle fibre must be significantly altered. The implications of these changes on the state of block are not simple, but it is clear that the reaction of the end-plate and of the muscle membrane adjacent to the end-plate will be radically conditioned by them. These rather "unphysiological" changes produced by a prolonged depolarisation reduce

---

[3] In a paper presented in Cambridge (September, 1975) during the "Sir Henry Dale Centennial Symposium" on "Post-synaptic actions of neurotransmitters".

the functional reserve at the neuromuscular junction and therefore the motor end-plate region becomes "vulnerable" to the actions of other drugs or to high frequencies of stimulation or to further high and prolonged exposure to depolarising drugs.

"Considering the two processes of neuromuscular block (a) competition with acetylcholine, (b) depolarisation, it may be said that study of a block produced by long-lasting depolarisation has provided a great deal of information not accessible through the study of a block produced by competition with acetylcholine. However, while the interpretation of results obtained with a competitive substance is relatively straight-forward, since the response of skeletal muscles to such substances is apparently uniform, the handling of a depolarising substance, or of a substance having a depolarising element, is much more difficult and the interpretation of the results obtained from different species and from different muscles needs great care. One other point should perhaps be considered, i.e. whether the classical definition of a neuromuscular blocking substance can be applied to substances blocking by long-lasting depolarisation. This definition requires that the substance should leave the nerve and muscle fibre unaffected. Information, however, is accumulating which indicates that a muscle cannot be subjected to repeated depolarisation without suffering some harm."

This question I myself posed as long ago as 1954, in a talk which I then gave in Philadelphia. After more than twenty-five years of experience with depolarising drugs in both animals and man, I consider that the problem is still with us.

Desensitisation

THESLEFF (1955a, b) questioned the existence of a block due solely to depolarisation and put forward the view that a major part of the block produced by decamethonium or suxamethonium was due to desensitisation even in the intact animal. Using various isolated muscle preparations he found that during the application of either acetylcholine, decamethonium or suxamethonium the motor end-plate region became depolarised, but after a few seconds this initial depolarising effect disappeared and the muscle membrane repolarised. This development of repolarisation in the continued presence of the depolarising drug was called desensitisation (or "receptor inactivation" by NASTUK et al., 1966) and was defined by ELMQVIST and THESLEFF (1962) as "a condition in which application of a depolarising drug has made chemoreceptors of the end-plate refractory to chemical stimulation". Since then this phenomenon of desensitisation has been widely studied and discussed (for further details, see Chapter 3; MICHELSON and ZEIMAL, 1973; RANG, 1975). Reading through the literature, however, one becomes aware that "desensitisation" means different things to different scientists. For example, there are pharmacologists and clinicians who describe as a "desensitisation" blockade, an interruption of neuromuscular transmission which is easily antagonised by anticholinesterase drugs or by a tetanus, and potentiated by tubocurarine. Others use the term desensitisation to refer to the reduced sensitivity to acetylcholine produced by drugs competing with it. These last two instances, however, are quite different from the phenomenon described as desensitisation by THESLEFF and his colleagues.

While desensitisation has been described by many workers in the course of *in vitro* experiments, we have always found that it is not a normal phenomenon in the whole animal or man. At the end of periods in excess of two hours, during which the muscles were kept paralysed with a continuous infusion of suxamethonium, the neuromuscular block still exhibits the well-known characteristics of a depolarisation block. Thus, anticholinesterase drugs are ineffective or deepen the block, while tubo-curarine antagonises it (ZAIMIS, 1959, 1962; CANNARD and ZAIMIS, 1959; MACLA-GAN, 1962; PATON and WAUD, 1962; DOUGLAS and PATON, 1954).

There are other findings which underline the mechanism of action of decame-thonium and suxamethonium in the intact animal and man. Temperature increases the magnitude and especially the duration of a block produced by a depolarising drug. In contrast, cooling reduces the magnitude of a block produced by tubocurar-ine. One of the consequences of the long-lasting depolarisation produced by decame-thonium and suxamethonium is an efflux of potassium from the depolarised area of the muscle cell. In both man and animals it was found that the amount of potassium released during a suxamethonium block is sufficient to raise the plasma potassium level. In patients with severe burns or with extensive injuries to soft tissues, an almost lethal efflux of potassium has been found after the administration of suxamethonium (for details, see Chapters 4 A and 5 B).

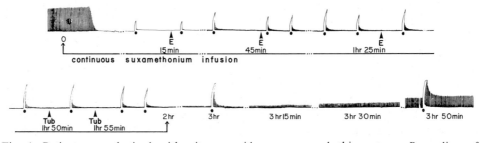

Fig. 1. Patient anaesthetised with nitrous oxide, oxygen and thiopentone. Recording of maximal twitches from the tibialis anterior muscle in response to indirect stimula-tion delivered one per 10 sec. At (E), edrophonium 5 mg I.V.; at (Tub), tubocurarine 4 mg I.V.; at (●), tetani 30 Hz for 10 sec. Total amount of suxamethonium, 1100 mg. Muscle temperature 37 to 38° C throughout. (From: CANNARD and ZAIMIS, 1959 — unpublished results)

Occasionally, when large concentrations of a depolarising drug are administered for long periods of time, a degree of desensitisation can be found. Dr. CANNARD and I came across one case in which the suxamethonium block had some of the charac-teristics of a true desensitisation block. This is illustrated in Fig. 1. The patient was anaesthetised with nitrous oxide, oxygen and thiopentone, and suxamethonium was administered in the form of a slow intravenous infusion. A few minutes after the beginning of the infusion the muscles of the patient became completely paralysed and remained paralysed not only for the two hours during which the drug was infused but also for a further one and a half hours after the infusion was stopped. The total amount of suxamethonium administered was 1100 mg. As Fig. 1 shows, the neuromuscular block did not respond to either edrophonium or tubocurarine. In most of the other clinical cases referred to in the literature as due to a desensitisation blockade, the paralysis was readily antagonised by anticholinesterase drugs and potentiated by tubocurarine.

That desensitisation cannot be a normal phenomenon is also shown by the finding that in isolated preparations it "may occur with acetylcholine concentrations that are within the range of concentrations normally produced at the end-plate by a motor nerve impulse" (ELMQVIST and THESLEFF, 1962). If such a situation were to occur in the intact animal, the margin of safety would be so narrow as to render transmission from motor nerve to skeletal muscle almost completely ineffective. THESLEFF (1959, 1961) also suggested that the block of neuromuscular transmission caused by high frequency stimulation of the motor nerve is caused by desensitisation of the end-plate receptors. OTSUKA et al. (1962) showed, however, that repeated stimulation of the motor nerve could significantly reduced the size of the e.p.p., while the sensitivity of the motor end-plate to the ionophoretically applied acetylcholine remained completely unchanged. They concluded, therefore, that the main cause of neuromuscular block during repeated stimulation was a gradual reduction of the amount of acetylcholine released by the nerve endings—in other words a pre-synaptic and not a post-synaptic change.

Nobody can deny the existence of desensitisation, but its importance has been exaggerated. Even in isolated muscle preparations, desensitisation is a concentration-dependent phenomenon. Differences in drug concentration might therefore explain the very substantial differences between the results of our own experiments and those of THESLEFF and his group. Using the same species (cat) and the same isolated muscle (tenuissimus) we were able to demonstrate a well-maintained depolarisation to acetylcholine, decamethonium and suxamethonium, while in the experiments of THESLEFF and his colleagues depolarisation was short-lived and desensitisation was put forward as the mechanism behind the neuromuscular block. In our experiments the concentration of the depolarising drug was very similar to that necessary to produce an almost complete block in the intact animal. In this way unnecessarily large concentrations were avoided. In contrast, in the studies of Thesleff and his colleagues the depolarising drugs were applied either ionophoretically or in concentrations much larger than those necessary to produce an interruption of neuromuscular transmission (see Chapter 4 A for details).

Scientists are interested in desensitisation because of the belief that the phenomenon may lead to an understanding of drug effects at molecular level. But they have a produce the right "atmosphere" for desensitisation to flourish: i.e. high concentrations of the depolarising drug, long or repeated applications, incubation of the receptor material with acetylcholine or other acetylcholine-like substance. In other words, it is almost a "hand-made" event, an experimental tool which can be useful in certain studies. Its importance in the intact animal or man is only marginal and it is a great pity that occasionally the terms "depolarising" and "desensitising" are used as synonyms to describe a neuromuscular blocking drug.

The Clinical Picture

In the 1960's certain confusing terms began to be used to describe the mechanism of action of depolarising neuromuscular blocking drugs in man.

"Initially, succinylcholine produces a depolarizing neuromuscular block. With increasing dosage and time, the block becomes non-depolarizing. There are at least three possible different names for the latter condition. One term is *Phase II* block. In this terminology, the Phase I block is synonymous with depolarization, and the Phase II block is sometimes referred to as Phase II, non-depolarizing. Another term which has been applied to this situation is *dual block*. A third term is *desensitization block*." (CHURCHILL-DAVIDSON and KATZ, 1966).

Three years later, KATZ and RYAN (1969) summed up the then existing situation as follows:

"The results and interpretation of previous studies have raised questions concerning the nature of the block, depolarizing (phase I) or desensitizing (phase II), produced by suxamethonium. One extreme is that the block is always depolarizing even with doses as large as 1000 mg (WHITE, 1963). Others have suggested that the block is initially depolarizing but changes to desensitizing: (a) in all patients (FOLDES et al., 1957); (b) in some patients after large doses of 500 to 1500 mg (CHURCHILL-DAVIDSON et al., 1960); (c) in most or all patients after small doses of 100 to 300 mg (KATZ et al., 1963; CRUL et al., 1966); or (d) in some patients depending upon how the drug is given (WALTS and DILLON, 1967). The other extreme is that the block is always desensitizing even with the first small dose (DE JONG and FREUND, 1967)."

In 1973, KATZ reviewed once more the situation in the clinical field and wrote:

"The effects of suxamethonium and tubocurarine on neuromuscular transmission in man were once regarded as simple. The block produced by tubocurarine was non-depolarizing and characterized by the presence of: (1) fade; (2) post-tetanic potentiation; and (3) antagonism by cholinesterase inhibitors. The block initially produced by suxamethonium was depolarizing and was characterized by the absence of: (1) fade; (2) post-tetanic potentiation; and (3) antagonism by cholinesterase inhibitors. With sufficient dosage and the passage of time the suxamethonium block came to resemble the tubocurarine block and was labelled desensitizing (dual, mixed, phase II non-depolarizing)."

KATZ (1973) concluded that the marked variation in the response of patients to neuromuscular blocking drugs possibly depends upon many factors such as: "muscle studied, rate of stimulation, the anaesthetic technique employed, the degree of block and whether electrical or mechanical responses were recorded". Before discussing the importance of these various factors let us see why our clinical colleagues have felt the need to use so many terms to describe a neuromuscular block produced by suxamethonium or decamethonium in man.

Reports on suxamethonium written in the fifties were full of praise for it as a neuromuscular blocking drug. For example, FOLDES et al. in 1952 wrote:

"The advantages of suxamethonium are its easy controllability; the absence of apnoea during, and of prolonged respiratory depression following, its administration; and the paucity of side-effects which accompany its use". Similarly, RICHARDS and YOUNGMAN (1952) found no side-effects "whatever" and described the recovery from a suxamethonium block as rapid, the time from the first sign of spontaneous respiration to full normality of all reflexes as being no more than a few minutes. Moreover, a quick recovery was found not only after a single dose but also after slow intravenous infusions.

Thus, during this period the advantages claimed were absence of any secondary effects and quick recovery of full muscle tone and reflex activity. At the same time, the block produced by decamethonium and suxamethonium was described as having all the characteristics of a depolarisation blockade: muscle fasciculations preceded the block; during a partial block a tetanus gave rise to a well-sustained contraction of the muscle and did not antagonise the block; anticholinesterase drugs were ineffective or potentiated the block; the action of competitive and depolarising drugs remained antagonistic.

Reviewing the literature of the last 25 years it becomes obvious that the pattern of neuromuscular block produced by depolarising drugs when administered to anaesthetised patients has changed. Slow recovery from a suxamethonium block and prolonged apnoea are now often present. At the same time the characteristics of the blockade appear to be different: a tetanus is not well-sustained and is followed by some recovery of the block; anticholinesterase drugs antagonise the block; competitive neuromuscular blocking drugs potentiate the block.

What is the reason for this changing pattern? The type of general anaesthetic used appears to me the most probable candidate. If one takes all the clinical results together it becomes clear that in unanaesthetised patients, or in those anaesthetised with nitrous oxide, oxygen and thiopentone, suxamethonium produces a neuromuscular block having all the characteristics of a depolarisation block. When, however, halothane or other fluorinated anaesthetics such as enflurane, isoflurane, Forane, are used to maintain anaesthesia the classical characteristics of a depolarisation block disappear. Table 1 refers to some publications which were chosen because the results described were based on actual measurements of events taking place at the neuromuscular junction.

Table 1. *The changing pattern of neuromuscular block produced by suxamethonium and decamethonium in man*

Anaesthesia	Suxamethonium and decamethonium	References
Without fluorinated anaesthetics (only nitrous oxide, oxygen, thiopentone) or in conscious volunteers	Muscle fasciculations precede the block; during a partial block a tetanus gives rise to a well-sustained contraction and does not antagonise the block; anticholinesterase drugs are ineffective or potentitate the block; the action of competitive and depolarising drugs remains antagonistic	CHURCHILL-DAVIDSON and RICHARDSON (1952) CANNARD and ZAIMIS (1959) ALI *et al.* (1970) MILLER and WAY (1971)
With fluorinated anaesthetics (halothane, enflurane, isoflurane, Forane)	Tetanus is not well-sustained and is followed by some recovery of the block; anticholinesterase drugs antagonise the block; competitive neuromuscular blocking drugs potentiate the block	GISSEN *et al.* (1966) CRUL *et al.* (1966) DE JONG and FREUND (1967) KATZ and RYAN (1969) FOGDALL and MILLER (1975)

The use of large doses of suxamethonium has played a part in the appearance of abnormal responses in man. For example, CHURCHILL-DAVIDSON (1961) reported that "with small doses of either suxamethonium or decamethonium both slow and fast rates of stimulation were well maintained and there was complete absence of post-tetanic facilitation. In contrast, when large or repeated doses of a depolarising drug were administered there was a gradual change in the pattern of the neuromuscular block until it finally resembled that seen after tubocurarine." The first signs of this change in pattern could be recognised after 500 to 1500 mg suxamethonium and after 6 to 20 mg of decamethonium. The author makes clear, however, that "a deliberate attempt was made to produce the signs of a full dual block. Occasionally" he adds, "to our bitter disappointment, the surgeon finished the operation before this goal could be achieved!"

That general anaesthetics can alter the response of the neuromuscular junction to drugs has been known for many years. For example, BROWN et al. (1936) had reported that ether raised the threshold of cat muscle to acetylcholine and abolished the repetitive response of the muscle to single nerve shocks after eserine. In 1960, FOLDES reviewed the effects of general anaesthetic agents in man and wrote:

"Of the commonly used inhalation anaesthetic agents, ether, chloroform and halothane influence the pharmacologic effects of relaxant drugs most markedly. The effect of cyclopropane is considerably less and that of nitrous oxide and of ethylene in clinically used concentrations is negligible. In general, inhalation anesthetic agents potentiate the neuromuscular effects of nondepolarizing drugs; those of depolarizing compounds are either not affected or are antagonized by ether or halothane."

Since then, many other reports have appeared but the discussion has concentrated on the ability of the general anaesthetic to increase, decrease or leave unchanged the magnitude and/or the duration of action of a neuromuscular blocking drug.

There is also evidence that the direct action of some anaesthetics on neuromuscular transmission, particularly the fluorinated ones, is by no means negligible. In patients anaesthetised with Forane (MILLER et al., 1971) and with enflurane or isoflurane (FOGDALL and MILLER, 1975) the muscles were unable to sustain a tetanus at more than 100 to 120 Hz. The effect was dose-related. Higher frequencies of stimulation could be maintained in the presence of halothane (MILLER et al., 1971; KATZ, 1971). ALI et al. (1970) showed, however, that halothane anaesthesia affected the mechanical response of the muscle even at low frequencies of stimulation. In patients anaesthetised with nitrous oxide there was no evidence of "fade" when stimulating at 2 Hz for 2 sec. In contrast, during halothane anaesthesia fade was present. COHEN et al. (1970) studied the effects of cyclopropane, diethyl ether, methoxyflurane and Ethrane in man. During a control period of nitrous oxide anaesthesia, tetanus was well maintained when elicited at a frequency of 30 and 300 Hz. During the administration of the other four anaesthetics, while a tetanus was sustained when elicited by a stimulus of 30 Hz, definite fade was evident in each of the patients examined when a 300 Hz tetanus was applied. This effect of Ethrane was also demonstrated by LEBOWITZ et al. (1970).

When PATON and I described the pharmacological actions of the methonium compounds for the first time, we gave the following description of the effect of ether on the neuromuscular block induced by decamethonium:

"With ether, decamethonium was less effective than with chloralose. Potentiation of the twitch and fasciculations were never seen, even with only feebly paralysing doses. Sparing of respiration was much less prominent than in the animal anaesthetized with chloralose. Tetani were sustained very poorly, as with d-tubocurarine chloride." (PATON and ZAIMIS, 1949).

As far as I am aware, this is the first observation of an anaesthetic actually changing the mechanism of action of a neuromuscular blocking drug. What we observed in the cat under ether anaesthesia is what happens in the anaesthetised man, particularly when fluorinated anaesthetics are used to maintain anaesthesia. We must infer, therefore, that in the presence of a particular type of anaesthetic agent a *change* takes place in the muscle membrane, a change which alters the mechanism of action of a depolarising drug.

Obviously this effect of fluorinated anaesthetics has played an important role and has clouded and confused the clinical picture, thus forcing the anaesthetist to borrow the terminology introduced by the animal worker—terminology based on results obtained from different animal species and from both *in vitro* and *in vivo* muscle preparations.

We have already discussed in some detail the phenomenon of "desensitisation", the conditions under which it is produced in isolated muscle preparations and how unlikely it is to have in man, or in the intact animal, a blockade produced only "by desensitisation".

Terms "phase I" and "phase II" have been borrowed by our clinical colleagues from a "two-phase" action of decamethonium which was described in isolated muscle preparations such as the rabbit lumbrical muscle, the guinea-pig diaphragm and human intercostal muscle (see Chapter 4A for details and references). The first phase consists of neuromuscular block of rapid onset which reaches a maximum in 4 to 6 min and then recovers spontaneously in spite of the continued presence of decamethonium in the same concentration. Maximum recovery occurs in 15 to 30 min, after which the second phase begins. This consists of a slowly progressing neuromuscular block which reaches a steady state after 3 to 6 hrs, and "remains constant for hours if undisturbed" (JENDEN, 1955). Suxamethonium and carbachol produce effects qualitatively similar to those of decamethonium. After 25 µg of neostigmine, acetylcholine also produces a similar action.

It appears, therefore, that attempts to express and explain effects occurring in man in terms of actions produced in isolated muscle preparations, immersed for hours in a solution containing a depolarising drug, can bring only confusion. A muscle separated from the body and kept for long periods of time in a "physiological" solution becomes pharmacologically a continuously changing piece of tissue while a muscle studied *in vivo* with its normal circulation intact is spared this gradual deterioration. So, as far as the animal studies are concerned, I feel that those that are most revealing for the anaesthetist are those which come closest to the conditions under which the drugs are being used clinically.

It is unfortunate that the term "dual" mode of action, which originally had a very precise meaning is now widely used in a number of different senses. The term was introduced (ZAIMIS, 1953) because the study of the effects produced by neuromuscular blocking drugs in various mammalian species had led to the discovery that whereas the response of all mammalian skeletal muscles to competitive neuromuscular blocking drugs is uniform, the response to depolarising drugs is not. As we have already seen, decamethonium and suxamethonium block neuromuscular transmission in man and cat by prolonged depolarisation. In many mammals, however, including the monkey, dog, rabbit, hare (ZAIMIS, 1953) and guinea-pig (HALL and PARKES, 1953) it was found that the two drugs initially exhibit a depolarising action but during the blocking process their action changes into that of a substance competing with acetylcholine. An analysis of the characteristics of the dual block shows that it has two components, one due to the initial 'acetylcholine-like' action, the other to a 'curare-like action (ZAIMIS, 1953). The block is preceded by potentiation of the maximal twitch, a feature peculiar to a substance capable of depolarising the motor endplates. However, a tetanus produced during the block is not well sustained and antagonises it. Finally, the block is deepened by tubocurarine and is readily antagonised by anticholinesterase drugs. In other words, one is confronted with a type of block which has some of the characteristics of a depolarisation block and some of the characteristics of a competitive one. Here it is the muscle membrane itself that is

Table 2. *Varieties of neuromuscular block produced by depolarising drugs*

	Decamethonium and suxamethonium	
Depolarisation block	"Dual block" having two components one depolarising, the other competitive (Zaimis, 1953)	Block *changing* from depolarising to "curare-like" (acutely)
Man: — unanaesthetised or anaesthetised with nitrous oxide and thiopentone Cat Avian muscle	Monkey, dog, rabbit, rat, guinea-pig, *from birth:* — present with first administered dose — no large or repeated doses necessary	Man: — anaesthetised with fluorinated anaesthetics Cat and avian muscle: — in the presence of certain drugs such as mecamylamine or SKF 525A

Desensitiation block (chemosensitivity lost)	Two-phase block (chemosensitivity present)
isolated preparations (very rare in vivo) acetylcholine or other depolarising drugs applied — ionophoretically — bath-applied in large concentrations — prolonged applications	isolated muscle preparations *1st phase:* rapid onset but block recovers spontaneously after which *2nd phase:* slow progressive block which reaches a steady state after 3 to 6 hrs and "remains constant for hours if undisturbed"

Table 3. *Conditions affecting the mechanism of action of suxamethonium in man*

Conditions	Characteristics of the neuromuscular block
Unanaesthetised or in the presence of drugs *not altering* the properties of the post-synaptic membrane	— all the characteristics of a depolarisation block even after repeated administrations or after long intravenous infusion
Diseased muscle (myasthenic patients)	— "dual" block
In the presence of certain general anaesthetics *altering* the properties of the post-synaptic membrane	— block *changing* acutely from depolarising to "curare-like"
With large and repeated doses	— pronounced tachyphylaxis, some desensitisation
With very high frequencies of stimulation (100 to 300 Hz) especially in the presence of certain anaesthetic agents	— anything may happen pre- and/or post-synaptically

different (by birth) from that in the human or in cat muscle. To demonstrate in these species a "dual" mechanism of action, one does not need to give a special anaesthetic or large and repeated doses of decamethonium or suxamethonium. With the first administered dose in monkey, dog, rabbit, hare and rat, a dose not larger than that producing a 90 to 95% neuromuscular block, the characteristics of a dual block are present.

I must admit, however, that of all the terms chosen (desensitisation block, phase I and phase II block) to describe the "changing pattern" of the neuromuscular block by suxamethonium and decamethonium in man in the presence of fluorinated anaesthetics, the most appropriate is "dual" block. This emerges from the information included in Table 2 in which I have attempted to summarise the known varieties of neuromuscular block produced by decamethonium and suxamethonium in different animal species or under differing conditions. In this case, however, dual block is produced because the depolarising drug finds a post-synaptic membrane whose properties have been changed by the presence of the anaesthetic drug. In Table 3 I have attempted to show the conditions which affect the mechanism of action of suxamethonium (or decamethonium) in man.

The Presence of Other Drugs

A *change* in the mechanism of action of depolarising neuromuscular blocking drugs has also been found in animals in the presence of other drugs.

MECAMYLAMINE

(a) *Mecamylamine* was introduced in the treatment of hypertension as a ganglionic blocking drug. However, mecamylamine, being a secondary amine, readily diffuses into cells and its effects are not restricted to the autonomic ganglia; the compound has a central nervous system action and a direct effect on the intestine, heart and neuromuscular junction (BENNETT et al., 1957). For example, mecamylamine potentiates the action of drugs competing with acetylcholine. The most interesting of all the results, however, were those obtained with depolarising drugs. After mecamylamine a dose of decamethonium, which previously produced an 80% block, became ineffective. A fourfold increase of the dose produced a 100% paralysis, which was then antagonised by neostigmine. This was an unexpected effect, since depolarisation block is not normally affected by neostigmine, and may even be prolonged by it; antagonism by neostigmine is characteristic only of substances competing with acetylcholine. This change in the mode of action of a depolarising drug in animals pretreated with mecamylamine was demonstrated even more clearly in avian muscle. When acetylcholine or acetylcholine-like drugs are injected into the gastrocnemius of a hen, they produce a contracture (ZAIMIS, 1954, 1959, and Chapter 4A). In contrast, substances competing with acetylcholine produce the usual flaccid paralysis. As Fig. 2 shows, in such a preparation suxamethonium produces a typical contracture. When it was given in the presence of mecamylamine, however, the drug developed a two-phase effect. The initial contracture was followed by a marked depression

(a)   (b)

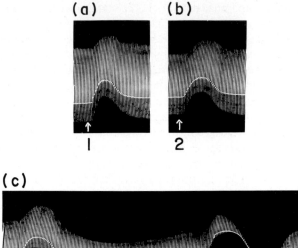

(c)

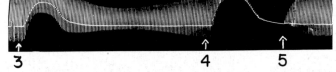

Fig. 2. Action of mecamylamine on depolarising drugs. Hen, 0.8 kg. Pentobarbitone anaesthesia. Contractions of the gastrocnemius muscle elicited by supramaximal shocks applied to the sciatic nerve every 10 sec. At (1), 20 µg; (2), (3) and (4) 40 µg of suxamethonium diiodide. At (5) 100 µg of neostigmine methylsulphate. Between (a) and (b) 0.5 mg of tubocurarine chloride. Between (b) and (c) 5 mg of mecamylamine hydrochloride. All injections made intravenously. (From: BENNETT et al., 1975)

of the maximal twitch, which was promptly reversed on administering neostigmine. This indicates that, as with the tibialis anterior of the cat, the mechanism of action of a depolarising drug was modified after mecamylamine to become that of a drug interrupting neuromuscular transmission by competing with acetylcholine. It follows that some change occurs at the post-synaptic membrane under the influence of mecamylamine.

(b) *SKF 525 A* is another compound altering the mechanism of action of depolarising neuromuscular blocking drugs. This drug is mainly known for its ability to potentiate the effect of many substances belonging to completely different groups (barbiturates, analgesics, amphetamines, antiepileptic drugs, etc.). It is supposed that this potentiation is the result of an inhibitory action of SKF 525 A on some liver enzymes. However, evidence is accumulating that the drug has direct effects on other structures in the body. For example, in the late fifties, we showed that in hearts

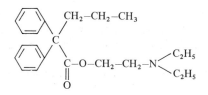

isolated from cats, rabbits and guinea-pigs the drug decreased the amplitude of the contractions and reduced the heart rate. The contractions of the isolated rabbit's intestine also slowly declined under the influence of SKF 525A. These effects were not prevented by atropine and not altered by the presence of hexamethonium. At the neuromuscular junction, SKF 525A markedly prolonged the action of tubocurarine and changed the mechanism of action of depolarising drugs. As Fig. 3 shows, suxamethonium produced a typical contracture in the gastrocnemius of a hen but in the presence of SKF 525A the drug after an initial contracture developed a curare-like effect. The contracture was followed by a marked depression of the maximal twitch which was promptly reversed by neostigmine and potentiated by tubocurarine[4].

(a)   (b)

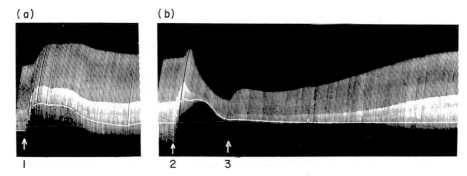

I   2   3

Fig. 3. Action of SKF525A on suxamethonium. Hen; pentobarbitone anaesthesia. Contractions of the gastrocnemius muscle elicited by supramaximal shocks applied to the sciatic nerve every 10 sec. At (1) and (2), 20 μg suxamethonium; at (3), 50 μg neostigmine. Between (a) and (b), 7 mg SKF525A. All drugs administered intravenously. (ZAIMIS, 1959; unpublished results)

Similar results were obtained by SUAREZ-KURTZ et al. (1969). As discussed in Chapter 3 by GINSBORG and JENKINSON, several workers have shown that SKF 525A increases the rate of desensitisation to ionophoretically-applied acetylcholine. The drug is also active when applied intracellularly and MAGAZANIK and VYSKOČIL (1972, 1973) suggested that a step beyond the binding site of the agonist may be affected. However, if we accept that desensitisation means a loss of chemosensitivity, the effect of SKF 525A on suxamethonium in the intact animal cannot be due to a "desensitisation" of the receptor sites. In the experiments just described the block produced by suxamethonium in the presence of SKF 525A is readily antagonised by edrophonium and potentiated by tubocurarine.

Other drugs can affect the action of depolarising neuromuscular blocking drugs without *changing* their mechanism of action. For example, it is well known that the magnitude and duration of the blockade can be reduced by substances which compete with acetylcholine, such as tubocurarine or gallamine.

Certain drugs known to affect adrenergic mechanisms produce changes in skeletal muscle resembling those observed in animals whose body temperature has been lowered. For example, by recording end-plate depolarisation together with the dura-

---

[4] The results formed the subject of a lecture given at the Research Institute of SMITH, KLINE and FRENCH (Philadelphia, Pa. U.S.A.) in 1959.

tion of the neuromuscular block produced by decamethonium, ZAIMIS et al. (1965) were able to show that in animals treated chronically with thyroxine there was a marked lengthening of the repolarisation phase and a parallel decrease in the rate of recovery of the twitch, the effect increasing progressively with the duration of the treatment (Fig. 4B). In these thyroxine-treated animals, the sensitivity of the muscles to anticholinesterase and depolarising drugs, including acetylcholine, was unchanged or increased. We have previously shown that at lowered muscle temperatures (BIGLAND et al., 1958) the duration of the process of repolarisation is very slow (Fig. 4A). It was interesting, therefore, to find that in the thyroxine-treated animals, whose body temperature was as a rule higher than that of the controls, the same slowing of the repolarisation phase occurred.

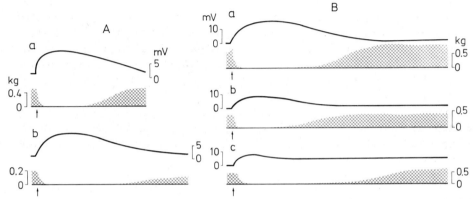

Fig. 4A and B. Cat, tibialis anterior muscle. Records of depolarisation of the end-plate region (measured with an external electrode) and of muscle contractions elicited by supramaximal shocks applied to the sciatic nerve every 10 sec.
(A) effect of cooling on a neuromuscular block produced by decamethonium (30 µg/kg I.V.): (a) muscle temperature 36° C; (b) muscle temperature 33° C.
(B) effect of thyroxine on a neuromuscular block produced by decamethonium (30 µg/kg I.V.): (a) control animal; (b) treated daily with thyroxine for 5 weeks; (c) treated daily with thyroxine for 10 months. (From: ZAIMIS et al., 1965)

Similar results were obtained in cats treated either acutely or chronically with guanethedine, amphetamine, ephedrine, bretylium, tyramine and dichloroisoprenaline (ZAIMIS, 1960; VERNIKOS-DANELLIS and ZAIMIS, 1960). Because of this striking resemblance between the changes produced by cooling alone and those produced by thyroxine and the other drugs, it has been suggested that the prolongation of the repolarisation is brought about by inhibition of metabolic processes—inhibition which results in a disturbance of the ionic shifts associated with the repolarisation of the muscle membrane (ZAIMIS, 1960).

The Importance of the Drug Structure and that of the Acetylcholine Receptor

One must not forget that differences in the chemical structures of the depolarising drugs affect their actions. Acetylcholine is known to be active at several sites, the ganglionic synapse, the neuromuscular junction, the effector cells innervated by postganglionic cholinergic nerve fibres, the central nervous system, producing what we call "different actions". It depolarises motor end-plates and ganglion cells, depresses some smooth muscle and stimulates others, stimulates glandular secretions, and so on. It seems almost incredible that one single molecule should produce so many different actions. One possible explanation is that its structure is such that it can fit and activate receptors with different properties. On the other hand, possibly the initial stage of the trigger mechanism of all these actions is the same but our methods are still too crude to detect it. Whatever be the explanation, the molecule of acetylcholine is a masterpiece and possesses to perfection the properties requisite for producing these actions. It is therefore not surprising that none of the innumerable synthetic compounds can really imitate acetylcholine in all its actions.

For both theoretical and practical reasons, the structural features that distinguish competitive from depolarising neuromuscular blocking drugs have received particular attention. The competitive substances, such as tubocurarine and gallamine, are for the most part relatively bulky, rigid molecules, whereas the depolarising neuromuscular blocking drugs, such as decamethonium and suxamethonium, have generally a more slender, flexible structure. This led BOVET (1951) to introduce the terms pachycurare and leptocurare, respectively.

PATON (1956) tried to estimate not the shape of the molecule but its tendency to be fixed in a fatty or a watery phase. He found a simple guideline by counting the carbon atoms in each molecule and comparing them with the number of hydrophilic quaternary groups. With an increasing ratio of hydrocarbon to hydrophilic material, the mode of action moves from depolarisation through mixed action to pure competition. Paton's scheme suggests that drugs with some measure of hydrocarbon loading may (through their lipoid affinity) develop an attachment to the membrane of a kind different from, additional to, and interfering with, the attachment which leads to end-plate activation. Although suxamethonium and decamethonium are less lipophilic than the other compounds, it seems possible, PATON concludes, that a latent competitive element in their action might develop, particularly if their action were sufficiently prolonged or if they were given in large doses so that lipoid fixation could occur. Quantitative measurements of this are not available, and indeed would be difficult to obtain.

To my mind, in order to understand how the various depolarising drugs produce their effects we need to have more clues about how the acetylcholine receptors function and how their chemical properties differ from animal to animal or from muscle to muscle in the same animal. For example, decamethonium and suxamethonium produce a depolarisation block in all the muscles of the cat, but a dual block in the soleus muscle. The same molecules produce a depolarisation block in man and avian muscle, but a dual block in monkey, dog and rat. Other substances can produce in the cat a neuromuscular block having right from the beginning all the characteristics of the dual block. For example, another member of the methonium series, tridecamethonium, produces in the cat the kind of block that decamethonium produces in the monkey and the dog. A muscle altered by disease can also respond differently from the normal muscle. For example, in myasthenic patients decamethonium produces a neuromuscular block having again all the characteristics of a dual block (for more details, see Chapters 4A and 5B). Thus it appears that the type of blockade produced by depolarising drugs depends on species and muscle differences, on the type of the depolarising substance, and finally on the condition of the muscle if it is normal or diseased. All these conditions are independent of the techniques used during the study of the depolarising drug. We can conclude, therefore, that the acetylcholine receptors at the muscle end-plate of different species and of different muscles have different properties, and that the mode of action of a quaternary molecule is determined not only by its own structure but also by the properties of the receptors concerned.

We have previously seen that certain general anaesthetics or drugs such as mecamylamine or SKF 525 A can actually *change* the mechanism of action of a depolarising neuromuscular blocking drug. The question is, how is this change produced? It has been suggested that the acetylcholine receptor is a protein and that the binding of acetylcholine is translated into a permeability change by means of a conformational change. According to one theory, drug molecules show different *efficacies* (the ability of a drug molecule to activate the receptors) because the nature of the conformational change they produce differs. Another theory (the two-state model) proposes that the activated state of the receptor is identical for all drugs—the difference between agonists of high and low efficacy lying in the fraction of occupied receptors that assume the active conformation. Other models have been proposed—they are all discussed in great detail by RANG in his 1975 review.

The acetylcholine receptor has been known for many years to contain an anionic site, since a quaternary ammonium or a similar group is the essential feature of all depolarising and competitive neuromuscular blocking drugs. Recently, attempts have been made to define other reactive groups within the receptor complex. One such group, a disulphide bond, was discovered by KARLIN and BARTELS (1966) in the eel electroplax preparation, where it is localized to within a few Ångstroms from the anionic receptor site. This disulphide bond could be reduced to free sulphydryl groups and reoxidized with concomitant inhibition and restoration of the response to acetylcholine and other monoquaternary depolarising agents. Very similar results have been demonstrated in frog (BEN-HAIM et al., 1973) and in chick muscle (RANG and RITTER, 1971). One of the striking findings of KARLIN (1969) was that after treatment with dithiothreitol, hexamethonium becomes an agonist with depolarising activity and decamethonium a more efficient agonist. This indicates that dithiothreitol treatment does not simply inactivate the acetylcholine receptor, but rather *changes* its structure in a specific manner. This occurs with the eel electroplax (KARLIN and WINNIK, 1968) and with chick biventer cervicis muscle (RANG and RITTER, 1971) but not with frog skeletal muscle (BEN-HAIM et al., 1973).

These results show that although a broad structural similarity exists between the acetylcholine receptors, a certain amount of differences can be found among various animal species. At the same time, the fact that hexamethonium becomes an agonist in the presence of dithiothreitol argues for the possibility that the receptor could actually *change* its structure in the presence of certain chemicals. The suggestion then could be made that some sort of structural alteration of the receptor takes place in the presence of fluorinated anaesthetics, mecamylamine or SKF 525 A and because of this decamethonium and suxamethonium produce a type of block which has some of the characteristics of a depolarisation block and some of the characteristics of a competitive one.

Pre-Synaptic or Post-Synaptic Action?

In the original evidence for the theory of chemical transmission at the neuromuscular junction there was nothing to suggest that acetylcholine or drugs such as tubocurarine or anticholinesterases might have a pre-synaptic action. In 1940, however, MASLAND and WIGTON showed that injection of acetylcholine into the popliteal artery of the anaesthetised cat, as well as exciting muscles gave rise to action potentials in the motor nerve which could be recorded antidromically in the ventral root. FENG and LI (1941) studied the phenomenon and demonstrated that while repetitive firing of nerve endings can arise from various other changes in the chemical environment, the effect produced by cholinesterase inhibitors is almost certainly due to local accumulation of acetylcholine around the axon terminals after each impulse. Discussing this repetitive "back-firing" of the motor nerve, BERNARD KATZ (1969) said that this rather puzzling phenomenon occurs in mammalian, but not in frog muscle and it apparently originates only at a very small percentage of end-plates in any one muscle. When he and MILEDI tried to elicit this effect by ionophoretic application of edrophonium, they succeeded only at a very small number of the many end-plates they tried. He concluded, therefore, that "the underlying depolarizing action in the nerve endings is weak and generally below threshold, and only at a few end-plates reaches the level required for re-excitation."

Several groups of scientists, however, (RIKER, HUBBARD, BARSTADT, BLABER and their co-workers—for references see Chapter 4C), working in this field insist that the main effects (if not all) of drugs such as anticholinesterases, competitive and depolarising neuromuscular blocking drugs, take place at the nerve ending and not on the post-synaptic membrane. On the other hand, by far the greatest number of neurophysiologists, pharmacologists and electrophysiologists have reached the conclusion that these drugs possess a large postsynaptic effect and only a relatively small presynaptic one (see also Chapters 2 and 3). The following assessment of the situation is a very clear and useful one:

"What seems to me the most probable explanation of the available, still rather incomplete, results is that there are ACh-receptors present in the presynaptic membrane, but at such low density that a release of ACh which almost completely depolarizes the muscle fibre, produces only a few millivolts change in the nerve. In general, the effect is below threshold and too weak to accelerate the rate of ACh release. In the frog this applies to all the myoneural junctions, in mammals to the majority. But at a few endings in mammalian muscle the potential change just reaches the threshold of re-excitation. The impulse coming from one nerve ending then spreads throughout the axon branches and re-excites the whole group of muscle fibres attached to them (cf. ECCLES, KATZ and KUFFLER, 1942). So, the final effect is quite powerful. On the other hand, anything which even slightly raises the threshold of excitation or interferes with ACh action (e.g., a subparalytic dose of curare) will abolish the 'back-firing' altogether. Now, it is on observations of just this kind that RIKER and his associates (see RIKER, 1966) have based the novel hypothesis that the *principal action* of substances like ACh, curare, anti-esterases etc. is presynaptic, and they have stated that there is no good evidence that these substances have a postsynaptic effect. RIKER (1966) chooses to disregard the fact that the end-plate sensitivity to ACh is as high after degeneration and disappearance of the nerve terminals as before. He dismisses as irrelevant the electrophysiological measurements of the end-plate activity, of the chemo-sensitivity of the junctional and peri-junctional parts of the muscle fibre, and of the local changes following denervation (MILEDI, 1960a, b); he has no use for the detailed studies of min. e.p.p.'s and, indeed, for all the other evidence which has been reviewed here. I agree that it is possible to entertain the hypothesis of Riker if, and only if, one is prepared to ignore everybody else's work on the subject." (KATZ, 1969).

Closing Remarks

Electron microscopy, biochemistry and electrophysiology have introduced very deli-
cate techniques and have produced an enormous amount of information at cellular
and even molecular level. As a result pharmacologists and clinical colleagues have
become almost apologetic about experiments *in vivo* and studies in man. Consequently, attempts are constantly made to express and explain effects occurring *in
vivo* in terms of actions produced in isolated muscles—muscles almost always removed from other species, or even other classes of animals; or to explain the action
of a drug in the intact animal by using results produced by large concentrations and
prolonged applications of drugs *in vitro*.

All the experimental techniques available to the research worker suffer from
inherent limitations. The *in vivo* studies, especially in man, can only be taken up to a
certain point, and the information obtained from experiments in the intact animal
has its limitations. Electrophysiology has concerned itself in the main with isolated
muscle preparations, usually from the frog. The maintenance of a suitable environment for the tissue, however, is extremely difficult. Therefore, results obtained *in
vitro* must be treated with caution, especially when they appear to differ from those
obtained *in vivo*. Biochemical studies involve the deliberate disruption of tissues and
the isolation of certain constituents. Electron microscopy has proved its worth in the
field of research, but here again the tissue is subjected to considerable insult during
preparation. It is thus impossible for a scientist belonging to any of these disciplines
to be absolutely sure that his results faithfully reflect the situation resulting from the
interaction of an active molecule with a cell in the intact body. It is only when we
bring all available information together and attempt to understand each other's
methods that the degree of existing disagreement between the results of various
investigators, and especially between results obtained in man and those reported
from animal experiments, will disappear.

References

ALI, H. H., UTTING, J. E., GRAY, C.: Stimulus frequency in the detection of neuromuscular block in
    humans. Brit. J. Anaesth. **42**, 967—978 (1970).
BEN-HAIM, D., LANDAU, E. M., SILMAN, I.: The role of a reactive disulphide bond in the function
    of the acetylcholine receptor at the frog neuromuscular junction. J. Physiol. (Lond.) **234**,
    305—325 (1973).
BENNETT, G., TYLER, C., ZAIMIS, E.: Mecamylamine and its mode of action. Lancet 1957 I, 218—
    222.
BIGLAND, B., GOETZEE, B., MACLAGAN, J., ZAIMIS, E.: The effect of lowered muscle temperature on
    the action of neuromuscular blocking drugs. J. Physiol. (Lond.) **141**, 425—434 (1958).
BOVET, D.: Some aspects of the relationship between chemical constitution and curare-like activ-
    ity. Ann. N.Y. Acad. Sci. **54**, 407—437 (1951).
BROWN, G. L., DALE, H. H., FELDBERG, W.: Reactions of the normal mammalian muscle to acetyl-
    choline and to eserine. J. Physiol. (Lond.) **87**, 394—424 (1936).
BURNS, B. D., PATON, W. D. M.: Depolarisation of the motor end-plate by decamethonium and
    acetylcholine. J. Physiol. (Lond.) **115**, 41—73 (1951).
CANNARD, T. H., ZAIMIS, E.: The effect of lowered muscle temperature on the action of neuromus-
    cular blocking drugs in man. J. Physiol. (Lond.) **149**, 112—119 (1959).
CHURCHILL-DAVIDSON, H. C.: The changing pattern of neuromuscular block. Canad. Anaesth.
    Soc. J. **8**, 91—98 (1961).

CHURCHILL-DAVIDSON, H. C., CHRISTIE, T. H., WISE, R. P.: Dual neuromuscular block in man. Anesthesiology 21, 144—149 (1960).
CHURCHILL-DAVIDSON, H. C., KATZ, R. L.: Dual, phase II, or desensitization block? Anesthesiology 27, 536—538 (1966).
COHEN, P. J., HEISTERKAMP, D. V., SKOVSTED, P.: The effect of general anaesthetics on the response to tetanic stimulus in man. Brit. J. Anaesth. 42, 543—547 (1970).
CRUL, J. F., LONG, G. J., BRUNNER, E. A., COOLEN, J. M. W.: The changing pattern of neuromuscular blockade caused by succinylcholine in man. Anesthesiology 27, 729—735 (1966).
DALE, H. H.: The beginnings and the prospects of neurohumoral transmission. Pharmacol. Rev. 6, 7—13 (1954).
DE JONG, R. H., FREUND, F. G.: Characteristics of the neuromuscular block with succinylcholine and decamethonium in man. Anesthesiology 28, 583—591 (1967).
DOUGLAS, W. W., PATON, W. D. M.: The mechanisms of motor end-plate depolarization due to a cholinesterase-inhibiting drug. J. Physiol. (Lond.) 124, 325—344 (1954).
ECCLES, J. C., KATZ, B., KUFFLER, S. W.: Effect of eserine on neuromuscular transmission. J. Neurophysiol. 5, 211—230 (1942).
ELMQVIST, D., THESLEFF, S.: Ideas regarding receptor desensitization at the motor end-plate. Rev. canad. Biol. 21, 229—234 (1962).
FENG, T. P., LI, T. H.: Studies on the neuromuscular junction. XXIII. A new aspect of the phenomena of eserine potentiation and post-tetanic facilitation in mammalian muscles. Chin. J. Physiol. 16, 37—56 (1941).
FOGDALL, R. P., MILLER, R. D.: Neuromuscular effects of enflurane, alone and combined with d-tubocurarine, pancuronium, and succinylcholine, in man. Anesthesiology 42, 173—178 (1975).
FOLDES, F.: The pharmacology of neuromuscular blocking agents in man. Clin. Pharmacol. Ther. 1, 345—395 (1960).
FOLDES, F. F., MACHAJ, T. S., HUNT, R. D., MCNALL, P. G., CARBERRY, P. C., IRVINGTON, M. J.: Synthetic muscle relaxants in anesthesia. J. Amer. med. Ass. 150, 1559—1566 (1952).
FOLDES, F. F., WNUCH, A. L., HAMER HODGES, R. J., THESLEFF, S., DE BEER, E. J.: The mode of action of depolarizing relaxants. Anesth. Analg. Curr. Res. 36, 23 (1957).
HALL, R. A., PARKES, M. W.: The effect of drugs upon neuromuscular transmission in the guinea-pig. J. Physiol. (Lond.) 122, 274—281 (1953).
JENDEN, D. J.: Effect of drugs upon neuromuscular transmission in the isolated guinea-pig diaphragm. J. Pharmacol. exp. Ther. 114, 398—408 (1955).
KARLIN, A.: Chemical modification of the active site of the acetylcholine receptor. J. gen. Physiol. 54, 245—264 (1969).
KARLIN, A., BARTELS, E.: Effects of blocking sulphydryl groups and of reducing disulfide bonds on the acetylcholine-activated permeability system of the electroplax. Biochim. biophys. Acta (Amst.) 126, 525—535 (1966).
KARLIN, A., WINNIK, M.: Reduction and specific alkylation of the receptor for acetylcholine. Proc. nat. Acad. Sci. (Wash.) 60, 668—674 (1968).
KATZ, B.: The release of neural transmitter substances. Liverpool: University Press 1969.
KATZ, R. L.: Modification of the action of pancuronium by succinylcholine and halothane. Anesthesiology 35, 602—606 (1971).
KATZ, R. L.: Electromyographic and mechanical effects of suxamethonium and tubocurarine on twitch, tetanic and post-tetanic responses. Brit. J. Anaesth. 45, 849—859 (1973).
KATZ, R. L., RYAN, J. F.: The neuromuscular effects of suxamethonium in man. Brit. J. Anaesth. 41, 381—390 (1969).
KATZ, R. L., WOLF, C. E., PAPPER, E. M.: The nondepolarizing neuromuscular blocking action of succinylcholine in man. Anesthesiology 24, 784—789 (1963).
LEBOWITZ, M. H., BLITT, C. D., WALTS, L. F.: Depression of twitch response to stimulation of the ulnar nerve during Ethrane anesthesia in man. Anesthesiology 33, 52—57 (1970).
LOEWI, O.: Über humorale Übertragbarkeit der Herznervenwirkung. Pflügers Arch. ges. Physiol. 189, 239—242 (1921).
MACLAGAN, J.: A comparison of the responses of the tenuissimus muscle to neuromuscular blocking drugs in vivo and in vitro. Brit. J. Pharmacol. 18, 204—216 (1962).

MAGAZANIK, L. G., VYSKOČIL, F.: The loci of α-bungarotoxin action on the muscle postjunctional membrane. Brain. Res. **48**, 420—423 (1972).

MAGAZANIK, L. G., VYSKOČIL, F.: Desensitization at the motor end-plate. In: RANG, H. P. (Ed.), Drug Receptors, pp. 105—119. London: Macmillan 1973.

MASLAND, R. L., WIGTON, R. S.: Nerve activity accompanying fasciculation produced by prostigmine. J. Neurophysiol. **3**, 269—275 (1940).

MICHELSON, M. J., ZEIMAL, E. V.: Acetylcholine: an approach to the molecular mechanism of action. Oxford: Pergamon Press 1973.

MILEDI, R.: The acetylcholine sensitivity of frog muscle fibres after complete and partial denervation. J. Physiol. (Lond.) **151**, 1—23 (1960a).

MILEDI, R.: Junctional and extra-junctional acetylcholine receptors in skeletal muscle fibres. J. Physiol. (Lond.) **151**, 24—30 (1960b).

MILLER, R. D., EGER, E. I., WAY, W. L., STEVENS, W. C., DOLAN, W. M.: Comparative neuromuscular effects of forane and halothane alone and in combination with d-tubocurarine in man. Anesthesiology **35**, 38—42 (1971).

NASTUK, W. L., MANTHEY, A. A., GISSEN, A. J.: Activation and inactivation of postjunctional membrane receptors. Ann. N.Y. Acad. Sci. **137**, 999—1014 (1966).

OTSUKA, M., ENDO, M., NONOMURA, J.: Presynaptic nature of neuromuscular depression. Jap. J. Physiol. **12**, 573—584 (1962).

PATON, W. D. M.: Mode of action of neuromuscular blocking agents. Brit. J. Anaesth. **28**, 470—480 (1956).

PATON, W. D. M., WAUD, D. R.: Drug-receptor interactions at the neuromuscular junction. In: DE REUCK, A. V. S. (Ed.): Curare and Curare-like Agents. Ciba Foundation Study Group No. 12, pp. 34—54. London: Churchill 1962.

PATON, W. D. M., ZAIMIS, E.: The pharmacological actions of polymethylene bistrimethylammonium salts. Brit. J. Pharmacol. **4**, 381—400 (1949).

RANG, H. P.: Acetylcholine receptors. Quart. Rev. Biophys. **7**, 283—399 (1975).

RANG, H. P., RITTER, J. M.: The effect of disulphide bond reduction on the properties of cholinergic receptors in chick muscle. Molec. Pharmacol. **7**, 620—631 (1971).

RICHARDS, H., YOUNGMAN, H. R.: The ultra-short-acting relaxants. Brit. med. J. **1**, 1334—1335 (1952).

RIKER, W. F., JR.: Actions of acetylcholine on mammalian motor nerve terminal. J. Pharmacol. exp. Ther. **152**, 397—416 (1966).

SUAREZ-KURTZ, G., PAULO, L. G., FONTELES, M. C.: Further studies on the neuromuscular effects of β-diethylaminoethyl-diphenyl propylacetate hydrochloride (SKF-525-A). Arch. int. Pharmacodyn. **177**, 185—195 (1969).

THESLEFF, S.: Neuromuscular block caused by acetylcholine. Nature (Lond.) **175**, 594—595 (1955a).

THESLEFF, S.: The mode of neuromuscular block caused by acetylcholine, nicotine, decamethonium and succinylcholine. Acta physiol. scand. **34**, 218—231 (1955b).

THESLEFF, S.: Motor end-plate "desensitization" by repetitive nerve stimuli. J. Physiol. (Lond.) **148**, 659—664 (1959).

THESLEFF, S.: Nervous control of chemosensitivity in muscle. Ann. N.Y. Acad. Sci. **94**, 535—546 (1961).

VERNIKOS-DANELLIS, J., ZAIMIS, E.: Some pharmacological actions of bretylium and guanethidine. Lancet 1960 2, 787—788.

WALTS, L. F., DILLON, J. B.: Clinical studies on succinylcholine chloride. Anesthesiology **28**, 372—376 (1967).

WHITE, D. C.: Dual block after intermittent suxamethonium. Brit. J. Anaesth. **35**, 305—312 (1963).

ZAIMIS, E.: Motor end-plate differences as a determining factor in the mode of action of neuromuscular blocking substances. J. Physiol. (Lond.) **122**, 238—251 (1953).

ZAIMIS, E.: The interruption of neuromuscular transmission and some of its problems. Pharmacol. Rev. **6**, 53—57 (1954).

ZAIMIS, E.: Mechanisms of neuromuscular blockade. In: BOVET, D., BOVET-NITTI, F., MARINI-BETTOLO, G. B. (Eds.): Curare and Curare-Like Agents, pp. 191—203. Amsterdam: Elsevier 1959.

ZAIMIS, E.: Parallelism of changes produced by cooling and by drugs known to affect adrenergic mechanisms. Nature (Lond.) **187**, 213—216 (1960).

ZAIMIS, E.: Experimental hazards and artefacts in the study of neuromuscular blocking drugs. In: DE REUCK, A. V. S. (Ed.): Curare and Curare-like Agents. Ciba Foundation Study Group No. 12, pp. 75—82. London: Churchill 1962.

ZAIMIS, E., METAXAS, N., HAVARD, C. W. H., CAMPBELL, E. D. R.: Cardiovascular and skeletal muscle changes in cats treated with thyroxine. In: Research in Muscular Dystrophy, pp. 301—311. Edited by Members of the Research Committee of the Muscular Dystrophy Group. London: Pitman Medical 1965.

CHAPTER 1

The Anatomy and Pathology
of the Neuromuscular Junction

Ruth E. M. Bowden and L. W. Duchen

A. Introduction

Knowledge of the structure of the neuromuscular junction is essential for an understanding of the processes of transmission and the interrelationship between the
nervous system and striated muscle. Correlation between morphological, physiological, pharmacological and biophysical research in experimental and clinical conditions has contributed fruitfully to present knowledge.

   This chapter is concerned with the morphology of the neuromuscular junction in
man and in animals commonly used in the laboratory. Since understanding has been
clarified by the study of clinical and experimental material both healthy and abnormal states will be described. Attention will be drawn to differences between species,
age groups and types of muscle and the effects of varying functional states.

   Important technical advances in elucidating anatomical features of the neuromuscular junction have included metallic impregnation of nerve fibres and the use of
intravital methylene blue. Histochemical and cytochemical techniques have demonstrated the subneural apparatus of Couteaux, the localization of cholinesterase and
the differentiation of various types of muscle fibre. More recently immunofluorescent
techniques have been used to locate receptor sites. Electron microscopy resolved the
longstanding controversy over the precise morphological relationship between nerve
and muscle and is essential for the critical analysis of the functional significance of
the various structural components of this particular cholinergic synapse.

B. Normal Muscle

I. The Motor Unit

The motor unit was defined by LIDDELL and SHERRINGTON (1925) and SHERRING-
TON (1930) as comprising a single lower motor neurone with all its processes and the
muscle fibres it innervates. It can be regarded as a functional entity (see BUCHTAL,
1960). Some implications of the concept of the motor unit are far-reaching. It has
been assumed that all branches of the axon terminate at neuromuscular junctions of
identical structure, and on muscle fibres with similar physiological and morphological characteristics. Supporting evidence for this has been put forward by KUGEL-
BERG and EDSTROM (1968) and EDSTROM and KUGELBERG (1968). The number of
muscle fibres innervated by a single motor axon varies. Estimates have been given of
about 13 fibres per unit in the human external rectus oculi and as many as 1700 in
the medial head of gastrocnemius (see BUCHTAL, 1960).

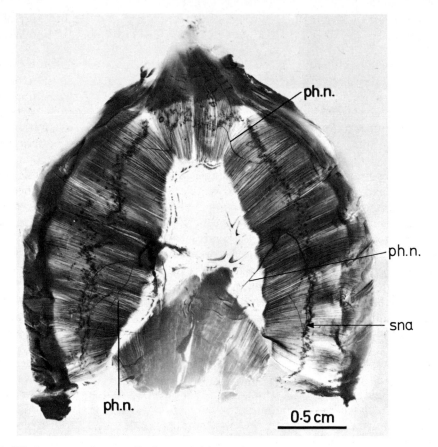

Fig. 1. Whole mount of mouse diaphragm (with attached costal margin) stained with osmic acid for myelinated nerve fibres, after which Lewis's (1958) diazo technique was used to demonstrate the bands of subneural apparatuses each of which lies at the mid-point of the muscle fibre. *sna* subneural apparatus, *ph.n.* phrenic nerve branches. (Preparation by Dr. H. A. El-Ramli). × 3.5

II. Pattern of Innervation and Distribution of Motor End-Plates

For many years the term "end-plate" (plaque terminale) introduced by Rouget in 1862 and "motor end-plate" (motorische Endplatte) introduced by Krause in the following year referred to all anatomical structures which participate in the complex known as the "neuromuscular junction": the motor nerve ending, the Schwann cell, the post-synaptic membrane and the sarcoplasm with its sole plate nuclei and cytoplasmic organelles. More recently, however, physiologists and pharmacologists use the term motor end-plate to designate the post-synaptic area only, and it is used in this sense in the subsequent chapters of this volume.

There is no general rule applicable to the point of entry of the nerve or nerves into the muscle belly although this is constant for any one individual muscle (Brash, 1955). The nerve may branch, form a plexus or a continuous band within the muscle. The distribution of motor end-plates is characteristic for each muscle and varies according to species, type of nerve and muscle fibre; and internal architecture of the muscle (FROHSE and FRÄNKEL, 1908; HINSEY, 1934; TIEGS, 1953; COËRS and WOOLF, 1959).

Mammalian extrafusal muscle fibres, *particularly those innervated by spinal nerves*, have a remarkable similarity in that the point of contact between axon and muscle fibre is usually midway between origin and insertion of the muscle fibre. The fact that there is normally a difference in excitability between different parts of a muscle was noted by LUCAS (1907); moreover, MARNAY and NACHMANSOHN (1938) found that in a muscle cut into segments the concentration of cholinesterase was highest in the central region. In a typical mammalian skeletal muscle intramuscular nerve bundles break up into a spray of single myelinated preterminal axons. Each preterminal axon innervates a single end-plate on a single muscle fibre. Since end-plates are found at the mid-point of every muscle fibre, each muscle will have a characteristically shaped and situated band of end-plates (Fig. 1). This is the general rule in the normal adult. However, the work of REDFERN (1970) and BAGUST et al. (1973) on the rat diaphragm and the flexor hallucis longus and soleus of the cat during development and early post-natal life revealed multiple end-plates on single muscle fibres which were possibly innervated by different motor neurones.

It is essential to use more than one technique of histological examination to obtain a valid picture of the innervation of a muscle, whether experimental or clinical. A full survey ideally should include fresh frozen sections for enzyme histochemistry, fixed frozen and paraffin sections as well as electron microscopy. From amongst the many methods used for light microscopy the following have proved valuable:- gold chloride (RANVIER's method and many subsequent modifications); silver impregnation of frozen sections (methods of CAJAL, BIELSCHOWSKY or SCHOFIELD, 1960); teased preparations (method of BARKER and IP, 1963) or paraffin sections (PALMGREN, 1948); intravital methylene blue (DOGIEL, 1890; COËRS and WOOLF, 1959) in teased or sectioned preparations; demonstration of cholinesterase activity in frozen sections (e.g. KOELLE and FRIEDENWALD, 1949) and the combined demonstration of cholinesterase and nerve fibres, e.g. by the method of NAMBA et al. (1967) or by a combination of the techniques of KOELLE and FRIEDENWALD with BIELSCHOWSKY's silver impregnation (Figs. 2 and 3).

The morphological studies of DOYÈRE (1840), KRAUSE (1863), RANVIER (1873) and KÜHNE (1887) (Fig. 4) laid the foundations for later work and are reviewed by BOEKE (1932), COUTEAUX (1947; 1960), ZACKS (1964) and COËRS (1967) amongst others. In 1931, TOWER established that every motor ending is derived from a myelinated axon and none is derived from sympathetic fibres.

The observation that myelinated preterminal axons rarely branch after they leave intramuscular nerve bundles, has given rise to the concept of the "functional terminal innervation ratio" i.e. the ratio between the number of muscle fibres and the number of preterminal axons innervating them. In normal human limb muscles (COËRS, 1955; COËRS, 1967; COËRS et al., 1973) only about 10% of preterminal axons supply more than one muscle fibre, and no muscle fibre is innervated by two different axons. Of the axons that branch, the majority innervate only two muscle fibres. The observations of FEINDEL et al. (1952) in the adult rabbit and monkey were similar in that when more than one end-plate was found on a single muscle fibre they were supplied by the same axon.

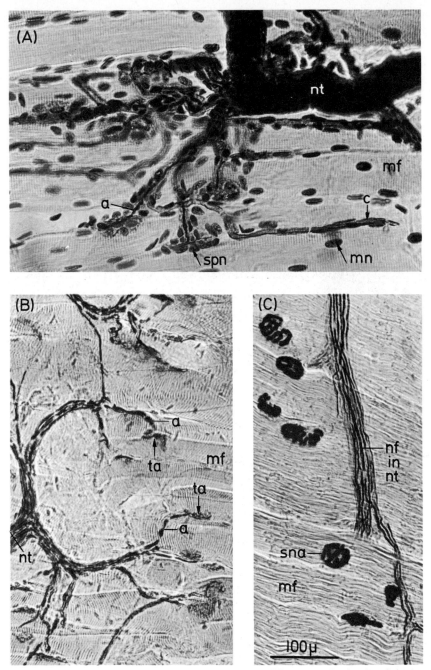

Fig. 2 A—C. Interosseus muscle of cat's hind paw. Three different methods of staining produce marked variations in the appearance of nerve endings. (A) Glees' silver impregnation. (B) Gold chloride (Bowden's modification). (C) Subneural apparatus stained by the technique of Koelle and Friedenwald followed by Bielchowsky's silver impregnation to demonstrate axons. *(nt)* intramuscular nerve trunk; *(nf)* nerve fibres; *(a)* preterminal axons; *(ta)* terminal arborizations; *(mf)* muscle fibre; *(c)* capillary; *(mn)* muscle nucleus; *(spn)* sole plate nuclei; *(sna)* subneural apparatus. ×180

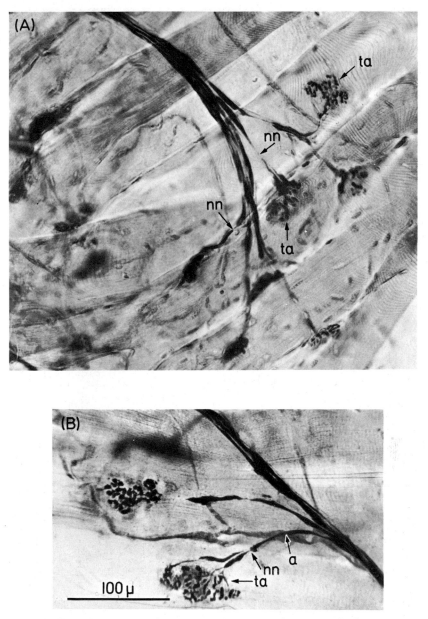

Fig. 3 A and B. Sartorius of normal rhesus monkey. Note the preterminal axons *(a)*, nodal narrowing *(nn)* and the marked variation in the morphology of terminal arborizations *(ta)*. Gold chloride, Bowden's modification (Bowden and Mahran, 1956). ×270

Mammalian muscle fibres innervated by *cranial nerves* have a more complex pattern of innervation which resembles that seen in some muscles of amphibia, birds and fish. The extraocular muscles have been studied extensively (Hines, 1931; Fein-del et al., 1952; Kupfer, 1960; Hess, 1961; Zenker and Anzenbacher, 1964; Terä-väinen, 1968 b; 1972). The intrinsic laryngeal muscles in man were studied by

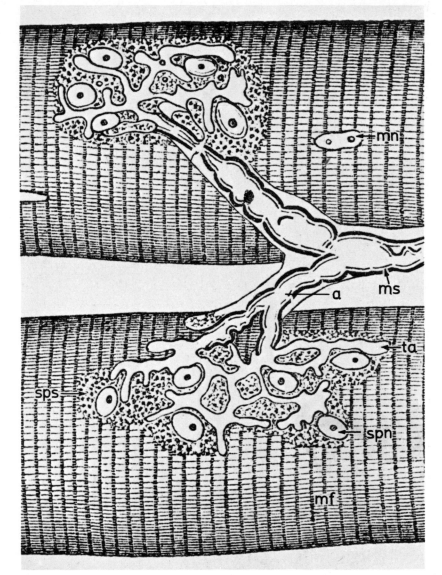

Fig. 4. KÜHNE's illustration of motor endings in lizard *(Lacerta viridis)* muscle fibres (two hours after death from curare). *(a)* preterminal axon; *(ms)* myelin sheath; *(ta)* terminal arborization; *(spn)* sole plate nucleus; *(sps)* sole plate sarcoplasm; *(mf)* muscle fibre and *(mn)* muscle nucleus

KEENE (1961) and in animals by WITHINGTON (1959), MANOLOV et al. (1963) and ABO-EL-ENENE (1967; see Fig. 5). Human facial muscles were studied by KADANOFF (1956) and those in the rat, rabbit and cat by BOWDEN and MAHRAN (1956). In these muscles the zone of innervation is not confined to a narrow band but is scattered, with great variation in the morphology of the terminal ramifications. Many muscle fibres have multiple end-plates, some derived from the same parent axon. In other

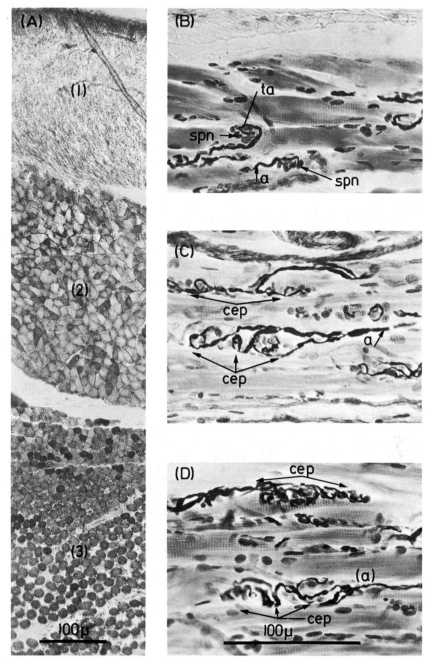

Fig. 5A—D. Larynx of cat. Thyroarytenoid muscle. (A) Montage showing: *(1)* the mucosa and submucosa; *(2)* the vocalis portion of the muscle; *(3)* the lateral portion of the muscle. Note the variation in the staining reaction of muscle fibres. Sudan Black-B ×180. (B) Simple end-plates in vocalis. (C) and (D) Compound end-plates in the lateral portion of thyroarytenoid muscle. (B), (C) and (D) Glees' silver stain ×360 (Preparations by M.A. ABO-EL-ENENE). *(a)* axon; *(ta)* terminal arborization; *(spn)* sole plate nuclei; *(cep)* compound end-plates

instances the possibility that these multiple nerve endings could be derived from
different neurones could not be excluded because of the plexiform arrangement of
intramuscular nerves. In a few cases the calibre of nerve fibres supplying a single end-
plate varies considerably. TERÄVÄINEN (1968b) has demonstrated unmyelinated axons (not containing catecholamines) innervating muscle fibres in extra-ocular muscles of the rat. In the extra-ocular muscles of all species studied two types of muscle
fibre have been identified; one type possessing a single end-plate, the other having
multiple end-plates, innervated by a single axon, scattered at intervals along its
length.

Fibres with a single end-plate are generally said to have *en plaque* innervation in
contrast to those with many end-plates whose innervation is described as *en grappe*.
This morphological differentiation of two types of innervation raises questions concerning the ultrastructural and functional differences between types of muscle fibre.

Focally and multiply innervated fibres have been demonstrated also in birds
(GINSBORG, 1960; SHEHATA and BOWDEN, 1960; KOENIG, 1970), the garter snake
(HESS, 1965), the frog (KATZ and KUFFLER, 1941) and fish (NAKAJIMA, 1969; KORNE-
LIUSSEN, 1973). In the multiply innervated fibres there are many small discrete end-
plates probably innervated by one axon. While the focally innervated, or fast, fibres
respond to a single motor impulse to give a propagated action potential followed by
a twitch, the multiply innervated (slow) fibres are unable to propagate action potentials and require a series of impulses to give a contraction (KUFFLER and VAUGHAN
WILLIAMS, 1953a; BURKE and GINSBORG, 1956; ORKAND, 1963). Both the development and the relaxation of tension are slower than in twitch fibres, whether the
contraction is initiated through nerve stimulation or by a uniform depolarisation of
the excitable membrane due to an increase of the potassium concentration in the
external fluid (KUFFLER and VAUGHAN WILLIAMS, 1953b; LÜTTGAU, 1963). KUF-
FLER and VAUGHAN WILLIAMS (1953b) showed by physiological means that these
slow fibres in the frog are innervated by motor axons of small diameter; support for
this was obtained by measurement of fibre size distributions in the adult fowl (SHE-
HATA, 1961; SHEHATA and BOWDEN, 1961).

III. The Structure of the Neuromuscular Junction

1. Axon Terminals

The axonal terminals lie distal to the last node of Ranvier of the myelin sheath. These
form an arborization, the spread of which is usually taken to indicate the size of the
neuromuscular junction. It is generally found that there is a direct relationship (see
Fig. 6) between the size of the end-plate region and the diameter of the muscle fibre it
innervates (HARRIS, 1954; COËRS, 1955; COËRS and WOOLF, 1959—human; SHEHATA,
1961—chick; ANZENBACHER and ZENKER, 1963—human, rhesus monkey, rat and
mouse; NYSTRÖM, 1968b—cat; RABERGER, 1971; KORNELIUSSEN and WAERHAUG,
1973—rat). As shown in Fig. 5 more than one myelinated preterminal axonal branch
may innervate a single end-plate (BARKER and IP, 1966; TUFFERY, 1971) and it has
been shown that the size and complexity of the terminal arborization varies according to the type of muscle fibre and according to age.

The morphology of axonal terminals appears to differ with different histological
techniques, fixation alone being responsible for some of these variations. Some stains

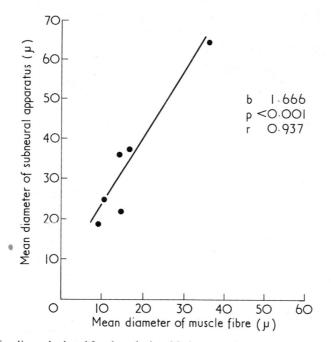

Fig. 6. Regression line calculated for the relationship between the mean diameter of the subneural apparatus and that of muscle fibres of chicks of different ages. *b* calculated slope of line, *r* correlation coefficient, *p* level of significance. (SHEHATA, 1961).

are selective for neurofilaments, mitochondria or vesicles of the axon, while others may stain elements of the synaptic space or of the subneural apparatus. Silver impregnations usually show fine tapering terminals. In contrast intravital methylene blue, gold chloride, or zinc iodide-osmium tetroxide produce swollen "terminal expansions" (COËRS and WOOLF, 1959; MAILLET, 1959; GRUBER and ECKERT, 1972) (Fig. 7 and cf. Figs. 2 and 3).

Electron microscopy finally demonstrated the anatomical discontinuity of nerve and muscle for which there was long-standing physiological and pharmacological evidence thus confirming the findings of COUTEAUX described in his classic paper of 1947. In 1954 REGER, ROBERTSON and PALADE independently described and illustrated the electron microscopic structure of the neuromuscular junction. Steady improvements in electron microscopic techniques have established the basic structural similarity of end-plates in all vertebrate species studied (REGER, 1958, 1959; DE HARVEN and COËRS, 1959; BIRKS et al., 1960). As shown in HUBBARD'S (1973) review recent work has concentrated on correlations between physiology and morphology and upon variations caused by alteration of function.

The electron microscopic appearance of the preterminal axon is shown in Fig. 8. The axon terminal (Fig. 9) is bounded by a membrane less than 10 nm thick. This axolemma is separated from the Schwann cell membrane by a space of similar width in which there is apparently no intervening substance. On the other hand, the space separating axolemma from the postsynaptic membrane of the muscle fibre is about

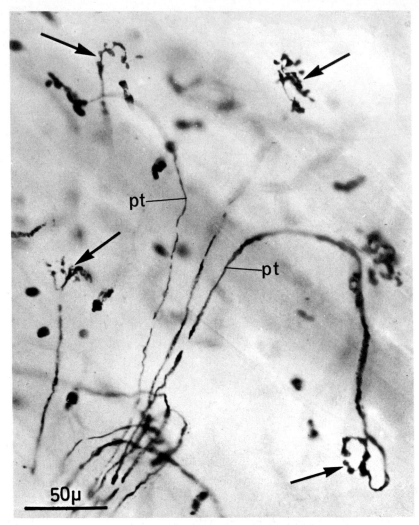

Fig. 7. Deltoid muscle biopsy from a female patient aged 24. Intravital methylene blue stain. The motor end-plates (arrows) are normal in appearance. Preterminal axons *(pt)* do not branch and there are no ultraterminal sprouts. (Preparation by Dr. D.G.F. Harriman, Department of Neuropathology, Medical School, University of Leeds). × 430

50 nm wide and contains amorphous basement membrane material. The appearance and thickness of axolemma is uniform throughout the neurone with the exception of thickenings in the part apposed to the synaptic gap. Possibly these thickenings are comparable with presynaptic thickenings in other sites in the nervous system (SOTE-LO, 1973). They have been found in all species studied electron microscopically but have been investigated most intensively in the frog (BIRKS et al., 1960; HEUSER and REESE, 1973). In the frog the axon terminals extend along the muscle fibres for up to 300 µm (KÜHNE, 1887). Because of their straightness and their length these terminals can be more predictably and accurately sectioned in either transverse or longitudinal

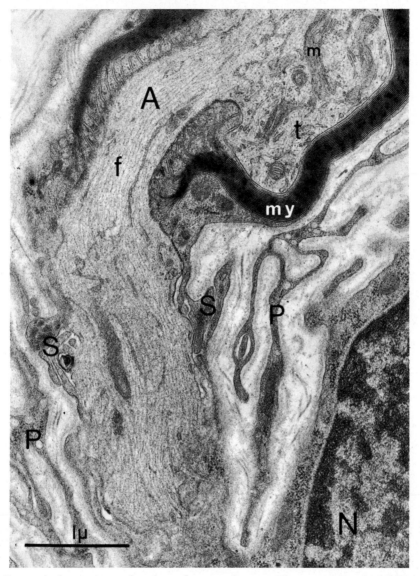

Fig. 8. Preterminal motor nerve in soleus of a normal mouse. The axon *(A)* contains neurofilaments *(f)* and neurotubules *(t)* and mitochondria *(m)*. The lamellae of the myelin sheath *(my)*
end at a node of Ranvier. The unmyelinated axons is covered by processes of Schwann cells *(S)*.
Processes of perineurial cells *(P)* coated by basement membrane are separated from the axon by
irregular spaces in which lie collagen fibres. N-muscle nucleus. × 27000

planes than is the case in other species. Further, the regularity of postsynaptic
folds of the sarcolemmal membrane and their orientation at right angles to the long
axis of the axonal terminal has facilitated the recognition of structural relationships
between intra-axonal constituents and the sarcolemmal folds. BIRKS et al. (1960)
noted that each thickening of the axonal membrane was usually situated opposite a

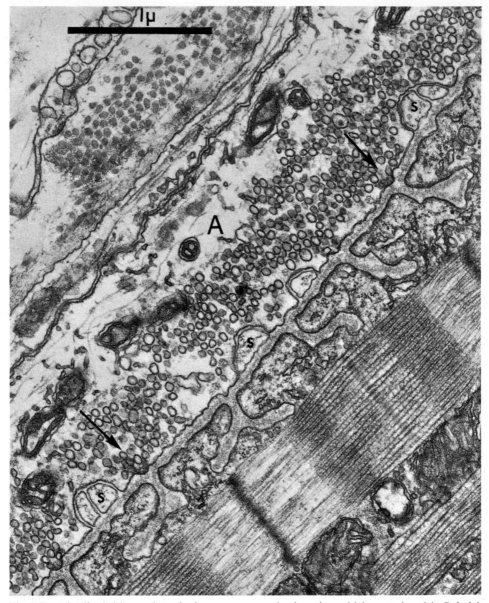

Fig. 9. Longitudinal thin-section of a frog neuromuscular junction which was placed in Palade's osmium tetroxide fixative while at rest. Vesicles are abundant in the axon terminal *(A)* and appear to cluster around presynaptic thickenings ("active zones") which are seen (arrows) opposite subneural folds. *S*-Schwann cell processes. (From HEUSER and REESE, 1973). × 37 500

post-synaptic fold and was associated with aggregations of synaptic vesicles within the axon terminal. In the rat diaphragm, HUBBARD and KWANBUNBUMPEN (1968) found localized thickenings of axolemmal membrane opposite 60% of postsynaptic folds. Synaptic vesicles touched or fused with axolemma at these points. HEUSER and

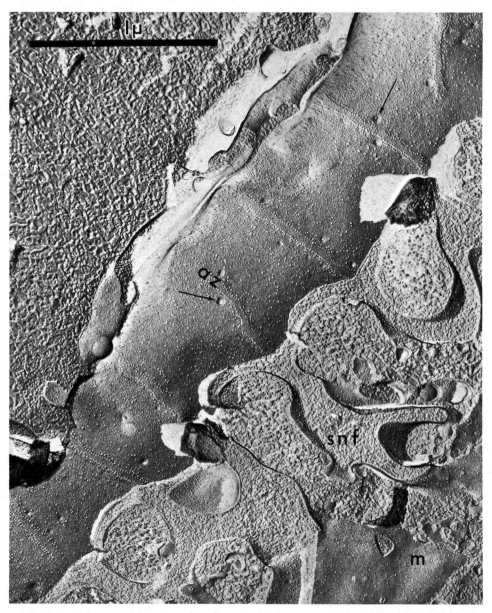

Fig. 10. Freeze-fracture replica of a motor nerve terminal stimulated in formaldehyde-glutaraldehyde fixative. Nerve stimulation at 10 Hz was begun immediately *after* placing the muscle in room-temperature fixative and continued for several minutes until the muscles were completely stiff. View of the cytoplasmic half, or A-face, of the plasmalemma of the axon terminal as seen from outside the terminal. Small dimples or pockets (arrows to some) beside the active zones *(az)* are present only in stimulated junctions and so probably represent synaptic vesicles coalescing with the plasmalemma during transmitter discharge. Subneural fold *(snf)*, muscle fibre *(m)*. (From HEUSER et al., 1974). ×49000

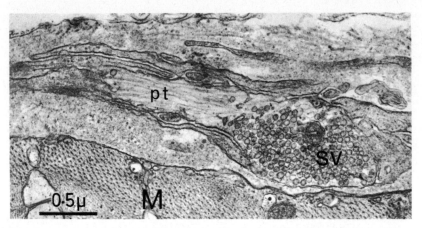

Fig. 11. Transverse section of pectoral fin muscle of normal goldfish showing the striking contrast between the preterminal *(pt)* and terminal parts of a motor axon. The terminal contains many synaptic vesicles *(SV)*. *M*-muscle fibre. × 27 500

Reese (1973) described axolemmal thickenings in greater detail in the frog (Fig. 9). They considered that the axon terminal, when sectioned longitudinally, can be differentiated into "synaptic units", each unit being centred upon a 100 nm wide band of dense material lining the plasma membrane. This dense band lies at right angles to the long axis of the terminal and invariably is located just above a postsynaptic fold of sarcolemma. Synaptic vesicles cluster about the dense band. Tongues of Schwann cell cytoplasm are found at regular intervals between axon and sarcolemma; and where axonal membrane contacts Schwann cell process the membrane is coated by filamentous dense material. Freeze-fracture studies by Heuser et al. (1974) have confirmed the presence of bands of thickened axolemmal membrane which are the sites of fusion of synaptic vesicles with the membrane (Fig. 10). These are probably sites of transmitter release, corresponding to the "active zones" of Couteaux and Pécot-Dechavassine (1970).

   Synaptic Vesicles are characteristic of axonal terminals throughout the central and peripheral nervous systems (De Robertis and Bennett, 1955; Palay, 1956; Gray and Guillery, 1966) and their presence distinguishes the terminal itself from the preterminal axon (Fig. 11 and 12). At the neuromuscular junction synaptic vesicles are almost certainly spherical, as shown by freeze-etching, though some vesicles with flattened profiles can often be seen in sections. Variation in shape of vesicles might well be the result of variations in the molarity of buffers particularly when aldehyde fixatives are used (Valdivia, 1971). In frog and mammalian nerve terminals the vesicles are bound by a unit membrane and normally are electron lucent, although a few dense core vesicles may also be seen. In fish up to 15% of vesicles in some nerve terminals may have a dense core (Korneliussen, 1973). "Coated vesicles" (Fig. 13) have a clear central core but their external surface is covered with small dense particles. Heuser and Reese (1973) suggested that coated vesicles represent a stage in membrane retrieval during transmitter release. In rat the average

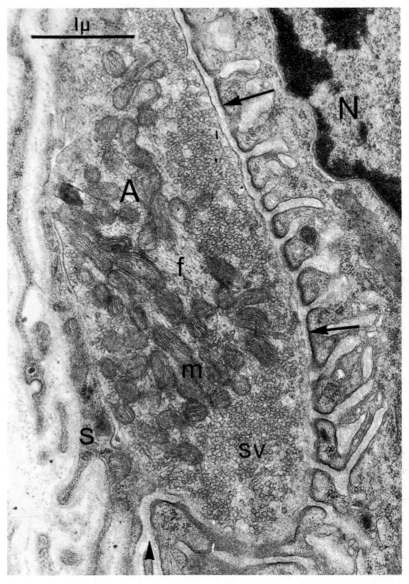

Fig. 12. Neuromuscular junction in soleus (slow, red muscle) of a normal adult mouse. In contrast with the preterminal axon (see Fig. 8) the terminal axon (A) contains many synaptic vesicles (SV). There are numerous mitochondria (m) but few neurofilaments (f). Note the thickened postsynaptic sarcolemmal membrane (arrows). The postsynaptic folds are mostly simple and have a mean depth of 0.5 μm. N-sole plate nucleus of muscle fibre. S-Schwann cell process. A-fusion of basement membrane of Schwann cell and muscle fibre. × 31500

volume of a synaptic vesicle was calculated to be about 5.2×10^4 cu.nm with an external diameter of about 45 nm and a wall 4 to 5 nm thick (HUBBARD, 1973). In the frog the mean external diameter of vesicles in resting nerve terminals is 52 nm (HEUSER and REESE, 1973). BIRKS et al. (1960) estimated the concentration of vesicles

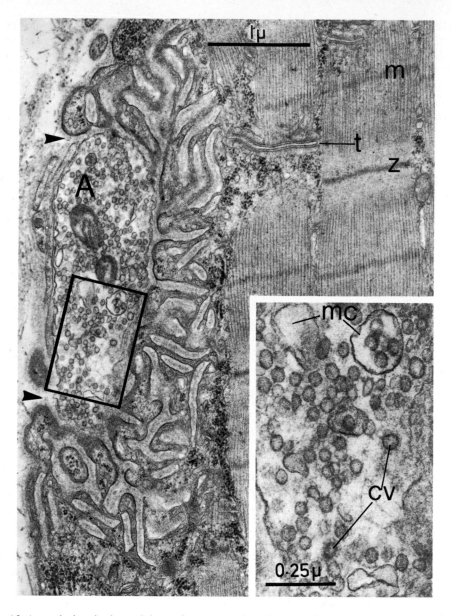

Fig. 13. An end-plate in the periphery of gastrocnemius of a normal mouse where fibres have been shown by other techniques to have the characteristics of fast, white muscle. When compared with soleus preparation (see Fig. 12) the axon terminal *(A)* is smaller in diameter (see GAUTHIER and PADYKULA, 1970) and the postsynaptic sarcolemmal folds are deeper, more numerous and branched. *m*-M line; *z*-Z line; *t*-transverse tubule of muscle fibre. A-fusion of basement membrane of Schwann cell and muscle fibre. Bar line = 1 μ. Inset is the area of axon terminal enclosed in the rectangle showing synaptic vesicles, coated vesicles *(cv)* and membrane-bound cisternae (mc)

in the frog terminals at about 1000 per cu.nm with about 3×10^6 vesicles per end-plate. These figures have been shown to vary with the type of muscle fibre and with the functional state of the nerve terminal, and the variations are discussed in a later section (p. 39 et seq). The distribution of vesicles within the axonal terminal is also of interest, and has been shown to vary with physiological function. BIRKS et al. (1960) observed that vesicles tend to occupy the synaptic region of the terminal. HUBBARD and KWANBUNBUMPEN (1968) reported that the vesicles were most concentrated in the region of the membrane thickenings lying opposite postsynaptic folds. Some vesicles appeared to touch or fuse with the membrane at these sites.

Mitochondria may be present in axonal terminals in large numbers and are often found in that part of the terminal adjacent to the Schwann cell. These mitochondria tend to be small and thin compared to those of the muscle cell in which they are larger and branched. Cristae tend to be fewer in number and less regularly arrayed than in other mitochondria. When fixation is delayed mitochondria in nerve terminals are particularly liable to undergo artefactual swelling and rarefaction even when those of the adjacent muscle fibre are well preserved. The appearance of mitochondria, and indeed of all cell organelles, varies to some extent with the fixative used and may also change with prolonged incubation in a bathing solution (TOH, 1971). Neurofilaments are usually not a prominent feature of normal terminals.

Localization of Transmitter. For many years acetylcholine has been known to be the transmitter at vertebrate neuromuscular junctions. The observations of DEL CASTILLO and KATZ (1954) led to general acceptance that transmitter is released in multi-molecular quanta. It is tempting to assume that vesicles are the site of transmitter packaging. At present there is no certain microscopic technique for the localization of acetylcholine (see BLOOM, 1972). The zinc iodide-osmium technique of MAILLET (1959) adapted by AKERT and SANDRI (1968) was thought to be specific for acetylcholine but the stain is also taken up by synaptic vesicles at non-cholinergic terminals. The electron histochemical demonstration of choline acetyltransferase (KASA et al., 1970) does not seem to be widely used and is at best an indirect method for identifying sites rich in acetylcholine. The association between synaptic vesicles and acetylcholine has been established biochemically after ultracentrifugation and separation of a vesicle-rich fraction from cerebral synaptosomes and from the electric organ of the *Torpedo* (see ISRAEL et al., 1973; WHITTAKER and DOWDALL, 1973). Other studies which have supported the suggestion that acetylcholine is stored in vesicles at the neuromuscular junction have been carried out. These take the form of physiological and morphological investigations on the same tissue under varying conditions.

2. Experimental Modifications of the Structure of the Axon Terminal

a) Electrical Stimulation

De ROBERTIS (1958) found that massive stimulation caused axonal terminals in the brain of the rat to become depleted of vesicles. JONES and KWANBUNBUMPEN (1970a; 1970b) studied the effect of nerve stimulation in the rat phrenic nerve-diaphragm preparation *in vitro* bathed in normal mammalian Ringer solution and in the presence and absence of hemicholinium. They found that in normal Ringer solution stimulation of the nerve for 2 or 4 min caused a significant reduction in the mean volume of synaptic vesicles and that more vesicles could be observed close to the axolemmal membrane. A reduction of vesicular volume and also of their number was found in axon terminals stimulated in bathing fluid containing hemicholinium. Intracellular recording with microelectrodes showed a fall in mean amplitude of miniature end-plate potentials (m.e.p.p.s) after nerve stimulation, particularly when the muscle was bathed in solutions containing hemicholinium. The amplitude of m.e.p.p.s in the preparations which had not been exposed to hemicholinium recovered to normal values within 7 to 8 min once nerve stimulation was stopped but when hemicholinium was present this only occurred after about 28 min. Although Jones and Kwanbunbumpen were able to correlate changes in volume and number of vesicles with the changes in the amplitude of m.e.p.p.s their conclusions about the effects of hemicholinium on vesicle size and numbers still require confirmation. Stimulation of the curarised nerve-muscle preparation of the frog (Ceccarelli et al., 1972) for 6 to 8 hrs caused nerve terminals to be severely depleted of stores of transmitter and of synaptic vesicles.

Experiments in which the rat nerve-diaphragm preparation was subjected to stimulation *in vitro* were reported by Korneliussen (1972). In these preparations it was also found that the striking feature of stimulated terminals was a drastic reduction in the numbers of vesicles and an increase in the numbers of elongated profiles and irregular membrane-bound spaces (cisternae) often enclosing vesicles within them. In all experiments some nerve endings contained virtually no vesicles. The frog neuromuscular junction was used in the experiments of Heuser and Reese (1973) who followed stimulation by immediate fixation in osmium tetroxide. After 1 min of stimulation at 10 Hz there was a 25% reduction in numbers of synaptic vesicles while coated vesicles increased in number. More cisternae were present than normal. After 15 min of nerve stimulation at the same frequency more than 60% of the vesicles were lost. Heuser and Reese measured the amounts of membrane in the terminals, including the axonal membrane, cisternae and vesicles and found that the loss of vesicle membrane was balanced by the increase in axonal plasma membrane and cisternae. They concluded that the membrane of the vesicles is incorporated into the plasma membrane by fusion during transmitter release and that the membrane is re-cycled by the formation of cisternae and its transformation back into vesicles (Fig. 14). Coated vesicles seem to be formed from the plasma membrane particularly at regions in contact with Schwann cells. Large miniature potentials were recorded by Pécot-Dechavassine and Couteaux (1973) after nerve-muscle preparations were exposed to acidified Ringer's solution. Heuser (1974) also found 'giant' spontaneous m.e.p.p.s after a period of rest following tetanic nerve stimulation for one hour. In both sets of experiments the axon terminals giving rise to these large potentials contained unusually large vesicles scattered amongst the normal-sized ones. If, as seemed likely the giant m.e.p.p.s were derived from the larger vesicles this provided further evidence for storage of transmitter in synaptic vesicles. The 'cisternae' described by Heuser and Reese (1973) in osmium fixed terminals are almost certainly the same kind of structure as those which appear as large vesicles after glutaraldehyde fixation. It seems likely that transmitter may be released from large vesicles even though they represent a stage in the formation of smaller vesicles.

b) Effects of Potassium

Raising the potassium concentration of the medium to 20 mmol/l causes the nerve terminals of an isolated muscle preparation to become depolarised. There is an outpouring of transmitter, detectable with microelectrodes as a great increase in the frequency of m.e.p.p.s. HUBBARD and KWANBUNBUMPEN (1968) showed that high concentrations of potassium chloride caused terminals to become severely depleted of synaptic vesicles. This change was prevented by raising the concentration of magnesium chloride which inhibits transmitter release.

c) Effects of Calcium

When frog sartorius muscles are bathed in isotonic solutions of calcium chloride (containing 83 mmol/l $CaCl_2$) the amplitude of spontaneous m.e.p.p.s is reduced. After prolonged exposure complete cessation of spontaneous transmitter release occurs (KATZ and MILEDI, 1969). HEUSER et al. (1971) found morphological changes in some terminals within $2\frac{1}{2}$ hrs of exposure to the high calcium-Ringer. These changes consisted of swollen mitochondria, dilated electron-lucent spaces in the axoplasm, clumped vesicles with dense membranes and clumped dense filaments. Over the next few hours abnormalities became more severe and terminals became fragmented and engulfed by Schwann cell processes. After 8 hrs exposure to high calcium levels restoration of the normal composition of the bathing solution resulted in only a small proportion of terminals regaining their normal structure. The changes caused by the high calcium were like those caused by nerve section but occurred more rapidly even when experiments were done at 4° C. Such experiments suggest a "final common path" of degeneration in axonal terminals in which the intracellular accumulation of calcium ions may be of importance.

d) Effects of Lanthanum

The effect of varying concentrations of lanthanum ions in the bathing solution has been studied in the frog by HEUSER and MILEDI (1971). Exposure to 1 mmol/l of lanthanum chloride caused a thousandfold increase in the frequency of m.e.p.p.s and led to irreversible block of transmission. After 2 hrs there was a great reduction in the numbers of synaptic vesicles and after 12 to 36 hrs all terminals were completely de void of synaptic vesicles, only coated vesicles and cisternae remaining. There were no spontaneous m.e.p.p.s at these end-plates.

e) Effects of Black Widow Spider Venom

The extract of the poison glands of the black widow spider (Latrodectus mactans tredecimgutatus) has a selective effect on axonal terminals. In muscles of the frog (LONGENECKER et al., 1970; CLARK et al., 1970; CLARK et al., 1972) and cat (OKA-MOTO et al., 1971) there is an increase in the frequency of m.e.p.p.s within a few minutes of exposure to the venom. The frequency may in fact rise to 1000/sec., the normal rate being 0.5 to 1.5/sec. After the peak frequency is reached the rate falls and spontaneous m.e.p.p.s finally cease. No effects were seen on the response of the muscle to direct stimulation. Omission of calcium from the bathing solution did not alter the action of the venom. Axon terminals were totally depleted of synaptic vesicles, and appeared swollen and disorganized. The pre-synaptic axonal membrane was lifted into a series of arches with the "active zones" remaining in position over the openings of the post-synaptic folds (Clark et al., 1972). These effects of black widow spider venom are not specific for cholinergic nerve terminals. Frontali (1972) found that the venom caused total depletion of catecholamine-dependent fluorescence from the rat iris, while Cull-Candy et al. (1973) observed the same effects in locust nerve-muscle synapses, where transmission is glutaminergic.

3. Transmitter Release and Synaptic Vesicles

Much interest has centred on the problem of the intracellular storage of neurotransmitters within vesicles (see Blaschko and Smith, 1971). The manner in which the arrival of the nerve action potential at the axonal terminal causes the changes in localization of vesicles and sets in motion the train of events associated with vesicle breakdown and formation is not entirely clear as yet. There is now abundant evidence that multimolecular packaging of acetylcholine occurs in vesicles and that each miniature potential is probably the result of the release of the contents of one vesicle. The evidence is derived from the correlations between the frequency of m.e.p.p.s and axonal depolarization by potassium, by electrical stimulation and by black widow spider venom and also from the relationship between vesicle size and the amplitude of potentials.

The morphological studies of Heuser and Reese (1973) and Heuser et al. (1974) showed that during stimulation, synaptic vesicles which normally lie in close contact with the axolemmal membrane of the terminal disappear while pits and dimples in the membrane develop. This change indicated that the vesicles coalesced with the axolemmal membrane, presumably discharging their contents of transmitter into the synaptic space by a process of exocytosis. The nerve terminal becomes depleted of vesicles but the number of coated vesicles and irregularly shaped cisternae is increased. If the stimulation is followed by a period of rest there is a gradual restoration of the morphology of the axonal terminal to normal, indicating that vesicles are being formed again. Heuser and Reese studied the problem of how vesicles are reformed by stimulating, *in vitro*, frog nerve-muscle preparations bathed in solutions containing horseradish peroxidase. They found that peroxidase, which does not permeate membranes, becomes localized within cisternae in the axonal terminal and then, when the period of stimulation is followed by a rest, peroxidase can be demonstrated within the vesicles. It was concluded that new vesicles are not formed directly from axolemmal membrane but that there is an intermediate stage of membrane retrieval involving the endocytosis of coated vesicles which coalesce to form the larger cisternae. Subsequent division of the cisternae seems to be the final stage in vesicle formation. When nerve terminals were stimulated after vesicles had become labelled with peroxidase there was a marked depletion of labelled vesicles. The findings of Heuser and Reese suggest very strongly that the release of transmitter at the neuromuscular junction is accomplished by fusion of vesicle and axolemmal membrane and that there is a cycle of membrane retrieval and reutilization resulting in the reformation of synaptic vesicles (Fig. 14).

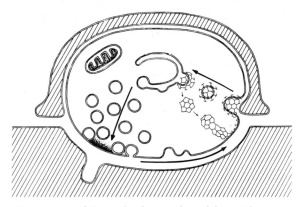

Fig. 14. Diagrammatic summary of the path of synaptic vesicle membrane recycling proposed by
HEUSER and REESE (1973): synaptic vesicles discharge their content of transmitter by coalescing
with the plasma membrane at specific regions adjacent to the muscle; then equal amounts of
membrane are retrieved by coated vesicles arising from regions of the plasma membrane adjacent
to the Schwann sheath; and then, the coated vesicles lose their coats and coalesce to form
cisternae which accumulate in regions of vesicle depletion and slowly divide to form new synaptic
vesicles

4. The Postsynaptic Region

The region under discussion is that part of the muscle membrane lying beneath the
axonal terminals. This region has many features, both structural and functional,
which distinguish it from the remainder of the muscle fibre; it is rich in sarcoplasm,
includes the sarcolemmal membrane and its folds, and contains nuclei and mitochondria in abundance (Fig. 15). The terminal branches of the nerve lie at the surface
of the muscle fibre in depressions known as synaptic gutters or troughs (the "primary
synaptic cleft"). The depth, shape and size of these gutters are very variable from
species to species and from muscle to muscle. There is a tendency for the gutter to be
deeper in mammalian muscle than in those of more primitive forms, and for the
sarcolemmal differentiation to be more complex in fibres with fast-twitch characteristics. In slow extrafusal muscle fibres of the frog, innervated by axons of small
diameter, the axon terminals lie in very shallow depressions (ROBERTSON, 1960;
PAGE, 1965), while in the fish (NAKAJIMA, 1969; KORNELIUSSEN, 1973) both shallow as
well as deeper gutters are present (Fig. 11). In extra-ocular muscle, nerve terminals
tend also to lie in shallow troughs whether or not they innervate fibres at single or
multiple end-plates. The depth of the synaptic gutter is of some importance since it
increases during the course of development and undergoes alteration in pathological
states. Effective, though not necessarily normal, transmission is known to occur
during embryological development and during regeneration of synapses when nerve-
muscle contacts are still superficial and immature (KOENIG and PÉCOT-DECHAVAS-
SINE, 1971; TONGE, 1974a, c, and d).

Mammalian muscle spindles contain two kinds of intrafusal muscle fibre—a
nuclear bag fibre and a nuclear chain fibre (BOYD, 1962; COOPER and DANIEL, 1963).
These intrafusal muscle fibres receive either "plate" or "trail" endings which somewhat resemble the two kinds of motor endings found on vertebrate "twitch" and

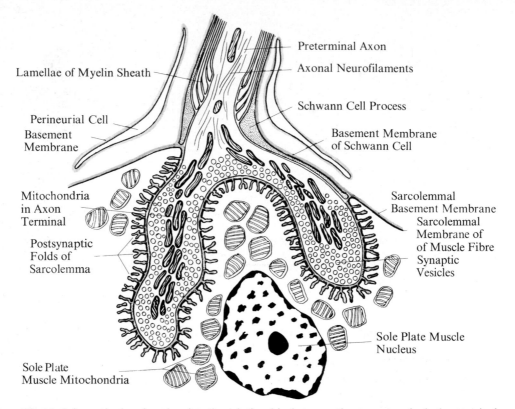

Preterminal Axon

Axonal Neurofilaments

Lamellae of Myelin Sheath

Schwann Cell Process

Perineurial Cell
Basement
Membrane

Basement Membrane
of Schwann Cell

Mitochondria
in Axon
Terminal

Sarcolemmal
Basement Membrane
Sarcolemmal
Membrane of
of Muscle Fibre
Synaptic
Vesicles

Postsynaptic
Folds of
Sarcolemma

Sole Plate Muscle
Nucleus

Sole Plate
Muscle Mitochondria

Fig. 15. Schematic drawing showing the relationship between the axon terminal, the terminal Schwann cell and the postsynaptic folds of the sarcolemma. Note also the characteristic distribution of the organelles

"slow" extrafusal fibres respectively (HESS, 1967; 1970). OVALLE (1972) has found that the "plate" endings on nuclear bag fibres are more superficially situated than those on nuclear chain fibres, and that "trail" type endings on both nuclear chain and nuclear bag fibres have little or no synaptic cleft. He points out, however, that extreme caution must be undertaken when attempts are made to compare extrafusal and intrafusal motor innervation, and when known physiological properties of extrafusal fibres are extrapolated to the intrafusal fibres. A given extrafusal fibre can only be innervated by one type of motor ending and the morphology of the muscle fibre can be directly correlated with the type of motor ending it receives. On the other hand, regardless of the morphology of the intrafusal muscle fibre, each kind of fibre (nuclear bag and nuclear chain) may receive the "plate" as well as the "trail" variety of motor ending.

    With the aid of certain vital stains and enzymatic histochemical techniques it is possible to render visible to the light microscope the "interface" between the terminal axoplasm and the sarcoplasm. In a section cut across a motor end-plate, this interface appears as a thin line to which lamellae are attached on the sarcoplasmic side. These lamellae extend in the form of ribbons which constitute Cou-

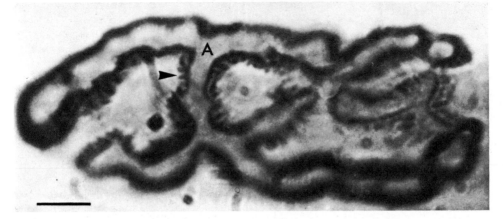

Fig. 16. Whole mount of guinea-pig serratus ant. showing a neuromuscular junction stained for cholinesterase (by a modification of KOELLE and FRIEDENWALD's method). The unstained axon terminal (A) lies in a gutter in the end-plate. The lamellae are in focus at arrow. Calibration: 5μ. (From L. M. BROWN, 1961)

TEAUX'S "sub-neural apparatus" (COUTEAUX, 1947, 1958, 1960, and 1963). Figure 16 shows a neuromuscular junction seen full face. The cholinesterase staining only reveals the interface between the axon and the end-plate and some of the lamellae (BROWN, 1961). The first observations of the neuromuscular junction carried out with the electron microscope (PALADE, 1954; REGER, 1954, 1958; ROBERTSON, 1954, 1960) revealed that the lamellae of the sub-neural apparatus were folds of the sarcolemmal membrane.

The postsynaptic membrane may or may not be infolded. Infolding seems to be of fundamental importance in the differentiation of some muscle fibres from others. The degree of postsynaptic differentiation can be correlated with other morphological and physiological features of the muscle fibre. Many of the characteristics of an individual muscle fibre are conferred on it by the particular type of axon innervating it (BULLER et al., 1960). The infolding of the sarcolemma at the end-plate (see Figs. 12 and 13) may therefore be regarded as one of the effects of the interaction between a muscle fibre and its particular type of nerve fibre (see GUTH, 1968). There are no postsynaptic folds in any type of skeletal muscle in fish (NAKAJIMA, 1969; KORNE-LIUSSEN, 1973), or in extrafusal slow muscle fibres of the frog (PAGE, 1965) and snake (HESS, 1965). More folds are present in the twitch muscle of the frog where there is a regular array at intervals of about 1 μm. These folds are parallel to each other, lie at right angles to the long axis of the nerve terminal perpendicular to the axon, and are about 0.5 μm deep. Beneath "plate" endings of mammalian intrafusal fibres there are few and simple folds, these being fewer on nuclear bag than on nuclear chain fibres (OVALLE, 1972). PILAR and HESS (1966) differentiated between the terminals of focally innervated extra-ocular fibres (which they identified as "twitch" fibres on morphological criteria) and those on multiply innervated ("slow") fibres in which the postsynaptic folds are virtually absent. Postsynaptic folds are a conspicuous feature in other mammalian muscle fibres studied with the electron microscope. ANDERSSON-

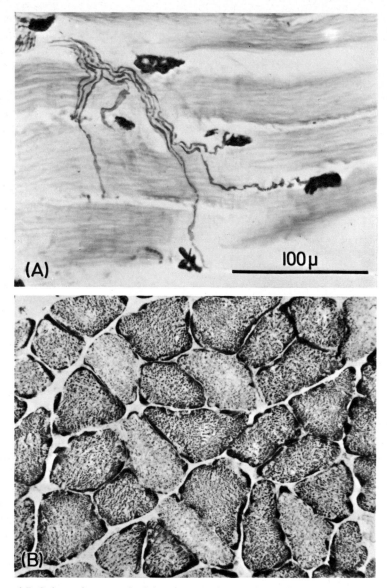

Fig. 17 A and B. Soleus of a normal adult mouse (a slow, red muscle). Compare with Fig. 18. (A) Longitudinal frozen section of formol-calcium fixed tissue stained by a modification of the method of Koelle and Friedenwald (1949) followed by silver impregnation for axons according to Namba et al. (1967). Note that each end-plate is innervated by a single preterminal axon. (B) Transverse section of fresh unfixed tissue stained to demonstrate the activity of succinate dehydrogenase (SDH), a mitochondrial enzyme. ×360

Cedergren (1959) and Fardeau (1973) reconstructed from serial sections a three-dimensional picture of the postsynaptic membrane in the mouse and guinea-pig respectively. In Andersson-Cedergren's reconstruction the folds appear as continuous intersecting strips whilst Fardeau (1973) showed a superficial cribriform layer with regular "holes" and a deeper part consisting of continuous intercommunicating spaces. The mammalian postsynaptic area is very complex. There is no clear indication that, apart from general features like the numbers, depth and branching of the folds, there is necessarily any regular pattern. It seems more likely that the membrane is thrown into a random series of folds.

Whatever the method of fixation, the postsynaptic membrane appears more electron dense than the extra-junctional sarcolemma (BIRKS et al., 1960; FARDEAU, 1973). This dense staining does not extend into the depths of the folds. Other specializations of the region include the localization of cholinesterase and of acetylcholine receptors.

Differences in end-plate structure and complexity have been observed in different types of fibre in mammalian skeletal muscles. Fibres may be distinguished by their colour (RANVIER, 1873) or by their speeds of contraction. Although all mammalian muscle fibres are twitch fibres they may be fast or slow contracting. Thus the slow mammalian fibres are unlike the slow fibres of the frog (see CLOSE, 1972). Histochemical differentiation has been studied by many including STEIN and PADYKULA (1962), GAUTHIER and PADYKULA (1966) and DUBOWITZ (1968). Slow fibres (Fig. 17) are generally identified by being rich in mitochondrial enzymes but poor in phosphorylase and myosin-ATPase. Fast fibres (Fig. 18) are rich in phosphorylase and ATPase but their mitochondria are smaller and fewer than in slow fibres and the reactions for mitochondrial enzymes are weaker. Fast fibres normally contain more glycogen than slow fibres and are of larger diameter. Fibres with enzyme reactions between the two extremes are also identifiable. Electron microscopy reveals that the internal structure of typical fast and slow mammalian muscle fibres differ from each other in a manner similar to that described in frog muscles by PEACHEY and HUXLEY (1962) and PAGE (1965). Characteristically there are larger and more numerous mitochondria in slow fibres (GAUTHIER, 1969). The Z-line in slow fibres is about 63 ± 3 nm thick, (PADYKULA and GAUTHIER, 1970), and the M-line absent or not well defined. On the other hand, fast fibres have a distinct M-line, and the Z-line is narrower, about 34 ± 3 nm. The tubules of the sarcoplasmic reticulum are more prominent than in slow fibres. In keeping with the general lack of complexity of the postsynaptic membrane in slow fibres of lower forms, the subneural apparatus of mammalian slow fibres has been observed to be less complex than in fast fibres (MURATA and OGATA, 1969—human; PADYKULA and GAUTHIER, 1970—rat; FARDEAU and ENGEL, 1970—guinea-pig; DUCHEN, 1971a—mouse; SANTA and ENGEL, 1973—rat). Quantitative studies on electron micrographs have confirmed and extended these observations. PADYKULA and GAUTHIER (1970) observed that axonal profiles at end-plates of red fibres of the rat diaphragm were relatively small and eliptical, measuring 2.8 to 4 μm by 1.1 to 1.7 μm. Postsynaptic folds were short, and about 0.5 μm in depth except at the periphery of the preparation near the muscle surface where they measured about 1.5 μm and the folds were seen to be about 0.33 μm apart. In white fibres the axonal terminals measured 4.6 to 8.4 μm by 1 μm, thus being longer and flatter than in red fibres, while folds were about 1 μm in depth, more regularly arranged and more numerous with only about 0.23 μm separating them. In a comparison of slow (soleus) and fast (periphery of gastrocnemius) fibres of the mouse DUCHEN (1971a) found that subneural folds were twice as numerous in fast fibres, an average of 2.6 folds opening into the primary synaptic cleft per μm of

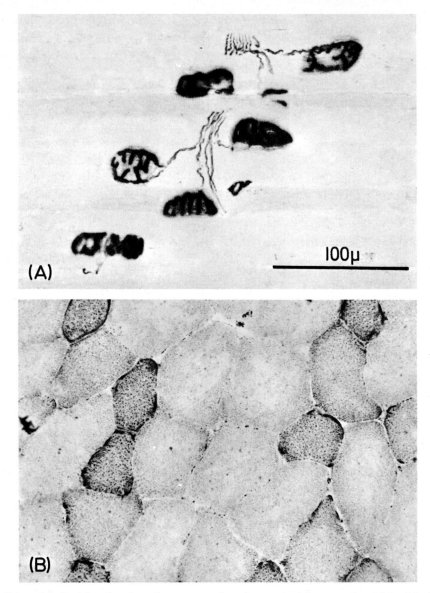

Fig. 18 A and B. Peripheral region of gastrocnemius of normal adult mouse in which white fibres preponderate. Comparison with Fig. 17 prepared by the same techniques shows that: (A) end-plates are larger in fast muscle fibres than in slow and have longer branching gutters around clear spaces. (B) Most muscle fibres are large in diameter with a weak SDH reaction. A few smaller fibres are present with an intermediate or strong SDH reaction. × 360

synaptic membrane. Folds were deeper in fast fibres (0.8 ± 0.1 μm) than in slow (0.5 ± 0.1 μm), and many more folds were branched. The quantitative analysis of electron micrographs by Santa and Engel (1973) compared the neuromuscular junction of red, white and intermediate fibres of the soleus and peripheral part of gastrocnemius of the rat. In the axonal terminals SANTA and ENGEL found no differences in mitochondrial content but observed that the vesicle content was about 1.4 times higher in red than in white fibres while the mean diameter of synaptic vesicles was slightly smaller in red fibres. The ratio of postsynaptic to presynaptic membrane length was 10.5 for white and 8.1 for red fibres. The intermediate fibres tended to have a complex postsynaptic membrane comparable to that of the white fibres though in other respects they were intermediate between the two extremes.

5. The Localization of Cholinesterase

The importance of cholinesterase in normal neuromuscular transmission is well established. The rapid hydrolysis of acetylcholine limits the duration of the action of transmitter and also provides a local source of choline for re-utilization within the nerve terminal. Cholinesterase activity is found in all vertebrate species in both the central and peripheral nervous systems as well as in red blood cells, serum and viscera. The main esterasic enzyme which is found in the nervous system, and partic-ularly at the neuromuscular junction, is acetylcholinesterase which is also found in red blood cells. In serum and viscera the predominant enzyme is nonspecific ('pseudo') cholinesterase. Its function is somewhat obscure and though it is found in growing nerve fibres (TERÄVÄINEN, 1968a; DUCHEN, 1970a) nerves and end-plates seem to form normally in the absence of this enzyme (LEHMANN et al., 1961).

The early report of MARNAY and NACHMANSOHN (1938) showed that cholinester-ase activity in muscles was greatest in the segment containing motor nerve endings. The development of a histochemical method of demonstrating cholinesterase in-creased knowledge of the detailed morphology of the neuromuscular junction and facilitated research into the innervation of healthy and disordered skeletal muscle since it allowed a clear histological distinction to be made between motor and sensory fibres (KOELLE and FRIEDENWALD, 1949). Subsequently other methods for the histochemical demonstration of cholinesterases have been developed for both light and electron microscopy. The theoretical basis and details of various methods are given by PEARSE (1960), and specificity, quantitative determination and enzyme kinetics are discussed by AUGUSTINSSON (1963). A critical review of the techniques developed for electron microscopy is given by FRIEDENBERG and SELIGMAN (1972). Nevertheless many problems remain in the study of ultrastructural localization. From light microscopical studies it is clear that the main enzyme activity at the normal adult end-plate is due to "specific" acetylcholinesterase (AChE) but weak "pseudo" cholinesterase (ChE) activity is also demonstrable (DENZ, 1953; NYSTRÖM, 1968a; TERÄVÄINEN, 1968a). Acetylthiocholine iodide is a convenient substrate for the demonstration of specific AChE, in a medium such as that described by LEWIS (1961). The nature of the enzyme can be further identified by using inhibitors which exert their action mainly, though not exclusively, on the specific enzyme. These inhibitors include di-isopropyl fluorophosphonate (DFP) used in a concentration of 1×10^{-6} mol/l and the compound known as 284C51 (Wellcome Laboratories) used in a concentration of 3×10^{-5} mol/l. When these inhibitors are used the specific AChE activity is largely abolished and the residual demonstrable activity is then mainly due to ChE. If the same substrate is used in conjunction with tetra-isopropylpyro-phospho-ramide (iso-OMPA) in a concentration of 3×10^{-6} mol/l, which inhibits ChE activity,

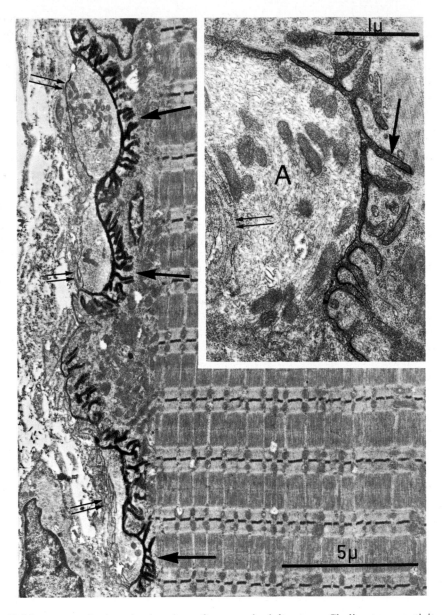

Fig. 19. Neuromuscular junction in soleus of a normal adult mouse. Cholinesterase activity has been demonstrated by the method of KOELLE and FRIEDENWALD (1949) after glutaraldehyde fixation. Blocks were post-fixed in osmium tetroxide, stained with uranyl acetate and embedded in epoxy resin. Sections were stained with lead citrate. The precipitate is most concentrated in the synaptic space and postsynaptic folds (single arrow) and is also present at axon-Schwann cell junctions and over membranes of Schwann cell processes (double arrows). × 7000. INSET is from a similar preparation. (Electron micrographs by Mr. A. J. DAVEY.) A-axon terminal. × 23000

the residual reaction product is due to ACh E. Conversely, butyrylthiocholine iodide as the substrate will reveal ChE more readily than AChE activity and the inhibitors will improve the specificity of the reaction and the validity of any interpretations. Many factors influence the final picture obtained with light microscopy; these include the fixative, length of fixation, temperature, the pH of the substrate and the duration of incubation. Reasonably reliable results can only be obtained by using several substrates each incorporating an inhibitor in parallel studies of numerous sections (COUTEAUX, 1958).

Electron microscopical localization of enzyme activity at the neuromuscular junction is even more capricious. The only trustworthy statement at present is that activity of cholinesterase is greatest in the synaptic cleft and in the postsynaptic folds (Fig. 19), facts already known from the light microscopical studies of COUTEAUX (1947) and COUTEAUX and TAXI (1952). The fixative and duration of fixation raise even more acute problems in electron microscopy. The inhibition of enzyme activity produced by fixation, which is necessary for morphological clarity and the prevention of diffusion artefacts, may itself produce other artefacts of molecular structure and localization (TERÄVÄINEN, 1969). Variations in the penetration of fixatives and substrates also lead to lack of reliability. The need to produce an electron-dense particle to allow identification of the site of enzyme action has usually involved several steps in the reaction, often with a crystalline sulphide deposit as the final visible molecule. These procedures do not guarantee that the final reaction product is located at the precise site of the original enzyme molecule. Shifts of variously charged particles and adsorption on to membranes are among the possible causes of artefact. The use of osmiophilic synthetic agents which incorporate an enzyme-susceptible thiolester group and a diazonium group within the same molecule, may lead to more reliable localization (see FRIEDENBERG and SELIGMAN, 1972). The exact site of enzyme synthesis may be of considerable importance in our understanding of mechanisms in nerve-muscle relationships in normal as well as in pathological states.

It is certain that AChE appears at the nerve-muscle interface after the arrival of the axon in the developing muscle both during normal embryological development (MUMENTHALER and ENGEL, 1961; TERÄVÄINEN, 1968a) and in tissue cultures (PETERSON and CRAIN, 1970). During embryological development considerable ChE activity is demonstrable in growing nerves (TERÄVÄINEN, 1968a). This disappears with the formation of the neuromuscular junction. The pattern of enzyme reactions reaches its mature state at about the time of birth with AChE apparently being the main enzyme at the synaptic interface while some ChE activity is always demonstrable at the axon-Schwann cell interface (DAVIS and KOELLE, 1967). An interesting comparison can be made with the effects of botulinum toxin (see DUCHEN, 1970a). LENTZ (1969) studied the formation of neuromuscular junctions in regenerating limb muscles of the newt and demonstrated the appearance of AChE in the synaptic gap concomitantly with the arrival of nerve fibres and the establishment of contacts, and also showed the association between the increase in enzyme activity and the development of postsynaptic folds. ChE activity is also found in non-innervated muscle from 13 day-old chick embryos after culture for 5 to 6 weeks (ENGEL, 1961). AChE activity can also be seen at myotendinous junctions (see MUIR, 1961), but its significance there is obscure. It is noteworthy that MILEDI (1960) demonstrated increased sensitivity of the muscle fibres to acetylcholine near their tendinous insertions.

More recent, non-histochemical methods for attempting to localize the exact site of AChE activity include the use of electron autoradiography (SALPETER, 1967; SALPETER et al., 1972). Tritium-labelled DFP was used and the DFP-binding sites were sought by subsequent autoradiography of ultrathin sections. These studies have confirmed the concentration of AChE sites in the junctional folds but the degree of resolution was not sufficient to distinguish between the presynaptic membrane, synaptic gap and postsynaptic membrane. SALPETER (1967) calculated that if enzyme activity is present within the axon terminal itself, it must be less than 10% of that present in the junctional region.

The search for the site of AChE synthesis and localization led a number of investigators to study the effects of denervation on the appearance of the end-plate in histochemical preparations with both light and electron microscopy. The results obtained by most studies of mammalian denervated muscle have been similar (e.g. SNELL and MCINTYRE, 1956; ELIAS, 1972). Even after disintegration of the axon, enzyme activity is readily demonstrable but the reaction becomes progressively weaker, finally disappearing after several weeks. Electron microscopically the results are essentially similar to those seen by light microscopy (CSILLIK and KNYIHAR, 1968) but enzyme activity can be demonstrated only in the postsynaptic folds, remaining for several weeks after denervation. It seems clear that the cholinesterase activity demonstrable after nerve section, and which was thought by some authors to indicate that the enzyme was synthesized by the muscle fibre, is merely residual enzyme which remains *in situ* because of the persistence of postsynaptic folds. Evidence indicates that the enzyme is concentrated within the basement membrane material which fills the postsynaptic folds. Such a conclusion is given credence by the recent experiments of HALL and KELLY (1971) and BETZ and SAKMANN (1973) in which *in vitro* nerve-muscle preparations were subjected to the action of trypsin, protease or collagenase. Exposure to protease caused the complete disappearance of the basement membrane of the muscle fibre and in the postsynaptic folds and the reduction or abolition of demonstrable cholinesterase activity at the end-plate. The physiological characteristics of nerve and muscle fibres were not altered nor was the muscle's sensitivity to acetylcholine (BETZ and SAKMANN, 1973). Incubation in 0.1% collagenase caused the preferential removal of basement membrane material from the synaptic cleft and folds and abolished AChE activity. HALL and KELLY (1971) found that collagenase caused the release of AChE into the bathing fluid. The results of these enzyme digestion experiments suggests that "end-plate acetylcholinesterase is situated in a relatively exposed position on the external nerve or muscle cell surface, either on the surface of the membrane or on the external lamina, and is not a structural component of the membrane" (HALL and KELLY, 1971).

An interesting development is the identification of three species of AChE all with apparently identical enzymic activity but with characteristic sedimentations in sucrose gradients (MASSOULIE et al., 1973; HALL, 1973). In the rat diaphragm one form, 16S, was found only in the end-plate region, while the others (4S and 10S) were found throughout the muscle fibre (HALL, 1973). The values for the three forms found in the electric organ of *Torpedo* were 8.5S, 4.2S, and 18.4S (MASSOULIE et al., 1973). Another interesting approach to the localization of AChE utilizes the production of anti-AChE antibody which can be labelled with fluoresceine (TSUJI et al., 1973). These recent developments in the study of AChE, an enzyme of vital importance in the functioning of the nervous system, may offer further insights into the pathogenesis of some neuro-muscular diseases.

Concentration of AChE at the myoneural junction and its eventual disappearance after denervation provide evidence for the "neurotrophic" control of its localization (see GUTH, 1968). DRACHMAN (1972) found a significant reduction in the enzyme after seven days' block of neuromuscular transmission produced by local injection of botulinum toxin in the sternomastoid of the rat and suggested that the induction of AChE is dependent upon the release of ACh into the synaptic gap.

6. The Basement Membrane

The surfaces of muscle fibres and Schwann cells are coated by an amorphous material of moderate electron density, seemingly the same as that found in renal glomeruli, around capillaries and larger blood vessels and known variously as surface coating, basement membrane, basal lamina, or, in muscle, ectolemma. It is a tough material since it may hold the contents of the sarcolemmal tube in place when the muscle fibre is necrotic (ALLBROOK, 1962; DUCHEN et al., 1974). When the muscle fibre is atrophied the basement membrane layer does not shrink but becomes thrown into folds where it is redundant (BIRKS et al., 1960; NASSAR, 1967; MILEDI and SLATER, 1968). The biochemical composition of basement membrane material was reviewed by KEFALIDES (1973). Although most work has been done on preparations derived from renal glomeruli the results might well apply to the material coating muscle and to the material within the synaptic cleft and postsynaptic folds. Morphologically all basement membrane material has the same appearance. It is rich in carbohydrates and contains a fraction with some of the characteristics of collagen. It is not found between Schwann cell and axolemmal membranes; and at the edge of the synaptic cleft, muscle and Schwann cell coats fuse together. The material fills the whole synaptic gap and extends down into the spaces formed by the postsynaptic folds of sarcolemma (see Figs. 8, 9, 11, 12, 13). Even after the sarcolemma disappears, the basement membrane of the postsynaptic folds persists when muscle fibres are necrotic (DUCHEN et al., 1974). The basement membrane is thought to function both as a structural support and a selective filter. At the neuromuscular junction it must allow for the rapid diffusion of acetylcholine, and it is also the material in which acetylcholinesterase is concentrated.

7. The Localization of Acetylcholine Receptors

The sensitivity of the sarcolemmal membrane to acetylcholine is greatest in the region of the neuromuscular junction. Normally extrajunctional sensitivity is low (MILEDI, 1960) but it increases after the loss of functional innervation (see THESLEFF, 1960b). There is good evidence for the existence of acetylcholine receptors which are concentrated at the neuromuscular junction, probably in the postsynaptic membrane. The localization of pharmacological agents, such as ^{14}C labelled curare, in end-plate regions has been demonstrated autoradiographically (WASER, 1965). Neurotoxic fractions of snake venoms have a curare-like action on muscle fibres (see LEE, 1972) and α-bungarotoxin, a fraction of the venom of *Bungarus multicinctus*, has proved of value for labelling and localizing receptors. α-bungarotoxin has been

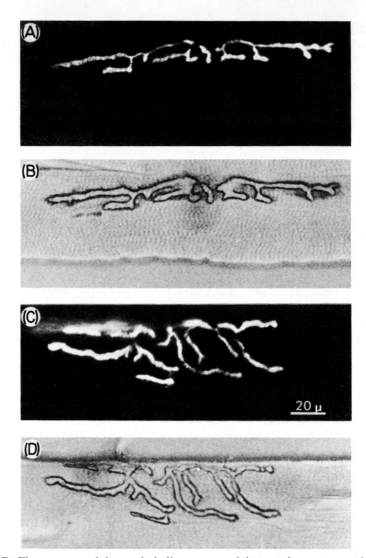

Fig. 20 A—D. Fluorescent staining and cholinesterase staining on the same muscle fibres. (A)
Xenopus sartorius muscle fibre stained with tetramethylrhodamine-labelled α-bungarotoxin. (B)
Same muscle fibre as in (A) stained for cholinesterase, the cholinesterase stain accumulating
preferentially at the edge of the neuromuscular junction and outlining it. Comparison of (A) and
(B) confirms that the fluorescent stain is confined to the neuromuscular junction. (C) and (D)
Muscle fibre from rectus femoris anticus of *Xenopus*, stained as in (A) and (B) respectively. (From
ANDERSON and COHEN, 1974, reproduced by permission of the Editorial Board of the Journal of
Physiology)

found to combine with cholinergic receptors at the neuromuscular junction (CHAN-
GEUX et al., 1970) and has been labelled with ^{131}I (MILEDI and POTTER, 1971) as well
as with ^{3}H (BARNARD et al., 1971), ^{125}I (FAMBROUGH and HARTZELL, 1972; HART-
ZELL and FAMBROUGH, 1972) and fluorescent dyes (ANDERSON and COHEN, 1974) in

attempts to calculate the concentration of receptor sites. The toxin is bound to sites strictly confined to the neuromuscular junction, and these cholinergic receptor sites are not identical with the sites of cholinesterase activity. The illustrations of ANDER-SON and COHEN (1974) very strongly support previously held views that the sites of receptors at which α-bungarotoxin is bound are confined to the postsynaptic membrane including the subneural folds (Fig. 20). More exact ultrastructural localization awaits electron microscopic methods of higher resolution than those available at present.

C. Development, Growth, and Plasticity of the Neuromuscular Junction

1. Development of the Neuromuscular Junction

The sequence of events occurring during the formation of the neuromuscular junction may be studied from three aspects—normal embryological development, the formation of new end-plates in adult muscle, and the formation of nerve-muscle contacts in tissue culture. Each of these fields of study offers a different set of environmental conditions which may not be strictly comparable, yet in all of them the sequence of events in the formation and maturation of the end-plate itself is closely similar.

The development of the neuromuscular junction in the normal intact embryo and the newborn has been described by several authors. One of the first was TELLO (1917) who illustrated by his beautiful silver preparations the histogenesis of motor innervation of muscle in the chick embryo. He showed the formation of simple connections between nerve and muscle, the subsequent elaboration of the terminal arborization and the aggregation of nuclei to form the sole-plate after the arrival of the axon. In new-born or immature mammalian muscle there may be only one slender axon terminal on a muscle fibre (TELLO, 1917; COËRS, 1955; NYSTRÖM, 1968 b). An important point to note is that in focally innervated muscle fibres the axon does not grow beyond the end-plate after contact is made (HEWER, 1935; CUAJUNCO, 1942; MA-VRINSKAIA, 1960). Any extension of the axon beyond the end-plate would be termed ultraterminal and HINSEY (1934) defined such an extension as an unmyelinated branch which arises from within the motor end-plate and which goes on to form another ending on the same or neighbouring fibre. In his review HINSEY concluded that "the literature seems to show that ultraterminal endings are more frequent in lower forms and in embryonic and young muscle, but they are seldom found in adult muscles of higher vertebrates: they appear to be more frequent in tongue muscles than in others". After it makes contact with the muscle fibre the axon grows only as a part of general somatic growth.

With advancing age arborization becomes more extensive and complex (SHE-HATA and BOWDEN, 1960; SHEHATA, 1961; BARKER and IP, 1966; HARRIMAN et al., 1970; TUFFERY, 1971) due to an increase in the number of small unmyelinated axonal branches within the end-plate. The exact mechanism of the production of these changes with normal ageing is not fully understood. It is of interest that polyphasic motor-unit action potentials which are characteristic of the early stages of recovery after peripheral nerve injuries (WEDDELL et al., 1944) are found in supposedly healthy adult muscles. These have been attributed to the regeneration of axons after repeated

minor traumata. Other factors which might be invoked are disturbances of neuromuscular transmission and structural changes in muscle fibres in the absence of overt
disease.

MUMENTHALER and ENGEL (1961) studied developing chick skeletal muscle and
found that some muscles were innervated by the 6th to 7th day. They observed
demonstrable cholinesterase activity in the whole muscle fibre, but after the 11th day
activity was concentrated in the end-plate areas. TERÄVÄINEN (1968c) in his study of
the developing end-plate in the rat tibialis anterior muscle found specific acetylcholinesterase visible at the junction in 18 day embryos. In the early stages of development the area of enzyme activity had a flat plate-like structure which deepened to
form a depression in the surface of the muscle fibre by the 2nd to 4th postnatal day.
Subneural lamellae could be seen by the 5th day. Nonspecific cholinesterase, but not
specific AChE, was seen in abundance along nerves in embryos but this enzyme
activity had disappeared by the 3rd week after birth.

Electron microscopic studies of the normal development of rat neuromuscular
junctions (TERÄVÄINEN, 1968a) showed close appositions between clusters of axons
and groups of myotubes. "Focal electron-opaque membrane specializations more
intimately connect axon and myotube membranes to each other" (KELLY and ZACKS,
1969). The depression of the muscle fibre membrane, the development of local thickening and the formation of postsynaptic folds occurred later. Primary clefts and
subneural folds are rudimentary at birth but by the 10th postnatal day the neuromuscular junction has a mature appearance similar to the adult, though the subneural folds are still shorter and less complicated than in the adult. Sole-plate
nuclei appear coincidentally with the peripheral migration of nuclei to the subsarco-
lemmal position (KELLY and ZACKS, 1969).

When we consider the stages in the formation of new end-plates in muscles of
adult animals the question arises of the resistance of innervated muscle to accessory
innervation. This property of innervated skeletal muscle has been recognized for
many years. TELLO (1917) compared the innervated muscle fibre which will not form
more end-plates to the fertilized ovum which is impervious to more spermatozoa. It
seems evident that the nerve fibre in some way has a "trophic" influence on the
muscle fibre which normally prevents it accepting additional innervation and forming new end-plates (for a review of this problem see GUTH, 1968). Any study of the
formation of new neuromuscular synapses in the adult must therefore involve
the creation of a region of muscle which is receptive to new innervation. Such a
receptive state can be induced either by denervation (GUTMANN and YOUNG, 1944),
by the creation of a non-innervated segment of muscle made by separating a non-
innervated segment near a tendon from the central innervated zone (AITKEN, 1950;
MILEDI, 1962; KOENIG, 1963, 1971; GWYN and AITKEN, 1966), or by paralysing the
muscle with a neuromuscular blocking agent such as botulinum toxin (FEX et al.,
1966; TONGE, 1974b). In all these situations the receptivity of the muscle to an
accessory (extra) nerve is associated with the development of supersensitivity of the
muscle fibre to acetylcholine, but how this association is controlled or whether other
factors are involved is not known. If a new nerve is implanted into a normally
innervated muscle it will not form new end-plates except for a few at the site of
implantation, presumably on fibres denervated by local trauma. However when FEX
and THESLEFF (1967) cut the original nerve as long as 12 weeks after implanting a new

one, within as short a period as 2 days stimulation of the implanted nerve elicited a twitch. This suggests that motor nerve terminals may exist within a muscle for a long time with no postsynaptic evidence of their existence. When new end-plates are forming in receptive muscle their appearance with both light (e.g. GWYN and AIT-KEN, 1966) and electron microscopy (KOENIG, 1971, 1973) resembles that seen in normal development. The first nerve-muscle contacts are superficial and devoid of synaptic gutters or postsynaptic differentiation. Thickening of the postsynaptic sar-colemma can be seen within 2 weeks and postsynaptic folds are formed by the third to fourth week in the rat. However, KOENIG and PÉCOT-DECHAVASSINE (1971) have produced evidence that neuromuscular transmission occurs well before the full ma-turation of the new neuromuscular junction thus confirming earlier observations in human foetuses and neonates (vide supra). The newly formed end-plates in pre-viously non-innervated segments of muscle never come to look entirely normal with light microscopy, either in silver impregnated sections or when stained to show cholinesterase activity. They consist of groups of oval or cuplike subunits, sometimes stretched out for long distances over the muscle fibre. The formation of new end-plates in muscles of regenerating limbs of the newt was studied by LENTZ (1969) and here again the sequence of events was similar to that seen during normal develop-ment and acetylcholinesterase activity appeared concomitantly with the differentia-tion of the postsynaptic sarcolemmal membrane.

2. Development in Tissue Culture

The use of tissue culture for the study of nerve-muscle interactions is a fairly recent development and offers the possibility of investigations which would be difficult or impossible to perform in the living animal. The ability of nerve cells from spinal cord explants to grow and establish contact with skeletal muscle is now well known (JAMES and TRESMAN, 1969; VENERONI and MURRAY, 1969; PETERSON and CRAIN, 1970). Although neuromuscular transmission across the junction thus formed and localized concentrations of AChE have been demonstrated, silver impregnation re-vealed ramifying axons and the absence of the orderly pattern of innervation seen in vivo. The sequence of events leading to the development of well-formed end-plates has been studied with electron microscopy by JAMES and TRESMAN (1969) and PAPPAS et al. (1971). The latter group, using muscle and spinal nerve cells of the rat, found indentation of the sarcolemma beneath axon terminals at 33 days, while at 60 days postsynaptic folds were deeper and by 80 days resembled those in adult muscles. Many dense-core vesicles were seen in nerve terminals in these preparations (Fig. 21).

The addition of tubocurarine in a concentration of 3×10^{-4} g/ml to the culture medium in which amphibian nerve and muscle tissue was growing did not prevent the formation of synaptic connections (COHEN, 1972). This observation has consid-erable bearing on the hypothesis that "trophic" attraction of axons to muscle fibres depends on the fibres' sensitivity to acetylcholine. A further step in the study of questions relating to the development of the neuromuscular junction was taken by STEINBACH et al. (1973). They showed that cells of clonal lines of mouse muscle and mouse neuroblastoma interact in tissue culture, the result being the production of an area of increased acetylcholine sensitivity on the muscle membrane. Addition of α-

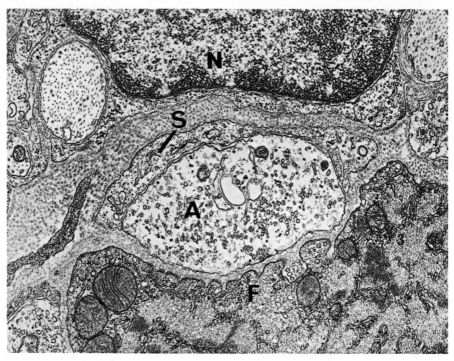

Fig. 21. Section through a neuromuscular junction of a 33-day-old muscle-cord culture. The axon
(A) contains many vesicles. The subjunctional portion of the sarcolemma of the muscle fibre
(F) shows some indentations. Schwann cell process *(S)* surrounds the axon, except at the
junctional contact area. *N*-nucleus of an adjacent Schwann cell ensheathing a small neurite (×
20 500). (From Pappas et al., 1971)

neurotoxin derived from the venom of *Naja naja* reversibly blocked the acetylcholine receptor sites on the muscle fibre but did not abolish the development of local
sensitivity. The addition of pyridinium, which blocks the synthesis and release of
acetylcholine in neuroblastoma cells, did not prevent the development of local sensitivity. It seems that neither the presence of acetylcholine in the nerve fibre nor
acetylcholine-sensitivity in the muscle fibre is necessary for the formation of neuromuscular junctions, though the importance of functioning motor nerve terminals in
the development of normal muscles is not in doubt. For example Drachman (1964)
showed that botulinum toxin, which blocks acetylcholine release, caused severe
muscular atrophy and deformity of the limbs in chick embryos.

3. Structural Denervation

The changes which take place in the morphology of the motor end-plate after section
of its nerve have been studied for many years (e.g. Tello, 1907), and are similar to the
changes following damage to the anterior horn cell (see Bowden, 1951). That portion of axon which is no longer in continuity with the perikaryon of the cell undergoes Wallerian degeneration. The rate of degeneration is more rapid in mammalian
than in amphibian nerve and there is some indirect evidence that it also varies with

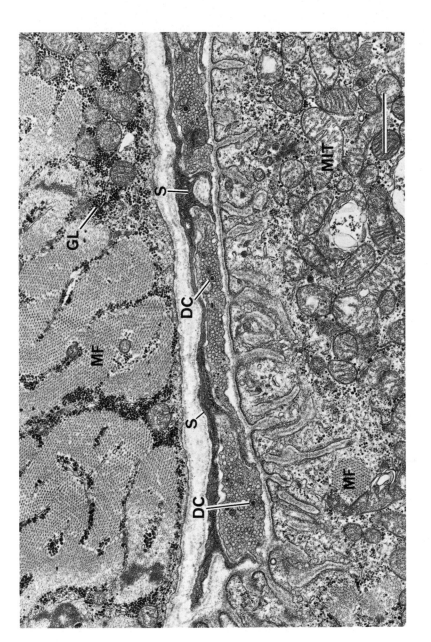

Fig. 22. Cross section of a portion of two muscle fibres from an 87-day-old muscle-cord culture. A section of a motor end-plate traversing the entire micrograph can be seen. The axonal terminals are filled with presynaptic vesicles, some of which are of the dense-core variety (DC). The postsynaptic or subjunctional infoldings of the sarcolemma, characteristic of neuromuscular junctions, are found along the entire region of synaptic contact. The axon terminals are ensheathed by Schwann cell processes (S), except at the synaptic contact surface. MIT-mitochondria: GL-glycogen particles; MF-myofilaments (×16300). (From PAPPAS et al., 1971). Calibration: 1μ

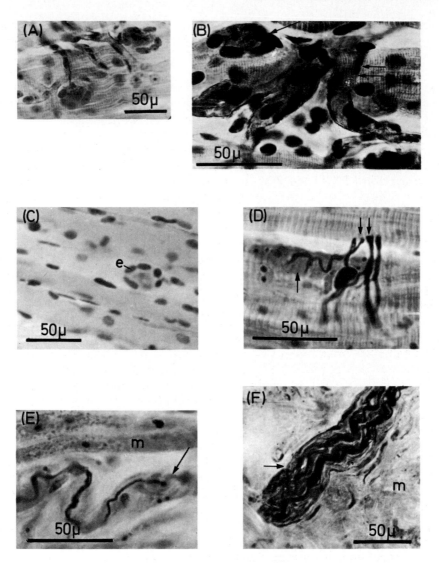

Fig. 23 A—F. Normal, denervated and reinnervated human muscle. (A) Motor end-plate in normal limb muscle. × 225. (B) 69 days after denervation. × 450 empty motor end-plate shown by
sole plate nuclei only (↑). Empty Schwann tube (↑↑). (C) 79 days after denervation. Note end-plate
(e) devoid of axon terminals. × 300. (D) 323 days after axonotmesis and 276 days after reinnervation was theoretically possible. An old end-plate ↑ has been reinnervated by thick nerve fibres ↑↑.
× 450. (E) 608 days after nerve injury, 408 days after suture and 298 days after it was theoretically
possible for nerves to reach the muscle. Muscle fibres (m) are atrophic [cf. (D)] and nerve fibres
run along and across muscle fibres for unusual distances and in this fig. one ends in a knob
(arrow) in connective tissue. × 450. (F) 3164 days after injury; 693 days after suture of the nerve.
Re-innervation of the nerve trunk (↑) is satisfactory, but no recovery is possible because of gross
atrophy of muscle (m) which is largely replaced by fat and connective tissue. × 300. Preparations
are all impregnated by BIELSCHOWSKY's silver technique by E. GUTMANN. (From BOWDEN and
GUTMANN, 1944, reproduced by permission of the Editor, Brain)

species and age (WEDDELL et al., 1943). After the axon and myelin sheath have
disappeared the end-plate region may be identified for several weeks by the persistence of demonstrable cholinesterase and by its collection of sole-plate nuclei for a
long time (Fig. 23 B and C), up to a year in human muscle (BOWDEN and GUTMANN,
1944). Cholinesterase activity in the end-plate decreases progressively and finally
disappears entirely. For a short time weak AChE activity may be seen in the terminal
part of the Schwann cell sheath (CSILLIK, 1967; ELIAS, 1972).

Electron microscopic changes at the end-plate after nerve section are very similar
in frog (BIRKS et al., 1960) and mammalian muscle (REGER, 1959; MILEDI and SLA-
TER, 1968; WASER and NICKEL, 1969). After nerve section both structure and transmission are normal for 8 to 12 hrs in the rat. In man nerve conduction may persist for as long as 2 to 3 days (BOWDEN, 1954). Then the mitochondria in the axon
terminals become swollen and spherical and synaptic vesicles become clumped together. Dense granular masses, membranous bodies and other organelles are found
in the degenerating nerve terminal which becomes fragmented, while processes of
hypertrophied Schwann cells extend around and between the axonal fragments.
Later the axon is replaced by Schwann cells whose cytoplasm then lies in direct
apposition to the post-synaptic membrane. Schwann cells remain in this position for
some days but later seem to become retracted away from the end-plate itself and
separated from it by collagen fibrils. Postsynaptic folds of the sarcolemmal membrane remain identifiable in denervated muscle fibres for many weeks (Fig. 24).

The pattern of innervation of a skeletal muscle is profoundly disturbed by any
condition causing a physical loss of some of its axons. An experimental situation in
which muscles were partially deprived of axons was described by WEISS and EDDS
(1945) and VAN HARREVELD (1945) who cut one of the spinal nerves supplying a
muscle. They found that after a time the atrophy caused by the partial denervation
was halted and thereafter the muscle regained its normal strength when tested elec-
trophysiologically. Since it was not possible for regenerating axons from the cut
spinal nerve to have reached the muscle by the time of recovery of function, this was
attributed to branching of the remaining axons. EDDS (1950), HOFFMAN (1950) and
EDDS and SMALL (1951) showed that if a muscle is partially denervated, the denervated muscle fibres become re-innervated. It was suggested that this process involved
collaterals sprouting at nodes of Ranvier of surviving intact axons. Both HOFFMAN
and EDDS detected newly formed fine fibres very soon after the partial denervation
and saw axonal branches arising mainly from the intact axons. The effectiveness of
this process would presumably depend in part upon the distribution of the muscle
fibres of the motor unit. If these fibres were scattered, the chances of reinnervation
would be greater than if the constituents of the unit were arranged in compact
bundles. Experimental partial denervation of muscle was studied by WOHLFART and
HOFFMAN (1956) who inoculated mice with THEILER's encephalomyelitis virus
(mouse poliomyelitis). This causes degeneration of anterior horn cells of the spinal
cord. Within a short time after the onset of paralysis in these mice, branching of
surviving axons was found.

In man diseases such as poliomyelitis, motor-neurone disease (amyotrophic lateral sclerosis) and WERDNIG-HOFFMANN disease (infantile motor neurone disease)
are all conditions in which there is a progressive loss of spinal anterior horn cells
with varying degrees of paralysis. In the *wobbler* mouse (DUCHEN and STRICH,

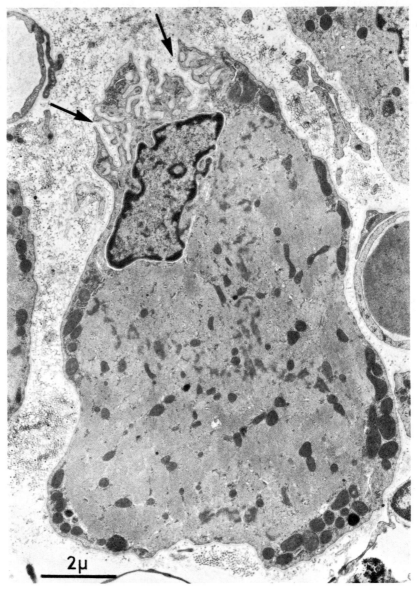

Fig. 24. Transverse section of a mouse gastrocnemius muscle fibre denervated for 10 weeks by excision of a segment of sciatic nerve. The postsynaptic folds of the original end-plate (arrows) are still identifiable in spite of the severe atrophy of the muscle fibre. The folds are shallower and wider than normal and contain collagen fibres. No Schwann cell processes are seen over the folds. × 10000

1968a) there is a progressive loss of motor axons due to an inherited degenerative disease of motor-neurones in the brainstem and spinal cord. In all these conditions muscles characteristically show a fascicular distribution of atrophy. The preterminal axons which survive are markedly branched so that each one innervates several or many muscle fibres instead of only one (WOHLFART, 1958; COËRS and WOOLF, 1959; DUCHEN and STRICH, 1968a). Axonal sprouting can be seen before the onset of clinically detectable muscle weakness and seems to be an early compensatory response to partial denervation. WEISS and EDDS (1945) calculated that muscle weakness became apparent only when more than 50% of motor axons had been lost. The exact mechanism initiating the branching and sprouting of axons in response to partial denervation is not known.

Many factors influence the possibility of re-innervation of existing sole plates after Wallerian degeneration. These include the nature of the lesion in the nerve trunk and the state of the muscle itself (BOWDEN and GUTMANN, 1944; BOWDEN, 1954). Examples of changes in human muscle are shown in Fig. 23.

D. The Neuromuscular Junction in Disorders of Transmission

1. Myasthenia Gravis

The best known human disease in which there is a disorder of neuromuscular transmission is myasthenia gravis. The relationship between myasthenia gravis and thymic hyperplasia or tumour is well known but not clearly understood. A disorder of immunological mechanisms has been suggested (see SIMPSON, 1969), while DESMEDT and BORENSTEIN (1973) regard it as a "metabolic motoneurone disease". The existence of a circulating neuromuscular blocking agent has not been demonstrated and the transient syndrome of neonatal myasthenia in some babies born to affected mothers is as yet unexplained.

Affected skeletal muscles were first studied histologically by BUZZARD (1905) who noted aggregations of lymphocytes ("lymphorrhages") particularly in extraocular muscles and noted that severe muscle atrophy may occur, albeit rarely. RUSSELL (1953) described muscle necrosis and atrophy of both single muscle fibres as well as of groups of fibres, while FENICHEL and SHY (1963) reported that half of the total number of biopsy specimens in myasthenia gravis showed no abnormality while the remaining ones showed single fibre atrophy. OOSTERHUIS and BETHLEM (1973) reviewed the problem of neurogenic muscular atrophy in myasthenia gravis. No satisfactory explanation for this phenomenon has yet been put forward.

COËRS (1955), COËRS and DESMEDT (1959), COËRS and WOOLF (1959), BICKERSTAFF (1960) and MACDERMOT (1960) all studied intramuscular nerve terminals in biopsies stained intravitally with methylene blue. They found areas in which there was much collateral sprouting of preterminal axons and elongation of the end-plates. WOOLF (1966) also found elongation of the synaptic region and considered that this was secondary to disordered neuromuscular transmission. These findings have been substantiated by other workers (Fig. 25) and similar changes have been shown in thick frozen sections of autopsy material impregnated by SCHOFIELD's (1960) silver technique (DANIEL and STRICH, 1966; BROWNELL et al., 1972). The tips of the enlarged and complex terminal arborizations showed small rings or knobs that are characteristic of growing axons stained with silver. These changes were most pronounced in extrinsic ocular muscles and those of tongue and larynx i.e. those muscles commonly most severely affected in myasthenia gravis.

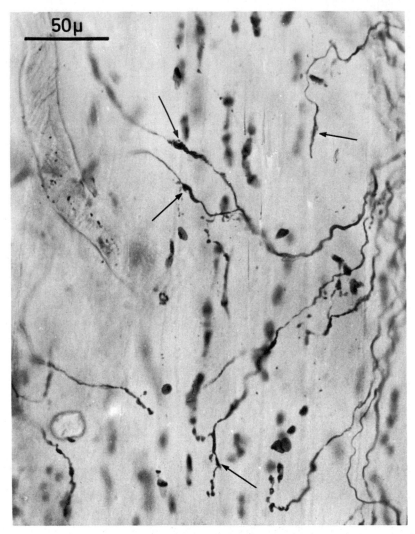

Fig. 25. Deltoid muscle biopsy from a female aged 32 with myasthenia gravis. Motor end-plates (arrows) are elongated and linear, terminal axonic expansions stunted or absent and preterminal branching as well as ultraterminal sprouts (i.e. beyond the end-plate) are present. (Preparation by Dr. D.G.F. HARRIMAN, Department of Neuropathology, Medical School, University of Leeds). Intravital methylene blue. × 430

Electron microscopic studies have been reported recently by ENGEL and SANTA (1971; 1973) and by FARDEAU et al. (1973). Although some normal-looking end-plates are invariably seen (Fig. 26), poor postsynaptic differentiation is the most usual abnormality (Fig. 27). Histometric analysis by ENGEL and SANTA showed that the ratio between lengths of postsynaptic and presynaptic membranes, normally about 10, was significantly reduced to about 8. Postsynaptic folds were sparse, shallow and often wide, and at many neuromuscular junctions no folds were seen. Many of the

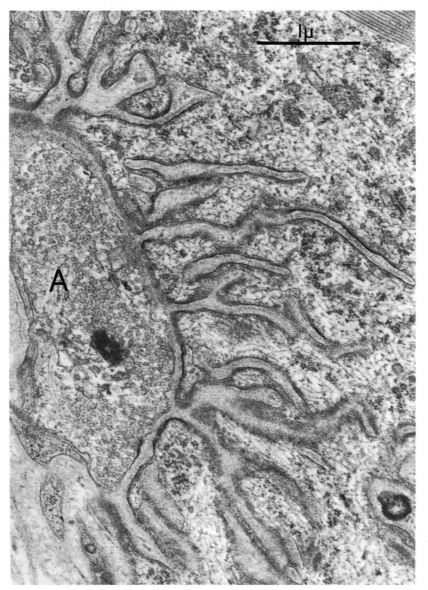

Fig. 26. Deltoid muscle biopsy from a 6 year-old male with myasthenia gravis of about a year's duration. This end-plate is normal in appearance. Compare with Fig. 28 from the same biopsy. × 27 000

axons were small and resembled immature growing axonal sprouts (Fig. 28). ENGEL and SANTA also illustrated rounded electron dense bodies lying in wide spaces between axon and muscle. They were unable to detect significant differences in the concentration or mean diameter of synaptic vesicles. These abnormalities seen in myasthenia gravis have many similarities to those found during the normal growth and development of end-plates, as well as during the recovery from the effects of

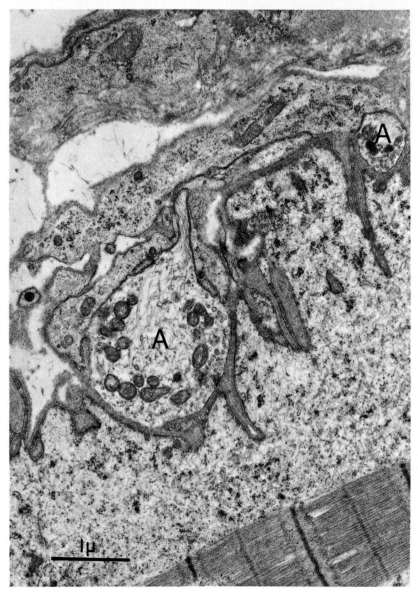

Fig. 27. Myasthenia gravis. A biopsy from a 15 year old male. Paucity and shallowness of sub-neural folds are commonly found in this disease. *A*-axon terminals. (Electron micrograph by Dr. M. Fardeau, Hôpital Salpêtrière, Paris). × 19000

botulinum and tetanus toxins. Therefore it seems that these changes are not the immediate cause of muscle weakness and fatigue but are more likely to be secondary to defective neuromuscular transmission.

    Other factors which merit consideration in the interpretation of these changes are those described as being due to long-term anticholinesterase administration (Engel

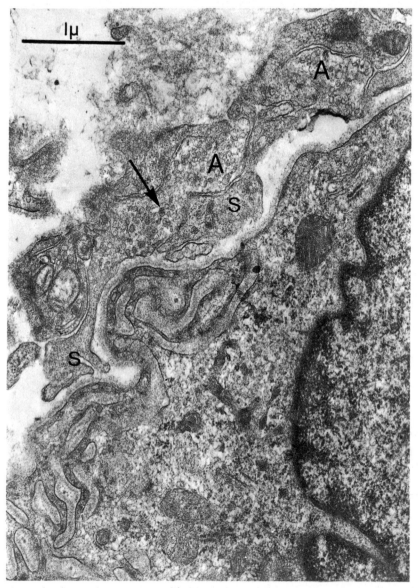

Fig. 28. Myasthenia gravis. Compare with Fig. 26 from the same biopsy. Unmyelinated axons (?sprouts) are seen in the vicinity of an end-plate (shown by the subneural folds). These little axons *(A)* contain vesicles, including one with a dense core (arrow), and do not make close synaptic contact with the muscle fibre. Note Schwann cell processes *(S)*. × 27000

et al., 1973). In rats given neostigmine subcutaneously daily for up to 20 weeks, changes were found to affect end-plates in soleus more than those in the superficial parts of gastrocnemius. Postsynaptic folds were irregularly widened and shallow and numerous dense granules were found in the synaptic gap, very like those seen at end-plates of soleus in the mouse following the local application of paralysing doses of

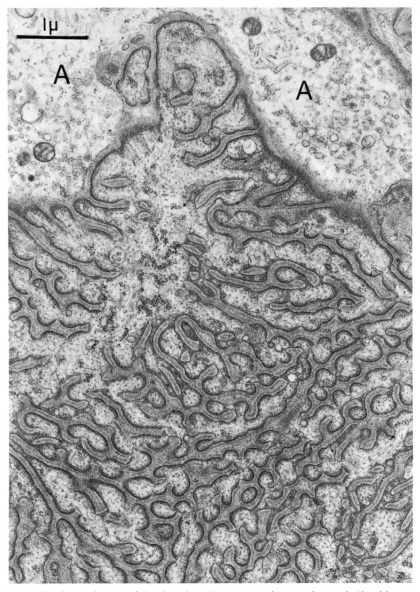

Fig. 29. Myasthenic syndrome of the Lambert-Eaton type in a male aged 60 with anaplastic bronchial carcinoma. The appearance of the axonal terminal *(A)* is probably within normal limits. Note the numerous and complex postsynaptic folds of sarcolemma. (Electron micrograph by Dr. M. Fardeau, Hôpital Salpêtrière, Paris). × 19000

tetanus toxin (Duchen, 1973a). Engel et al. (1973) considered that the changes found in experimental animals given the anticholinesterase drug resembled those found in myasthenia gravis and that such changes might be in part responsible for the physiological alterations in that disease. However, the primary defect remains undetected and of itself may not produce morphological changes. Experimental observations with neuromuscular blocking agents have demonstrated that completely silent synapses may not be abnormal in appearance.

A syndrome characterised by severe muscle weakness may be induced in animals by the injection of cholinergic receptor protein combined with complete Freund's adjuvant. The protein is derived from the electric organs of *Torpedo* or *Electrophorus* (KARLSSON et al., 1972: SUGIYAMA et al., 1973) and antibodies to it seem to react with the immunised animal's own receptor proteins, causing muscle weakness or paralysis (PATRICK and LINDSTROM, 1973; HEILBRONN and MATTSSON, 1974; HEILBRONN et al., 1975; GREEN et al., 1975). A study of the skeletal muscles of rats immunised with receptor protein plus adjuvant has been made by ENGEL et al. (in the press) who found that abnormalities were present only at the end-plates or in their immediate vicinity. Seven to eleven days after the immunising injection focal degeneration of the superficial tips of the subneural folds can be seen, accompanied by an inflammatory reaction during which macrophages invade the muscle fibre and separate the postsynaptic region from the remainder of the muscle cell. Nerve terminals remain intact and come to lie directly on the macrophages and then, at a later stage, on a simplified sarcolemmal membrane which is deficient in subneural folds. The electron microscopic appearance comes to resemble closely the appearances found in human myastenia gravis but it remains to be determined whether a similar pathogenesis operates in the human disease.

2. The Myasthenic Syndrome

A condition characterised by muscular weakness and fatiguability seen in association with bronchogenic carcinoma was reported by EATON and LAMBERT (1957). Detailed electrophysiological studies of the defect in neuromuscular transmission were performed by LAMBERT and ELMQVIST (1971). The morphological findings in the neuromuscular junction have been reported by ENGEL and SANTA (1971), FUKUHARA et al. (1972), FARDEAU et al. (1973). There is a remarkable increase in the depth and complexity of the postsynaptic folds (Fig. 29) together with an unusually large number of pinocytotic vesicles at the postsynaptic sarcolemmal membrane. Quantitative analysis of the electron micrographs by ENGEL and SANTA (1971) showed the ratio between postsynaptic and presynaptic membrane lengths to be much increased (17 instead of the normal 10). FUKUHARA et al. (1972) also observed changes which they interpreted as evidence for repeated degeneration and regeneration of axon terminals. As yet no investigation appears to have included any light microscopic study of the pattern of innervation of affected muscles. Such a study, and careful autopsy investigations are essential for fuller understanding of this syndrome which has the symptoms of myasthenia gravis but shows an uncharacteristic increase in the length of the postsynaptic membrane.

3. Hereditary Motor End-Plate Disease in the Mouse

The development and progression of pathological neuromuscular states can be studied in successive generations of mice with hereditary diseases of the nervous system. Several of these conditions have been recognised (SIDMAN et al., 1965; GREEN, 1966). The clinical features of hereditary motor end-plate disease, first described by

Searle (1962), are increasing muscular weakness and wasting, death occurring by the third to fourth week after birth. Some of the histological features were described by Duchen et al. (1967), and a more detailed account, including the genetics was given by Duchen (1970 b). Electrophysiological findings were described by Duchen and Stefani (1971) and Harris and Ward (1974). All the evidence indicates that the primary abnormality is in the motor nerve terminals, and is associated with progressive failure of neuromuscular transmission. The symbol *med* was given to the autosomal recessive gene by which the disease is transmitted.

The heterozygous carriers of the *med* gene are clinically normal and about 25% of the offspring of heterozygous matings are homozygous (*med/med*) and develop the disease. At birth and for the next 8 to 10 days homozygous *med* mice appear normal. Unsteadiness of gait then appears, and is followed over the next few days by rapidly progressive weakness and wasting in proximal muscles. By the 18th to 19th day the mouse can scarcely make effective movements. The disease is fatal, usually by the 19th to 23rd day. Death is probably due in part to lack of food and water which the animal is too weak to take.

The atrophy and paralysis of skeletal muscle is due to a progressive failure of neuromuscular transmission. Motor axons, axon terminals and muscle fibres are all normal in appearance even at about the 14th day, when muscle weakness is already severe. Muscle fibres then become progressively atrophied though some muscles are affected more than others. Axonal sprouts from the nerve terminals in the end-plate are found after the 12th to 15th day. These grow along muscle fibres, often branching and extending for some distance from the end-plate. The original end-plate can be readily distinguished by the presence of postsynaptic folds of sarcolemma but when axonal sprouts grow along the muscle fibres their contact with the sarcolemma is very superficial (i.e. there is no gutter) and no postsynaptic folds can be found beneath them (Fig. 30). The sprouts usually contain vesicles and mitochondria and look very like any other nerve terminal. They are always enclosed by Schwann cell cytoplasm on their external surface and sometimes Schwann cell processes lie between axon and muscle fibre.

Electrophysiological examination of the most severely affected muscles in the proximal forelimb (e.g. biceps brachii) shows a progressive failure of muscle fibres to respond to stimulation of their nerves with an action potential although they are still capable of responding to direct stimulation. The fibres fibrillate and become supersensitive to acetylcholine. By the 19th day, practically every muscle fibre fails to respond to nerve stimulation, and the whole muscle is supersensitive to ACh. On direct stimulation the time-course of the twitch is slower. These physiological changes are considered pathognomonic of denervation but in fact nerve fibres are present in greater abundance than normal. The myelinated axons look normal and conduct normally, and, most significantly m.e.p.p.s can be recorded intracellularly in every muscle fibre tested. The persistence of m.e.p.p.s indicates that axon terminals are still in contact with muscle fibres and contain transmitter, which correlates with the presence of synaptic vesicles within the terminals. The electrophysiological observations of Duchen and Stefani (1971) have been confirmed by Harris and Ward (1974) who found in addition that paralysed *med* muscle fibres could generate action potentials in the presence of 1×10^{-6} mol/l tetrodotoxin, which provides further evidence of their state of "functional denervation".

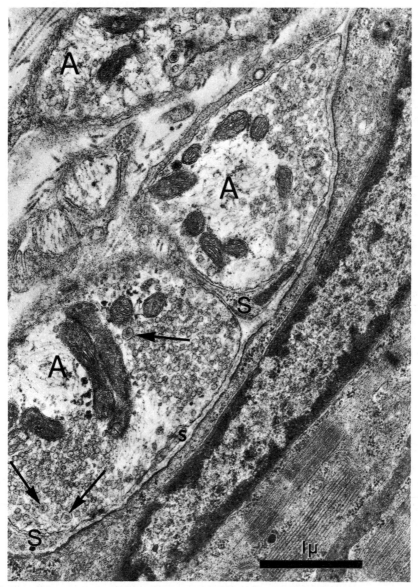

Fig. 30. Hereditary motor end-plate disease (med). Biceps brachii of a 23 day-old *med* mouse. This muscle was totally paralysed to stimulation of its nerve. Axon terminals *(A)*, contain vesicles, some with a dense core (arrows). Schwann cell processes *(S)* interpose between axon and muscle fibre at several places. No postsynaptic folds are seen. The interposition of Schwann cell processes and absence of postsynaptic folds indicate that these axons have sprouted beyond the confines of the motor end-plate. × 27000

The exact cause of the failure of transmission in the *med* mouse is not yet clear. Since it seemed certain that the nerve terminals still contained transmitter, several tests were performed to see whether the frequency of m.e.p.p.s could be influenced by the same factors as those affecting the normal neuromuscular junction. Repetitive stimulation of the nerve fails to increase m.e.p.p. frequency but a raised concentration of potassium in the bathing fluid does so. The tentative hypothesis that the nerve action potential does not invade the terminals cannot be tested without intra- or extracellular recording with microelectrodes placed at the terminals themselves under direct vision. This disease points to the fact that a single gene is in some way able to control the events in motor nerve terminals which link the arrival of the nerve action potential with the synchronous release of acetylcholine. It also suggests the possible importance of heredity in the development of disorders of neuromuscular transmission in man.

4. The Effects of Botulinum Toxin

Any review of the pathology of the neuromuscular junction would be incomplete without reference to this powerful toxin which exercises its effects with such precise selectivity that it has become a useful tool in the experimental study of the morphology and physiology of motor end-plates.

The clinical syndrome of Botulism was known in the late 18th century and its association with the ingestion of spoiled food, especially sausage, is recognized in the name, derived from the Latin *botulus*, a sausage. It is characterised by apyrexial progressive development of symmetrical weakness or paralysis of skeletal muscles especially those innervated by cranial nerves, disturbances of the secretion of saliva and buccopharyngeal mucus, mydriasis and loss of accommodation, obstinate constipation and retention of urine, all in the absence of any impairment of intellectual and sensory functions. Those interested in historical reviews should consult MÜLLER (1869), VAN ERMENGEM (1896, 1897), DICKSON (1918), HEWLETT (1929) and LEIGHTON (1923). VAN ERMENGEM's outstandingly thorough and classical investigation merits particular attention. He discovered the causative organism, isolated its toxin and demonstrated that after inoculation the organism failed to multiply in animal tissues. He also observed a species variation in susceptibility to the toxin.

VAN ERMENGEM's findings were soon confirmed and the organism has been found all over the world (DUBOVSKY and MEYER, 1922a, 1922b; MEYER and DUBOVSKY, 1922a, 1922b). BURKE (1919a, 1919b) isolated two strains types A and B and subsequently at least 6 strains with characteristic toxins have been isolated. Their bacteriology and chemistry have been reviewed by BOROFF and DASGUPTA (1971).

Until the experiments of DICKSON and SHEVKY (1923a, 1923b) demonstrated the action of the toxin at cholinergic nerve terminals of the peripheral nervous system many sought to explain the paralysis on the basis of various microscopic alterations of nerve cells in the motor nuclei of the brainstem and of vascular thrombosis, which were probably of a secondary nature (cf. myasthenia gravis). MOTT (1900), who worked in the laboratories of the Maudsley Hospital, wrote that "there are a number of poisons—diphtheria, botulismus—in which the fatty degeneration of the muscle is far in excess of what could be reasonably attributed to the changes found in the nerves. Probably the vulnerable point of the neuro-muscular mechanism is at the junction of the nerve with the muscle. Comparative studies which would show degenerative changes in the motor end-plates are extremely difficult and it is rather by inference than direct observation that we must believe the poison to act upon this structure." In guinea pigs which had survived for 8 days after the administration of botulinum toxin he found "the most noteworthy change was extreme fatty degenera-tion of the heart and striped muscles of the body. Seeing that the peripheral nerves showed no degenerative changes one may conclude that the poison acted more particularly upon the muscles or the nerve endings in muscle."

DICKSON and SHEVKY (1923a, 1923b) established that the effects of botulinum toxin are due to its peripheral and not to a central action. As a result of previous histological investigations (DICKSON, 1918) which had not established the mode of action of the toxin, they administered it to cats and rabbits and observed the physio-logical changes in autonomic function and in skeletal muscle. They noted a progres-sive block of the vagus to stimulation and a rise in the threshold for cardiac slowing and movement of the small intestines: a failure of secretion of saliva in response to stimulation of the chorda tympani: a failure of contraction of the bladder and erection of the penis on stimulation of the nervae erigentes, and abolition of pupil-lary constriction on stimulation of the oculomotor nerve. No effects on vasomotor or splanchnic nerves were observed. A progressive fatiguability of skeletal muscle was manifested by the rise in the threshold to stimulation which progressed to complete failure of neuromuscular transmission. They concluded that sensory fibres of peri-pheral nerve and the reflex arc were not affected and that "it had not been deter-mined whether the damage is in the anatomical nerve endings of the somatic motor fibres or in the myoneural junction but it is not of the nature of an organic destruc-tion of tissue".

BURGEN et al. (1949) investigated the *in vitro* action of botulinum toxin on the isolated rat diaphragm. They used the isolated phrenic nerve-diaphragm preparation of BÜLBRING and found that after the addition of toxin (large doses of type A and B) there was a latent period, varying slightly with the dose, before paralysis began to be evident. The toxin became "fixed" to the muscle within 5 min and the latent period was shortened and the progress of the paralysis more rapid at 38° C than at 17° C. This temperature effect was also observed with frogs. BURGEN et al. (1949) observed that nerve conduction was normal and that the muscle contracted in response to direct stimulation and to close arterial injection of acetylcholine. Effects of the toxin were not prevented by the anti-cholinesterase drugs (eserine, neostigmine and tetra-ethyl pyrophosphate), and there was no augmentation of contraction by potas-sium chloride. All these indicated differences between the mechanisms of action of curare and botulinum toxin. A most important observation of BURGEN et al. was that the amount of acetylcholine released from terminals by stimulation of the phrenic nerve was greatly reduced when the diaphragm had become paralysed.

AMBACHE (1949) showed that cholinergic transmission to the sphincter pupillae was blocked by intra-ocular injection of the toxin. The muscle did not react to oculomotor stimulation or to light but still responded to intra-arterially injected acetylcholine. Sensory and adrenergic nerve fibres were unaffected, and the pupil dilated on stimulation of cervical sympathetic trunks. Subconjunctival injection of toxin produced paralysis of the extrinsic muscles of the eye, which however con-tracted on intra-carotid injection of acetylcholine. AMBACHE found that local injec-tions of toxin into tibialis anterior of one leg in the cat led to the development of paralysis within 48 hrs. Stimulation of the peroneal nerve failed to elicit contraction, and again the muscle responded to intra-arterial injections of ACh. AMBACHE (1951, 1952) also demonstrated the effects of the toxin on preganglionic sympathetic synapses while HILTON and LEWIS (1955) and KUPFER (1958) extended the study of its effects on the autonomic system.

BROOKS (1956) showed that botulinum toxin suppressed the spontaneous release of transmitter and suggested that its site of action was localized at the tips of motor nerve terminals. It is now accepted that the toxin exerts its effects by inhibiting the release of ACh. Evidence for an additional weak action on adrenergic terminals has been presented (RAND and WHALER, 1965; HOLMAN and SPITZER, 1973). A few published reports of experiments in which central effects were sought did not give any clear indication of a central action. However this does not rule out the possibility of some action on central cholinergic terminals such as those of collaterals of anterior horn cells within the spinal cord, though as yet no adequate test has been devised.

The physiological effects of the toxin on structures innervated by cholinergic nerves are comparable to those caused by denervation. GUYTON and MacDONALD (1947) also showed that "in every way the muscle in botulinum poisoning was found to be comparable to a denervated muscle". Other similarities between muscle treated with the toxin and denervated muscle include muscular atrophy (JIRMANOVA et al. 1964; DRACHMAN, 1964), supersensitivity to ACh (THESLEFF, 1960a), fibrillation (JOSEFSSON and THESLEFF, 1961) and the ability of the muscles to accept innervation by an implanted nerve (FEX et al. 1966).

In *acutely* paralysed muscles electron micrographs of nerve terminals from which acetylcholine release is totally blocked contain what appears to be a normal complement of synaptic vesicles and other organelles; the Schwann cells, as well as the anatomical relationships between nerve and muscle and the postsynaptic sarcolemma also show no sign of changes (THESLEFF, 1960a; ZACKS et al., 1962; DUCHEN, 1971b).

However changes occur at motor end-plates in muscles *chronically* paralysed by botulinum toxin, although it is difficult to demonstrate these effects because the toxin is the "most poisonous poison" known to man (LAMANNA, 1959). Cases of poisoning in man, fortunately rare, still carry a high mortality rate, but a patient who survives will eventually recover completely, although this is a very slow process. Recovery takes several months, with cranial muscles, particularly extra-ocular muscles, being the last to regain normal function. The chronic effects can only be studied adequately experimentally by injecting a sublethal dose directly into a muscle group. The toxin is rapidly bound, presumably to motor nerve terminals in a manner comparable to that demonstrated *in vitro* by BURGEN et al. (1949). The little that is absorbed into the systemic circulation is diluted out and more distant cholinergic terminals are affected to a lesser extent than the local ones which can be saturated with toxin. In guinea pigs GUYTON and MacDONALD (1947) combined a high dose of toxin injected locally into gastrocnemius with an intraperitoneal injection of antitoxin given some hours later when the action of the toxin on the local nerve terminals was already irreversible. They achieved complete paralysis of gastrocnemius with the animal otherwise generally healthy. Muscle contraction in these animals recovered very slowly, reaching only 50% of normal in 5 months and 90% in a year. DUCHEN and STRICH (1967, 1968b) reported changes in the innervation of the leg muscles of mice given sublethal local paralysing doses of toxin. As the muscle fibres become atrophied a profuse sprouting of motor axons develops. Axonal growth continues for several weeks with sprouts ramifying along and across adjacent muscle fibres.

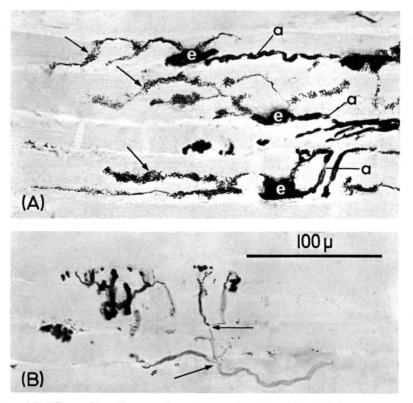

Fig. 31 A and B. Effects of botulinum toxin on innervation of muscle of adult mouse. (A) Soleus, (B) Gastrocnemius. A-After 18 days of paralysis original end-plates *(e)* are identifiable. Long branching axonal sprouts (arrows) extend beyond each end-plate. The reaction product along the sprouts can be shown to be due to pseudocholinesterase activity (DUCHEN, 1970a). Preterminal axons *(a)* appear normal and are unbranched. B-40 weeks after the injection of toxin when recovery from paralysis is well-established, motor end-plates are morphologically abnormal with cholinesterase activity scattered and irregular. Axonal branching (arrows) now appears to be preterminal and not ultraterminal. (Method of NAMBA et al.). × 360

DUCHEN (1970a) showed that the axonal sprouts grow from the motor nerve terminals in which transmitter release has been blocked, and as these axons grow and branch they establish new contacts with muscle fibres at random (Fig. 31). Some new contacts are formed on the same fibre which the axon previously innervated but some are clearly on other fibres. Subsequently spots of cholinesterase activity can be detected along the new axons. Cholinesterase activity becomes stronger and more sharply localized forming end-plates of varying size and shape which often consist of collections of rounded cup-like subunits. Much preterminal axonal branching also occurs. DUCHEN (1971b) showed that the sprouts which grow out from pre-existing nerve terminals contain vesicles, mitochondria and filaments and are always enclosed within a layer of Schwann cell cytoplasm. The site of the original neuromuscular junctions can be identified from the position of postsynaptic folds but many axons lying in immediate apposition to these folds no longer have the characteristics of

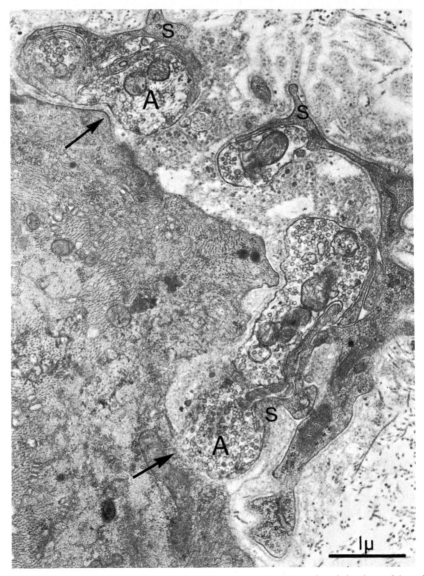

Fig. 32. Transverse section of gastrocnemius of a mouse 7 weeks after injection of botulinum toxin. Note the small axon terminals (A) making superficial and irregular contacts (arrows) with an atrophied and disorganized muscle fibre. There are no subneural folds. S-Schwann cell processes. × 20 000

terminals but look more like part of a preterminal axon in that very few or no vesicles but many neurofilaments are seen. This appearance strongly suggests that as the axonal sprouts have grown well beyond the original end-plate this site may no longer be an end-plate in the strict sense because the axon terminal is at some point distal to it. It is not known whether transmission is ever restored at the original end-plate. An important point is that no axonal degeneration occurs and that sprouts take origin from intact terminals with a normal appearance. The new contacts formed by growing axons with the sarcolemma of atrophied and supersensitive muscle fibres are at first superficial, with little or only shallow indentation of the sarcolemma (Fig. 32). The indentation deepens forming new "primary synaptic clefts" but postsynaptic folds are not seen until some weeks later. Eventually mature motor end-plates are formed but they remain distinguishable from the normal because they are mostly smaller and often scattered in a manner reminiscent of multiply innervated muscle fibres. Postsynaptic sarcolemmal folds are sometimes sparse and shallow. Often these new axon "terminals" are not situated on raised hillocks of sarcoplasmic organelles and typical sole-plate nuclei may not be seen beneath them. DUCHEN (1970d) also showed that if nerves to a muscle are crushed after the muscle is paralysed by botulinum, axons regenerate and rapidly re-innervate the original site of the end-plate. This shows that the toxin does not become fixed to the postsynaptic membrane.

Functional recovery from botulinum toxin has been studied *in vitro* by TONGE (1974c) who found that although nerve stimulation failed to elicit muscle contraction within 6 hrs of the administration of toxin, occasional subthreshold end-plate potentials (e.p.p.s) could be evoked over the next few weeks. These e.p.p.s gradually increased in amplitude until action potentials and feeble muscle twitching returned. Supersensitivity to acetylcholine became marked and persisted for a long time after the return of neuromuscular transmission. The onset of fatigue is abnormally rapid in these mouse muscles during repetitive nerve stimulation, and this phenomenon persists for months after the administration of the toxin. TONGE (1974c) considered that the fatigue was due to marked reduction of the mean quantal content of the end-plate potential. Only when the mean quantal content rose to approximately 20 or above (i.e. about one-third of normal) did the rate of fatigue become normal. The distribution of acetylcholine sensitivity on the muscle fibre also returned to normal when the quantal content rose to about 20.

One curious phenomenon is that the axonal sprouting does not begin at the same time at all end-plates in the mouse. DUCHEN (1969, 1970a) found that in the red soleus almost every end-plate shows axonal sprouting within 6 to 8 days of the onset of paralysis. In muscles such as gastrocnemius, extensor digitorum longus and the peronei sprouting begins about 3 weeks after the onset of paralysis. Soleus is composed entirely of slow type fibres, while the outer part of gastrocnemius and most fibres of extensor digitorum are fast in type and other muscles have a mixture of slow and fast fibres in varying proportions. It seems that for some reason axonal sprouting begins sooner in slow than in fast fibres after transmission is blocked. Judging from the restoration of muscle fibre size and from the enzyme histochemical reactions (DUCHEN, 1970c), the fibres in soleus, and in regions of other muscles where slow fibres predominate, recover first (Fig. 33). This is an unexpected finding at first sight, since slow fibres are numerous in the extrinsic ocular muscles and in the muscles of the larynx, which are the last to recover clinically. However, their pattern of innervation is unlike that of limb muscles, since many fibres have double or multiple end-plates. This apparent discrepancy merits further investigation. The more prolonged functional denervation of fast muscle fibres may be a cause of the more severe ultrastructural pathological changes observed in them than in slow fibres (DUCHEN, 1971c).

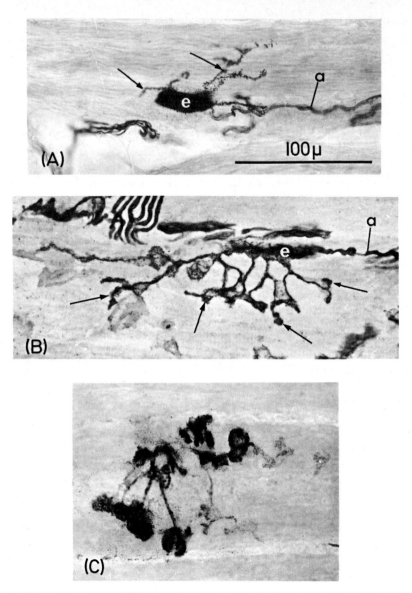

Fig. 33 A—C. Soleus of mouse. (A) 8 days (B) 4 weeks and (C) 7 weeks after the local injection of tetanus toxin. The preterminal axons *(a)*, end-plates *(e)* and ultraterminal axonal sprouts (arrows) are shown. In C there are scattered areas of cholinesterase activity linked together by axonal sprouts. Method of Namba et al. × 360. (From Duchen and Tonge, 1973, reproduced by permission of the Editorial Board, Journal of Physiology)

All these changes can be found after a single injection of botulinum toxin. There are a number of points about both the normal and abnormal which are revealed by the changes induced by botulinum toxin. These include the occurrence of renewed axonal growth in response to the block of transmitter release at nerve terminals, the variation in the time of onset of axonal growth in different sites, the variation in pathological changes in different types of muscle fibres, the effect on muscle fibres of an apparently permanent disturbance of the normal pattern of innervation and the sequence of events during the formation of new end-plates. There must be many more facts to be learned from the use of botulinum toxin concerning the interactions between axons and muscle fibres at the neuromuscular junction.

5. The Effects of Tetanus Toxin

The exotoxin produced by *Clostridium tetani* was first discovered by CARLE and RATTONE (1884) who inoculated rabbits with tissue from a primary lesion of a patient who had died of tetanism. The bacillus was described by NICOLAIER in 1884 and isolated in pure culture by KITASATO (1889) and by TIZZONI and CATTANI (1890). The biochemistry and physiology of the toxin is reviewed comprehensively by VAN HEYNINGEN and MELLANBY (1971).

The clinical syndrome of tetanism, well described by WILSON (1940) is dominated by overactivity of muscle with intermittent spasms, often with opisthotonus, and carrying a high mortality. Earlier physiologists sought to explain the phenomenon by postulating the facilitation of the release of transmitter at nerve terminals. The investigation of BROOKS et al. (1957) and CURTIS and DE GROAT (1968) indicated that the toxin blocked inhibitory mechanisms within the spinal cord, thus leading to overactivity of motor neurones. This provided an explanation for the muscular spasms. However, in 1948 AMBACHE et al. had found that intraocular injection of toxin into the rabbit's eye produced peripheral effects similar to those of botulinum toxin, suppressing transmitter release at cholinergic nerve terminals. Further it has long been known that gross muscular weakness, sometimes amounting to flaccid tetraplegia with wasting of muscles, may occur in patients who survive the tetanic spasms (see KAESER et al., 1968).

Further evidence for a peripheral action of the toxin was provided by KAESER and SANER (1970), DIAMOND and MELLANBY (1971) and MELLANBY and THOMPSON (1972) who all demonstrated a presynaptic block of neuromuscular transmission. This evidence for blockade of transmitter release seemed irreconcilable with the dramatic motor hyperactivity in clinical tetanism, but the apparent contradiction was resolved by correlative morphological and physiological studies of motor end-plates in limb muscles of mice with experimental local tetanus (DUCHEN and TONGE, 1973; DUCHEN, 1973a, 1973b).

Direct local injection of a sublethal dose of the toxin into the leg muscles causes intense but local muscle spasm after 48 hrs ("local tetanus"). This tetanic spasm may persist up to 4 weeks during which time the muscles remain rigid and hard. The slow type fibres of affected muscles become severely atrophied (e.g. in soleus and the deeper parts of gastrocnemius) and in mixed muscles like plantaris, single atrophic fibres lie among the fast fibres which are normal in size or are only slightly atrophied. Within about 8 to 10 days of the injection of toxin axonal sprouting is seen at end-plates of slow muscle fibres, the growth of axons continuing for up to 4 weeks when new neuromuscular junctions are formed outside the original area of the end-plate (Fig. 33). No sprouting is seen at end-plates of fast muscles. Although neuromuscular transmission is blocked within 48 hrs, even at the third day (Fig. 34) no pathological

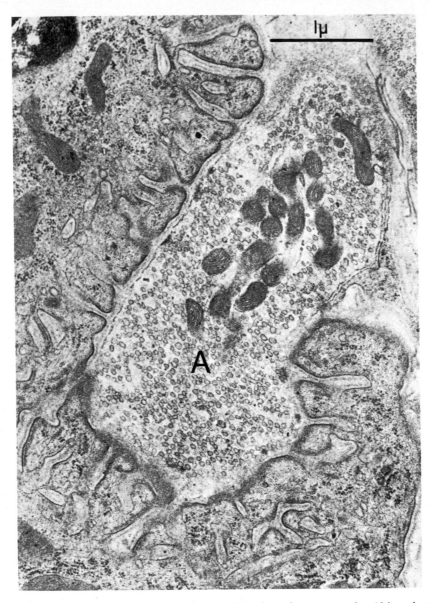

Fig. 34. Soleus of a mouse 3 days after the local injection of tetanus toxin. Although totally paralysed and unresponsive to nerve stimulation miniature end-plate potentials were recorded in this muscle, providing evidence for continued spontaneous release of transmitter. *A*-axonal terminal. No pathological changes are apparent in the myoneural junction. × 27000

changes were seen at the myoneural junction with electron microscopy. The sprouts could be seen after about 8 days. These sprouts which contain vesicles, filaments and mitochondria, are enclosed within Schwann cells and establish contact with the sarcolemma in an apparently random way. The new end-plates are at first superficial

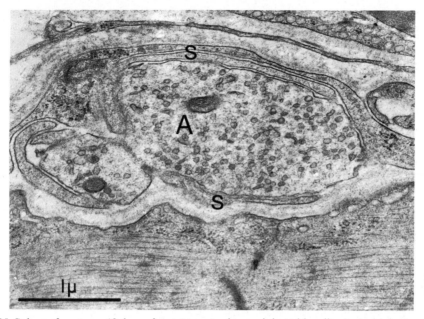

Fig. 35. Soleus of a mouse 12 days after tetanus toxin was injected locally. An axonal sprout *(A)* contains mitochondria and vesicles but does not make close contact with the muscle fibre. Unmyelinated vesicle-containing axons are not found normally. *S*-Schwann cell processes. ×27000

and show no postsynaptic differentiation (Fig. 35) but with longer time of survival the new junctions show deeper primary clefts and more and better postsynaptic folds. Numerous rounded electron-dense bodies accumulate at end-plates between axon and muscle fibre (Fig. 36).

DUCHEN and TONGE (1973) found that soleus (composed wholly of slow, or red, muscle fibres) was paralysed to nerve stimulation and showed all the physiological characteristics of denervated muscle, i.e. atrophy, fibrillation, and supersensitivity to acetylcholine. However, the fibres were clearly still innervated since m.e.p.p.s could be recorded from every muscle fibre tested. Therefore the fibres were functionally denervated by the toxin. Neuromuscular transmission was slowly restored to normal after about 4 or 5 weeks. In contrast, when fast muscles were examined (extensor digitorum longus) no paralysis and very little other abnormality was found.

Thus we may conclude that tetanus toxin causes a presynaptic block of neuromuscular transmission at cholinergic nerve terminals, but that nerve terminals of different types of muscle fibre differ in their sensitivity to the action of the toxin. If the amount of toxin to which the nervous system is exposed is not large the central effects will predominate, with resultant clinical tetanism, and only slow muscle fibres will be paralysed. Most muscles contain a mixture of slow and fast fibres, soleus being one of the very few composed largely of slow. In muscles of the cat (GORDON and HOLBOURN, 1949) and of mouse and rat (YELLIN, 1969) which contain a mixture of slow and fast fibres, the more superficial layers are composed mainly of fast fibres and slow fibres are more concentrated in deeper parts of the muscle so that the

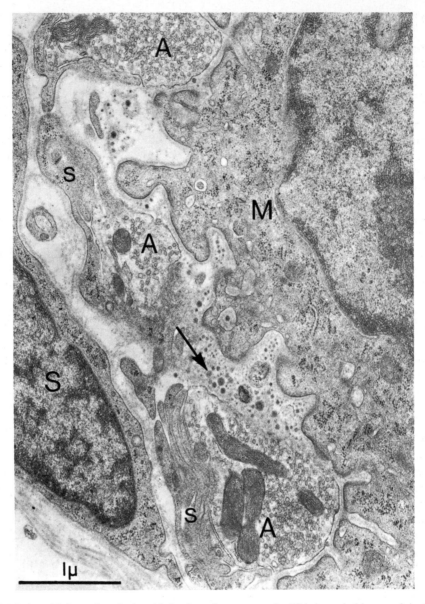

Fig. 36. Soleus 20 days after the local injection of tetanus toxin. This is probably an original end-plate because of the well-formed subneural folds. Lying between axon *(A)* and muscle *(M)* and within some of the folds are numerous rounded dense bodies (arrow). *S*-Schwann cell. × 20000

paralysis of slow fibres is masked by the intense overactivity of the other non-paralysed fibres. As the amount of tetanus toxin is increased and nerve terminals innervating fast fibres become affected a progressively greater proportion of muscle will become paralysed masking the central effects of the toxin.

E. The Neuromuscular Junction in Disorders of the Muscle Fibre

The term *myopathy* signifies a disease primarily affecting muscle fibres. As yet there is no clear answer to the crucial question as to whether or not there is an associated disorder of the nervous system and in particular of the lower motor neurone. Criteria for the pathological diagnosis of myopathy are changes such as muscle fibre necrosis, an excessive variation in fibre size with occasional very large fibres in some forms of dystrophy, fibre splitting, interstitial cell infiltrations and fibrosis, and, of great importance diagnostically, the absence of groups of many atrophied muscle fibres (the so-called fascicular distribution) which is characteristic of neurogenic muscular atrophy. In most discussions of the rôle of the nervous system in the production of disease of skeletal muscle the main emphasis is placed on whether or not the muscle shows evidence of neurogenic disease, but in this context neurogenic muscle disease is usually equated with partial motor denervation—i.e. the loss of some axons innervating a muscle. In man such partial denervation occurs in motor neurone disease, poliomyelitis, peripheral neuropathies or traumatic nerve or spinal cord lesions, and it is also found in hereditary motor neurone disease in the *wobbler* mouse (DUCHEN and STRICH, 1968a). All these conditions can usually be distinguished histologically from the myopathies and this distinction has been largely responsible for the belief that in the myopathic diseases the primary site of pathology lies within the muscle fibre. However, there is no positive evidence available that the lower motor neurone and neuromuscular transmission are normal in all respects in the myopathies. The suggestion that they are not normal (McCOMAS et al., 1971) is based on indirect electrophysiological evidence which may be open to question.

There have been few published studies of the neuromuscular junction in the myopathic diseases. In 1946 BOWDEN and GUTMANN compared the clinical, electro-diagnostic and biopsy findings in one adult with so-called late onset dystrophy and an adolescent with peroneal muscular atrophy. A variety of staining techniques was used and nerves were impregnated with a modified Bielschowsky-Gros silver method. In the dystrophic case no empty nerve trunks were found in any muscle; in some muscles the motor end-plates were apparently normal but where muscle fibres were grossly affected the axons ran for long distances along the muscle fibres. In the second case changes were patchy, ranging from normal innervation to complete denervation with empty or partially empty nerve trunks and signs suggesting early regeneration of axons. Other studies have been made by means of intravital methylene blue staining of motor point biopsies (COËRS, 1955; COËRS and WOOLF, 1959; WOOLF, 1969). No very clear picture emerges from these studies. COËRS (1955) remarked that the end-plates may be smaller or larger than normal according to the degree of atrophy or hypertrophy of the muscle fibres, and that these variations cause a shrinkage or an enlargement of the terminal arborization. If degeneration of muscle fibres is very marked the terminal arborizations may become very complex and widely spread. A quantitative electron microscopic study of end-plates in cases of Duchenne-type muscular dystrophy was made by JERUSALEM et al. (1974). They found that the area of nerve terminals, the mitochondrial and synaptic vesicle content of nerve terminals and the mean diameter of vesicles were all within normal limits. No degenerating nerve terminals were found. A consistent abnormality was that postsynaptic folds were shallower than normal (they referred to this change as "focal atrophy") thus significantly decreasing the ratio of postsynaptic to presynaptic membrane lengths. JERUSALEM et al. concluded that there was no morphological evidence for an abnormality of motor neurones in muscular dystrophy. COERS (1955) points out that the changes remain limited to the most distal part of the terminal axons (i.e. are limited to the end-plates themselves) and that preterminal axons show little or no excess branching. When branching of the preterminal axons is found the innervation ratio is increased and this finding is said to be indicative of a muscle disease of neurogenic origin. This argument breaks down when the disease *dystrophia myotonica* is considered, since the skeletal muscles have all the histopathological characteristics of a primary myopathic disease and yet the terminal arborizations are much enlarged and complex and there is abundant preterminal axonal branching. The difficulties of nomenclature, and the problems of identification of disease processes by limited histological techniques are exemplified by the hereditary so-called muscular dystrophy of the mouse (MICHELSON et al., 1955). In this inherited disease changes occur which are similar to those seen in the myopathies and a voluminous body of literature has accumulated based on a premise that the nervous system in normal in this animal. Recently more complete and careful neuropathological examinations have shown the existence of pathological changes, particularly involving both motor and sensory nerve roots (BRADLEY and JENKISON, 1973; SALAFSKY and STIRLING, 1973), and the pathogenesis of the disease is in doubt. Few studies of the innervation of muscle of the dystrophic mouse have been made, electron microscopy showing various abnormalities such as unusually large gaps between nerve and muscle, the interposition of Schwann cell processes into such gaps, variations in the numbers and depth of postsynaptic folds and unusual amounts of neurofilamentous material, (RAGAB, 1971; GILBERT et al., 1973).

Experimentally it is possible to induce pathological changes within the muscle cell while leaving the motor nerves and nerve terminals intact. DUCHEN et al. (1974) used the depolarizing fraction ("cardiotoxin") of the venom of the snake *Dendroaspis jamesoni* (EXCELL and PATEL, 1972) injecting small quantities directly into leg muscles of the mouse. Severe lesions of muscle fibres developed very rapidly and the sarcolemmal membrane was lost, the debris within the muscle fibre being held in place by the basement membrane alone. Beneath the nerve terminals the postsynaptic folds of sarcolemma were lost but the basement material normally filling them remained *in situ*. The muscle fibres were then invaded by phagocytic cells and myoblastic cells proliferated. Next the axonal terminals became enveloped in processes of Schwann cell cytoplasm which separated them from the muscle fibre. Within 2 to 3 weeks regeneration of the muscle fibres was complete, but the morphology of the neuromuscular junction had become abnormal, remaining so permanently. The abnormality was caused by irregular and discrete small areas of synaptic contact formed between the expanding regenerating muscle cell and the axonal terminals. Muscle function was restored to normal within a few weeks in spite of the persistent abnormality of the morphology of the end-plates. A curious phenomenon is that the postsynaptic membrane seemed to remain "undifferentiated" at many points, with poorly formed or absent postsynaptic folds. An important finding with light microscopy was that changes in motor nerves were strictly localized to the terminal arborizations. No changes were seen in preterminal axons, there was no axonal sprouting and, in the final state, no preterminal axonal branching could be seen. These experiments have shown that a lesion primarily affecting the muscle fibre, leaving the nerve terminal structurally and, probably, functionally intact, may lead to a very abnormal appearance of the neuromuscular junction.

F. Conclusion

This review has drawn attention to the numerous techniques now available for the study of the morphology of the motor end-plate and to the powerful and selective tools provided by the localised use of sublethal doses of various toxins, which may affect the release of transmitter or exert their action on the muscle fibre itself. The need to use a variety of histological and cytological methods cannot be overstressed. In experimental material these should be combined wherever possible with electro-physiological investigations. A similar approach to the investigation of human neuromuscular disorders is much needed. The use of biopsies suffers from limitations common to all sampling techniques. In any study of the neuromuscular junction, particularly in pathological states, extensive sampling of numerous blocks and many sections prepared by a variety of techniques for demonstrating nerve endings and different features of the muscle fibre is necessary. The morphology of end-plates varies with species and in any one species with the age of the individual and with the type of muscle fibre. Endings supplied by cranial nerves may differ from those of trunk and limb musculature. Appearances may even vary in different parts of the same end-plate.

The trophic relationship between nerve and muscle fibre remains a major topic of investigation. The relationship between morphological and functional completion is ill understood; apparently normal function is consistent with simple endings in young animals and with bizarre endings after regeneration of nerves. Disturbances of the preterminal pattern of innervation as well as of the spatial relationship between axonal terminals and sarcolemmal membrane and of the postsynaptic folds may be of diagnostic significance. Valid conclusions can only be drawn by careful appraisal of the "total morphological picture" in conjunction with a full clinical investigation including, when possible, neurophysiological studies.

References

ABO-EL-ENENE, M. A.: Functional anatomy of the larynx. Ph. D. Thesis, University of London, 1967.

AITKEN, J. T.: Growth of nerve implants in voluntary muscles. J. Anat. (Lond.) **84**, 38—49 (1950).

AKERT, K., SANDRI, C.: An electron-microscopic study of zinc iodide-osmium impregnation of neurons. I. Staining of synaptic vesicles at cholinergic junctions. Brain Res. **7**, 286—295 (1968).

ALLBROOK, D.: An electron microscopic study of regenerating skeletal muscle. J. Anat. (Lond.) **96**, 137—152 (1962).

AMBACHE, N.: The peripheral action of *Cl. Botulium* toxin. J. Physiol. (Lond.) **108**, 127—141 (1949).

AMBACHE, N.: A further study of the action of *Clostridium Botulinum* toxin upon different types of autonomic nerve fibre. J. Physiol. (Lond.) **113**, 1—17 (1951).

AMBACHE, N.: Effect of botulinum toxin upon the superior cervical ganglion. J. Physiol. (Lond.) **116**, 9P (1952).

Ambache, N., Morgan, R. S., Wright, G. P.: The action of tetanus toxin on the rabbit's iris. J. Physiol. (Lond.) **107**, 45—53 (1948).

Anderson, M. J., Cohen, M. W.: Fluorescent staining of acetylcholine receptors in vertebrate skeletal muscle. J. Physiol. (Lond.) **237**, 385—400 (1974).

Andersson-Cedergren, E.: Ultrastructure of motor end plate and sarcoplasmic components of mouse skeletal muscle fiber as revealed by three-dimensional reconstructions from serial sections. J. Ultrastruct. Res., Suppl. **1**, 5—181 (1959).

Anzenbacher, H., Zenker, W.: Über die Größenbeziehung der Muskelfasern und ihrer Endplatten. Z. Zellforsch. **60**, 860—871 (1963).

Augustinsson, K. B.: Classification and comparative enzymology of the cholinesterases and methods for their determination. In: Koelle, G. B. (Ed.): Handbuch der experimentellen Pharmakologie, Vol. 15, pp. 89—128. Cholinesterases and Anticholinesterase Agents. Berlin-Heidelberg-New York: Springer 1963.

Bagust, J., Lewis, D. M., Westerman, R. A.: Polyneuronal innervation of kitten skeletal muscle. J. Physiol. (Lond.) **229**, 241—255 (1973).

Barker, D., Ip, M. C.: A silver method for demonstrating the innervation of mammalian muscle in teased preparations. J. Physiol. (Lond.) **169**, 73—74 P (1963).

Barker, D., Ip, M. C.: Sprouting and degeneration of mammalian motor axons in normal and de-afferented skeletal muscle. Proc. roy. Soc. B **163**, 538—554 (1966).

Barnard, E. A., Wieckowski, J., Chiu, T. H.: Cholinergic receptor molecules and cholinesterase molecules at mouse skeletal muscle junctions. Nature (Lond.) New Biol. **234**, 207—209 (1971).

Betz, W., Sakmann, B.: Effects of proteolytic enzymes on function and structure of frog neuro-muscular junctions. J. Physiol. (Lond.) **230**, 673—688 (1973).

Bickerstaff, E. R., Woolf, A. L.: The intramuscular nerve endings in myasthenia gravis. Brain **83**, 10—23 (1960).

Birks, R., Huxley, H. E., Katz, B.: The fine structure of the neuromuscular junction of the frog. J. Physiol. (Lond.) **150**, 134—144 (1960).

Birks, R., Katz, B., Miledi, R.: Physiological and structural changes at the amphibian myo-neural junction in the course of nerve degeneration. J. Physiol. (Lond.) **150**, 145—168 (1960).

Blaschko, H. K. F., Smith, A. D.: A discussion on subcellular and macromolecular aspects of synaptic transmission. Phil. Trans. B **261**, 273—437 (1971).

Bloom, F. E.: Localization of neurotransmitters by electron microscopy. Res. Publ. Ass. nerv. ment. Dis. **50**, 25—57 (1972).

Boeke, J.: Nerve endings, motor and sensory. In: Penfield, W. (Ed.): Cytology and Cellular Pathology of the Nervous System, Vol. I, pp. 243—315. New York: Hoeber 1932.

Boroff, D. A., Dasgupta, B. R.: Botulinum toxin. In: Kadis, S., Montie, T. C., Ajl, S. J. (Eds.) Microbial Toxins, Vol. IIA, pp. 1—68. New York, Academic Press 1971.

Bowden, R. E. M.: Some recent studies of skeletal muscle in anterior poliomyelitis and other neuromuscular disorders in man and the experimental animals. In Poliomyelitis, 2nd International Poliomyelitis Conference. Philadelphia: Lipincott 1951.

Bowden, R. E. M.: Electromyography. In: Seddon, H. J. (Ed.): Peripheral Nerve Injuries, M.R.C. Special Report Series No. 282, pp. 263—297. London: H.M.S.O. 1954.

Bowden, R. E. M., Gutmann, E.: Denervation and re-innervation of human voluntary muscle. Brain **67**, 273—313 (1944).

Bowden, R. E. M., Gutmann, E.: Observations in a case of muscular dystrophy with reference to diagnostic significance. Arch. Neurol. Psychiat. (Chic.) **56**, 1—19 (1946).

Bowden, R. E. M., Mahran, Z. Y.: The functional significance of the pattern of innervation of the muscle quadratus labii superioris of the rabbit, cat and rat. J. Anat. (Lond.) **90**, 217—227 (1956).

Boyd, I. A.: The structure and innervation of the nuclear bag muscle fibre system and the nuclear chain muscle fibre system in mammalian muscle spindles. Phil. Trans. B **245**, 81—136 (1962).

Bradley, W. G., Jenkison, M.: Abnormalities of peripheral nerves in murine muscular dystrophy. J. neurol. Sci. **18**, 227—247 (1973).

Brash, J. C.: Neuro-vascular hila of limb muscles. Edinburgh: Livingstone 1955.

Brooks, V. B.: An intracellular study of the action of repetitive nerve volleys and of botulinum toxin on miniature end-plate potentials. J. Physiol. (Lond.) **134**, 264—277 (1956).

BROOKS, V. B., CURTIS, D. R., ECCLES, J. C.: The action of tetanus toxin on the inhibition of moto-neurones. J. Physiol. (Lond.) **135**, 655—672 (1957).

BROWN, L. M.: A Thiocholine method for locating cholinesterase activity by electron microscopy. Bibl. anat. (Basel) **2**, 21—33 (1961).

BROWNELL, B., OPPENHEIMER, D. R., SPALDING, J. M. K.: Neurogenic muscle atrophy in myasthenia gravis. J. Neurol. Neurosurg. Psychiat. **35**, 311—322 (1972).

BUCHTAL, F.: The general concept of the motor unit. Res. Publ. Ass. nerv. ment. Dis. **38**, 3—30 (1960).

BULLER, A. J., ECCLES, J. C., ECCLES, R. M.: Interactions between motoneurones and muscles in respect of the characteristic speeds of their responses. J. Physiol. (Lond.) **150**, 417—439 (1960).

BURGEN, A. S. V., DICKENS, F., ZATMAN, L. J.: The action of botulinum toxin on the neuro-muscular junction. J. Physiol. (Lond.) **109**, 10—24 (1949).

BURKE, G. S.: The occurence of bacillus botulinus in nature. J. Bact. **4**, 541—553 (1919a).

BURKE, G. S.: Notes on bacillus botulinus. J. Bact. **4**, 555—565 (1919b).

BURKE, W., GINSBORG, B. L.: The electrical properties of the slow muscle fibre membrane. J. Physiol. (Lond.) **132**, 586—598 (1956).

BUZZARD, E. F.: The clinical history and post-mortem examination of five cases of myasthenia gravis. Brain **28**, 438—483 (1905).

CARLE, A., RATTONE, G.: Studio sperimentale sull'eziologia del tetano. G. Accad. Med. Torino **32**, 174—180 (1884).

CECCARELLI, B., HURLBUT, W. P., MAURO, A.: Depletion of vesicles from frog neuromuscular junctions by prolonged tetanic stimulation. J. Cell Biol. **54**, 30—38 (1972).

CHANGEUX, J.-P., KASAI, M., LEE, C.-Y.: Use of a snake venom toxin to characterize the cholinergic receptor protein. Proc. nat. Acad. Sci. (Wash.) **67**, 1241—1247 (1970).

CLARK, A. W., HURLBUT, W. P., MAURO, A.: Changes in the fine structure of the neuromuscular junction of the frog caused by black widow spider venom. J. Cell Biol. **52**, 1—14 (1972).

CLARK, A. W., MAURO, A., LONGENECKER, H. E., HURLBUT, W. P.: Effects of black widow spider venom on the frog neuromuscular junction. Nature (Lond.) **225**, 703—705 (1970).

CLOSE, R. I.: Dynamic properties of mammalian skeletal muscles. Physiol. Rev. **52**, 129—197 (1972).

COËRS, C.: Les variations structurelles normales et pathologiques de la jonction neuromusculaire. Acta neurol. belg. **55**, 741—866 (1955).

COËRS, C.: Structure and organization of the myoneural junction. Int. Rev. Cytol. **22**, 239—267 (1967).

COËRS, C., DESMEDT, J. E.: Mise en évidence d'une malformation caractéristique de la jonction neuromusculaire dans la myasthénie. Acta neurol. belg. **59**, 539—561 (1959).

COËRS, C., RESKE-NIELSEN, E., HARMSEN, A.: The pattern of terminal motor innervation in healthy young adults. J. neurol. Sci. **19**, 351—356 (1973).

COËRS, C., WOOLF, A. L.: The innervation of muscle. Oxford: Blackwell 1959.

COHEN, M. W.: The development of neuromuscular connexions in the presence of D-tubocurarine. Brain Res. **41**, 457—463 (1972).

COOPER, S., DANIEL, P. M.: Muscle spindles in man: their morphology in the lumbricals and the deep muscles of the neck. Brain **86**, 563—586 (1963).

COUTEAUX, R.: Contribution à l'étude de la synapse myoneurale. Rev. canad. Biol. **6**, 563—711 (1947).

COUTEAUX, R.: Morphological and cytochemical observations on the post-synaptic membrane at motor end-plates and ganglionic synapses. Exper. Cell Res., Suppl. **5**, 294—322 (1958).

COUTEAUX, R.: Motor end-plate structure. In: BOURNE, G. H. (Ed.): Structure and Function of Muscle Vol. I, pp. 337—380. New York: Academic Press 1960.

COUTEAUX, R.: The differentiation of synaptic areas. Proc. roy. Soc. B **158**, 457—480 (1963).

COUTEAUX, R., PÉCOT-DECHAVASSINE, M.: Vésicules synaptiques et poche au niveau des "zones actives" de la jonction neuromusculaire. C. R. Acad. Sci. (Paris) **271**, 2346—2349 (1970).

COUTEAUX, R., TAXI, J.: Recherches histochimiques sur la distribution des activités cholinestérasiques au niveau de la synapse myoneurale. Arch. Anat. micr. Morph. exp. **41**, 352—392 (1952).

CSILLIK, B.: Functional structure of the post-synaptic membrane in the myoneural junction. Budapest: Akadémiai Kiado 1965.

Csillik,B., Knyihar,E.: On the effect of motor nerve degeneration on the fine-structural localization of esterases in the mammalian motor end-plate. J. Cell Sci. **3**, 529—538 (1968).
Cuajunco,F.: Development of the human motor end plate. Contr. Embryol. Carneg. Instn. **30**,
127—152 (1942).
Cull-Candy,S.G., Neal,H., Usherwood,P.N.R.: Action of black widow spider venom on an
aminergic synapse. Nature (Lond.) New Biol. **241**, 353—354 (1973).
Curtis,D.R., DeGroat,W.C.: Tetanus toxin and spinal inhibition. Brain Res. **10**, 208—212
(1968).
Daniel,P.M., Strich,S.J.: Skeletal muscle. In: Wright,G.P. Symmers,W.St.C. (Eds.): Systemic Pathology, Vol. II, pp. 1331—1346. London: Longmans Green 1966.
Davis,R., Koelle,G.B.: Electron microscopic localization of acetylcholinesterase and nonspecific cholinesterase at the neuromuscular junction by the gold-thiocholine and gold-thiolacetic acid methods. J. Cell. Biol. **34**, 157—171 (1967).
DeHarven,E., Coërs,C.: Electron microscopic study of the human neuromuscular junction. J.
biophys. biochem. Cytol. **6**, 7—10 (1959).
DeRobertis,E.: Submicroscopic morphology and function of the synapse. Exp. Cell Res., Suppl.
5, 347—369 (1958).
DeRobertis,E., Bennett,H.S.: Some features of the submicroscopic morphology of the syn-
apses in frog and earthworm. J. biophys. biochem. Cytol. **1**, 47—58 (1955).
DelCastillo,J., Katz,B.: Quantal components of the end-plate potential. J. Physiol. (Lond.)
124, 560—573 (1954).
Denz,F.A.: On the histochemistry of the myoneural junction. Brit. J. exp. Path. **34**, 329—339
(1953).
Desmedt,J.E., Borenstein,S.: The myasthenic neuromuscular disorder. In: La Transmission
Cholinergique de L'excitation, pp.275—280. Paris: INSERM 1973.
Diamond,J., Mellanby,J.: The effect of tetanus toxin in the goldfish. J. Physiol. (Lond.) **215**,
727—741 (1971).
Dickson,E.C.: Botulism: A clinical and experimental study. New York: Rockefeller Institute for
Medical Research Monograph No.8 (1918).
Dickson,E.C., Shevky,R.: Botulism. Studies on the manner in which the toxin of *Clostridium
botulinum* acts upon the body. I. The effect upon the autonomic nervous system. J. exp. Med.
37, 711—731 (1923a).
Dickson,E.C., Shevky,E.: Botulism. Studies on the manner in which the toxin of *Clostridium
botulinum* acts upon the body. II. The effect upon the voluntary nervous system. J. exp. Med.
38, 327—346 (1923b).
Dogiel,A.S.: Methylenblautinktion der motorischen Nervenendigungen in den Muskeln der
Amphibien und Reptilien. Arch. mikr. Anat. **35**, 305—320 (1890).
Doyère,L.: Mémoire sur les Tardigrades. Ann. Sci. Natur. Ser.2, Zoologie **14**, 269—361 (1840).
Drachman,D.B.: Atrophy of skeletal muscle in chick embryos treated with botulinum toxin.
Science **145**, 719—721 (1964).
Drachman,D.B.: Neurotrophic regulation of muscle cholinesterase: effects of botulinum toxin
and denervation. J. Physiol. (Lond.) **226**, 619—627 (1972).
Dubovsky,B.J., Meyer,K.F.: An experimental study of the methods available for the enrich-
ment, demonstration and isolation of B. Botulinus in specimens of soil and its products, in
suspected foods, in clinical and in necropsy material. J. infect. Dis. **31**, 501—540 (1922a).
Dubovsky,B.J., Meyer,K.F.: The distribution of the spores of B. Botulinus in the territory of
Alaska and the Dominion of Canada. J. infect. Dis. **31**, 595—599 (1922b).
Dubowitz,V.: Developing and diseased muscle: a histochemical study. Spastics International
Medical Publications Research Monograph No.2. London: Heinemann 1968.
Duchen,L.W.: Histological differences between soleus and gastrocnemius muscles in the mouse
after the local injection of botulinum toxin. J. Physiol. (Lond.) **204**, 17—18P (1969).
Duchen,L.W.: Changes in motor innervation and cholinesterase localization induced by botu-
linum toxin in skeletal muscle of the mouse: differences between fast and slow muscles. J.
Neurol. Neurosurg. Psychiat. **33**, 40—54 (1970a).
Duchen,L.W.: Hereditary motor end-plate disease in the mouse: light and electron microscopic
studies. J. Neurol. Neurosurg. Psychiat. **33**, 238—250 (1970b).

DUCHEN, L. W.: The effects of botulinum toxin on the distribution of succinate dehydrogenase and phosphorylase in fast and slow skeletal muscles of the mouse. J. Neurol. Neurosurg. Psychiat. **33**, 580—585 (1970c).

DUCHEN, L. W.: The effects in the mouse of nerve crush and regeneration on the innervation of skeletal muscles paralysed by *Clostridium botulinum* toxin. J. Path. **102**, 9—14 (1970d).

DUCHEN, L. W.: An electron microscopic comparison of motor end-plates of slow and fast skeletal muscle fibres of the mouse. J. neurol. Sci. **14**, 37—45 (1971a).

DUCHEN, L. W.: An electron microscopic study of the changes induced by botulinum toxin in the motor end-plates of slow and fast skeletal muscle fibres of the mouse. J. neurol. Sci. **14**, 47—60 (1971b).

DUCHEN, L. W.: Changes in the electron microscopic structure of slow and fast muscle fibres of the mouse after the local injection of botulinum toxin. J. neurol. Sci. **14**, 61—64 (1971c).

DUCHEN, L. W.: Motor nerve growth induced by botulinum toxin as a regnerative phenomenon. Proc. roy. Soc. Med. **65**, 196—197 (1972).

DUCHEN, L. W.: The effects of tetanus toxin on the motor end-plates of the mouse: an electron microscopic study. J. neurol. Sci. **19**, 153—167 (1973a).

DUCHEN, L. W.: The local effects of tetanus toxin on the electron microscopic structure of skeletal muscle fibres of the mouse. J. neurol. Sci. **19**, 169—177 (1973b).

DUCHEN, L. W., EXCELL, B. J., PATEL, R., SMITH, B.: Changes in motor end-plates resulting from muscle fibre necrosis and regeneration: a light and electron microscopic study of the effects of the depolarizing fraction (cardiotoxin) of *Dendroaspis jamesoni* venom. J. neurol. Sci. **21**, 391—417 (1974).

DUCHEN, L. W., SEARLE, A. G., STRICH, S. J.: An hereditary motor end-plate disease in the mouse. J. Physiol. (Lond.) **189**, 4—6 P (1967).

DUCHEN, L. W., STEFANI, E.: Electrophysiological studies of neuromuscular transmission in hereditary "motor end-plate disease" in the mouse. J. Physiol. (Lond.) **212**, 535—548 (1971).

DUCHEN, L. W., STRICH, S. J.: Changes in the pattern of motor innervation of skeletal muscle in the mouse after local injections of *Clostridium botulinum* toxin. J. Physiol. (Lond.) **189**, 2—4 P (1967).

DUCHEN, L. W., STRICH, S. J.: An hereditary motor neurone disease with progressive denervation of muscle in the mouse. The mutant "wobbler". J. Neurol. Neurosurg. Psychiat. **31**, 535—542 (1968a).

DUCHEN, L. W., STRICH, S. J.: The effects of botulinum toxin on the pattern of innervation of skeletal muscle in the mouse. Quart. J. exp. Physiol. **53**, 84—89 (1968b).

DUCHEN, L. W., TONGE, D. A.: The effects of tetanus toxin on neuromuscular transmission and on the morphology of motor end-plates in slow and fast skeletal muscle of the mouse. J. Physiol. (Lond.) **228**, 157—172 (1973).

EATON, L. M., LAMBERT, E. H.: Electromyography and electric stimulation of nerves in diseases of motor unit: observations on myasthenic syndrome associated with malignant tumours. J. Amer. med. Ass. **163**, 1117—1124 (1957).

EDDS, M. V.: Collateral regeneration of residual motor axons in partially denervated muscles. J. exp. Zool. **113**, 517—552 (1950).

EDDS, M. V., SMALL, W. T.: The behaviour of residual axons in partially denervated muscles of the monkey. J. exp. Med. **93**, 207—216 (1951).

EDSTRÖM, L., KUGELBERG, E.: Histochemical composition, distribution of fibres and fatiguability of single motor units. J. Neurol. Neurosurg. Psychiat. **31**, 424—433 (1968).

ELIAS, E. R.: Histological and histochemical studies of red and white mammalian muscles, anterior horn cells and related bouton terminaux following denervation and reinnervation Ph.D. Thesis, University of London, 1972.

ENGEL, A. G., LAMBERT, E. H., SANTA, T.: Study of long-term anticholinesterase therapy. Neurology (Minneap.) **23**, 1273—1281 (1973).

ENGEL, A. G., SANTA, T.: Histometric analysis of the ultrastructure of the neuromuscular junction in myasthenia gravis and in the myasthenic syndrome. Ann. N.Y. Acad. Sci. **183**, 46—63 (1971).

ENGEL, A. G., SANTA, T.: Motor endplate fine structure. In: DESMEDT, J. E. (Ed.): New Developments in Electromyography and Clinical Neurophysiology, Vol. I, pp. 196—228. Basel: Karger 1973.

Engel,A.G., Tsujihata,M., Lindstrom,J., Lennon,V.A.: End-plate fine structure in myasthenia gravis and in the experimental auto-immune myasthenia. Ann. N.Y. Acad. Sci. (in the press).

Engel,W.K.: Cytological localization of cholinesterase in cultured skeletal muscle cells. J. Histochem. Cytochem. 9, 66—72 (1961).

Excell,B.J., Patel,R.: Characterization of toxic fractions from Dendroaspis jamesoni venom. J. Physiol. (Lond.) 225, 29—30 P (1972).

Fambrough,D.M., Hartzell,H.C.: Acetylcholine receptors: number and distribution at neuromuscular junctions in rat diaphragm. Science 176, 189—191 (1972).

Fardeau,M.: Ultrastructure des jonctions neuro-musculaires dans la musculature squelettique du cobaye. In: La Transmission Cholinergique de L'excitation, pp.29—50. Paris: INSERM 1973.

Fardeau,M., Engel,W.K.: Relation entre la morphologie des plaques motrices et le type des fibres musculaires squelletiques (chez le cobaye). In: VIth International Congress of Neuropathology Proceedings 740. Paris: Masson 1970.

Fardeau,M., Godet-Guillain,J., Chevallay,M.: Modifications ultrastructurales des plaques motrices dans la myasthenie et les syndromes myastheniques. In: La Transmission Cholinergique de L'excitation, pp.247—256. Paris: INSERM 1973.

Feindel,W., Hinshaw,J.R., Weddell,G.: The pattern of motor innervation in mammalian striated muscle. J. Anat. (Lond.) 86, 35—48 (1952).

Fenichel,G.M., Shy,G.M.: Muscle biopsy experience in myasthenia gravis. Arch. Neurol. (Chic.) 9, 237—243 (1963).

Fex,S., Sonesson,B., Thesleff,S., Zelena,J.: Nerve implants in botulinum poisoned mammalian muscle. J. Physiol. (Lond.) 184, 872—882 (1966).

Fex,S., Thesleff,S.: The time required for innervation of denervated muscles by nerve implants. Life Sci. 6, 635—639 (1967).

Friedenberg,R.M., Seligman,A.M.: Acetylcholinesterase at the myoneural junction: cytochemical ultrastructure and some biochemical considerations. J. Histochem. Cytochem. 20, 771—792 (1972).

Frohse,F., Fränkel,M.: Die Muskeln des menschlichen Armes. Jena: G. Fischer 1908.

Frontali,N.: Catecholamine—depleting effect of black widow spider venom on iris nerve fibres. Brain Res. 37, 146—148 (1972).

Fukuhara,N., Takamori,M., Gutmann,L., Chou,S.-M.: Eaton-Lambert syndrome. Ultrastructural study of the motor end-plates. Arch. Neurol. (Chic.) 27, 67—78 (1972).

Gauthier,G.F.: On the relationship of ultrastructural and cytochemical features to color in mammalian skeletal muscle. Z. Zellforsch. 95, 462—482 (1969).

Gauthier,G.F., Padykula,H.A.: Cytological studies of fiber types in skeletal muscle. J. Cell. Biol. 28, 333—354 (1966).

Gilbert,J.J., Steinberg,M.C., Banker,B.Q.: Ultrastructural alterations of the motor end plate in myotonic dystrophy of the mouse (dy^{2J}/dy^{2J}). J. Neuropath. exp. Neurol. 32, 345—364 (1973).

Ginsborg,B.L.: Some properties of avian skeletal muscle fibres with multiple neuromuscular junctions. J. Physiol. (Lond.) 154, 581—598 (1960).

Gordon,G., Holbourn,A.H.S.: The mechanical activity of single motor units in reflex contractions of skeletal muscle. J. Physiol. (Lond.) 110, 26—35 (1949).

Gray,E.G., Guillery,R.W.: Synaptic morphology in the normal and degenerating nervous system. Int. Rev. Cytol. 19, 111—182 (1966).

Green,D.P.L., Miledi,R., Vincent,A.: Neuromuscular transmission after immunization against acetylcholine receptors. Proc. roy. Soc. B 189, 57—68 (1975).

Green,E.L.: Biology of the laboratory mouse. 2nd Ed. New York: McGraw-Hill 1966.

Gruber,D., Eckert,K.: Die motorischen Endplatten in der Schlundmuskulatur von Katze und Hund, dargestellt mit dem Osmiumsäure-Zinkjodid-Verfahren nach Maillet. Anat. Anz. 131, 406—413 (1972).

Guth,L.: "Trophic" influences of nerve on muscle. Physiol. Rev. 48, 645—687 (1968).

GUTMANN, E., YOUNG, J.Z.: The reinnervation of muscle after varying periods of atrophy. J. Anat. (Lond.) **78**, 15—43 (1944).

GUYTON, A.C., MACDONALD, M.A.: Physiology of botulinus toxin. Arch. Neurol. Psychiat. (Chic.) **57**, 578—592 (1947).

GWYN, D.G., AITKEN, J.T.: The formation of new endplates in mammalian skeletal muscle. J. Anat. (Lond.) **100**, 116—126 (1966).

HALL, Z.W.: Multiple forms of acetylcholinesterase and their distribution in endplate and non-endplate regions of rat diaphragm muscle. J. Neurobiology **4**, 343—361 (1973).

HALL, Z.W., KELLY, R.B.: Enzymatic detachment of endplate acetylcholinesterase from muscle. Nature (Lond.) New Biol. **237**, 62 (1971).

HARRIMAN, D.G.F., TAVERNER, D., WOOLF, A.L.: Ekbom's syndrome and burning paraesthesiae: a biopsy study by vital staining and electron microscopy of the intramuscular innervation with a note on age changes in motor nerve endings in distal muscles. Brain **93**, 393—406 (1970).

HARRIS, C.: The morphology of the myoneural junction as influenced by neurotoxic drugs. Amer. J. Path. **30**, 501—519 (1954).

HARRIS, J.B., WARD, M.R.: A comparative study of "denervation" in muscles from mice with inherited progressive neuromuscular disorders. Exp. Neurol. **42**, 169—180 (1974).

HARTZELL, H.C., FAMBROUGH, D.M.: Acetylcholine receptors. Distribution and extrajunctional density in rat diaphragm after denervation correlated with acetylcholine sensitivity. J. gen. Physiol. **60**, 248—262 (1972).

HEILBRONN, E., MATTSSON, C.: The nicotinic cholinergic receptor protein: Improved purification method, preliminary amino acid composition and observed auto-immune response. J. Neurochem. **22**, 315—317 (1974).

HEILBRONN, E., MATTSSON, C., STALBERG, E., HILTON-BROWN, P.: Neurophysiological signs of myasthenia in rabbits after receptor antibody development. J. neurol. Sci. **24**, 59—64 (1975).

HESS, A.: The structure of slow and fast extrafusal muscle fibers in the extraocular muscles and their nerve endings in guinea pigs. J. cell. comp. Physiol. **58**, 63—79 (1961).

HESS, A.: The sarcoplasmic reticulum, the T system, and the motor terminals of slow and twitch muscle fibers in the garter snake. J. Cell Biol. **26**, 467—476 (1965).

HESS, A.: The structure of vertebrate slow and twitch muscle fibers. Invest. Ophthal. **6**, 217—228 (1967).

HESS, A.: Vertebrate slow muscle fibers. Physiol. Rev. **50**, 40—62 (1970).

HEUSER, J.E.: A possible origin of the "giant" spontaneous potentials that occur after prolonged transmitter release at frog neuromuscular junctions. J. Physiol. (Lond.) **239**, 106—108 P (1974).

HEUSER, J.E., KATZ, B., MILEDI, R.: Structural and functional changes of frog neuromuscular junctions in high calcium solutions. Proc. roy. Soc. B **178**, 407—415 (1971).

HEUSER, J.E., MILEDI, R.: Effect of lanthanum ions on function and structure of frog neuromuscular junctions. Proc. roy. Soc. B **179**, 247—260 (1971).

HEUSER, J.E., REESE, T.S.: Evidence for recycling of synaptic vesicle membrane during transmitter release at the frog neuromuscular junction. J. Cell. Biol. **57**, 315—344 (1973).

HEUSER, J.E., REESE, T.S., LANDIS, D.M.D.: Functional changes in frog neuromuscular junctions studied with freeze-fracture. J. Neurocytol. **3**, 109—131 (1974).

HEWER, E.E.: The development of nerve endings in the human foetus. J. Anat. (Lond.) **69**, 369—379 (1935).

HEWLETT, R.T.: Bacillus botulinus. In: A system of Bacteriology in Relation to Medicine (Medical Research Council), Vol. 3, p. 373. London: H.M.S.O. 1929.

HILTON, S.M., LEWIS, G.P.: The cause of the vasodilatation accompanying activity in the submandibular salivary gland. J. Physiol. (Lond.) **128**, 235—248 (1955).

HINES, M.: Studies on the innervation of skeletal muscle. III. Innervation of the extrinsic eye muscles of the rabbit. Amer. J. Anat. **47**, 1—54 (1931).

HINSEY, J.C.: The innervation of muscle. Physiol. Rev. **14**, 514—585 (1934).

HOFFMAN, H.: Local re-innervation in partially denervated muscle: a histophysiological study. Aust. J. exp. Biol. med. Sci. **28**, 383—397 (1950).

HOLMAN, M.E., SPITZER, N.C.: Action of botulinum on transmission from sympathetic nerves to the vas deferens. Brit. J. Pharmacol. **47**, 431—433 (1973).

Hubbard, J. I.: Microphysiology of vertebrate neuromuscular transmission. Physiol. Rev. **53**, 674—723 (1973).

Hubbard, J. I., Kwanbunbumpen, S.: Evidence for the vesicle hypothesis. J. Physiol. (Lond.) **194**, 407—420 (1968).

Israel, M., Gautron, J., Lesbats, B.: Fractionnement de l'organe electrique de le Torpille. In: La Transmission Cholinergique de L'excitation, pp. 61—69. Paris: INSERM 1973.

James, D. W., Tresman, R. L.: An electron-microscopic study of the de novo formation of neuromuscular junctions in tissue culture. Z. Zellforsch. **100**, 126—140 (1969).

Jerusalem, F., Engel, A. G., Gomez, M. R.: Duchenne dystrophy II. Morphometric study of motor end-plate fine structure. Brain **97**, 123—130 (1974).

Jirmanova, I., Sobotkova, M., Thesleff, S., Zelena, J.: Atrophy in skeletal muscles poisoned with botulinum toxin. Physiol. bohemslov. **13**, 467—472 (1964).

Jones, S. F., Kwanbunbumpen, S.: The effects of nerve stimulation and hemicholinium on synaptic vesicles at the neuromuscular junction. J. Physiol. (Lond.) **207**, 31—50 (1970a).

Jones, S. F., Kwanbunbumpen, S.: Some effects of nerve stimulation and hemicholinium on quantal transmitter release at the mammalian neuromuscular junction. J. Physiol. (Lond.) **207**, 51—61 (1970b).

Josefsson, J.-O., Thesleff, S.: Electromyographic findings in experimental botulinum intoxication. Acta physiol. scand. **51**, 163—168 (1961).

Kadanoff, D.: Die Sensiblen Nervenendigungen in der Mimischen Muskulatur des Menschen. Z. mikr.-anat. Forsch. **62**, 1—15 (1956).

Kaeser, H. E., Müller, H. R., Friedrich, B.: The nature of tetraplegia in infectious tetanus. Europ. Neurology **1**, 17—27 (1968).

Kaeser, H. E., Saner, A. A.: The effect of tetanus toxin on neuromuscular transmission. Europ. Neurology **3**, 194—205 (1970).

Karlsson, E., Heilbronn, E., Widlund, L.: Isolation of the nicotinic acetylcholine receptor by biospecific chromatography on insolubilized *Naja naja* neurotoxin. FEBS Letters **28**, 107—111 (1972).

Kasa, P., Mann, S. P., Hebb, C.: Localization of choline acetyltransferase. Nature (Lond.) **226**, 812—814 (1970).

Katz, B., Kuffler, S. W.: Multiple motor innervation of the frog's sartorius muscle. J. Neurophysiol. **4**, 209—223 (1941).

Katz, B., Miledi, R.: Spontaneous and evoked activity of motor nerve endings in calcium Ringer. J. Physiol. (Lond.) **203**, 689—706 (1969).

Keene, Lucas M. F.: Muscle spindles in human laryngeal muscles. J. Anat. (Lond.) **95**, 25—29 (1961).

Kefalides, N. A.: Structure and biosynthesis of basement membranes. Intern. Rev. of Connective Tissue Res. **6**, 63—104 (1973).

Kelly, A. M., Zacks, S. I.: The fine structure of motor endplate morphogenesis. J. Cell Biol. **42**, 154—169 (1969).

Kitasato, S.: Über den Tetanusbacillus. Z. Hyg. Infekt.-Kr. **7**, 225—233 (1889).

Koelle, G. B., Friedenwald, J. S.: A histochemical method for localizing cholinesterase activity. Proc. Soc. exp. Biol. (N.Y.) **70**, 617—622 (1949).

Koenig, J.: Innervation motrice expérimentale d'une portion de muscle strié normalement dépourvue de plaques motrice chez le rat. C. R. Acad. Sci. (Paris) **256**, 2918—2920 (1963).

Koenig, J.: Contribution á l'étude de la morphologie des plaques motrices des grands dorsaux anterieur et posterieur du poulet après innervation croisée. Arch. Anat. micr. Morph. exp. **59**, 403—425 (1970).

Koenig, J.: Contribution a l'étude de la néoformation expérimentale des plaques motrices de rat. Arch. Anat. micr. Morph. exp. **60**, 1—26 (1971).

Koenig, J.: Morphogenesis of motor end-plates "*in vivo*" and "*in vitro*". Brain Res. **62**, 361—365 (1973).

Koenig, J., Pécot-Dechavassine, M.: Relations entre l'apparition des potentiels miniatures spontanes et l'ultrastructure des plaques motrices en voie de réinnervation et de néoformation chez le rat. Brain Res. **27**, 43—57 (1971).

Korneliussen, H.: Ultrastructure of normal and stimulated motor endplates. Z. Zellforsch. **130**, 28—57 (1972).

KORNELIUSSEN, H.: Ultrastructure of motor nerve terminals on different types of muscle fibers in the Atlantic Hagfish *(Myxine glutinosa)*. Z. Zellforsch. **147**, 87—105 (1973).

KORNELIUSSEN, H., WAERHAUG, O.: Three morphological types of motor nerve terminals in the rat diaphragm, and their possible innervation of different muscle fiber types. Z. Anat. Entwickl.-Gesch. **140**, 73—84 (1973).

KRAUSE, W.: Über die Endigung der Muskelnerven. Z. f. rationelle Med. **18**, 136—160 (1863).

KÜHNE, W.: Neue Untersuchungen über die motorische Nervendigungen. Z. Biol. **23**, 1—148 (1887).

KUFFLER, S. W., VAUGHAN WILLIAMS, E. M.: Small-nerve junctional potentials. The distribution of small motor nerves to frog skeletal muscle, and the membrane characteristics of the fibres they innervate. J. Physiol. (Lond.) **121**, 289—317 (1953a).

KUFFLER, S. W., VAUGHAN WILLIAMS, E. M.: Properties of the "slow" skeletal muscle fibres of the frog. J. Physiol. (Lond.) **121**, 318—340 (1953b).

KUGELBERG, E., EDSTRÖM, L.: Differential histochemical effects of muscle contractions on phosphorylase and glycogen in various types of fibres: relation to fatigue. J. Neurol. Neurosurg. Psychiat. **31**, 415—423 (1968).

KUPFER, C.: Selective block of synaptic transmission in ciliary ganglion by type A botulinus toxin in rabbits. Proc. Soc. exp. Biol. (N.Y.) **99**, 474—476 (1958).

KUPFER, C.: Motor innervation of extraocular muscle. J. Physiol. (Lond.) **153**, 522—526 (1960).

LAMANNA, C.: The most poisonous poison. Science **130**, 763—772 (1959).

LAMBERT, E. H., ELMQVIST, D.: Quantal components of end-plate potentials in the myasthenic syndrome. Ann. N.Y. Acad. Sci. **183**, 183—199 (1971).

LEE, C. Y.: Chemistry and pharmacology of polypeptide toxins in snake venoms. Ann. Rev. Pharmacol. **12**, 265—286 (1972).

LEHMANN, H., SILK, E., LIDDELL, J.: Pseudo-cholinesterase. Brit. med. Bull. **17**, 230—233 (1961).

LEIGHTON, G.: Botulism and food preservation. The Loch Maree tragedy. London: Collins 1923.

LENTZ, T. L.: Development of the neuromuscular junction. I. Cytological and cytochemical studies on the neuromuscular junction of differentiating muscle in the regenerating limb of the newt *Triturus*. J. Cell Biol. **42**, 431—443 (1969).

LEWIS, P. R.: A simultaneous coupling azo dye technique suitable for whole mounts. Quart. J. micr. Sci. **99**, 67—72 (1958).

LEWIS, P. R.: The effect of varying the conditions in the Koelle technique. Bibl. anat. (Basel) **2**, 11—20 (1961).

LIDDELL, E. G. T., SHERRINGTON, C. S.: Recruitment and some other features of reflex inhibition. Proc. roy. Soc. B **97**, 488—518 (1925).

LONGENECKER, H. E., HURLBUT, W. P., MAURO, A., CLARK, A. W.: Effects of black widow spider venom on the frog neuromuscular junction. Nature (Lond.) **225**, 701—703 (1970).

LUCAS, K.: The excitable substances of amphibian muscle. J. Physiol. (Lond.) **36**, 113—135 (1907).

LÜTTGAU, H. C.: The action of calcium ions on potassium contractures of single muscle fibres. J. Physiol. (Lond.) **168**, 679—697 (1963).

MACDERMOT, V.: The changes in the motor endplate in myasthenia gravis. Brain **83**, 24—36 (1960).

MAILLET, M.: Modifications de la technique Champy au tètraoxyde d'osmium-iodure de potassium. Résultats de son application a l'etude des fibres nerveuses. C. R. Soc. Biol. (Paris) **6**, 939—940 (1959).

MANOLOV, S., PENEV, D., ITCHEV, K.: Innervation multiple des fibres musculaires extrafusales du muscle vocal du chat. Comptes. Rend. Acad. Bulgare Sci. **16**, 849—852 (1963).

MARNAY, A., NACHMANSOHN, D.: Choline esterase in voluntary muscle. J. Physiol. (Lond.) **92**, 37—47 (1938).

MASSOULIE, J., RIEGER, F., BON, S., POWELL, J.: Les différentes formes moléculaires de l'acétylcholinesterase. In: La Transmission Cholinergique de L'excitation, pp. 143—144. Paris: INSERM 1973.

MAVRINSKAIA, L. F.: On the relationship between the development of the nerve endings of the skeletal muscles and the appearance of movement activity in the human foetus. Arkh. Anat. Gistol. Embriol. **38**, 61—68 (1960).

McCOMAS, A. J., SICA, R. E. P., CAMPBELL, M. J.: "Sick" motoneurones. A unifying concept of muscle disease. Lancet **1971**, **I**, 321—325.

MELLANBY, J., THOMPSON, P. A.: The effect of tetanus toxin at the neuromuscular junction in the goldfish. J. Physiol. (Lond.) **224**, 407—419 (1972).

MEYER, K. F., DUBOVSKY, B. J.: The distribution of the spores of B. botulinus in California. J. infect. Dis. **31**, 541—555 (1922a).

MEYER, K. F., DUBOVSKY, B. J.: The distribution of the spores of B. Botulinus in the United States. J. infect. Dis. **31**, 559—594 (1922b).

MICHELSON, A. M., RUSSELL, E. S., HARMAN, P. J.: Dystrophia muscularis: a hereditary primary myopathy in the house mouse. Proc. nat. Acad. Sci. (Wash.) **41**, 1079—1084 (1955).

MILEDI, R.: Junctional and extra-junctional acetylcholine receptors in skeletal muscle fibres. J. Physiol. (Lond.) **151**, 24—30 (1960).

MILEDI, R.: Induced innervation of end-plate free muscle segments. Nature (Lond.) **193**, 281—282 (1962).

MILEDI, R., POTTER, L. T.: Acetylcholine receptors in muscle fibres. Nature (Lond.) **233**, 599—603 (1971).

MILEDI, R., SLATER, C. R.: Electrophysiology and electron-microscopy of rat neuromuscular junctions after nerve degeneration. Proc. roy. Soc. B **169**, 289—306 (1968).

MOTT, F. W.: The degeneration of the neurone. London: John Bale, Sons and Danielsson 1900.

MÜLLER: Das Wursgift. Dtsch. Klin. **21**, 321 et seq; **22, 27** et seq; (26 sections) (1869).

MUIR, A. R.: Observations on the attachment of myofibrils to the sarcolemma at the muscle-tendon junction. In: Histochemistry of Cholinesterase, p. 182. Basel: Karger 1961.

MUMENTHALER, M., ENGEL, W. K.: Cytological localization of cholinesterase in developing chick embryo skeletal muscle. Acta anat. (Basel) **47**, 274—299 (1961).

MURATA, F., OGATA, T.: The ultrastructure of neuromuscular junctions of human red, white and intermediate striated muscle fibers. Tohoku J. exp. Med. **99**, 289—301 (1969).

NAKAJIMA, Y.: Fine structure of red and white muscle fibers and their neuromuscular junctions in the snake fish (*Ophiocephalus argus*). Tissue and Cell **1**, 229—246 (1969).

NAMBA, T., NAKAMURA, T., GROB, D.: Staining for nerve fiber and cholinesterase activity in fresh frozen sections. Amer. J. clin. Path. **47**, 74—77 (1967).

NASSAR, A. M.: Structural changes of fast and slow mammalian muscle after tenotomy, denervation and reinnervation. Ph.D. Thesis, University of London, 1967.

NICOLAIER, A.: Über infectiosen tetanus. Dtsch. med. Wschr. **10**, 842—844 (1884).

NYSTRÖM, B.: Histochemical studies of end-plate bound esterases in "slow-red" and "fast-white" cat muscles during post-natal development. Acta neurol. scand. **44**, 295—318 (1968a).

NYSTRÖM, B.: Postnatal development of motor nerve terminals in "slow-red" and "fast-white" cat muscles. Acta neurol. scand. **44**, 363—383 (1968b).

OKAMOTO, M., LONGENECKER, H. E., RIKER, W. F., SONG, S. K.: Destruction of mammalian motor nerve terminals by black widow spider venom. Science **172**, 733—736 (1971).

OOSTERHUIS, H., BETHLEM, J.: Neurogenic muscle involvement in myasthenia gravis: a clinical and histopathological study. J. Neurol. Neurosurg. Psychiat. **36**, 244—254 (1973).

ORKAND, P. M.: Light and electron microscopic studies of skeletal and cardiac muscle in the normal state and in drug-induced myopathies in the cat. Ph.D. Thesis, University of London, 1964.

OKRAND, R. K.: A further study of electrical responses in slow and twitch muscle fibres of the frog. J. Physiol. (Lond.) **167**, 181—191 (1963).

OVALLE, W. K.: Motor nerve terminals on rat intrafusal muscle fibres, a correlated light and electron microscopic study. J. Anat. (Lond.) **111**, 239—252 (1972).

PADYKULA, H. A., GAUTHIER, G. F.: The ultrastructure of the neuromuscular junction of mammalian red, white and intermediate skeletal muscle fibers. J. Cell Biol. **46**, 27—41 (1970).

PAGE, S. G.: A comparison of the fine structures of frog slow and twitch muscle fibres. J. Cell Biol. **26**, 477—497 (1965).

PALADE, G. E.: Electron microscope observations of interneuronal and neuromuscular synapses. Anat. Rec. **118**, 335—336 (1954).

PALAY, S. L.: Synapses in the central nervous system. J. biophys. biochem. Cytol., Suppl. **2**, 193—202 (1956).

PALMGREN, A.: A rapid method for selective silver staining of nerve fibres and nerve endings in mounted paraffin sections. Acta zoologica Stockholm **29**, 377—392 (1948).

PAPPAS,G.D.,PETERSON,E.R.,MASUROVSKY,E.B.,CRAIN,S.M.:Electron microscopy of the *in vitro* development of mammalian motor end-plates. Ann. N.Y. Acad. Sci. **183**, 33—45 (1971).

PATRICK,J., LINDSTROM,J.: Autoimmune response to acetylcholine receptor. Science **180**, 871—872 (1973).

PEACHEY,L.D., HUXLEY,A.F.: Structural identification of twitch and slow striated muscle fibres of the frog. J. Cell Biol. **13**, 177—180 (1962).

PEARSE,A.G.E.: Carboxylic esterases. In: Histochemistry. Theoretical and Applied, 2nd Ed., pp.456—490. London: Churchill 1960.

PÉCOT-DECHAVASSINE,M., COUTEAUX,R.:Potentiels miniatures d'amplitude anormale obtenus dans des conditions experimentales et changements concomitants des structures presynaptiques. In: La Transmission Cholinergique de L'excitation, pp.177—185. Paris: INSERM 1973.

PETERSON,E.R., CRAIN,S.M.: Innervation in cultures of fetal rodent skeletal muscle by organotypic explants of spinal cord from different animals. Z. Zellforsch. **106**, 1—21 (1970).

PILAR,G., HESS,A.: Differences in internal structure and nerve terminals of the slow and twitch muscle fibres in the cat superior oblique. Anat. Rec. **154**, 243—251 (1966).

RABERGER,E.: Innervationsunterschiede zwischen roten und weißen Muskelfasern der Ratte. Verh. anat. Ges. (Jena) **66**, 431—434 (1971).

RAGAB,A.H.M.F.: Motor end-plate changes in mouse muscular dystrophy. Lancet **1971 II**, 815—816.

RAND,M.J., WHALER,B.C.: Impairment of sympathetic transmission by botulinum toxin. Nature (Lond.) **206**, 588—591 (1965).

RANVIER,L.: Proprietes et structures differentes des muscles rouge et des muscles blancs, chez les lapins et chez les raies. C.R. Acad. Sci. (Paris) **77**, 1030—1034 (1873).

REDFERN,P.A.: Neuromuscular transmission in new-born rats. J. Physiol. (Lond.) **209**, 701—709 (1970).

REGER,J.F.: Electron microscopy of the motor end plate in intercostal muscle of the rat. Anat. Rec.**118**, 344 (1954).

REGER,J.F.: The fine structure of neuromuscular synapses of gastrocnemii from mouse and frog. Anat. Rec. **130**, 7—24 (1958).

REGER,J.F.: Studies in the fine structure of normal and denervated neuromuscular junctions from mouse gastrocnemii. J. Ultrastruct. Res. **2**, 269—282 (1959).

ROBERTSON,J.D.: Electron microscope observations on a reptilian myoneural junction. Anat. Rec. **118**, 346 (1954).

ROBERTSON,J.D.: Electron microscopy of the motor end-plate and the neuromuscular spindle. Amer. J. phys. Med. **39**, 1—43 (1960).

ROUGET,M.: Note sur la terminaison des nerfs moteurs dans les muscles chez les reptiles, les oiseaux et les mammifères. J. de la physiol. de l'homme, Par., **5**, 574—593 (1862).

RUSSELL,D.S.: Histological changes in the striped muscles in myasthenia gravis. J. Path. Bact. **65**, 279—289 (1953).

SALAFSKY,B., STIRLING,C.A.: Altered neural protein in murine muscular dystrophy. Nature. (Lond.) New Biol. **246**, 126—128 (1973).

SALPETER,M.M.: Electron microscope radioautography as a quantitative tool in enzyme cytochemistry. I. The distribution of acetylcholinesterase at motor end plates of a vertebrate twitch muscle. J. Cell Biol. **32**, 379—389 (1967).

SALPETER,M.M., PLATTNER,H., ROGERS,A.: Quantitative assay of esterases in end plates of mouse diaphragm by electron microscope autoradiography. J. Histochem. Cytochem. **20**, 1059—1068 (1972).

SANTA,T., ENGEL,A.G.: Histometric analysis of neuromuscular junction ultrastructure in rat red, white and intermediate muscle fibres. In: DESMEDT,J.E. (Ed.): New Developments in Electromyography and Clinical Neurophysiology, Vol.I, pp.41—54. Basel: Karger 1973.

SCHOFIELD,G.C.: Experimental studies on the innervation of the mucous membrane of the gut. Brain **83**, 490—514 (1960).

SEARLE,A.G.: Mouse News Letter **27**, 34 (1962).

SHEHATA,S.H.: The innervation of avian muscle. Ph.D. Thesis, University of London, 1961.

SHEHATA,S.H., BOWDEN,R.E.M.: The innervation of avian striated muscle. J. Anat. (Lond.) **94**, 574—575 (1960).

SHEHATA,S.H., BOWDEN,R.E.M.: Further observations on the innervation of avian muscles. J. Anat. (Lond.) **95**, 601 (1961).

SHERRINGTON,C.S.: Some functional problems attaching to convergence. Proc. roy. Soc. B **105**, 332—362 (1930).

SIDMAN,R.L., GREEN,M.C., APPEL,S.H.: Catalog of the neurological mutants of the mouse. Cambridge: Harvard Univ. Press 1965.

SIMPSON,J.A.: Myasthenia gravis and myasthenic syndromes. In: WALTON,J.N. (Ed.): Disorders of Voluntary Muscle, 2nd Ed., pp. 541—578. London: Churchill 1969.

SNELL,R.S., MCINTYRE,N.: Changes in the histochemical appearances of cholinesterase at the motor end-plate following denervation. Brit. J. exp. Path. **37**, 44—48 (1956).

SOTELO,C.: Morphologie des synapses centrales. In: La Transmission Cholinergique de L'excitation, pp. 5—27. Paris: INSERM 1973.

STEIN,J.M., PADYKULA,H.A.: Histochemical classification of individual skeletal muscle fibers of the rat. Amer. J. Anat. **110**, 103—123 (1962).

STEINBACH,J.H., HARRIS,A.J., PATRICK,J., SCHUBERT,D., HEINEMANN,S.: Nerve-muscle interaction in vitro. *Role of acetylcholine.* J. gen. Physiol. **62**, 255—270 (1973).

SUGIYAMA,H., BENDA,P., MEUNIER,J.-C., CHANGEUX,J.-P.: Immunological characterisation of the cholinergic receptor protein from *Electrophorus electricus*, FEBS Letters **35**, 124—128 (1973).

TELLO,F.: Dégéneration et régéneration des plaques motrices après la section des nerfs. Trab. Inst. Cajal Invest. biol. **5**, 117—149 (1907).

TELLO,F.: Genesis de las terminaciones nerviosas motrices y sensitivas. Trab. Inst. Cajal Invest. biol. **15**, 101—199 (1917).

TERÄVÄINEN,H.: Development of the myoneural junction in the rat. Z. Zellforsch. **87**, 249—265 (1968a).

TERÄVÄINEN,H.: Electron microscopic and histochemical observations on different types of nerve endings in the extraocular muscles of the rat. Z. Zellforsch. **90**, 372—388 (1968b).

TERÄVÄINEN,H.: Carboxylic esterases in developing myoneural junctions of rat striated muscles. Histochemie **12**, 307—315 (1968c).

TERÄVÄINEN,H.: Localization of acetylcholinesterase in the rat myoneural junction. Histochemie **17**, 162—169 (1969).

TERÄVÄINEN,H.: Effect of unilateral electrocoagulation of the oculomotor nucleus on the ultrastructure of small multiple myoneural junctions present in the extraocular muscles. Acta neurol. scand. **48**, 321—329 (1972).

THESLEFF,S.: Supersensitivity of skeletal muscle produced by botulinum toxin. J. Physiol. (Lond.) **151**, 598—607 (1960a).

THESLEFF,S.: Effects of motor innervation on the chemical sensitivity of skeletal muscle. Physiol. Rev. **40**, 734—752 (1960b).

TIEGS,O.W.: Innervation of voluntary muscle. Physiol. Rev. **33**, 90—144 (1953).

TIZZONI,G., CATTANI,G.: Über das Tetanusgift. Zbl. Bakt. **8**, 69—73 (1890).

TOH,H.T.: Biochemical, structural and functional changes in isolated heart and skeletal muscle preparations. Ph.D. Thesis, University of London, 1971.

TONGE,D.A.: Reinnervation of skeletal muscle in the mouse. J. Physiol. (Lond.) **236**, 22—23P (1974a).

TONGE,D.A.: Synaptic function in experimental dually innervated muscle in the mouse. J. Physiol. (Lond.) **239**, 96—97P (1974b).

TONGE,D.A.: Chronic effects of botulinum toxin on neuromuscular transmission and sensitivity to acetylcholine in slow and fast skeletal muscle of the mouse. J. Physiol. (Lond.) **241**, 127—139 (1974c).

TONGE,D.A.: Physiological characteristics of reinnervation of skeletal muscle in the mouse. J. Physiol. (Lond.) **241**, 141—153 (1974d).

TOWER,S.S.: Further study of the sympathetic innervation to skeletal muscle: anatomical considerations. J. comp. Neurol. **53**, 177—203 (1931).

TSUJI,S., RIEGER,F., PELTRE,G.: La localisation immunologique de l'acetylcholinesterase. In: La Transmission Cholinergique de l'excitation, pp. 129—130. Paris: INSERM 1973.

TUFFERY,A.R.: Growth and degeneration of motor end-plates in normal cat hind limb muscles. J. Anat. (Lond.) **110**, 221—247 (1971).

VALDIVIA, O.: Methods of fixation and the morphology of synaptic vesicles. J. comp. Neurol. **142**, 257—274 (1971).

VAN ERMENGEM, E.: Recherches sur des empoisonnements produit a Ellezelles (Hainaut) par du jambon et sur les causes du botulisme, de l'ichthyosisme, et en general. Arch. Pharmacodyn. **2**, 355—357 (1896).

VAN ERMENGEM, E.: Contribution à l'étude des intoxications alimentaires. Recherches sur des accidents a caractères botuliniques par du jambon. Arch. de Pharmacodyn. **3**, 213—350 (1897).

VAN HARREVELD, A.: Reinnervation of denervated muscle fibers by adjacent functioning motor units. Amer. J. Physiol. **144**, 477—493 (1945).

VAN HEYNINGEN, W. E., MELLANBY, J.: Tetanus toxin. In: KADIS, S., MONTIE, T. C., AJL, S. J. (Eds.): Microbial Toxins, Vol. II A, pp. 69—108. New York: Academic Press 1971.

VENERONI, G., MURRAY, M. R.: Formation *de novo* and development of neuromuscular junctions *in vitro*. J. Embryol. exp. Morph. **21**, 369—382 (1969).

WASER, P. G.: Autoradiographic investigations of curarizing and depolarizing drugs in the motor endplate. In: ROTH, L. J. (Ed.): Isotopes in Experimental Pharmacology, pp. 99—115. Chicago: Chicago University Press 1965.

WASER, P. G., NICKEL, F.: Electronmicroscopic and autoradiographic studies of normal and denervated endplates. In: AKERT, K., WASER, P. G. (Eds.): Mechanisms of Synaptic Transmission, pp. 157—169. Amsterdam: Elsevier 1969.

WEDDELL, G., FEINSTEIN, B., PATTLE, R. E.: The clinical application of electromyography. Lancet **1943 I**, 236—239.

WEDDELL, G., FEINSTEIN, B., PATTLE, R. E.: The electrical activity of voluntary muscle in man under normal and pathological conditions. Brain **67**, 178—257 (1944).

WEDDELL, G., ZANDER, E.: A critical evaluation of methods used to demonstrate the tissue neural elements, illustrated by reference to the cornea. J. Anat. (Lond.) **84**, 168—195 (1950).

WEISS, P., EDDS, M. V.: Spontaneous recovery of muscle following partial denervation. Amer. J. Physiol. **145**, 587—607 (1945).

WHITTAKER, V. P., DOWDALL, M. J.: Constituents of cholinergic vesicles. In: La Transmission Cholinergique de L'excitation, pp. 101—117. Paris: INSERM 1973.

WILSON, S. A. K.: Tetanus. In: Neurology, pp. 625—638. London: Arnold 1940.

WITHINGTON, J. L.: Comparative studies of the nerve supply of the larynx with special reference to the afferent innervation of the musculature. Ph.D. Thesis, University of London, 1959.

WOHLFART, G.: Collateral regeneration in partially denervated muscles. Neurology (Minneap.) **8**, 175—180 (1958).

WOHLFAHRT, G., HOFFMAN, H.: Reinnervation of muscle fibers in partially denervated muscles in Theiler's encephalomyelitis of mice (mouse poliomyelitis). Acta psychiat. scand. **31**, 345—365 (1956).

WOOLF, A. L.: Morphology of the myasthenic neuromuscular junction. Ann. N.Y. Acad. Sci. **135**, 35—56 (1966).

WOOLF, A. L.: Pathological anatomy of the intramuscular nerve endings. In: WALTON, J. N. (Ed.): Disorders of Voluntary Muscle, 2nd Ed., pp. 203—237. London: Churchill 1969.

YELLIN, H.: A histochemical study of muscle spindles and their relationship to extrafusal fiber types in the rat. Anat. Rec. **125**, 31—46 (1969).

ZACKS, S. I.: The motor endplate. Philadelphia: Saunders 1964.

ZACKS, S. I., METZGER, J. F., SMITH, C. W., BLUMBERG, J. M.: Localization of ferritin-labelled botulinus toxin in the neuromuscular junction of the mouse. J. Neuropath. exp. Neurol. **21**, 610—633 (1962).

ZENKER, W., ANZENBACHER, H.: On the different forms of myo-neural junction in two types of muscle fiber from the external ocular muscles of the rhesus monkey. J. cell. comp. Physiol. **63**, 273—285 (1964).

CHAPTER 2

Neurochemistry of Cholinergic Terminals

F. C. MacIntosh and B. Collier

A. Introduction

This chapter is concerned with the metabolism of acetylcholine (ACh) at synapses where it functions as the neurotransmitter. The vertebrate neuromuscular junction has been studied more closely than any other synapse, but most of the studies have made use of biophysical or morphological techniques rather than biochemical ones; relatively few investigators have attempted to measure the ACh content of skeletal muscle, or the rate of its release or its synthesis. For such neurochemical experiments other tissues, especially the brain, sympathetic ganglia and the electric organ, are generally chosen. These tissues are much richer in cholinergic synapses, and therefore in ACh, so the technical difficulties of estimating submicrogram amounts of ACh are less formidable. Each of the three tissues provides advantages for particular types of experiment, and together they have furnished most of the available neurochemical data. There is now, however, both direct and indirect evidence that ACh metabolism in muscle is similar in many respects to ACh metabolism in the tissues in which it has been studied in more detail. With this justification, a great deal of information obtained from tissues other than muscle will be discussed in this chapter.

The first detailed studies of ACh metabolism were made about 40 years ago by Brown and Feldberg (1936 b) on the perfused superior cervical ganglion of the cat, and by Quastel and his co-workers (Quastel et al., 1936; Mann et al., 1938) on rat brain tissue respiring *in vitro*. During the next 20 years the subject received little further attention, though much was learned, especially through analysis of the muscle end-plate potential (e.p.p.), about the processes involved in the release and the action of ACh. Towards the end of that period three new techniques appeared that were destined to revolutionize the study of cholinergic transmission. With remarkably little delay, the introduction of intracellular microelectrodes was followed by the discovery of quantal transmission at the neuromuscular junction, while the introduction of thin-section electron microscopy was followed by the discovery of synaptic vesicles. The introduction of cell-fractionation technology led, after a longer interval, to the harvesting of isolated nerve endings (synaptosomes) and synaptic vesicles, and thus to information about the subcellular localization of ACh and of the enzymes involved in its synthesis and breakdown, namely choline acetyltransferase (ChAc) and acetylcholinesterase (AChE) respectively. When studies of ACh metabolism were resumed, the hemicholinium base HC-3 became a useful tool, because it was found to inhibit ACh synthesis by blocking the trans-membrane transport of choline. During the last decade, the availability of radioactive choline and ACh, and the development of equipment for their routine measurement, have been a further stimulus to work on the turnover of ACh. A recent development has been the advent of new methods for the chemical assay of ACh and choline; the traditional biological assay procedures will no doubt continue to be used by some investigators.

Neurochemical studies of ACh storage and turnover have made it necessary to postulate the existence of several intracellular compartments or pools of ACh, which differ in their availability for release and in their turnover rates during rest or activity. Further efforts have been made using neurochemical techniques with the object of specifying the properties and sites of these pools, if possible, in terms of (a) the quanta of the biophysicists, (b) the nerve-endings and vesicles of the electron microscopists and (c) the various populations of subcellular particles biochemists have separated from tissue homogenates. These efforts have not been wholly success-ful and no fully satisfactory scheme incorporating all the available information can as yet be put forward. Among the many uncertainties that remain, the biggest and most embarrassing is still, after more than 20 years of experiment and speculation, the role of the synaptic vesicles. There is no doubt that the vesicles store ACh, and that the ACh they store is eventually set free by nerve impulses. However, the "vesicle hypothesis", namely that a transmitter quantum consists of the ACh released by exocytosis of a single vesicle, though it is still plausible, is unproven. The principal alternative hypothesis, which has not yet been excluded, is that the vesicles are only a reservoir, and that a quantum is not preformed, but represents the ACh that escapes from the nerve-ending cytosol when a gate or channel in the plasma membrane opens transiently.

The chapter, after a note on the chemical assay of ACh, deals successively with the neurochemical aspects of ACh synthesis, storage, release, turnover and inactiva-tion, and ends with short accounts of axonal transport and synaptic plasticity as related to cholinergic junctions. Under each of the major headings attention is given to the various tissues which have been the principal objects of study. Each of the tissues has advantages and disadvantages: preparations involving skeletal muscle or ganglia permit precise control of synaptic activity but are unsuited for cell-fractiona-tion studies; brain, besides its obvious importance, gives the best yield of synapto-somes, of which however an unknown and probably a rather small fraction is choli-nergic; electric organ is an excellent source of vesicles and synaptic proteins, but its ACh metabolism is relatively slow. Several interesting and important topics are not discussed: they include invertebrate cholinergic mechanisms, the embryonic devel-opment of cholinergic neurones and receptors, cholinergic postsynaptic mechanisms, and clinical applications. Among recent reviews that cover much of the same ground as the present one, those of Potter (1970b, c), Hebb (1972) and Hubbard (1974) may be especially recommended.

B. Methods for Extracting and Measuring Acetylcholine

1. Preparation of Tissues for Extraction of ACh

No elaborate precautions are required for *peripheral tissues* except when it is neces-sary to determine the effect of high-frequency stimulation (20 Hz and upwards) on the ACh content of the tissue. Though ACh turnover occurs during rest, and is accelerated by activity, synthesis of the transmitter normally keeps pace with its release and destruction, so that the level of stored ACh never falls much below the maximum. This is at least true for ganglia (BROWN and FELDBERG, 1936 b; BIRKS and MACINTOSH, 1961; FRIESEN and KHATTER, 1971 a), for diaphragm (POTTER, 1970 a), and for intestinal muscle (PATON et al., 1971). For these peripheral tissues there is no evidence that a short delay (less than one minute) between the excision of the tissue and its immersion in the cold extraction medium affects the amount of ACh that can be extracted from it; but data are sparse, and it is obviously sensible to keep the interval short and to ensure that no stimulation or injury of the tissue occurs during this period. High-frequency cholinergic nerve stimulation reversibly reduces stored ACh in ganglia (ROSENBLUETH et al., 1939; MACINTOSH, 1963; FRIESEN and KHATTER, 1971 a; BOURDOIS et al., 1975) and in muscles (ROSENBLUETH et al., 1939; BHATNAGAR and MACINTOSH, 1960); the ACh content tends to recover even while the stimulation continues, and it rebounds above the initial level after the stimulation is over. When the effect of such high-frequency excitation on ACh content is to be observed, additional precautions to shorten the delay between excision and extraction are necessary (e.g. maintaining blood flow or perfusion as long as possible, and cutting the nerve last of all).

In *brain*, the level of stored ACh fluctuates much more than it does in the periphery, and the question of how to sample the tissue is harder to answer. The ACh content of this tissue varies inversely with the rate at which ACh is released and destroyed; as that rate becomes faster the rate of synthesis lags further behind. Thus ACh content rises during anaesthesia and natural sleep, and falls during excitement and convulsions (RICHTER and CROSSLAND, 1949). It is therefore not surprising that the absolute levels reported for ACh content in brain vary according to the method used to kill the animal. In general, ACh content is reported as lower when animals are killed by decapitation, higher when the brain is frozen quickly by immersion into liquid nitrogen, and highest when the animal is killed by microwave irradiation (RICHTER and CROSSLAND, 1949; TORU and APRISON, 1966; STAVINOHA et al., 1973). It is not certain, however, that the method of choice is the one that provides the highest value. Often the purpose of the experiment dictates the method to be used. For example the dissection of discrete areas of brain is difficult with frozen brain; and frozen tissue or tissue heated by microwave irradiation is likely to be less suitable for the preparation of subcellular fractions than is tissue obtained by decapitation. High values for ACh content have been obtained using a "near freezing" technique (TAKAHASHI and APRISON, 1964), and tissue recovered using this procedure can readily be dissected and is suitable for subcellular fractionation; however, the technique requires care to avoid any loss of ACh (cf. TAKAHASHI and APRISON, 1964 with HANIN et al., 1970).

2. Extraction of ACh

A number of procedures are available that satisfactorily extract all the ACh from a tissue, and there is little evidence to suggest that any one is better than another. Extractants include trichloroacetic acid, perchloric acid, formic acid mixed with acetone, acetic acid mixed with ethanol, and acetonitrile. Before such tissue extracts can be used for ACh assay, it is often necessary to separate ACh from other materials in the extract. This can be achieved by precipitation of an insoluble complex, or by extraction into an organic phase as a soluble complex. Precipitation of ACh from aqueous solutions can be done as reineckate (e.g. Hanin and Jenden, 1969) or as periodide (e.g. Schmidt et al., 1970); in both cases it is necessary to add a co-precipitant, such as tetramethylammonium or tetraethylammonium, unless relatively large amounts of quaternary compounds are already present. Extraction of ACh from aqueous solution into an organic medium can be achieved using tetraphenylboron (Fonnum, 1969) or hexanitrodiphenylamine (Potter, 1970a; Eksborg and Persson, 1974). In all of these procedures, choline is recovered together with ACh.

3. Assay of ACh

Until quite recently, most measurements of ACh used some method of bioassay; a few investigators estimated choline also, after converting it to ACh. The choice of bioassay preparation is largely dependent upon the investigator's preference and experience, the availability of animals, and the degree of sensitivity required. The preparations available have been fully described and their relative merits discussed elsewhere (Table I: cf. also MacIntosh and Perry, 1950; Whittaker, 1963). During the last few years, several chemical methods which assay ACh have been developed, and some of these are sensitive enough to replace techniques of bioassay. In principle, chemical assays ought to provide better reproducibility, and perhaps specificity, than bioassays do; furthermore, they avoid the tedious and often exasperating aspects of bioassays. The chemical assays available are described with considerable practical detail in a recent book (Hanin, 1974). A major point for consideration in most chemical assays for ACh is the presence of choline with the ACh in the sample to be assayed; choline is extracted from tissues with ACh, and it is collected together with ACh in tissue washings or perfusates.

The main methods available for non-biological assay of ACh include: (a) *Gas chromatography*. The quaternary bases ACh and choline are demethylated to their corresponding tertiary amines, which are volatile; these can be separated by gas-liquid chromatography and measured with a flame-ionization detector. The quantitative demethylation uses benzenethiolate (Hanin and Jenden, 1969) or pyrolysis of a halide salt (Szilagyi et al., 1968). With a standard detector, the sensitivity of these methods is about 20 to 50 pmol, but this can be appreciably increased by using a mass spectrometer as the detector. (b) *Hydrolysis and measurement based upon acetate*. For large amounts of ACh, the acetyl moiety can be measured colorimetrically as the ferric hydroxamate (Hestrin, 1949). A more sensitive procedure depends upon reacting acetyl hydrazide with salicylaldehyde to form a fluorescent derivative (Fellman, 1969); this method can detect about 200 to 500 pmol of ACh. Similar, or somewhat better, sensitivity has been achieved by O'Neill and Sakamoto (1970), in an NADH-linked procedure that converts acetate to citrate enzymatically. (c) *Hydrolysis and measurement based upon choline*. These methods require that endogenous choline in the sample is first removed. Choline can be separated from ACh by paper electrophoresis, the ACh then hydrolysed to choline, and this choline determined by radioenzymic assay with the aid of either choline acetyltransferase and radioactive acetyl-CoA (Feigenson and Saelens, 1969), or choline kinase and radioactive ATP

Table 1. Comparison of sensitivity of various methods for determination of ACh.

Method	Sensitivity (pmol)	Reference
Bioassay—frog rectus	25	CHANG and GADDUM (1933)
leech muscle	5; 0.5	MINZ (1932); SZERB (1961)
guinea-pig ileum	2	PATON and VIZI (1969)
Venus heart	0.5	WELSH and TAUB (1948)
cat blood pressure	10	MACINTOSH and PERRY (1950)
toad lung	0.01	NISHI et al. (1967)
Gas chromatography	50	HANIN and JENDEN (1969)
	20	SCHMIDT et al. (1970)
Fluorimetry	200	FELLMAN (1969)
	100	O'NEILL and SAKAMOTO (1970)
	100	BROWNING (1972)
Radio-enzymic	5	GOLDBERG and MCCAMAN (1973)
	20	SHEA and APRISON (1973)
	20	FEIGENSON and SAELENS (1969)
	80	REID et al. (1971)

(REID et al., 1971). In other procedures choline kinase is first used to remove choline from the sample containing ACh, the ACh is then hydrolysed to choline and this choline is measured by a radioenzymic method using either choline acetyltransferase (SHEA and APRISON, 1973) or choline kinase (GOLDBERG and MCCAMEN, 1973). In yet another procedure (BROWNING, 1972), choline is first removed by the action of choline kinase; ACh is then hydrolysed to choline, which in turn is phosphorylated by the kinase with the liberation of ADP from ATP. The ADP so formed is reacted with phosphoenolpyruvate in the presence of pyruvate kinase to yield pyruvate, which is reduced in a reaction that oxidizes NADH; this is then the basis for a fluorimetric assay for ACh.

There is, therefore, a variety of methods now available for measuring ACh and the choice of method will depend largely upon available equipment and the sensitivity required. Table 1 summarizes the methods and indicates the approximate sensitivity of each.

C. Acetylcholine Synthesis

HEBB's 1972 review of the current status of this topic is comprehensive and critical, and includes a valuable discussion of the methods available for assaying choline acetyltransferase. The present section will deal more briefly with most of the problems considered by Hebb, but will refer to more recent findings of significance, especially in relation to choline transport.

1. Choline Acetyltransferase: Its Location and Physical Properties

ACh synthesis *in vivo* depends on the enzymatic transfer of acetyl from coenzyme A to choline:

$$\text{Choline} + \text{acetyl-CoA} \rightleftharpoons \text{ACh} + \text{CoA}.$$

The enzyme that catalyses the transfer is choline acetyltransferase (ChAc; acetyl-CoA-choline-O-transferase; EC 2.3.1.6), formerly called choline acetylase (Nach-mansohn and Machado, 1943). In vertebrates ChAc is presumed to be located almost entirely in neural elements, since it disappears from tissues when they have been chronically denervated (Banister and Scrase, 1950; Hebb et al., 1964; Potter, 1970a). The enzyme is absent, or nearly so, from Schwann cells and other glial elements (Hebb, 1961; Kása et al., 1970a, b; Cotman et al., 1971). Thus there is no reason to question the long-held belief (cf. Feldberg, 1945) that ChAc is contained mainly within cholinergic neurones and is present in highest concentration at their terminals. There are a few exceptions to this rule, one being the human placenta, which is rich in ChAc though it contains no nerve terminals (Comline, 1946; Morris, 1966); the function of the enzyme in this tissue is unknown. In the nervous system as a whole, the distribution of ChAc corresponds well with that of ACh; on the other hand AChE has a somewhat wider distribution than either (cf. Hebb and Morris, 1969).

ChAc preparations obtained from various species and tissues have generally similar properties. When extracted from ox brain and partially purified, the enzyme appears to be a stable, relatively basic protein, whose molecular weight estimated by gel filtration is about 65000 daltons (Glover and Potter, 1971). When freed from other proteins it tends to become less stable (White and Cavallito, 1970a), and it has been suggested (Chao and Wolfgram, 1973) that the native enzyme of some 120000 daltons can dissociate into two sub-units of unequal size and activity.

Although ChAc appears always to be a basic protein, the net positive charge on the molecule varies considerably from species to species, as is shown by the affinity of different preparations for negatively charged surfaces (Fonnum, 1970; Fonnum and Malthe-Sørenssen, 1972, 1973). Indeed, a single tissue may yield several isoenzymes with different isoelectric points (Fonnum and Malthe-Sørenssen, 1972, 1973; White and Wu, 1973b). As a result of these variations preparations of ChAc, especially when obtained from different species, may exhibit marked differences in terms of the solubility of the enzyme and its affinity for natural membranes (Tuček, 1966a, b). These differences are accentuated when the enzyme is extracted into a medium of low pH or low ionic strength: both conditions make it less soluble (Fonnum, 1967, 1968a).

Such differences caused temporary confusion when the first successful attempts were made to fractionate brain synaptosomes with the aid of osmotic lysis: thus one laboratory (De Robertis et al., 1963) found most of the ChAc associated with a particulate fraction rich in synaptic vesicles, while another (Whittaker et al., 1964) found most of the enzyme in the supernatant or soluble fraction. Eventually the situation was clarified on the basis of the solubility differences mentioned above, and there is now general agreement that most, though not all, of the enzyme must exist free in the nerve-terminal cytoplasm. It has been suggested (cf. Whittaker, 1970; Hebb, 1972) that some of the membrane-bound enzyme may be attached to the outer surface of the vesicles, and so, perhaps, strategically located for assisting vesicular uptake of newly-synthesized ACh, a process which occurs but is poorly understood. Histochemical visualization of ChAc has not been able to decide this issue: the approximate intracellular location of the enzyme can be revealed by precipitation (Burt, 1969, 1970; Kása, 1970; Kása et al., 1970a, b; Burt and Dettbarn, 1972) or immunofluorescence (ENG et al., 1974; McGEER et al., 1974) techniques, but such methods can hardly provide the spatial resolution necessary for detecting a protein adsorbed at the vesicular surface.

2. Choline Acetyltransferase: Its Chemistry, Substrates, and Inhibitors

Because of the difficulty of purifying ChAc little has been learned about its amino acid composition, or about the chemistry of the active site where its two substrates are bound. REISBERG (1957) and several later workers (POTTER et al., 1968; MANNER-VIK and SÖRBO, 1970; ROSKOSKI, 1974) reported inhibition by sulfhydryl reagents, but there have been some inconsistent findings, and it seems possible that the sensitive SH group may be distant from the sites of substrate attachment (WHITE and CAVAL-LITO, 1970b; HEBB, 1972). Another candidate for participation at the active site is the imidazole group (SEVERIN and ARTENIE, 1968; WHITE and CAVALLITO, 1970b; CUR-RIER and MAUTNER, 1974). This proposal is supported by the finding (BURT and SILVER, 1973) that free imidazole in the absence of any enzyme can transfer the acetyl moiety from CoA to choline. It is of interest that imidazole itself can catalyse the hydrolysis of many esters, and that the imidazole group has been implicated as a component of the active centre of AChE (vide COHEN and OOSTERBAAN, 1963, for references).

ChAc has been clearly distinguished from other acetyltransferases, and it seems safe to assume that the neuronal enzyme normally catalyses no reaction other than the acetylation of choline. The reason for this, however, is that neuronal ChAc is not normally in contact with substrates other than acetyl-CoA and choline. In non-nervous tissue and in invertebrates the presence of choline esters other than ACh has been reported, and of these, the propionylcholine of ox spleen (BANISTER et al., 1953), is no doubt a product of ChAc. The ability of ChAc to transfer propionyl groups to choline has been demonstrated (BERMAN et al., 1953; BERRY and WHITTAKER, 1959). Choline itself may be replaced as the acetyl acceptor by many other bases, including some non-quaternaries (BERMAN et al., 1953; BURGEN et al., 1956; DAUTERMAN and MEHROTRA, 1963; HEMSWORTH and MORRIS, 1964; HEMSWORTH and SMITH, 1970a,b; FRANKENBERG et al., 1973; CURRIER and MAUTNER, 1974). One substrate of interest, although it is not known to occur naturally, is the triethyl analogue of choline, usually referred to as triethylcholine: its pharmacological effects will be discussed later.

A specific inhibitor of ChAc that is active in vivo would be a very useful research tool, but the search for compounds of this type has not been well rewarded. The styrylpyridine derivatives synthesized and tested by CAVALLITO and his colleagues (SMITH et al., 1967; CAVALLITO et al., 1969, 1970; WHITE and CAVALLITO, 1970a, b; see also BAKER and GIBSON, 1971), especially the compound designated NVP$^+$, are strong non-competitive inhibitors when tested in vitro but are ineffective in the intact animal unless applied locally (HEMSWORTH and FOLDES, 1970; AQUILONIUS et al., 1971; GOLDBERG et al., 1971, 1972; ROSS et al., 1971; ROSENBERG et al., 1972; GLICK et al., 1973; JENDEN et al., 1974; SAELENS et al., 1974; STEVENSON and WILSON, 1974). Several halogenated derivatives of choline are also more effective in vitro than in vivo: these include chloroacetylcholine and its bromo- and iodo-analogues, whose reversible inhibitory action is limited in practice by the instability of the compounds

(Hebb, 1963; Morris and Grewaal, 1969). An analogue of ACh, 3-bromoacetonyl-trimethylammonium bromide, is an irreversible inhibitor (Persson et al., 1967; Aquilonius et al., 1971). Unlike the hemicholiniums, which do not act on ChAc but inhibit ACh synthesis by a different mechanism, none of these compounds has been shown, when given systemically, to deplete tissue ACh or to produce effects that can be ascribed to impaired cholinergic transmission. It has recently been reported that an opened-chain hemicholinium derivative, acetylseco-hemicholinium-3, shows some *in vivo* as well as *in vitro* activity as a ChAc inhibitor (Domino et al., 1973), but the possibility that the *in vivo* inhibition of ACh synthesis resulted mainly from decreased choline transport into nerve terminals was not excluded.

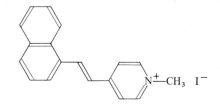

trans–N–Methyl–4(1–Naphthylvinyl)pyridinium iodide (NVP$^+$)

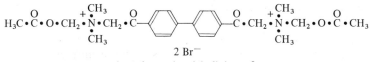

2 Br$^-$

Acetylseco–hemicholinium–3

3. Choline Acetyltransferase: Its Kinetics

There is general agreement that the reaction catalysed by ChAc is reversible and that acetyl-CoA has a higher affinity for the enzyme than has choline: most of the estimates of K_m are in the order of 8 to 25 µmol/l for acetyl-CoA and 400 to 1100 µmol/l for choline (e.g. McCaman and Hunt, 1965; Schuberth, 1966; Kaita and Goldberg, 1969; White and Cavallito, 1970a; Glover and Potter, 1971; Henderson and Sastry, 1971; Morris et al., 1971; White and Wu, 1973a). The isoenzymes obtained from rat brain do not differ in their affinity for choline (Fonnum and Malthe-Sørenssen, 1972). Most studies have concluded that ACh inhibits the enzyme competitively with respect to choline but non-competitively with respect to acetyl-CoA, whereas the reverse is true of CoA (White and Cavallito, 1970b; Morris et al., 1971; Sastry and Henderson, 1972). This and other evidence is consistent with the conclusion that the transacetylation is an ordered reaction of the Theorell-Chance type, in which the two substrates combine with the enzyme and the two products leave, all in a set order (Fig. 1). There remain, however, some puzzling discrepancies between results from different laboratories, and other types of mechanism have not been finally excluded (for discussion see Hebb, 1972).

Studies of ChAc *in vitro* have not determined the factors that limit ACh synthesis rates *in vivo*. In peripheral nerve endings ACh synthesis occurs at a measurable rate

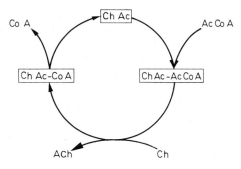

Fig. 1. Diagrammatic representation of the synthesis of ACh. An ordered bi-bi reaction of the Theorell-Chance type is illustrated

during rest and is accelerated during activity, but in both situations some regulatory process normally maintains ACh stores at a nearly constant level (BIRKS and MACINTOSH, 1961; COLLIER and MACINTOSH, 1969; POTTER, 1970a). Product inhibition by ACh would be a convenient control for ACh synthesis, but this can hardly be a major factor since even isotonic ACh has been shown to inhibit synthesis by less than 50% (KAITA and GOLDBERG, 1969; GLOVER and POTTER, 1971). GLOVER and POTTER (1971) consider that the level of free ACh may be set by mass action, in which case the CoA/acetyl-CoA ratio and the ACh/choline ratio would equally determine the rate and direction of transacetylation. Unfortunately we have no reliable information about any of these concentrations, or their ratios, in nerve endings.

4. Supply of Acetyl Groups for ACh Synthesis

The immediate source of acetyl groups for ACh is certainly acetyl-CoA. The ultimate source, at least in the brain, appears to be glucose, which generates pyruvate through the Embden-Meyerhof pathway; pyruvate is converted to acetyl-CoA by pyruvate dehydrogenase. That this route is the main one, at least in the brain, was concluded from experiments in which labelled ACh of high specific activity was formed from radioactive glucose or pyruvate by slices of brain (CHENG et al., 1967; BROWNING and SCHULMAN, 1968; NAKAMURA and CHENG, 1969; NAKAMURA et al., 1970; SOLLENBERG and SÖRBO, 1970; GREWAAL and QUASTEL, 1973; LEFRESNE et al., 1973) or by intact brain after intracisternal administration of the precursor (TUČEK and CHENG, 1970, 1974). These results confirmed the conclusions reached much earlier by QUASTEL and his colleagues (QUASTEL et al., 1936; MANN et al., 1938), who measured the formation and release of ACh by brain slices incubated in the presence of various substrates. KAHLSON and MACINTOSH (1939) reached similar conclusions from measurements of ACh synthesis and release in stimulated sympathetic ganglia, but it now seems likely that the decreased ACh release in glucose-deprived ganglia was due in part to reduction of the presynaptic spike (DUNANT and DOLIVO, 1968).

In some species or tissues glucose and pyruvate may not be the main sources of the acetyl moiety: thus acetate is preferentially used for ACh synthesis in rabbit corneal epithelium (FITZGERALD and COOPER, 1967), lobster nerve (CHENG and NAKAMURA, 1970) and *Torpedo* electroplaques (ISRAËL and TUČEK, 1974). Whatever the precursor, be it acetate or pyruvate, acetyl-CoA is generated within the mitochondria, for both acetyl-CoA-synthetase (which forms acetyl-CoA from acetate) and the pyruvate dehydrogenase complex (which forms acetyl-CoA from pyruvate) are located within mitochondria.

Much labour and thought have been devoted to the question of how acetyl-CoA, made from acetate or pyruvate in the mitochondrial inner compartment, can give rise to the acetyl-CoA that becomes available to ChAc in the cytosol. The mitochondrial wall is supposedly impermeable to acetyl-CoA, but Tuček (1970) has suggested that enough acetyl-CoA to support ACh synthesis might diffuse out. On the other hand Sollenberg and Sörbo (1970) and Hebb (1972) have suggested that acetyl-CoA produced in the mitochondria might be converted to citrate, which then leaves, perhaps as a metabolite, and regenerates acetyl-CoA with the aid of the extra-mitochondrial enzyme citrate ATP lyase. However, extracellular citrate is ineffective as a sourse of acetyl groups for ACh synthesis under conditions in which glucose or pyruvate is well utilized (Quastel, 1962; Sollenberg and Sörbo, 1970; Nakamura et al., 1970; Tuček and Cheng, 1974). It is clear that more information is needed before firm conclusions can be drawn about this important point.

5. Supply of Choline for ACh Synthesis

It is now established that choline for the synthesis of ACh comes from three principal sources: (a) free choline in plasma, (b) an internal source, presumably phospholipid breakdown, and (c) re-use of choline produced by the action of AChE on released ACh.

(a) It is obviously desirable teleologically that the level of free choline in plasma should be high enough to support both ACh and phospholipid synthesis, but not high enough to activate cholinergic receptors. In fact, the plasma of most mammals contains choline at a concentration of 10 to 20 μmol/l (Bligh, 1952). How its level is regulated is not well understood. The kidney may be presumed to play a part, since the renal tubules of mammals and birds can both reabsorb and excrete choline: reabsorption predominates unless the plasma level is artificially raised (Rennick, 1958; Vander, 1962; Gardiner and Paton, 1972; Acara and Rennick, 1973; Trimble et al., 1974). Injected choline leaves the circulation quickly (Hunt, 1915; Kahane and Lévy, 1950; Bligh, 1953a), for the half-time of disappearance is about 1 to 2 min; with continued infusion of choline a steady level is approached with a half-time of 7 min or less (Gardiner and Paton, 1972). Much of the infused choline is disposed of by the liver and kidneys (Bligh, 1953a; Gardiner and Paton, 1972). These organs besides providing possible routes of excretion, contain most of the body's choline dehydrogenase (EC 1.1.99.1, choline oxidase). The abdominal viscera, lung and brain are also important extraction sites (Gardiner and Paton, 1972), and infused choline can be disposed of after the removal of both liver and kidneys, though more slowly than in the intact animal (Bligh, 1953a).

It has been shown in man that the plasma choline level is unaffected by feeding or by exercise (Bligh, 1952), or by the presence of various hepatic or renal diseases (Bligh, 1952) or myasthenia gravis (Birks and MacIntosh, 1961). The circulating free choline concentration falls by about 50% in rats placed on a severely choline-deficient diet (Bligh, 1953b), although such animals have no apparent impairment of neuromuscular transmission (LI, 1941). Plasma choline is also lowered for an hour or so in dogs given a single dose of cortisone, and for days in human patients after major surgery (MACINTOSH, 1963), but the mechanism responsible for the lowering is unknown. Hydrocortisone does not have such an effect in rodents (GWEE and LIM, 1972).

The dietary intake of choline is supplemented by a limited biosynthesis, which occurs mainly in the liver but to some extent in a few other tissues (BREMER and GREENBERG, 1961). The product of this reaction is phosphatidylcholine rather than choline itself, the raw material being phosphatidylethanolamine with the methyl groups supplied by 5-methyl adenosyl-methionine. DROSS and KEWITZ (1972) have recently proposed on the basis of somewhat indirect evidence that brain can synthesize choline, but other workers have found no evidence for this (ANSELL and SPANNER, 1971), and at present it seems more likely that circulating choline is the source of neuronal ACh.

Some attention has been given to the idea that choline reaches the nerve terminals in the form of one of its esters. ANSELL and SPANNER (1971) suggested that choline is transferred from blood to brain in the form of phosphatidyl- or lysophosphatidylcholine, because after injecting labelled choline intraperitoneally into rats they found little or no labelled free choline or phosphorylcholine in the blood, while radioactivity accumulated in the brain. It appears that choline in the form of phospholipid can cross the blood-brain interface (HOEZL and FRANCK, 1969), but free choline can also do so (see below). There is no direct evidence that circulating phospholipid can readily transfer its choline to the pools of ACh and free choline in the brain. Such a possibility seems unlikely in the case of peripheral synapses (COLLIER and MACINTOSH, 1969). When ganglia were perfused with plasma to which [^{3}H] choline had been added, the specific radioactivity of the ACh formed during preganglionic stimulation agreed well with the specific activity of the free choline (labelled + endogenous) in the plasma; this would not have been so if the plasma phospholipid had contributed much of the choline for ACh synthesis.

Another choline ester which might provide choline for ACh synthesis is phosphorylcholine. HANIN et al. (1972a, b) showed that following the intravenous injection of [^{14}C] phosphorylcholine labelled ACh could be found in the salivary glands. However, whether nerve endings can use unhydrolysed phosphorylcholine for this purpose has not been tested: the injected ester may have to be broken down to choline extracellularly before it can be used for ACh synthesis.

In contrast to these uncertainties it is well established that circulating free choline readily enters brain tissue and becomes available for conversion to ACh (POTTER et al., 1968; SCHUBERTH et al., 1969; DIAMOND, 1971; ROSS and JENDEN, 1973; SAELENS et al., 1973; JENDEN et al., 1974). It also enters the cerebrospinal fluid (GARDINER and DOMER, 1968), and from either the inner or the outer surface of the brain it can gain access to the tissue and be metabolized to ACh (CHAKRIN et al., 1972; BARKER et al., 1972). That choline though a quaternary base can move between blood, brain and CSF need cause no surprise, for it was shown long ago that ACh can do this (for references see BURGEN and MACINTOSH, 1955). The speed with which ACh or choline passes from the blood into the brain shows that its principal route is the direct one across the capillary walls, rather than the indirect one via the choroid plexuses and cerebrospinal fluid. Whether the passage is assisted by some special carrier mechanism is unknown; it is not blocked by HC-3 (Ross and Jenden, 1973), and in that way it differs from choline uptake processes at many other sites.

(b) Cholinergic terminals can use endogenous sources of choline to support ACh synthesis, at least when no choline is supplied to them from outside. This was demonstrated by Brown and Feldberg (1936b), who showed that a ganglion perfused with a medium containing eserine but no choline could release more ACh, in response to preganglionic nerve stimulation, than its normal ACh content. In parallel experiments, Quastel and his colleagues (Quastel et al., 1936; Mann et al., 1938) found that the turnover of ACh by brain slices or mince placed in an eserinized choline-free medium could greatly exceed the ACh originally present. It is now known that the endogenous choline that is used for ACh synthesis in such tests with brain tissue is not stored as free choline (Browning, 1971; Collier et al., 1972), and the same is probably true of ganglia, which contain little free choline (Friesen et al., 1967).

Phospholipid turnover is presumably the source of most of the choline converted into ACh by tissues deprived of exogenous choline. In the absence of choline a perfused ganglion can maintain an ACh output that amounts to about 1.5% of its resting ACh content per minute (Perry, 1953; Birks and MacIntosh, 1961). This figure may be taken as a rough estimate of the rate at which choline is liberated by turnover of the ganglion's phosphatidylcholine, which on a molar basis is 50 to 100 times greater than its store of either ACh or free choline (Friesen et al., 1967). A second rough estimate of phospolipid choline turnover is given by the rate at which labelled choline supplied at a physiological concentration is incorporated into phosphorylcholine and phospholipid. The two estimates nearly coincide (Collier and Lang, 1969).

When synaptic activity is prolonged, ACh output and synthesis are better maintained if choline is present in the extracellular medium: for a perfused ganglion the maximum turnover rate is then at least 4 to 5 times higher than in the absence of choline (Birks and MacIntosh, 1961; Matthews, 1963). The "physiological" concentration of choline, about 10 µmol/l, is sufficient for optimal synthesis (Birks and MacIntosh, 1961). The volume of medium used to perfuse a ganglion is very large compared to the volume of the tissue, so there can be no accumulation of endogenous choline in the extracellular compartment; in this situation, as just noted, the rate of ACh turnover during stimulation depends on whether or not choline has been added to the medium. The situation is quite different in some of the other preparations that have been used for studying turnover. For example, free choline in substantial amounts soon diffuses into the fluid in which brain slices or minces are suspended (Bhatnagar and MacIntosh, 1967; Browning, 1971; Collier et al., 1972; Lefresne et al., 1973). In such tests the concentration of choline in the medium may rise high enough to support ACh synthesis at the optimal rate, though in some cases the addition of further choline causes a moderate increase of ACh synthesis (Mann et al., 1938; Bhatnagar and MacIntosh, 1967). In most of the other cases that have been studied ACh synthesis is not accelerated by supplying the tissue with additional choline. In the rat phrenic-diaphragm preparation, raising the choline level of the medium does not alter ACh release (Straughan, 1960) or ACh turnover (Potter, 1970a). Bennett and McLachlan (1972b) estimated ACh synthesis in isolated ganglia by measuring the size of the intracellularly-recorded excitatory postsynaptic potentials, and observed no change when choline (30 µmol/l) was added to the bathing medium. They used no anticholinesterase drug in most of their experiments, and this favoured the recapture of choline derived from released ACh [see (c), below]. However, in one experiment in the presence of neostigmine, the successive stimuli evoked diminishing responses, as if the level of transmitter in the releasable pool were critically dependent on the re-use of choline made available by ACh hydrolysis. Finally PATON and his colleagues (PATON, 1963; PATON and ZAR, 1968; PATON et al., 1971) have reported that innervated preparations of intestinal smooth muscle maintained steady rates of ACh release and synthesis in response to electrical stimulation, even without the addition of choline and in the presence of an anticholinesterase agent. In such cases, presumably, enough choline to support ACh synthesis is released by the tissue. In general, however, it seems wise that choline at the concentration normally present in plasma (10 µmol/l) should be present in the extracellular medium throughout any experiment that involves the repetitive activation of cholinergic synapses. This precaution is particularly necessary in studies of ACh turnover made with radioactive choline. Data on the uptake and transformation of labelled choline when nothing is known about the specific activity of the choline in the medium are likely to create confusion rather than add to our knowledge.

(c) It has already been indicated that the choline derived from just-released ACh is an important source of substrate for ChAc action. That this might be so was first proposed by PERRY (1953), who had observed that ganglia subjected to prolonged stimulation during perfusion with a choline-free fluid retained their ability to release ACh unless an anticholinesterase drug had been present during the stimulation. A possible explanation was that the nerve endings could re-cycle choline but not ACh; in support of this, Perry showed that the amount of ACh discharged by a given preganglionic stimulation in the presence of eserine was much greater than the amount of choline discharged in the absence of eserine under otherwise identical conditions.

Further direct and indirect evidence to support PERRY's proposal has accumulated in recent years (COLLIER and MACINTOSH, 1969; POTTER, 1970a; BENNETT and MCLACHLAN, 1972b; COLLIER and KATZ, 1974). There is reason to believe that normally more than half of the choline set free by a single impulse is immediately recaptured by the same or nearby nerve terminals. This implies, as COLLIER and MACINTOSH noted, that choline uptake must be greatly facilitated for a few msec after the impulse has invaded the terminals. Presumably the mechanism helps to maintain transmitter output, especially when synaptic traffic is brisk.

6. Transport of Choline

Choline, like other quaternary bases, is generally believed to enter most kinds of cell very slowly, and for that reason it is used for experiments in which an isolated tissue is to be exposed to a medium in which sodium has been replaced by an inert nonpermeant cation. Nevertheless most if not all cells can take up choline at a measurable rate, and whenever the kinetics of the uptake has been examined, it has been found to involve at least in part a saturable, i.e. carrier-mediated, process. This is true for example of skeletal muscle fibres (RENKIN, 1961), which take up choline more or less evenly along their whole length (POTTER, 1970a); of squid axons (HODGKIN and

Martin, 1965); and of erythrocytes (Askari, 1966; Martin, 1968). Various other quaternary compounds, including ACh, can be taken up by the same, or at least a closely related, mechanism (see also Saelens and Stoll, 1965; Taylor et al., 1965), although in general the carrier has been found to have a higher affinity for choline (K_m usually in the range 20 to 100 µmol/l; see Table 2) than for the other bases tested. In addition to this carrier-mediated uptake of choline into cells, passive uptake can be detected when choline or another quaternary compound is applied at high external concentrations; uptake is then proportional to concentration and non-saturable, and is therefore not carrier-mediated. Only the carrier-mediated uptake is competitively inhibited by compounds structurally related to choline; the hemicholinium base HC-3 (Long and Schueler, 1954; Schueler, 1955) being an especially potent inhibitor.

A different mechanism is involved in the uptake of nicotinic agonists and antagonists by skeletal muscle, and perhaps by other cholinergically innervated tissues. These compounds are bound at motor end-plates (Waser and Lüthi, 1957), and some of the depolarizing agents such as decamethonium (though not carbaminoylcholine) penetrate more rapidly there than elsewhere in the fibre (Taylor et al., 1965; Creese and MacLagan, 1967). The mechanisms of uptake in such cases presumably involves cholinergic postsynaptic receptors, for it is blocked by tubocurarine, and the area where uptake occurs has been shown to spread from the end-plate to the rest of the fibre after motor denervation (Taylor et al., 1965). Potter (1970a) has reported that virtually no choline enters muscle by this mechanism, which is not surprising since choline is a very weak nicotinic agonist.

The uptake of labelled choline by brain tissue was first studied by Schuberth et al. (1966, 1967) and Schuberth and Sundwall (1967, 1968), working with slices, and by Potter (1968), Marchbanks (1968b) and Diamond and Kennedy (1969), using synaptosomes. These studies showed that at least some nerve endings have a considerable capacity for carrier-mediated choline uptake, as experiments on ganglia (Perry, 1953; MacIntosh et al., 1956, 1958) had suggested. The uptake mechanism appeared to be very similar to that in squid axons and mammalian erythrocytes, for it was concentrative, sodium- and temperature-dependent, and competitively inhibited by HC-3.

In these early experiments on brain tissue less than 20% of the choline taken up was converted to ACh, and the kinetic data (cf. also Cooke and Robinson, 1971) showed the carrier to have no greater affinity for choline than had been reported for squid axons and erythrocytes. The calculated K_m values were in the range 40 to 200 µmol/l, which was somewhat surprising since Birks and MacIntosh (1961) had been unable to accelerate ACh synthesis in ganglia by raising the extracellular choline above its physiological concentration (about 10 µmol/l). However an additional transport system with much higher affinity for choline has now been demonstrated in brain, especially in synaptosomes (see Fig. 2, for example): K_m values in the range 1 to 5 µmol/l have been reported from several laboratories (Yamamura and Snyder, 1972, 1973; Dowdall and Simon, 1973; Guyenet et al., 1973; Haga and Noda, 1973; Kuhar et al., 1973). There is good evidence that this high-affinity system is located in cholinergic nerve terminals, whereas the low-affinity system appears to be located in all neurones and probably in other kinds of cells also. Three groups of studies provide the evidence. First, it has been shown that most of the choline

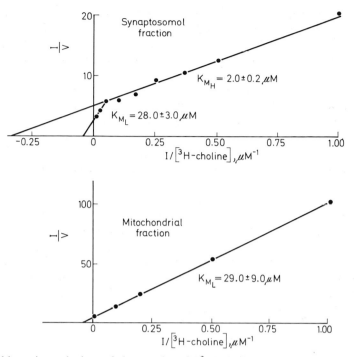

Fig. 2. Double-reciprocal plots of the uptake of [³H] choline by purified synaptosomal and mitochondrial fractions of the corpus striatum. Data for the synaptosomal fraction (upper graph) are best described by two straight lines with positive ordinate intercepts indicating a two component system. Data for the mitochondrial fraction (lower graph) describe a straight line with a positive ordinate intercept typical of Michaelis-Menten single system kinetics. K_m values and their standard errors were determined from the respective computed equations. Velocity (V) is expressed as micromoles of [³H] choline accumulated per g of protein in 4 min. Each point is the mean of triplicate determination. The experiment was replicated three times. (From YAMAMURA and SNYDER, 1973)

transported by the high-affinity system becomes acetylated (YAMAMURA and SNYDER, 1973; GUYENET et al., 1973); the ACh thus formed is available for release (MULDER et al., 1974). Second, the high-affinity uptake is characteristically observed in brain areas that are rich in ACh and ChAc (SORIMACHI and KATAOKA, 1974), whereas low-affinity uptake is widely distributed (DIAMOND and MILFAY, 1972). Finally, a brain lesion that causes selective degeneration of cholinergic fibres to the hippocampus sharply reduces the high-affinity choline uptake by hippocampal synaptosomes, but has little effect on their low-affinity uptake (KUHAR et al., 1973). The high affinity choline uptake mechanism also has a high affinity for HC-3 (Table 2). Its functional significance is undoubtedly to provide choline for ACh synthesis during synaptic activity. The function of the low-affinity system is more dubious: it may be related to phospholipid synthesis.

Little information is at present available on the substrate specificity of the high-affinity choline transport system, or on how it operates at the molecular level. Speculation about the mechanism must await a fuller account of the system's proper-

Table 2. Data for choline uptake measured *in vitro*

Preparation	Apparent Michaelis Constants (µmol/l)				Authors
	K_m choline		K_i HC-3		
	high affinity	low affinity	high affinity	low affinity	
Axon					
squid		100		20	Hodgkin and Martin (1965)
Brain slices					
rat		226			Schuberth et al. (1966)
rat		57			Cooke and Robinson (1971)
mouse (cortex)		83		5	Schuberth and Sundwall (1967)
Brain synaptosomes					
rat (cortex)		40—80		19	Potter (1968)
rat		83			Diamond and Kennedy (1969)
rat (cortex)	4—8	40	0.05—0.1	40—50	Haga and Noda (1973)
rat (striatum)	3.5		0.025		Guyenet et al. (1973)
rat (striatum)	1.4	93	1.1	122	Yamamura and Snyder (1973)
squid	2—4	>24			Dowdall and Simon (1973)
Erythrocytes					
human		20			Askari (1966)
		30			Martin (1968)
		48		4	Martin (1969)
		23			Martin (1972)

ties, comparable to the account MARTIN (1968, 1969, 1972) has given of the low-affinity system in erythrocytes. Choline transport in erythrocytes shows pronounced exchange-flux features and is differentially sensitive to the levels of sodium and potassium on either side of the membrane; moreover inhibitors that can be transported by the carrier will slow the efflux, as well as the influx, of the substrate. It is important to determine whether the high-affinity system shares these properties, and whether the trans-membrane potential in nerve endings, which favours the concentrative accumulation of any permeant base, can also affect the directionality of the carrier. Other factors that might well affect the kinetics of transport include intracellular ACh and the presence of further carrier systems operating between synaptic vesicles and the cytosol. Until these factors are better understood even the most recent affinity constants cited in Table 2 should be regarded with some reserve. A final point of uncertainty is whether the high-affinity choline transport is active, in the sense of being directly coupled to an energy transducer such as an ATPase. Metabolic inhibitors reduce choline uptake (SCHUBERTH et al., 1966; MARCHBANKS, 1968b; ABDEL-LATIF and SMITH, 1972), but these might act indirectly, for example by reducing the transmembrane potential.

7. Inhibitors of Choline Transport

A number of quaternary ammonium bases can competitively inhibit choline uptake. Their pharmacology was competently reviewed by BOWMAN and MARSHALL (1972), and with the exception of the recognition of high-affinity choline uptake no new principles have emerged since then. The inhibitor that has received most attention is still the bis-quaternary base HC-3 (hemicholinium-3), the compound whose toxicity as a respiratory paralysant attracted the attention of F. W. SCHUELER (1955) to the group of choline derivatives that possess the characteristic hemicholinium structure. Another inhibitor of great interest is the triethyl analogue of choline (2-hydroxy-ethyl-triethylammonium or triethylcholine: TEC).

The *hemicholiniums*, first synthesized by LONG and SCHUELER (1954), are characterized (SCHUELER, 1955) by the presence of a choline or choline-like moiety cyclized through hemiacetal formation. Pharmacologically their common property is the ability to cause delayed paralysis at repetitively activated cholinergic synapses: the block is due to the depletion of stored ACh, and can be prevented or relieved by choline. HC-3 is the only member of the group to have received extensive study, but there is no reason to suppose that the other hemicholiniums differ from it in their basic action.

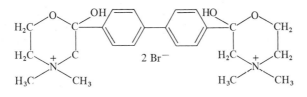

HC–3 (Hemicholinium–3: Schueler, 1955)

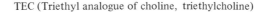

$$HO \bullet CH_2 \bullet CH_2 \overset{+}{N} (C_2H_5)_3$$
$$Cl^-$$

TEC (Triethyl analogue of choline, triethylcholine)

The diphenyl bridge of HC-3 can be replaced by other non-polar groupings without much qualitative change in pharmacological activity (MARSHALL and LONG, 1959; POWERS et al., 1962; THAMPI et al., 1966; GARDINER and SUNG, 1969). The monoquaternary half-molecule (HC-15: SCHUELER, 1955) retains activity against choline transport as measured by tests on synaptosomes (HEMSWORTH et al., 1971) but this is not apparent from *in vivo* observations (SCHUELER, 1955; BOWMAN et al., 1967). Minor changes affecting the rings, e.g. N-ethylation instead of methylation, or methylation of any one of the carbons, also allow part or all of the activity to be retained. Analogues without ring closure via hemiacetal formation do not act like the hemicholiniums, though they may have potent anticholinesterase, ganglion-blocking or tubocurarine-like activity (SCHUELER, 1955; LONG et al., 1967; DIAUGUSTINE and HAARSTAD, 1970). As noted earlier (p. 106), the acetyl ester of one opened-ring tautomer of HC-3 inhibits ChAc (DOMINO et al., 1973). Further information about structure-activity relationships within the hemicholinium series is given by BENZ and LONG (1969a, b), BOWMAN and HEMSWORTH (1965b) and BOWMAN and MARSHALL (1972).

Though the high potency of HC-3 and its close relatives depends on the closed choline ring with its hemiacetal linkage, a number of quaternary bases which lack this structure show biological activity resembling that of hemicholinium. Triethylcholine (Keston and Wortis, 1946; Bowman and Rand, 1962; Bowman and Hemsworth, 1965a) is the best known of such compounds, but its parent compound tetraethylammonium also appears to be a weak inhibitor of choline transport (Bhatnagar and MacIntosh, 1967). Certain other quaternary bases have been found to be between HC-3 and triethylcholine in potency: they include the *bis*-pyridazine derivative WIN 4981 (Gesler et al., 1959; Gesler and Hoppe, 1961), troxonium and other basic esters of trimethoxybenzoic acid (Bhatnagar et al., 1964, 1965), and a number of *bis*-choline derivatives (Bowman and Hemsworth, 1965b). A recent addition to the list is the naphthylvinylpyridinium group, whose members, in addition to inhibiting ChAc by direct action, have been shown to suppress choline uptake into isolated synaptosomes (Barker and Mittag, 1973).

All of the compounds mentioned above, including HC-3, have side-effects that are unrelated to their action on choline transport. Thus HC-3 can produce an immediate neuromuscular block of the tubocurarine type (i.e. postsynaptic and competitive) when given in high doses (Martin and Orkand, 1961; Thies and Brooks, 1961); this effect is easily distinguished from the gradual block of presynaptic origin that occurs during repetitive excitation and is the drug's most characteristic effect (Reitzel and Long, 1959). Most of its other side-effects are insignificant. It has been reported to interfere with peripheral adrenergic transmission in some cases but not in others (for references see Bowman and Marshall, 1972); but in ordinary dosage it has little if any action on ganglion cells (Birks and MacIntosh, 1961), on muscarinic receptors (Wilson and Long, 1959; Carlyle, 1963; Harry, 1963; Lewartowski and Bielecki, 1963; Vincenzi and West, 1965), on cholinesterase (Schueler, 1955; Domino et al., 1968) or on axonal conduction when applied externally (Frazier et al., 1969; Dunant, 1972). A finding whose significance is not yet clear is that HC-3 inhibits choline kinase (Ansell and Spanner, 1974), the enzyme which catalyses the first step in the incorporation of choline into phospholipid. Triethylcholine, unlike HC-3, has little tubocurarine-like activity (Bowman and Rand, 1961), but like its parent base tetraethylammonium (Koketsu, 1958; Collier and Exley, 1963) it increases ACh release from motor nerve terminals (Bowman and Hemsworth, 1965a), and thus can antagonize neuromuscular block caused by tubocurarine (Bowman and Rand, 1961; Roberts, 1962). Triethylcholine also has postsynaptic ganglion-blocking activity, as does troxonium (Bowman and Rand, 1961; Bhatnagar et al., 1965). Further references to the best-documented effects and side-effects of the more potent blockers of choline transport may be found in the reviews by Schueler (1960) and Bowman and Marshall (1972).

It has generally been assumed that the presynaptic action of HC-3 is at the level of the plasma membrane, and that it thus reduces the rate at which choline is supplied to ChAc. This assumption may be an over-simplification. The effects of HC-3 on ACh turnover in muscles and ganglia are only slowly reversed by removing the drug from the medium (cf. Cheymol et al., 1962; Matthews, 1966), in contrast to the effects of sodium deprivation (Quastel, 1962; Birks, 1963) or postsynaptic blockers, which quickly disappear when the medium is made drug-free. For this and other reasons it has been tempting to suppose that HC-3 and its congeners might have a second action on ACh metabolism, this time at the intracellular level: for example it might be stored and released as a false transmitter, either as the free base (MacIntosh, 1961) or as its acetyl ester (Rodriguez de Lores Arnaiz et al., 1970); Bow-

MAN and RAND (1961) have in fact made a similar suggestion for acetyltriethylcholine. However, although HC-3 is taken up by nervous tissue (SELLINGER et al., 1969; CSILLIK et al., 1970; KNYIHÁR and CSILLIK, 1970; RODRIGUEZ DE LORES ARNAIZ et al., 1970), this is not by the mechanism that transports choline, nor does HC-3 replace ACh stoichiometrically (COLLIER, 1973; SLATER and STONIER, 1973a, b). Moreover captured HC-3 cannot be released by nerve stimulation (COLLIER, 1973). Triethylcholine can be taken up and acetylated by isolated synaptosomes (POTTER, 1968; HEMSWORTH and SMITH, 1970a); the acetyl ester is pharmacologically rather inert (BOWMAN et al., 1962), but it has not yet been shown to be released by nerve impulses. Exclusion of the false-transmitter hypothesis still leaves open the possibility that HC-3 and/or triethylcholine can inhibit the transfer of ACh from the cytosol to the synaptic vesicles, a process about which almost nothing is known. Unfortunately this is not easy to test, because the process has not been demonstrated *in vitro* (scc pp. 169—170).

8. ACh Uptake

In the presence of certain anticholinesterase agents, brain slices and other isolated tissue can take up ACh added to the medium in which they are suspended (cf. POLAK and MEEUWS, 1966; SCHUBERTH and SUNDWALL, 1967; LIANG and QUASTEL, 1969a, b; POLAK, 1969). This uptake occurs against a concentration gradient, and appears to involve a low affinity transport system (apparent K_m about 100 µmol/l). ACh uptake, like choline uptake, can be inhibited by HC-3, but the two transport mechanisms are readily distinguishable pharmacologically; ACh uptake is inhibited by drugs such as eserine, atropine, tubocurarine and hexamethonium in concentrations that do not affect choline transport. The uptake of ACh is not specifically associated with cholinergic nerves (KATZ et al., 1973; KUHAR and SIMON, 1974) and, as will be discussed later (pp. 172—173), the phenomenon appears to have no physiological significance.

9. Control of ACh Synthesis

At least in mammalian cholinergic synapses, the synthesis and the release of ACh are closely linked. During rest, ACh synthesis is slow, and it is increased during activity, so that tissue levels of ACh are maintained fairly constant (e.g., MANN et al., 1938; BIRKS and MACINTOSH, 1961; BROWNING and SCHULMAN, 1968; COLLIER and MACINTOSH, 1969; POTTER, 1970a; GREWAAL and QUASTEL, 1973). The mechanism by which ACh synthesis is regulated is not yet known with any ccrtainty; several hypotheses have been proposed.

a) Product Inhibition

It has been suggested (KAITA and GOLDBERG, 1969; SHARKAWI and SCHULMAN, 1969; SHARKAWI, 1972) that ACh regulates its own synthesis by feed-back inhibition upon choline acetyltransferase. However, ACh inhibits choline acetyltransferase by less than 50% even when present in a concentration greater than 100 mmol/l (POTTER et al., 1968; KAITA and GOLDBERG, 1969; GLOVER and POTTER, 1971). High concentrations of ACh probably occur in synaptic vesicles, but, as discussed above, these are not the site of ACh synthesis, for choline acetyltransferase appears to be outside synaptic vesicles. Concentrations of ACh that would be capable of inhibiting choline acetyltransferase are not likely to be achieved in the nerve terminal cytoplasm, and, therefore, regulation of ACh synthesis by feed-back inhibition of the transmitter itself is not likely. The second product of the choline acetyltransferase reaction, CoA, is a more effective inhibitor of ACh synthesis than is ACh (White and Cavallito, 1970b; Glover and Potter, 1971; White and Wu, 1973a). However, for CoA to regulate ACh synthesis, the ratio of CoA to acetyl-CoA would have to decrease when ACh release occurs, which would not be expected.

b) Availability of Substrates

As discussed earlier, our knowledge about the availability of acetyl-CoA at the site of ACh synthesis is incomplete. However, it is not likely that the supply of cytoplasmic acetyl-CoA limits the activity of choline acetyltransferase: for in the first place, acetyl-CoA is required for metabolic reactions other than ACh synthesis; and secondly, the availability of acetyl-CoA to choline acetyltransferase would have to be increased by synaptic activity, and it is not clear how this could occur. The demonstration of a high-affinity uptake mechanism for choline in cholinergic nerve endings has led to the suggestion that the availability of choline inside the nerve terminal might regulate ACh synthesis. Most of the choline transported into isolated synaptosomes by this high-affinity mechanism is metabolized to ACh (Yamamura and Snyder, 1973), and the amount of choline transported is linearly related to the amount of ACh synthetized (Guyenet et al., 1973). If choline transport does limit ACh synthesis, the mechanism must be accelerated either by the arrival of nerve impulses in the nerve terminal or by the release of ACh. In sympathetic ganglia at least, choline uptake occuring selectively in cholinergic nerve terminals appears to be increased as the result of synaptic activity (Collier and Katz, 1974). Thus, choline availability provides a possible mechanism whereby ACh synthesis might be regulated, but much more information will be required before this can be accepted as the physiological control mechanism.

c) Mass Action

Potter and his colleagues (Potter et al., 1968; Glover and Potter, 1971) have suggested that the rate of ACh synthesis depends upon the relative concentration of both substrates, choline and acetyl-CoA, and both products, ACh and CoA. From the equilibrium constant for choline acetyltransferase measured in vitro, from estimates of the ratio of acetyl-CoA:CoA based upon reported values in extracts of whole tissue, and by assuming the intracellular concentration of choline to be equal to the extracellular concentration, the limiting ACh concentration was calculated to be around 1 mmol/l. It is possible that the ACh concentration in the cytoplasm could reach this value, in which case ACh synthesis would be increased by any process that mobilized ACh from the cytoplasm; physiologically this stimulus is presumed to be the uptake of ACh from the nerve-terminal cytoplasm into synaptic vesicles to replace released transmitter. Potter's hypothesis is attractive, but remains to be tested.

D. Acetylcholine Storage

With a few exceptions (e.g. human placenta, ungulate spleen, corneal epithelium) most of the ACh in vertebrate tissue is located in cholinergic neurones, where it is found throughout their length. From early measurements of ACh in nerve trunks and tissues (e.g. BARSOUM, 1935; LOEWI and HELLAUER, 1939; MacINTOSH, 1941) it was apparent that ACh concentrations might reach 0.1 mmol/l or more in the interior of cholinergic axons and be much higher than that in cholinergic terminals (BROWN and FELDBERG, 1936a). As yet there are no estimates for ACh in the perikarya of mammalian neurones, but measurements of the concentration of perikaryal ACh in identified cholinergic neurones of the mollusc *Aplasia* (0.35 mmol/l, McCAMAN et al., 1973) are similar to the concentrations calculated for ACh in the axoplasm of mammalian cholinergic axons (0.3 mmol/l, EVANS and SAUNDERS, 1967). As discussed later in this section, ACh is present in still higher concentration in cholinergic nerve terminals.

Besides these differences in the anatomical location of stored ACh, there is also evidence that tissue ACh is held in several "pools". This evidence has been obtained in two ways. First, biochemical cell-fractionation techniques applied to tissue homogenates allow at least three ACh-containing subcellular fractions to be prepared: two from inside nerve endings and one from outside. Second, studies of ACh content and ACh release made on intact tissues during neuronal activity or at rest suggest the existence of distinct ACh pools differing in their availability for release: two or three of which are located inside nerve endings and one outside. Unfortunately, it is not always clear whether the ACh pools defined by a particular set of criteria applied to one tissue correspond to the ACh pools defined by different criteria applied to another tissue. In this section an attempt is made to summarize, and so far as possible to correlate, the results obtained on different tissues and with different techniques. The tissues that have been most extensively studied are mammalian brain, autonomic ganglia and skeletal muscles, and electroplaques from the fish *Torpedo*.

1. Brain

ACh is found in both grey and white matter (MacINTOSH, 1941). Evidence that the ACh of brain is compartmentalized comes from observations made over many years on the distribution of ACh in homogenates of brain in isotonic salt solution (CORTEGGIANI et al., 1936; TRETHEWIE, 1938; TOBIAS et al., 1946; ELLIOTT and HENDERSON, 1951; STONE, 1955; CROSSLAND and SLATER, 1968; RICHTER and GOLDSTEIN, 1970; HRDINA and MANECKJEE, 1971; SLATER, 1971). In these experiments brain ACh was separated into two fractions. "Free" ACh, which accounted for 13—30% of the total, was released into the homogenizing medium and could be measured only if the medium contained an anticholinesterase agent, while "bound" ACh, which was retained in the homogenized tissue, was protected from cholinesterase, but could be extracted by acid or heat. "Free" ACh must in part arise from leakage of "bound" ACh during homogenization (TRETHEWIE, 1938; ELLIOTT and HENDERSON, 1951; STONE, 1955), but the two pools are not entirely artefacts of that procedure, because treatment of animals with certain drugs affects "free" and "bound" ACh differently (CROSSLAND and SLATER, 1968; RICHTER and GOLDSTEIN, 1970; SLATER, 1971).

A similar partitioning of brain ACh was found when the tissue was homogenized in isotonic sucrose containing eserine (Hebb and Whittaker, 1958); 20 to 25% of the ACh could be recovered in a high-speed supernatant while 75 to 80% remained particle-bound. On differential centrifugation, the bound ACh sedimented with the "mitochondrial" fraction (Hebb and Whittaker, 1958; Bellamy, 1959), and when this was further fractionated by centrifuging it into a discontinuous sucrose gradient (Whittaker, 1959) most of the ACh was recovered in a particulate fraction that was lighter than mitochondria but heavier than myelin. Electronmicroscopic observation of this fraction showed it to be rich in pinched-off nerve endings, called "synaptosomes" (Gray and Whittaker, 1962). De Robertis and his colleagues (1961) independently demonstrated the presence of pinched-off nerve endings in the mitochondrial fraction prepared from sucrose homogenates of cerebral cortex.

The synaptosomal fraction prepared from brain is also rich in putative neurotransmitters other than ACh (De Robertis et al., 1962; Michaelson and Whittaker, 1963; Magnan and Whittaker, 1966; Fuxe et al., 1067; Fonnum, 1968b; Masuoka, 1968; Bradford, 1970; Gfeller et al., 1971; Rassin, 1972). The heterogeneity of brain synaptosomal preparations rather limits their usefulness for studies of cholinergic mechanisms. Several of the authors cited have achieved partial separation of the synaptosomes that contain different neurotransmitters, and the complete separation of cholinergic and noradrenergic synaptosomes from immature rat brain has recently been described (McGovern et al., 1973).

Synaptosomes can be lysed osmotically (De Robertis et al., 1963; Whittaker et al., 1964) or mechanically (Takeno et al., 1969). Lysis releases the cytoplasmic constituents, together with about half of the synaptosomal ACh, which can then only be preserved if the medium contains an anticholinesterase agent. In contrast to this "labile-bound", and presumably cytoplasmic, ACh, the rest of the ACh is "stable-bound", remaining attached to particles and protected from cholinesterase. In the experiments of Whittaker et al. (1964) the stable-bound ACh became bimodally distributed on a sucrose density gradient: about 40% was recovered in a fraction composed mainly of monodispersed synaptic vesicles, while the rest appeared to be associated with incompletely disrupted synaptosomes. Whittaker and his colleagues suggested that the ACh of the second fraction might be in vesicles that had not been released during lysis, but this may be an oversimplification, for Barker et al. (1972) have reported that the ACh of this fraction turns over more rapidly than does the ACh of the monodispersed synaptic vesicles. Figure 3 illustrates the approximate distribution of ACh in fractions of brain.

Presumably the ACh that can be harvested with the synaptic vesicle fraction must have been located in the vesicles *in situ*. It is very probable that some of the ACh changes its distribution during the preparation and fractionation of the tissue homogenates, particularly through leakage from the stable-bound (mainly vesicular) into the labile-bound and free pools; vesicular ACh could thus be seriously underestimated. Nevertheless, there is now convincing evidence that the three pools do exist *in vivo*, and that they are not artefacts of homogenization.

(a) When brain slices are incubated in the presence of an anticholinesterase, the three pools are affected differently. In the experiments of Collier et al. (1972), free ACh showed a four-fold increase, ACh in the nerve-ending cytosol fraction doubled, but the ACh content of the purified vesicular fraction remained unchanged.

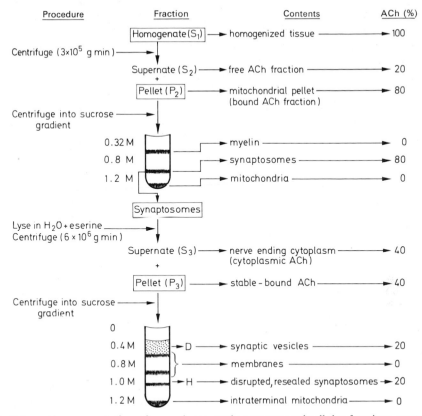

Fig. 3. Schematic representation of procedures used to prepare subcellular fractions containing ACh from a brain homogenate (prepared in the presence of eserine). The distribution of ACh is approximate, and for the purpose of simplicity, recoveries are assumed to be 100% and contamination of one fraction by material from another is assumed to be zero. The ACh content of a fraction is expressed as a percentage of that contained in the S_1 fraction, which would be the supernatant obtained by centrifuging the original homogenate at low speed (10^4 gmin) to remove undisrupted tissue

(b) When brain slices are incubated with radioactive choline in a medium containing a high concentration of potassium, ACh becomes labelled to a higher specific activity in the cytoplasm than in the vesicles (RICHTER and MARCHBANKS, 1971 b).

(c) When radioactive choline is injected into the brain (CHAKRIN and WHITTAKER, 1969) or reaches the brain from the circulation (AQUILONIUS et al., 1973), the free, cytoplasmic and vesicular ACh pools become labelled to different specific activities, free ACh being labelled to the lowest specific activity when the period of exposure is short.

(d) Treatment in vivo with certain drugs affects the level of ACh in the three pools differently (BEANI et al., 1969), and may also alter the relative rate of incorporation of labelled choline into each ACh pool (AQUILONIUS et al., 1973).

These experiments prove that there is more than one ACh pool in vivo, but they give no precise information about the location or functional significance of the pools.

"Free ACh" is generally believed (cf. Whittaker, 1969) to come mainly from disrupted nerve cell bodies and axons. This seems plausible, because there is evidence (Carlini and Green, 1963; Hebb, 1963; Evans and Saunders, 1974) that most of the axonal ACh is freely diffusible *in vivo*, though a little is probably particle-bound (Häggendal et al., 1973). Thus most axonal ACh would be expected to appear in the supernatant after centrifugation of a brain homogenate. Most of the limited information available indicates that axonal ACh *in vivo* turns over much more slowly than synaptic ACh, and the slow incorporation of choline into "free ACh" as determined by the sucrose-homogenate technique (Chakrin and Whittaker, 1969; Aquilonius et al., 1973) supports that conclusion. On the other hand Slater (1968) has reported that "free ACh" as separated by the saline-homogenate technique of Crossland and Slater is more readily depleted than "bound ACh" when triethylcholine is given intraventricularly to conscious rats. This suggests that the "free" ACh isolated by this technique is not the same as axonal ACh; its morphological compartment can not be identified on the basis of available evidence. At present there is no method of estimating axonal ACh in brain grey matter. Indeed its concentration may not be the same in all regions of a given axon, for there is a proximodistal gradient of ACh in peripheral cholinergic axons (Evans and Saunders, 1967).

The *"labile-bound"* fraction of synaptosomal ACh is not easily equated with a single morphologically identifiable compartment. It presumably contains the ACh originally present in the nerve-ending cytoplasm (including some ACh recently synthesized by the ChAc located there), but it must also contain ACh that has been released into the cytosol from vesicles or other structures as a result of preparative techniques. This artefactual release is a real hazard: for brain and other tissues there is evidence that a part of vesicular ACh is relatively loosely bound and can transfer during fractionation from the stable-bound into the labile-bound fraction (cf. Barker et al., 1970; Richter and Marchbanks, 1971b; Marchbanks and Israël, 1972). If this is so the former fraction would be underestimated and the latter overestimated. This loss could indicate the presence of a population of particularly fragile vesicles, or it could indicate that ACh within a single vesicle is heterogeneous. Of these two possibilities Marchbanks and Israël (1972) prefer the second (see also Marchbanks, 1973).

It is widely agreed that the *"stable-bound"* ACh obtained from synaptosomes is held within synaptic vesicles, and was therein *in situ*; though there is little evidence that this fraction contains the ACh that is most readily released during synaptic activity. Whittaker (1965) and Whittaker and Sheridan (1965) made estimates of vesicle numbers in this fraction, and on the assumption that 10 to 15% of the synaptosomes in a brain homogenate might be cholinergic, they calculated that the number of ACh molecules per *cholinergic vesicle* might be 1650 to 2500. If ACh were the principal cation and accounted for half or more of the osmolarity, the interior of the vesicle would be approximately isotonic with the nerve-ending cytosol. The roughness of the calculation was admitted and should be stressed, especially because the proportion of cholinergic synaptosomes in a fraction prepared from the brain can only be guessed. Nevertheless, the estimated values agree well with estimates based on preparations in which most of the synaptosomes were probably cholinergic (Wilson et al., 1973).

To estimate the *number of ACh molecules in a released quantum* one must have estimates of both the quantity of ACh and the number of quanta released per junction and per impulse, and these values are not available for ACh release in brain.

When sliced or minced brain is incubated in a balanced salt solution, tissue ACh gradually increases to several times the highest level found *in vivo* (McLennan and Elliott, 1950; Elliott and Henderson, 1951; Bhatnagar and MacIntosh, 1967). Nothing is known about the location of the additional ACh, except that it is not in the vesicular (stable-bound) fraction (Collier et al., 1972). The presence of an anticholinesterase agent, which enables peripheral cholinergic nerve endings (Birks and MacIntosh, 1961; Potter, 1970a; Collier and Katz, 1971) and peripheral nerve trunks (Evans and Saunders, 1974) to double their resting ACh content by accumulating "surplus ACh" (pp. 124, 127), has little or no effect on the accumulation of ACh by incubated brain (Bhatnagar and MacIntosh, 1967; Bourdois and Szerb, 1972). Apparently the elimination of intracellular AChE creates additional ACh storage capacity in peripheral tissue but not in brain, whereas some abnormality under *in vitro* conditions creates additional ACh storage capacity in brain, though not in excised nerves (Evans and Saunders, 1974), muscles (Potter, 1970a) or ganglia (Sacchi and Perri, 1973).

2. Ganglion

A superior cervical ganglion contains about 1500 pmol of ACh in the cat (Birks and MacIntosh, 1961) and about 150 pmol in the rat (Sacchi and Perri, 1973), the overall concentration of ACh in these ganglia being about 0.1 mmol/l, roughly the same as in the preganglionic trunk. The presynaptic elements account for most of a ganglion's ACh but no more than 1% (0.1 to 0.2% in varicosities alone: Birks, 1974) of its mass, and thus the mean ACh concentration in nerve terminals must be at least 10 mmol/l; presumably the concentration of ACh is higher than that in the vesicles, and lower in the cytoplasm. It is harder to isolate synaptosomes from ganglia than from brain, but Wilson et al. (1973), who prepared a relatively pure fraction of vesicles from bovine ganglia, made corrections for contamination and losses, and calculated the ACh content to be 1630 molecules per vesicle; this is close to Whittaker's estimate for cholinergic vesicles from the cortex of the brain. Assuming all the ACh of a vesicle to be free in the internal compartment, with a diameter of 30 nm, the concentration there would be about 190 mmol/l.

In the presence of HC-3, prolonged preganglionic stimulation will reduce the stored ACh of a cat's or a rat's superior cervical ganglion to about 15% of the initial level but no farther (Birks and MacIntosh, 1961; Sacchi and Perri, 1973). The residual 15% has been called "*stationary ACh*", in contrast to the "*depot ACh*" which constitutes most of the store and can be released by nerve impulses. In the cat's superior cervical ganglion, it is also found that 15% of the ACh remains after perfusion with a sodium-free medium (Quastel, 1962; Birks, 1963) and 15% of the ACh resists labelling from radioactive choline (Collier and MacIntosh, 1969). Birks and MacIntosh (1961) suggested that most of the stationary ACh might be axonal, and that some is also contained in the small number of perikarya and outgoing axons that are cholinergic. Thus stationary ACh in ganglia is probably equivalent to part of the "free" ACh measured in sucrose-homogenates of brain.

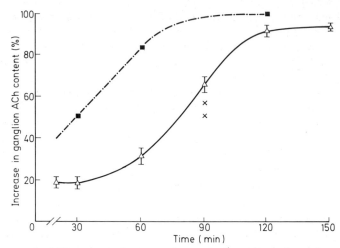

Fig. 4. The increase in ACh content of cat superior cervical ganglia perfused for varying periods of time with choline-Locke solution containing one of the following anticholinesterase drugs: ■, eserine sulphate (each point represents the result of a single experiment); △, neostigmine bromide (each point represents the mean ±s.e. of at least three experiments), or ×, ambenonium chloride (each point represents the result of a single experiment). (From Collier and Katz, 1971)

Depot ACh appears not to be a single compartment. The time course of its release during prolonged synaptic activity suggested that it might be distributed between two rather distinct pools, the smaller of which can be more readily released than the larger. Birks and MacIntosh considered that the smaller pool might be refilled from the larger one. This undoubtedly happens to some extent; but more recent studies, in which part of the ganglionic ACh was labelled with radioactive choline, shows that much of the ACh that enters the readily-releasable pool is newly synthesized rather than derived from a reserve pool (Collier and MacIntosh, 1969; Collier, 1969). There are now some electrophysiological data that provide information about ACh synthesis and storage in the superior cervical ganglion. Most of these data refer to the declining responses of the ganglion cells during repetitive preganglionic excitation in the presence of HC-3: McCandless et al. (1971) recorded postsynaptic spikes in situ in cats and Bennett and McLachlan (1972a, b) and Sacchi and Perri (1973) recorded excitatory postsynaptic potentials in isolated ganglia from the guinea-pig and rat respectively. The results of these studies were in general agreement with those from the more direct measurements, except that there was no evidence to suggest more than one pool of releasable ACh. Some sort of dual- or multiple-pool scheme for the depot must, however, be postulated to account for the behaviour of labelled choline and ACh in turnover studies (Collier and MacIntosh, 1969; Collier, 1969), even though the earlier models are incorrect in detail (cf. also Birks and Fitch, 1974).

A further pool of ACh appears in a ganglion exposed to a lipid-soluble cholinesterase inhibitor such as eserine or tetraethylpyrophosphate: this has been named "*surplus ACh*" (Birks and MacIntosh, 1961). Surplus ACh accumulates slowly, and can double tissue ACh levels, but its presence does not increase the amount of ACh released by a nerve impulse. Surplus ACh formation occurs, but is delayed (Fig. 4), when a lipid-insoluble cholinesterase inhibitor such as neostigmine or ambenonium is used (COLLIER and KATZ, 1971). This and other evidence indicates that surplus ACh is located in an intracellular compartment where its accumulation is normally prevented by AChE. The compartment appears to be a presynaptic one, for chronically decentralized ganglia have little ability to accumulate surplus ACh or to take up ACh from an exogenous source (COLLIER and KATZ, 1971; KATZ et al., 1973). At present there is no evidence to suggest that any of the major cellular elements in such ganglia (e.g. adrenergic neurones or glial cells) are deprived of ChAc or of ACh-binding sites when they have lost their preganglionic input.

If surplus ACh is free in the presynaptic cytosol, where most of the ganglion's regular ACh is presumably synthesized, this suggests the existence of presynaptic AChE which faces inwards or is attached to intracellular structures. There is some evidence that this is so, but it comes from tissues other than ganglia and is inconclusive. In particular: (a) LEWIS and SHUTE (1966) found some nerve-terminal AChE associated with reticulum, though none with vesicles; (b) ROBINSON and BELL (1967), using KARNOVSKY'S stain which may be less specific for this purpose, showed some AChE apparently within autonomic axons in bladder, though most of the axonal enzyme was shown to be outward-facing; (c) MORRIS (1973) found that a small part of the AChE in electroplaque homogenates was soluble and may originally have been intracellular; (d) the ACh content of cholinergic nerve trunks, whose AChE has been inhibited, gradually increases until it is twice its initial concentration, much as is seen with ganglia (EVANS and SAUNDERS, 1974); and (e) preganglionic AChE is presumably made in the region of the cell body and is transported distally to reach the synapse; it is not easy to see how this could be accomplished while maintaining complete spatial separation of the enzyme from the axoplasm. However it must be stressed again that the ability to form surplus ACh may not be characteristic of all cholinergic terminals. In fact the evidence that this is so in the brain is at best tenuous (COLLIER et al., 1972) or negative (BOURDOIS and SZERB, 1972; MARCHBANKS, 1973). The availability of ganglionic synaptosomes (WILSON and COOPER, 1972) may help to determine the location of surplus ACh at peripheral junctions, where evidence in favour of the presynaptic cytosol is already strong. It is still possible that the inward-facing AChE may be in the non-synaptic parts of the axon rather than in the boutons or varicosities.

Two further facts must be mentioned in relation to ACh storage in ganglia, though their significance is not clear at present. (a) SACCHI and PERRI (1973) have shown that preganglionic terminals depleted of ACh by stimulation in the presence of HC-3, or in the absence of thiamine, release ACh in the form of quanta that are of normal size but are greatly diminished in number; this is exactly the opposite of what appears to occur in muscle (ELMQVIST and QUASTEL, 1965a: see p. 171 for further discussion). (b) The report by ROSENBLUETH et al. (1939) that prolonged high-frequency excitation increases the ACh stores in ganglia has been confirmed by more recent studies (FRIESEN and KHATTER, 1971a; BIRKS and FITCH, 1974; BOURDOIS et al., 1975). The extra store is presynaptic and releasable, but its precise location is a matter for speculation (BOURDOIS et al., 1975; see pp. 188—189).

For *parasympathetic ganglia* the only data available are those of PILAR et al. (1970, 1973), who found a high concentration of ACh, approaching 1 mmol/l, in pigeon ciliary ganglia; the ACh levels in the postganglionic nerves were similar to those in other cholinergic nerve trunks. An unexpected finding was that preganglionic denervation caused the disappearance of ACh within a few days from both the ganglion and the preganglionic branches, as if the ability of the postsynaptic elements to store ACh was somehow dependent on the presence of the presynaptic elements. There seems to be no such dependence in the case of other parasympathetic neurones: thus decentralized salivary glands retain much of their ACh and ChAc, and these are almost certainly contained in postganglionic axons and their endings (Chang and Gaddum, 1933; Nordenfelt, 1963; Ekström and Holmberg, 1972). The role of presynaptic elements in the maintenance of postsynaptic ACh may be peculiar to avian ciliary ganglia, which are unlike most parasympathetic ganglia in other important respects (Martin and Pilar, 1963a).

The upper limit for the size of an ACh quantum released onto a parasympathetic ganglion cell in the frog's interatrial septum has been given by Dennis et al. (1971); it was found that a miniature excitatory postsynaptic potential can be matched by the electrophoretic application of about 6×10^5 molecules of ACh. It is of interest that Nishi et al. (1967) obtained the same value for the release of ACh onto a sympathetic ganglion cell in the frog, but in the latter case more than a single quantum would usually be released.

3. Skeletal Muscle

Most skeletal muscles in mammals have a low ACh content on a weight basis, about 0.3 to 2.0 pmol/g (for references see Hebb et al., 1964). The concentration is much higher in diffusely innervated muscles such as the tongue and external eye muscles (Bhatnagar and MacIntosh, unpublished). In rat diaphragm, the only muscle that has been closely examined, almost all of the ACh is in the end-plate region of the muscle (Hebb et al., 1964; Potter, 1970a), but a significant fraction of this, about 25% (Hebb et al., 1964) may be in intramuscular nerve trunks rather than the axonal terminations. Six weeks after motor denervation of the diaphragm or a leg muscle only a few percent of the total store remains; some of this may be in the Schwann cells (Miledi and Slater, 1968).

Most of the ACh in a normal diaphragm can be replaced with radioactive ACh when the diaphragm is placed in a medium containing [^{14}C]choline (Potter, 1970d). Replacement is much more rapid when the phrenic nerve is stimulated (Fig. 5), but some 20% of the ACh is more slowly labelled. A similar percentage of the ACh remains in the muscle during prolonged stimulation in the presence of HC-3 (Potter, 1970a); this is analogous to "stationary" ACh in ganglia. The 80% of muscle ACh that is releasable is presumably "depot" ACh in the motor terminals, and Potter (1970a) showed that the newly synthesized transmitter is preferentially released, as in ganglia.

Except for Potter's (1970a) experiments, neurochemical experiments have not provided much information about pools of depot ACh with differing rates of release from motor nerve terminals. Neurophysiological observations, on the other hand, do generally support a two-pool system, for they show that the fractional release rate during repetitive stimulation falls from a high initial value to a lower steady value, (see for example Thies, 1965; Elmqvist and Quastel, 1965b; Martin, 1966; Čapek et al., 1971; Ginsborg and Jenkinson, this volume). This suggests that in motor

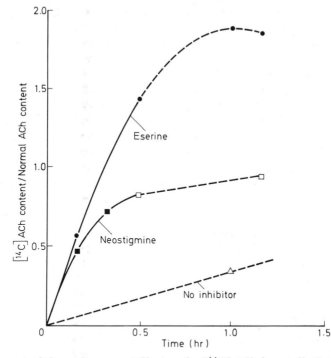

Fig. 5. Replacement of the endogenous ACh store by $[^{14}C]$ ACh in rat diaphragm incubated with $[^{14}C]$ choline. Continuous lines represent nerve stimulation at 20/sec for the first 9 min of each 10 min period; dashed lines represent unstimulated muscles. Open symbols: esterase inhibitor absent or removed at preceding point. Each point represents the mean result of assays of the end-plate regions of six or more muscle segments. Standard errors were less than $\pm 15\%$ of the mean values for muscles not in eserine, and less that $\pm 20\%$ for those in eserine $[^{14}C]$ choline and the esterase inhibitors were introduced 5 min befor zero time. (From POTTER, 1970a)

nerve terminals, as in preganglionic nerve endings, a reserve fraction of the depot is being mobilized to replenish a more readily releasable fraction. In these experiments, however, the readily available fraction was so small (about 10^3 quanta per junction, and less than 1% of the total depot) that it would not be detected by the usual neurochemical measurements. Thus the replenishment mechanism, whatever its nature, may well be different in motor nerve terminals from the one deduced from data on ganglia. A single report, by CECCARELLI et al. (1973), gives ACh output plots from frog muscle that resemble those obtained from ganglia (e.g. their Fig. 4), but ACh turnover in their experiments might have been influenced by choline deficiency. Surplus ACh accumulates in the junctional region of a diaphragm whose acetylcholinesterase has been inactivated (POTTER, 1970a). As in ganglia (BIRKS and MACINTOSH, 1961; COLLIER and KATZ, 1971), the accumulation takes about an hour when eserine is used and can about double total ACh content; surplus ACh disappears when eserine is removed and is not formed if neostigmine is applied to the muscle instead (Fig. 5), and its presence does not add to the amount of ACh released by nerve stimulation. POTTER (1970a) reported that when the stimulation is prolonged surplus ACh can contribute to release. Surplus ACh in muscle seems even more unlikely than surplus ACh in ganglia to have a postsynaptic location, for (a) ChAc is a predominantly neural enzyme in muscle (Hebb et al., 1964; Potter, 1970a) and (b) surplus ACh accumulates equally well in resting muscles and in muscles that are actively releasing ACh (Potter, 1970a).

Muscle is not an easy tissue to homogenize in a way that might preserve nerve endings, and it is not surprising that muscle homogenates have yielded no synapto- somes or other particles that retained sedimentable ChAc (Potter, 1970a). Potter found however that the microsomal fraction of a homogenate from eserine-treated muscle contained about 20% of the ACh originally present; this might have been associated with vesicles. It is significant that Potter recovered about as much ACh in this microsomal fraction from muscles incubated with neostigmine as with eser- ine: since only the eserine-treated muscles would have formed surplus ACh, this is further evidence that surplus ACh is not found in vesicles. Potter's vesicular frac- tions were not pure enough to allow estimates of ACh per vesicle, and no estimates based on muscle fractionation tests are available. The literature however offers sev- eral estimates of the amount of ACh per quantum of transmitter, based on experi- ments in which quanta were counted and other experiments in which ACh release was measured. The earliest calculation, by Birks (cited by MacIntosh, 1959), gave 900 molecules per quantum, but all subsequent estimates have been much higher (see Table 3, p. 135). Elmquist and Quastel (1965a) using two different methods of calculation obtained values of 57000 and 62000, close to the maximum number of ACh molecules that could be packed into a vesicle (Canepa, 1964: for further infor- mation and discussion see Ginsborg, 1970). We consider later the possibility that a quantum is released from an extravesicular pool of ACh, or from a vesicular cluster. It is also conceivable that many quanta are released from non-synaptic regions of the nerve terminal and cannot be recorded, or that quantal and non-quantal release go on together. Our present estimates of the number of ACh molecules per vesicle or per quantum are not of much help in enabling us to prefer one or another scheme for ACh storage, release and turnover.

4. Electric Organ

This structure, in species of *Torpedo* and a number of other fish, can be regarded as a voltaic pile made up of modified motor end-plates stacked in series. Feldberg and Fessard (1942) showed that the electric organ of Torpedo is innervated by cholin- ergic nerves, and that the tissue is extremely rich in ACh, with an overall concentra- tion of about 0.5 mmol/l. More recently, beginning with the studies of Sheridan et al. (1966), ACh storage in the electric organ has been studied with the techniques of subcellular fractionation. There are two important points of difference between hom- ogenates of electroplaques and homogenates of brain: the Torpedo material yields few if any synaptosomes, and so much AChE is present that any ACh that is not bound is destroyed, even if an anticholinesterase drug has been added. About half of the tissue ACh, in fact, survives homogenization, and some 85% of this can be recovered in a purified synaptic-vesicle fraction obtained by density-gradient centri- fugation (Israël et al., 1970). No "free" (cytoplasmic) ACh is recovered, but its level is given by the difference between total tissue ACh and particle-bound ACh. As in experiments on brain, the free ACh behaves differently from the bound ACh, being preferentially labelled when radioactive choline is supplied to the tissue and preferentially released when the tissue is stimulated (DUNANT et al., 1971, 1972). The vesicular ACh itself appears not to be homogeneous, since any recently-synthesized ACh that is present tends to be removed when the fraction is subjected to isotonic gel filtration (MARCHBANKS and ISRAËL, 1972). Further purification of the vesicular fraction was achieved by WHITTAKER and his colleagues (WHITTAKER, 1971; WHITTAKER et al., 1972a, 1974; DOWDALL et al., 1974). The vesicles are large but not very uniform in size, with a mean diameter of 84 nm and a membrane thickness of 8 nm. They are estimated to contain 6.6×10^4 molecules of ACh on the average, with a calculated ACh concentration of 650 mmol/l, which if the ACh were free and accounted for half the osmolarity would be isotonic with sea-water. Synaptic vesicles from the electroplaques do not contain AChE (MORRIS, 1973), but they are rich in ATP (WHITTAKER et al., 1972b; BOHAN et al., 1973; DOWDALL et al., 1974), and contain a low-molecular weight (about 10^4 daltons) acidic protein, called "vesiculin" (WHITTAKER, 1971; WHITTAKER et al., 1974). The molar ratio of ACh to vesiculin is about 12, and of ACh to ATP about 11. There is no evidence so far that either vesiculin or a vesiculin-ATP complex can bind ACh, but vesiculin and ATP can bind to each other, and vesiculin may for that reason be present *in vivo* as a dimer (WHITTAKER et al., 1974). At least four other proteins were found in purified Torpedo vesicle fractions (ULMAR and WHITTAKER, 1974; WHITTAKER et al., 1974), but their function is unknown: they may of course be concerned with ACh transport or vesicle-vesicle or vesicle-membrane interactions. The most recent experiments (ZIMMERMANN and WHITTAKER, 1974a, b) showed that ACh, ATP and vesiculin contents do not change in parallel when the tissue is activated *in vivo*: ACh is depleted earlier than the others, and recovers more quickly during a period of rest.

5. Other Tissues

Interesting preliminary studies on the myenteric-plexus-longitudinal-muscle preparation of the guinea-pig ileum (PATON et al., 1971; GILBERT et al., 1973; SZERB and SOMOGYI, 1973), on salivary glands *in situ* (HANIN et al., 1972a, b) and on turtle photoreceptors (LAM, 1972), suggest that each of these preparations may provide useful data on ACh storage and release, but more information will be required before ACh turnover in these tissues can be compared with that in others.

E. Acetylcholine Release

ACh release can be studied in two ways: (a) directly, by collecting released ACh for measurement, and (b) indirectly, by recording postsynaptic events. In (a), the ACh is measured biologically or chemically, and radiometric measurements may be included if the ACh has been isotopically labelled. In such studies, an anticholinesterase agent must be present to preserve ACh after its release: these drugs may have unknown effects on the processes leading up to release. In (b), the recorded events are nearly always electrical transients, and in most cases the released ACh is measured as quanta. Its discharge can then be timed with millisecond precision, which is impossible when ACh release is measured directly. The use of an anticholinesterase drug can generally be avoided, but to facilitate the observations some other abnormality is frequently introduced, such as a change in the medium's calcium/magnesium ratio, to reduce ACh release, or the addition of an ACh antagonist, to reduce its action. Direct and indirect measurements of release made in parallel usually agree qualitatively, but may not give quantitatively equivalent results even if allowance is made for the disturbing factors just mentioned.

1. Correlation of Neurochemical and Electrophysiological Data

a) Skeletal Muscle

The ACh released by an isolated rat diaphragm at rest may be measured as picomoles, by assay of the bathing fluid if an anticholinesterase drug is present, or as quanta, by counting m.e.p.p.s at single end-plates and multiplying by the number of end-plates. Estimates of the ACh in a quantum obtained by comparing the two measurements appear to be too high, but such a comparison gives more plausible values when the output of transmitter is increased by exposure of the muscle to a medium containing raised potassium, or by nerve stimulation.

The reported values for spontaneous ACh release by hemidiaphragms in an eserine-containing medium are in fair agreement: values in pmol/min: 2.4 (STRAUGHAN, 1960); 2.7 (MITCHELL and SILVER, 1963); 2.3 (KRNJEVIĆ and STRAUGHAN, 1964) and 3.6 (POTTER, 1970a; output corrected for use of only 36% of the muscle.) The mean of these values is 2.7 pmol/min, which corresponds to about 2.7×10^{-16} mol/min per junction, because the hemidiaphragm contains about 10^4 end-plates. The mean frequency of m.e.p.p.s recorded from the diaphragm is usually about 60 to 150/min (LILEY, 1956a; HUBBARD et al., 1968). Thus, if the ACh that is released spontaneously is the ACh that generates m.e.p.p.s, each m.e.p.p. would result from the release of about 3×10^{-18} mol of ACh, or about 1.8×10^6 molecules. KRNJEVIĆ and MILEDI (1958) found that an e.p.p. could be matched fairly closely by applying ACh iontophoretically near the end-plate. About 10^5 molecules were required to produce depolarization similar to that of a m.e.p.p., and this must be considered the upper limit of the amount of ACh responsible for a m.e.p.p. since the nerve-ending must be in closer apposition to the ACh receptors than a pipette tip can be. The figures given above suggest that no more than 10% of the measured resting release of ACh can represent ACh that generates m.e.p.p.s. The remaining 90% or more could have come from structures other than the motor nerve endings, for chronically denervated muscles release 50 to 70% as much ACh as normal muscles do under similar experimental conditions (MITCHELL and SILVER, 1963; KRNJEVIĆ and STRAUGHAN, 1964; POTTER 1970a). Another possible source of non-quantal ACh is surplus ACh, since POTTER (1970a) found that resting ACh release from neostigmine-treated diaphragms (which do not accumulate surplus ACh) was 40% less than that measured from eserine-treated diaphragms (which do accumulate surplus ACh). ACh overflow from the extrajunctional portions of the phrenic nerve (cf. EVANS and SAUNDERS, 1974) may also contribute to measured ACh release.

When a diaphragm is exposed to 30 mmol/l potassium, ACh release increases by a factor of no more than 3, to about 5.5 pmol/min (MITCHELL and SILVER, 1963); however, m.e.p.p. frequency rises by a factor of several hundred, to about 700/sec (LILEY, 1956b). If m.e.p.p. frequency and size can be as well maintained in the presence of eserine as in its absence (which has not been tested), and if all the additional ACh were used to generate the additional m.e.p.p.s, then the output of ACh per m.e.p.p. would be about 9×10^{-21} pmol or 5400 molecules.

The ACh content of a quantum can also be estimated from measurements of the ACh released by nerve stimulation, provided the number of quanta per impulse and per junction is known. Estimates of ACh release by indirectly stimulated hemidiaphragms agree rather well: considering only those experiments in which the frequency of stimulation was 5 Hz or less and a reasonable correction (about 40%) could be made for resting output, values for ACh release per volley and end-plate are 7×10^{-18} mol (KRNJEVIĆ and MITCHELL, 1961), 5×10^{-18} mol (BOWMAN and HEMSWORTH, 1965a), and 4×10^{-18} mol (POTTER, 1970a). Unfortunately the number of quanta released per impulse at a single end-plate is less well established for these experimental conditions, though an early estimate of 20 by KRNJEVIĆ and MITCHELL (1961) is probably much too low. HUBBARD and WILSON (1973) observed that tubocurarine could reduce the quantum content of an e.p.p in their repetitively stimulated hemidiaphragms, and they considered that data from cut-muscle preparations would be more appropriate. Their own experiments showed much variability between individual junctions but suggested a mean value of about 200 for stimulation frequencies of 5 Hz or less. Accepting that value for quantum content, and 5×10^{-18} mol for the volley output at a single junction, the amount of ACh per quantum can be estimated at about 15000 molecules. [For slightly different calculations and conclusions see POTTER (1972) and HUBBARD and WILSON (1973). The earliest estimate of this sort, based by BIRKS (cited by MACINTOSH, 1959) on data from cat leg muscles, was only 6% of the above value; the reason for this discrepancy is not entirely clear.]

During continued stimulation of a motor nerve, the quantum content of an e.p.p. is not maintained unless the frequency is less than 1 Hz. At higher frequencies there is an initial fall, which is steepest during the first few impulses, after which e.p.p. size is fairly well maintained at a level that is frequency-dependent: the higher the frequency the lower the quantum content (BROOKS and THIES, 1962; ELMQVIST and QUASTEL, 1965b; THIES, 1965; ČAPEK et al., 1971; CECCARELLI et al., 1973; HUBBARD and WILSON, 1973). A very similar relationship between the frequency and duration of stimulation is shown by neurochemical observations. These studies cannot detect the decline of ACh output during the first few impulses, but they show that the volley output of ACh is nearly independent of frequency during brief periods of stimulation (e.g. 360 volleys: POTTER, 1970a), while it declines with increasing frequency during longer periods of stimulation (STRAUGHAN, 1960; KRNJEVIĆ and MITCHELL, 1961; BOWMAN and HEMSWORTH, 1965a; POTTER, 1970a).

b) Ganglion

ACh is released *spontaneously* from eserine-treated ganglia. The rate of ACh release in both the perfused superior cervical ganglion of the cat (BIRKS and MACINTOSH, 1961) and the isolated superior cervical ganglion of the rabbit (DAWES and VIZI, 1973) is 1 to 2 pmol/min, or about 0.1% of the store. Its source has not been determined. Spontaneous quantal release may account for part of this measured ACh release, but spontaneous junctional potentials (the ganglionic equivalent of m.e.p.p.s) are rather infrequent in mammalian ganglion cells at rest (Blackman and Purves, 1969; Sacchi and Perri, 1973) though their frequency rises after stimulation. Such quantal release may go unrecorded if the quanta are released onto dendritic sites too remote for a clear signal to be received at the soma. However, it is likely that a good deal of the ACh that can be collected from resting ganglia represents ACh that has not been released quantally but has overflowed from surplus ACh, or has leaked from axons. In the case of the perfused superior cervical ganglion of the cat, extraganglionic tissue included in the perfusion may contribute to the observed ACh release.

The unipolar autonomic ganglion cells of amphibia exhibit spontaneous junctional potentials and are well suited for experiments on the quantal aspects of ganglionic transmission. Quantitative data for the spontaneous and evoked release of ACh quanta have been obtained by several groups of workers. Raising extracellular potassium accelerates the discharge of quanta, as at the neuromuscular junction (Blackman et al., 1963c; Dennis et al., 1971), but the simple logarithmic relationship established by Liley (1956b) for the mammalian neuromuscular junction has not been shown to hold for the synapses in amphibian ganglia. Dennis and his colleagues (1971), recording from vagal ganglion cells in the frog heart, were able to mimic a spontaneous junctional potential by the microapplication of as little as 10^{-18} mol of ACh; as in the case of the neuromuscular junction this figure can be regarded as an upper limit for the size of an ACh quantum in this situation. Nishi and his colleagues (1967), in a remarkable investigation on frog sympathetic ganglia, were the first to provide parallel data for ACh release and quantum release in the same preparation. In their experiments a single nerve volley released 80 to 130 quanta onto an average ganglion cell. The corresponding amount of ACh released, assayed on the toad lung, was about 1.5×10^{-18} mol. On that basis a quantum would contain 8000 to 12000 molecules.

Sacchi and Perri (1973) attempted the awkward task of getting comparable data about quantum size at mammalian ganglionic synapses. They recorded intracellularly from the multipolar neurones in the isolated rat superior cervical ganglion, and succeeded in estimating the quantum content of responses to impulses in a single preganglionic axon. In all their successful experiments quantum content declined towards zero during repetitive stimulation in the presence of HC-3; there was no apparent change in quantum size. By integrating the declining quantal output curve Sacchi and Perri calculated the number of quanta initially present in one axon's endings on a ganglion cell to be about 8000. If similar axons represent the mean preganglionic input to each of the 4×10^4 ganglion cells, it can be calculated that the total initial store of transmitter would be contained within about 2×10^9 quanta. Sachhi and Perri also measured ganglionic ACh, and found that 85% of it (about 150 pmol) was lost while the quanta were being depleted; dividing this loss by the number of quanta discharged would lead to the conclusion that there are about 45000 molecules in a quantum. Sacchi and Perri did not draw this conclusion themselves, no doubt because they had reservations about the assumptions on which it was based; but they noted that their data were compatible with previous estimates (Hubbard, 1970).

There are no data yet about the relationship between potassium concentration and spontaneous junctional potential frequency at mammalian ganglionic synapses.

Several workers have provided bioassay data indicating that the cat superior cervical ganglion perfused with 25 to 50 mmol/l potassium released ACh at about the same rate as when stimulated at 10 to 20 Hz (BROWN and FELDBERG, 1936b; HUTTER and KOSTIAL, 1955; BIRKS, 1963; DESIRAJU, 1966); and DAWES and VIZI (1973) have obtained similar results on the isolated superior cervical ganglion of the rabbit.

Though experiments on ganglia have thus supplied only scanty results on the absolute size of an ACh quantum, they have provided quantitative information about a number of the factors that influence the process of release. In most cases the neurochemical and neurophysiological observations are in satisfactory agreement, but there are occasional exceptions.

The release of ACh during preganglionic nerve stimulation is strictly *calcium-dependent* (HARVEY and MACINTOSH, 1940; HUTTER and KOSTIAL, 1954; DOUGLAS et al., 1961) and is inhibited by excess of magnesium (HUTTER and KOSTIAL, 1954), and the same is true of the discharge of quanta (BLACKMAN et al., 1963b; MARTIN and PILAR, 1963b; DENNIS et al., 1971). In the perfused superior cervical ganglion of the cat, as in the hemidiaphragm (POTTER, 1970a), the volley-output of ACh during *brief preganglionic stimulation* (500 volleys) was found to be independent of the *frequency* of stimulation over the range 1 to 64 Hz (BIRKS and MACINTOSH, 1961). Electrical recording has given similar results (BENNETT and MCLACHLAN, 1972b; SACCHI and PERRI, 1973). Changes in quantum output during the first few impulses of a series cannot usually be detected by neurochemical methods, though they may be striking in electrical records (for references see KUNO, 1971). It has been reported, however, (DAWES and VIZI, 1973), that the volley-output of ACh in rabbit ganglia is 2.5 times higher at 0.3 Hz than at 1 to 10 Hz, recalling similar observations in ileal muscle (COWIE et al., 1968; PATON and ZAR, 1968; KOSTERLITZ and WATERFIELD, 1973). This might reflect better filling of the available ACh store at the lowest frequency, but other explanations have not been excluded; for example, there could be a presynaptic block of impulses at the higher frequencies in the isolated ganglion. With more *prolonged stimulation*, the volley-output of ACh is well maintained at physiological frequencies of activation, provided ACh synthesis is unimpeded (BIRKS and MACINTOSH, 1961; BIRKS and FITCH, 1974). At higher frequencies, however, e.g. 20 Hz or more, the output rate falls over 8 to 12 min from a high initial value to a lower steady-state value (BROWN and FELDBERG, 1936b; KAHLSON and MACINTOSH, 1939; PERRY, 1953; BIRKS and MACINTOSH, 1961; MATTHEWS, 1963; BIRKS and FITCH, 1974). In a typical experiment on ganglia perfused with Locke solution supplemented with choline, BIRKS and MACINTOSH (1961) found the steady-state output rate at 20 Hz to be 40 to 45% of the initial output rate. A biophysical experiment on guinea-pig ganglia (BENNETT and MCLACHLAN, 1972b) gave a very similar result (Fig. 6A): the recorded e.p.s.p.s. diminshed during the first 10 min of stimulation and then remained steady at about 40% of the initial size. The agreement between electrical and bioassay data is not always as good as this, however (Fig. 6B). When ganglia exposed to HC-3 are subjected to high-frequency stimulation, both ACh output and quantum output progressively fall. However, ACh release measured directly shows a two-phase decline, as if two distinct transmitter pools were being depleted (BIRKS and MACINTOSH, 1961; MATTHEWS, 1966); whereas e.p.s.p. size declines monophasically (BENNETT and MCLACHLAN, 1972a; SACCHI and PERRI, 1973) with a time-course like that of the more rapidly depleted pool in the neurochemical

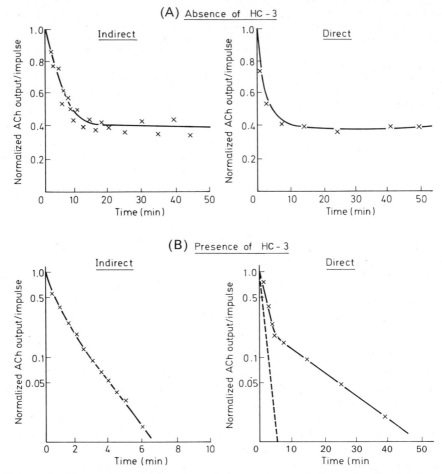

Fig. 6 A and B. Comparison of ACh release from superior cervical ganglia stimulated continuously at 20 Hz; release measured directly by bioassay from perfused superior cervical ganglion
of cat (from Birks and MacIntosh, 1961) or indirectly by recording excitatory postsynaptic
potentials from isolated superior cervical ganglion of guinea-pig (from Bennett and McLachlan, 1972a, b). In A, release was measured in the absence of HC-3; in B, release was measured in
the presence of HC-3. The two measures of the time-course of ACh release agree in the absence of
HC-3, but in the presence of HC-3 direct measure of ACh shows two components. The dotted
line in B (direct) represents the first exponential obtained by correcting the first component for
the presence of the second component; this first exponential approximates to the time-course of
the electrophysiological data

experiments. The reason for the discrepancy between these direct and indirect measures of ACh release is not yet entirely clear.

BIRKS and MACINTOSH (1961) reported that normal plasma contains a factor that
helps to maintain ACh output during prolonged high-frequency stimulation. This
factor appeared to promote mobilization of ACh already in the depot, rather than
synthesis or release *per se*. The factor has not been identified, and no attempt has
been made to examine its action by electrophysiological methods.

Table 3

Estimated ACh content[a]	(molecules)	Reference
(a) Synaptic vesicles		
(i) cerebral cortex	1650—2500	WHITTAKER (1965)
		WHITTAKER and SHERIDAN (1965)
(ii) superior cervical ganglion	1630	WILSON et al. (1973)
(b) Quanta		
(i) neuromuscular junction	900	BIRKS (cited by MACINTOSH, 1959)
	57000—62000	ELMQVIST and QUASTEL (1965a)
	15000	See page 131: calculated from data of KRNJEVIĆ and MITCHELL (1961), BOWMAN and HEMSWORTH (1965a), POTTER (1970a), and HUBBARD and WILSON (1973)
	15000—30000	POTTER (1972)
	40000—50000	HUBBARD (1970)
	12000—21000	HUBBARD and WILSON (1973)
(ii) ganglia (frog)	8000—12000	NISHI et al. (1967)
superior cervical ganglion (rat)	45000	See page 132: calculated from data of SACCHI and PERRI (1973)

[a] Data from mammalian tissues except where noted.

2. ACh Content: Vesicles vs. Quanta

The available estimates for both quantities are assembled in Table 3; reference has already been made to most of them. Except for the early estimate by BIRKS (cited by MACINTOSH, 1959), the values for the ACh content of a quantum are higher than the values for the ACh content of a vesicle. The discrepancy is awkward for the vesicle theory of ACh release, but cannot yet be considered fatal for it. The following are possible explanations for the discrepancy.

(a) ACh release as measured directly might overestimate quantal release. As yet there is no evidence that nerve impulses accelerate non-quantal release. It is possible that the anticholinesterases, which must be used whenever ACh has to be measured directly, might increase ACh release and thus cause quantum size to be overestimated. This appears unlikely at least in ganglia, because the release of ACh in the presence of an anticholinesterase agent is not greater than is the release of choline in the presence of hemicholinium (COLLIER and KATZ, 1974). (In such experiments, HC-3 was used to prevent the recapture of choline derived from released ACh.)

(b) Quanta released at a distance from the postsynaptic membrane might be underestimated by electrophysiological techniques. The process would presumably be teleologically wasteful, and there is no evidence that it can occur in the case of boutons that have characteristic zones of contact with their postsynaptic cells.

(c) The ACh that is released from one vesicle might release more ACh to make one quantum. The hypothesis that ACh can release ACh in this way has had some currency. It is discussed, and rejected, in part 4 of this section (pp.137—139).

(d) Quanta might result from the coupled exocytosis of the contents of a number of vesicles. No morphological or other evidence for such a suggestion has been offered, but it cannot be excluded.

(e) Exocytosis involving a single vesicle might provide a temporary channel or pore through which ACh from contiguous vesicles, or from the cytosol, could diffuse outward. Such a hypothesis could accommodate most of the morphological data, and the process would have the teleological virtue of economizing vesicle-bound materials (protein and ATP) of higher molecular weight than ACh. Unfortunately there is no obvious way to test the hypothesis.

(f) The ACh content of vesicles might be underestimated by present methods. This is certainly possible, as discussed in Section D. Better methods of preserving vesicles can probably be devised.

(g) Vesicles might not be the source of releasable ACh. Transmitter release might than be from the cytoplasmic ACh, or from ACh in structures that are as yet not identified. The problem of whether ACh can be released from the nerve-ending cytosol is discussed in the following paragraphs and is referred to elsewhere; the possibility certainly cannot be ruled out.

3. Is ACh Released from the Nerve-Terminal Cytoplasm?

The principal alternative to the vesicle hypothesis is the possibility that nerve impulses release transmitter from the cytoplasmic store of ACh: this may be called the cytosol hypothesis. Quantal release of ACh is then postulated to be the result of stepwise changes in the permeability of the presynaptic membrane at transmitter release sites; i.e., the opening of ACh "gates" for a set time to allow diffusion of ACh quanta out of the nerve ending.

Perhaps the most impressive single piece of evidence supporting the cytosol hypothesis was obtained by Tauc et al. (1974). They injected purified AChE into cholinergic interneurones of buccal ganglia in *Aplysia* and found that after a delay, corresponding to the time needed for axonal transport of the enzyme to the nerve terminals, transmission at the axonal terminals was abolished although axonal conduction was unimpaired. This is certainly a result one might expect if the cytosol hypothesis were true, because the injected enzyme would not be expected to reach the vesicle interior; but there are other possible explanations. For example, exchange diffusion of ACh across the vesicular membrane might cause loss of vesicular as well as extravesicular ACh; or the pH change resulting from the rapid hydrolysis of cytoplasmic ACh might have important local effects. Unfortunately Tauc and his colleagues did not test whether the synaptic block produced by the enzyme can be prevented or reversed by anticholinesterases. Nevertheless, the experiments of Tauc et al., and those of Dunant et al. (1972, 1974) and Birks (1974), which are referred to later, are not easy to reconcile with the vesicle hypothesis in its simplest form.

The arguments against the cytosol hypothesis all have counter-arguments. The principal arguments and counter-arguments are the following:

(a) Quantum size is not altered by depolarization: depolarization of the nerve terminal increases the frequency but not the size of m.e.p.p.s (Del Castillo and Katz, 1954 b; Boyd and Martin, 1956), whereas it might be expected that the efflux of ACh^+ ions from the cytosol during the opening of a membrane gate would be a function of the transmembrane potential. However, it could be argued that the transmembrane potential determines how far the gate is opened, or that calcium influx during nerve terminal depolarization determines how many gates are opened.

(b) Surplus ACh is not released by nerve impulses (BIRKS and MACINTOSH, 1961; POTTER, 1970a; COLLIER and KATZ, 1971). The idea that surplus ACh is in the presynaptic cytosol is attractive, because decentralized ganglia accumulate little or no surplus ACh when their AChE is inactivated (COLLIER and KATZ, 1971), and there is no other presynaptic compartment that would be an obvious candidate. However, it is still possible that surplus ACh forms in a postsynaptic or glial structure whose ability to synthesize or store ACh disappears if the presynaptic fibres degenerate.

(c) Accumulated exogenous ACh cannot be released by physiological stimuli. Brain slices accumulate exogenous ACh when they are incubated in a medium containing a suitable anticholinesterase (POLAK and MEEUWS, 1966; SCHUBERTH and SUNDWALL, 1967; LIANG and QUASTEL, 1969a; POLAK, 1969; HEILBRONN, 1970), and part of this ACh has been recovered in nerve endings (SCHUBERTH and SUNDWALL, 1968), though not in synaptic vesicles (S. H. SALEHMOGHADDAM and B. COLLIER, unpublished); ACh thus accumulated is not released by potassium ions (KATZ et al., 1973). Although these results are consistent with the vesicle hypothesis, they do not eliminate the cytosol hypothesis, because most of the accumulated exogenous ACh is not found in nerve endings (LIANG and QUASTEL, 1969a), and the uptake of ACh is not specifically into cholinergic tissue (KATZ et al., 1973).

(d) Choline is not released by nerve impulses. If ACh is released through presynaptic "gates", other cytoplasmic constituents such as choline might be expected to escape during the process of transmitter release. When tissue ACh has been labelled using radioactive choline, and the subsequent release of ACh measured in the presence of an anticholinesterase agent, increased release of labelled ACh is not accompanied by a significantly increased release of choline (COLLIER and MACINTOSH, 1969; POTTER, 1970a; HAGA, 1971; CHAKRIN et al., 1972). However, in these experiments, only a small proportion of the residual label is likely to have remained as free choline in the cytoplasm of the cholinergic nerve terminals. Moreover it is not impossible that an ACh "gate" might be able to distinguish ACh from choline.

Thus it must be concluded that the cytosol hypothesis has not been shown to be incorrect; and indeed it must also be realized that direct evidence for the release of ACh from vesicles by exocytosis is not much more compelling. It will be readily understood that it is not easy to design a crucial experiment that might distinguish between the rival hypotheses, because it is quite clear that vesicular ACh must have originated in the cytoplasm (Section C), and one can hardly doubt that in some circumstances, as yet poorly defined, it can return there. Furthermore it is likely that there are subpopulations of vesicles that differ from other vesicles in terms of their fragility and may be differently affected by procedures designed to label or harvest them.

4. Is Release of ACh Regenerative?

It has been suggested (KOELLE, 1961, 1962) that the amount of ACh released by a nerve impulse is in itself too small to effect synaptic transmission, but that this ACh quickly releases more ACh, so that there is enough transmitter to evoke a postsynaptic response. A corollary of this hypothesis is that ACh and ACh-like drugs act presynaptically to release ACh, and that a large part of their action depends upon such a mechanism; this has been proposed for drugs acting on autonomic ganglia

(Fellman, 1969) and on the neuromuscular junction (Riker et al., 1957, 1959; Riker, 1960; Chiou and Long, 1969; Chiou, 1970, 1973).

There is good electrophysiological evidence that ACh depolarizes cholinergic nerve terminals (Hubbard et al., 1965; Koketsu and Nishi, 1968; Pilar, 1969), but the concentrations required are rather high, and the action appears to reduce transmitter release (Ciani and Edwards, 1963; Hubbard et al., 1965; Pilar, 1969) rather than increase it. The physiological and pharmacological significance of drug-induced depolarization of motor nerve terminals will be discussed by others in this volume. The present discussion will be concerned with neurochemical experiments related to the regenerative release of ACh.

McKinstry and Koelle (1967a, b) tested the positive feedback hypothesis of Koelle (1961) by measuring ACh release from the perfused superior cervical ganglion and injecting carbachol into the perfusion stream. Carbachol released ACh, but there were some differences between the release of ACh by carbachol and the release of ACh by nerve impulses. For example, hexamethonium blocked ACh release by carbachol but not by nerve stimulation, while perfusion with a calcium-deficient medium reduced ACh release by nerve impulses but not that by carbachol. The experiments of Collier and Katz (1970) provided a possible explanation for the results of McKinstry and Koelle (1967a), and supplied evidence that exogenous ACh does not release ACh from the transmitter depot. In these experiments, Collier and Katz labelled the ganglion's transmitter store by perfusing the tissue during nerve stimulation with [^{3}H] choline but without an anticholinesterase; subsequent nerve stimulation released a good deal of radioactivity, but injected or perfused ACh or carbachol released little. A similar result was obtained by Brown et al. (1970). In parallel experiments, Collier and Katz (1970) labelled ganglionic ACh by perfusion with [^{3}H] choline and eserine, but without nerve stimulation; this allowed the accumulation of surplus [^{3}H] ACh, but little of the ACh in the ganglion's pre-existing store became labelled. Under these conditions, nerve stimulation released little radioactivity, but injected or perfused ACh or carbachol effectively released radioactive ACh. The amount of surplus ACh released by carbachol injected close to the ganglion (Collier and Katz, unpublished) was 198 pmol by 2.7 nmol of carbachol and 247 pmol by 5.5 nmol of carbachol, which was more than enough to account for all of the ACh released by carbachol in the experiments of McKinstry and Koelle. These findings show that ACh-like drugs, and exogenous ACh itself, can release surplus ACh but not depot ACh.

The mechanism by which a regenerative release mechanism might be terminated has never been fully explained. Koelle originally (1961) based his hypothesis, in part, on the presynaptic localization of ganglionic acetylcholinesterase, and it was implied that the enzyme terminated the process by destroying the ACh. More recently, Koelle (1971) has suggested that the pre-synaptic release sites rapidly become desensitized to ACh, and that this terminates release; he suggested, further, that the failure of exogenous ACh to release transmitter ACh in Collier and Katz's (1970) experiments was due to such desensitization. However, if this were so, exogenous ACh applied during nerve stimulation ought to reduce transmitter release, because the ACh-induced desensitization would be expected to interfere with the feedback mechanism. This was not observed in the experiments of Collier and Katz (1970); when

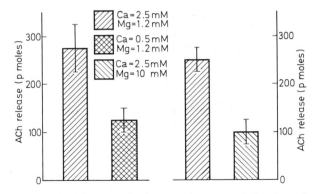

Fig. 7. The effect of reduced calcium or raised magnesium upon ACh release from rat diaphragm during phrenic nerve stimulation (20 Hz for 15 min). Results expressed as mean ±s.e. (4 experiments)

endogenous ACh stores had been [³H]-labelled, the release of radioactivity during nerve stimulation was not reduced by exogenous ACh in a concentration that effectively blocked synaptic transmission.

5. Calcium and ACh Release

Many secretory and neurosceretory processes are now known to be calcium-dependent (RUBIN, 1970), and the release of ACh at synapses was the first of these to be identified. Detailed information about the action of calcium and the antagonistic action of magnesium has come mainly from electrophysiological studies which are discussed in Chapter 3 of this volume. As noted earlier, there is good general agreement between the results of neurochemical experiments on perfused ganglia (HARVEY and MACINTOSH, 1940; HUTTER and KOSTIAL, 1954; see also DOUGLAS et al., 1961; DESIRAJU, 1966) and those of neurophysiological experiments on muscles (FENG, 1937; BROWN and HARVEY, 1940; COWAN, 1940; DEL CASTILLO and STARK, 1952; FATT and KATZ, 1952; DEL CASTILLO and ENGBAEK, 1954; DEL CASTILLO and KATZ, 1954a) and ganglia (BRONK et al., 1938; BRONK, 1939; BLACKMAN et al., 1963c,d). There have been few direct studies of the effects of calcium or magnesium on ACh release in muscle, but Fig. 7 (B. COLLIER and D. R. WOOD, unpublished) offers an example. Further evidence that ACh release in ganglia is calcium-dependent has come from quantal analysis of postsynaptic responses in mammalian (BLACKMAN et al., 1963d) and avian (MARTIN and PILAR, 1964) ganglia. Changes in calcium or magnesium concentrations also affect ACh release in smooth muscle (GERHARDS et al., 1964a,b; PATON et al., 1971; KOSTERLITZ and WATERFIELD, 1973).

   The idea that the action of calcium on the process of transmitter release depends on its uptake into nerve endings is an old one (cf. BIRKS and MACINTOSH, 1957; HODGKIN and KEYNES, 1957), and there is now some experimental support for it. Following the demonstration by HODGKIN and KEYNES (1957) that calcium influx into squid axons is accelerated by depolarization and by nerve impulses, LIPICKY et al. (1963) in similar experiments on rabbit ganglia found that treatment with high potassium increased ^{45}Ca influx by 25 to 70%. Lipicky et al. also measured ACh efflux and found that the ratio of ACh release to ^{45}Ca uptake was about 1:1. Blaustein (1971) observed still larger changes in his experiments on the superior cervical ganglion of the rat: ^{45}Ca influx rose by 300% when $[K^+]$ was increased, and by about 100% when the preganglionic trunk was stimulated at 12 Hz. Blaustein did not measure ACh release, but calculation of its probable rate from the data of others (Birks and MacIntosh, 1961; Saċchi and Perri, 1973) suggests that in his experiments also the ratio of ACh efflux to calcium influx might have been about 1:1. It might be supposed that the calcium influx in such tests would have been mainly into ganglion cells, but that apparently was not the case, since the influx was unaffected by ganglion-blocking agents, and was completely blocked by magnesium in a concentration (21 mmol/l) that suppresses ACh release by preganglionic stimulation. Measurements like those by Lipicky et al. (1963) and Blaustein (1971) do not distinguish net calcium uptake from calcium exchange, but they are certainly consistent with the idea that the movement of calcium into nerve terminals is the trigger for the ACh release mechanism. Studies of calcium uptake at the neuromuscular junction may present even greater difficulty. Such studies have been initiated by Lièvremont et al. (1969), who detected calcium uptake histochemically, and by Evans (1973), who examined the distribution of radioactive calcium. Selective accumulation of calcium at the neuromuscular junction was demonstrated in both investigations, but much of the uptake may have been postsynaptic. Recent experiments on *Torpedo* electroplaques (Babel-Guérin and Dunant, 1972; Babel-Guérin, 1974), in which uptake of calcium could be correlated with release of ACh, offer hope that the effects of intracellular calcium at cholinergic terminals can be studied more directly than in the past.

Most of the numerous speculations about the molecular mechanisms of calcium action have been put forward to account for various biophysical data on the release of ACh quanta at the neuromuscular junction. One of the exceptions is the hypothesis of Üvnäs (1973), which is perhaps the simplest one stated so far. He suggested that ACh is bound within storage vesicles to a sulphomucopolysaccharide-protein complex, and that release occurs by simple cation exchange, i.e. the exchange of calcium ions for ACh. Üvnäs based this suggestion upon experiments that measured the binding of drugs and ions to a sulphomucopolysaccharide complex isolated from mast cells, but he found that such complexes were present also in a synaptic-vesicle fraction from *Torpedo* electric organ and that ACh bound to them could be displaced by calcium. He calculated that the influx of sodium and calcium present within the synaptic cleft might suffice to account for the observed rates of ACh release, and following Folkow et al. (1967), he argued that a quantum of transmitter is probably less than the amount stored in one vesicle. On this and other grounds Üvnäs considered that partial displacement of the transmitter in a vesicle was more likely than the total loss of its content by exocytosis. Üvnäs's hypothesis has attractive features, but at present there appears to be more evidence against it than in its favour. For example ACh and ACh-like agents do not release transmitter (see part 4 of this section), as might be expected if a simple cation-exchange process were to operate. Also a reduction in extracellular calcium concentration does not reduce the size of a quantum but only the probability that it will be released. Thirdly, it is most unlikely that a quantum contains less ACh than does a vesicle. It may also be significant that calcium does not release ACh from isolated vesicles (WHITTAKER, 1959).

Several hypotheses about the release mechanism concern the relationship between the vesicles and the presynaptic membrane. BURTON et al. (1964) and BURTON and HOWARD (1967) proposed that gangliosides in the vesicle membrane enable it to fuse with the presynaptic membrane as a preliminary to ACh release. SIMPSON (1968), extending the hypothesis, suggested that calcium influx causes ganglioside to be redistributed between a membrane phase and an aqueous (cytosol) phase. However his model, based on the experiments of QUARLES and FOLCH-PI (1965), would seem to require that the concentration of intra-axonal calcium should rise to exceed 5 mmol/l during invasion of the terminal by an impulse, which seems improbable. There appears also to be some doubt whether synaptic vesicles contain gangliosides (EICHBERG et al., 1964; WHITTAKER, 1966; WIEGANDT, 1967; TROTTER and BURTON 1969). BLIOCH et al. (1968) propose that calcium ions, entering the terminal axoplasm during the action potential, mask fixed negative charges on the inner surface of the presynaptic membrane and thus allow the approach and adhesion of synaptic vesicles, whose surfaces are negatively charged; a further mechanism, not described, then leads to exocytosis. Synaptic vesicles are indeed negatively charged (VOS et al., 1968; RYAN et al., 1971) and their surface properties may well be altered by calcium, but evidence is lacking that the calcium transients at the inner face of the presynaptic membrane are large enough to produce such a change. Although other cations can substitute for calcium and allow ACh release, the theory cannot easily account for the relative effectiveness of calcium as compared with other divalent ions (cf. DODGE et al., 1969; MEIRI and RAHAMIMOFF, 1971; LASKOWSKI and THIES, 1972). Moreover calcium, but not other divalent cations, can induce the release of transmitter after direct injection into presynaptic terminals of the squid giant synapse (MILEDI, 1973).

A promising new approach to the role of calcium in release mechanisms is the identification of specific calcium-binding proteins (WOLFF and SIEGEL, 1972; ALEMA et al., 1973). One such protein is found in cholinergically innervated tissues (SIEGEL et al., 1973), and a recent report (POLITOFF et al., 1974) suggests that a similar substance may be present on the surface of synaptic vesicles in frog motor terminals.

That extracellular sodium is not necessary for ACh release by potassium has been known for some time (HUTTER and KOSTIAL, 1954). Intracellular sodium, however, has important effects on ACh binding and release by intact nerve terminals, and these are largely or entirely mediated by competition between sodium and calcium for intracellular binding sites (BIRKS and COHEN, 1965, 1968a, b; GAGE and QUASTEL, 1966; BIRKS et al., 1968; COLOMO and RAHAMIMOFF, 1968; KELLY, 1968). Accordingly, any large change in the rate of sodium pumping can be expected to influence both resting and depolarization-coupled release of ACh, even apart from the changes in calcium flux that are likely to occur at the same time. On the basis that calcium is an inhibitor of membrane-bound (Na^+–K^+–Mg^{++})-activated ATPase, PATON et al. (1971) and VIZI (1972) have suggested that calcium uptake may promote ACh release by its action on this enzyme; the inhibition of ATPase is postulated to induce some change in the membrane that would favour exocytosis. At present the suggestion does not seem a very attractive model for ACh release under physiological conditions. The release of ACh quanta evoked by inhibitors of ATPase, such as the cardiac glycosides, only reaches a high frequency after a delay that is long enough for intracellular sodium levels to be considerably elevated (cf. Elmqvist and Feldman, 1965b; Birks and Cohen, 1968a, b).

There is a striking difference in the time-course of the effect of drugs like ouabain on ACh release measured directly from smooth muscle or brain slices (Paton et al., 1971; Vizi, 1972), and indirectly from the frequency of m.e.p.p.s recorded from skeletal muscle (Elmqvist and Feldman, 1965b; Birks and Cohen, 1968a, b). Direct measurement showed ACh release to be increased within a few seconds of adding the drug, but the frequency of m.e.p.p.s was not increased until many minutes after adding ouabain. It is possible that the inhibition of membrane-bound ATPase allows non-vesicular ACh to leak out of nerve terminals, but does not induce the release of vesicular ACh; such non-quantal release of ACh would be of doubtful physiological significance.

ACh is also released from tissues that are exposed to a sodium-free medium (Quastel, 1962; Birks, 1963; Bhatnagar and MacIntosh, 1967; Paton et al., 1971; Vizi, 1972). In this case the release is accelerated by the simultaneous withdrawal of calcium, and it fails to trigger an increase in ACh synthesis. There is no evidence that the release is quantal, or that it has anything to do with ACh release as it occurs normally; more probably, it is a sign that some sodium-dependent transport or storage process has been inactivated.

Certain agents or procedures promote the release of ACh quanta even when the external calcium concentration is greatly reduced or zero. The most fully documented example of this is the acceleration of m.e.p.p.s that is induced by prolonged repetitive stimulation or depolarization of the motor terminals (Miledi and Thies, 1967, 1971; Hurlbut et al., 1971). In this case the process that controls m.e.p.p. frequency does appear to be calcium-dependent, but it is nearly saturated at calcium concentrations in the micromolar range, in contrast to the process that controls e.p.p. quantum content, whose effectiveness varies with calcium concentrations over the range 0.1 to 2 mmol/l (Cooke and Quastel, 1973). Examples of apparently calcium-independent acceleration of m.e.p.p.s include: raised osmolarity (Blioch et al., 1968); cardiac glycosides (Birks, 1963; Elmqvist and Feldman, 1965b; Birks and Cohen, 1965, 1968a, b; cf. also Vizi, 1972); ethanol and other compounds with a high affinity for membrane lipids (Quastel et al., 1971); lanthanum (DeBassio et al., 1971; Heuser and Miledi, 1971); black widow spider venom (Longenecker et al., 1970) and β-bungarotoxin (Chang et al., 1973a). Whether each of these treatments causes the release of ACh by a mechanism that is entirely independent of calcium is not clear; they might cause the release of calcium from intracellular stores. Black widow spider venom depletes motor terminals of synaptic vesicles (Clark et al., 1972; Ceccarelli et al., 1973), and presumably of ACh as well, since it causes depletion of stored ACh in ganglia and in brain (Paggi and Rossi, 1971; Frontali et al., 1972). However β-bungarotoxin (see next section) can apparently block ACh release without producing either kind of depletion (Chang et al., 1973a).

6. Neurotoxins and ACh Release

Most of the animal toxins that are known to affect ACh release are non-specific, in that their action is not confined to cholinergic synapses. This seems to be the case with black widow spider venom, which also poisons mammalian adrenergic and insect glutaminergic terminals (FRONTALI, 1972; CULL-CANDY et al., 1973); with batrachotoxin (ALBUQUERQUE et al., 1971), whose depolarizing action on motor nerve terminals increases m.e.p.p. frequency with subsequent junctional block, but also acts on end-plates; and with tityustoxin from scorpion venom, whose action resembles that of batrachotoxin in many ways. Tityustoxin can release ACh from brain slices (GOMEZ et al., 1973) but it also releases other mediators (see MOSS et al., 1974). Black widow spider venom, which seems to have little postsynaptic action, may well prove a useful experimental tool for studying the turnover of quanta at nerve terminals (CECCARELLI et al., 1973), especially if direct measurements of ACh are made in parallel. In muscles exposed to the venom, the progressive depletion of vesicles in the terminals seems to match the cumulative m.e.p.p. count, and can be correlated with the junctional block that develops as the depletion approaches completion (CECCARELLI et al., 1973). In ganglia exposed to this venom the correlation between vesicle depletion and synaptic block is less obvious, for it has been reported (CHMOULIOVSKY et al., 1972) that though transmission is blocked within an hour the number of synaptic vesicles does not fall significantly until two hours later. It should be noted that all the experiments mentioned above were made with crude venom, which contains at least 5 proteins (FRONTALI and GRASSO, 1964); the purified principle (or principles) is not yet available. Crotactin, a purified protein toxin (HABERMANN, 1957) from the venom of *Crotalus durissus terrificus*, the South American rattlesnake, appears to act very much like black widow spider venom (VITAL BRAZIL and EXCELL, 1971). The action of cobra venom, which releases ACh from brain tissue (BRAGANÇA and QUASTEL, 1952) is probably less specific; the venom is a rich source of phospholipase A, which also releases ACh, but the effect of this enzyme seems to be secondary to partial lysis of nerve endings (HEILBRONN and CEDERGREN, 1970).

Two far more specific agents, botulinum toxin and β-bungarotoxin, have as their principal effect the lasting inhibition of ACh release; they have little postsynaptic effect, and little effect on other synapses. The astonishing potency of botulinum toxin remains as mysterious as ever, though some interesting new facts have emerged. This toxin causes no obvious change in synaptic ultrastructure (THESLEFF, 1960; ZACKS et al., 1962), does not deplete tissue ACh (HART et al., 1965), and does not (as was once thought) prevent invasion of the motor terminals by nerve impulses (HARRIS and MILEDI, 1971). Ferritin-labelled toxin tends to be localized within the synaptic clefts of the neuromuscular junction, but is not seen in association with synaptic vesicles (ZACKS et al., 1962). The material inside the clefts is thought to be rich in gangliosides, and SIMPSON and RAPPORT (1971 a, b) found that only ganglioside, out of a variety of lipids tested, was able to bind botulinum toxin; tetanus toxin, whose actions include presynaptic blockade of the neuromuscular junction (MELLANBY and THOMPSON, 1972; DUCHEN and TONGE, 1973, see also Chapter 1) is also bound by ganglioside. However, the significance of these morphological and chemical observations is rather dubious, for it is not known whether labelled toxin binds at other kinds of cholinergic junction, or at non-cholinergic junctions, nor has any difference been detected between the gangliosides of cholinergic synapses and other synapses.

HUGHES and WHALER (1962) showed that nerve stimulation hastened the onset of paralysis in phrenic-diaphragm preparations exposed to botulinum toxin, and SIMPSON (1971, 1973), extending that finding, observed that the stimulation was effective only if it released transmitter: with low calcium or high magnesium there was no acceleration of the blockade. Simpson (1973) suggested that the process of ACh release might help to uncover fresh toxin-binding sites, but an obvious alternative hypothesis would be that vesicle exocytosis and recycling permits uptake of toxin into the nerve ending, where it might interfere with the transfer of cytoplasmic ACh into vesicles, as Hubbard and Quastel (1973) have suggested. Some support for such an idea is provided by the experiments of Boroff et al. (1974), who report that the onset of paralysis in botulinum-poisoned frogs is presaged by a fall in quantum (m.e.p.p.) size, while e.p.p. quantum content, where it can be measured, stays normal. Experiments on the turnover of labelled choline and ACh in poisoned nerve-endings, if found to be technically feasible, could hardly fail to improve our understanding of the toxin's mode of action, but no report of such experiments has yet been published.

In contrast to α-bungarotoxin's affinity for ACh receptors, which makes it a potent postsynaptic blocking agent, β-bungarotoxin appears to act only presynaptically (Chang and Lee, 1963): after a period of accelerated quantal release (Chang et al., 1973a) transmission at the neuromuscular junction is irreversibly blocked. The blocking action is very similar to that of botulinum toxin, and in fact the two toxins are mutually antagonistic on the rat phrenic-diaphragm preparation (Chang et al., 1973b; Chang and Huang, 1974). The early report of Chang and Lee (1963) suggested that β-bungarotoxin, unlike botulinum toxin, has no action on cholinergic terminals other than those in skeletal muscle: if true this is of great interest, but confirmatory studies are needed. It is also uncertain whether β-bungarotoxin reduces the number of vesicles in the motor terminals. Chen and Lee (1970) reported a reduction, but Chang et al. (1973a) with different experimental conditions found none, and as already mentioned observed no loss of stored ACh.

7. Drugs and ACh Release

The literature on this topic is voluminous and is considered from a different point of view in Chapter 3. No comprehensive summary is attempted here: instead, a few examples are given of the principal types of action.

a) Drugs that Increase Evoked ACh Release

These act in various ways: it is reasonable to suppose that in each case (as also in post-tetanic potentiation: Hubbard, 1974) there is an increase in some presynaptic store of calcium available to the release process. (i) *Cardiac glycosides* (Birks and Cohen, 1965) and *metabolic inhibitors* such as cyanide or dinitrophenol (Katz and Edwards, 1973) increase e.p.p. quantum content. Evoked ACh release in the presence of these agents does not appear to have been measured directly, but they increase the spontaneous discharge of m.e.p.p.s from motor terminals and of ACh from ganglia, intestine and cortical slices (Birks, 1963; Birks and Cohen, 1965; Paton et al., 1971; Vizi, 1972; Katz and Edwards, 1973). (ii) *Tetraethylammonium* increases evoked, but not spontaneous, ACh release from muscles and ganglia (Stovner, 1957; Koketsu, 1958; Douglas and Lywood, 1961; Blackman, 1963; Collier and Exley, 1963; Matthews and Quilliam, 1964; Kuperman and Okamoto, 1965; Katz and Miledi, 1967), almost certainly because of the drug's ability to prolong the axonal spike by blocking potassium efflux. *Triethylcholine*, which acts on nerves like its close relative tetraethylammonium (Lorente de No, 1949), also increases the evoked release of ACh quanta in muscles and ganglia during brief periods of stimulation (ROBERTS, 1962; BLACKMAN, 1963). Gallamine, which can also be regarded as a tetraethylammonium derivative, may have a comparable effect (JONES and LAITY, 1965). Under carefully selected conditions, even tubocurarine and decamethonium may have a weak effect of this sort (JONES and LAITY, 1965; HUBBARD et al., 1969; BLABER, 1970, 1973; GALINDO, 1971). Cesium ions may also be mentioned here, as being capable of increasing the presynaptic spike and hence ACh release in mammalian ganglia (DUNANT, 1969) as well as at the neuromuscular junction (GINSBORG and HAMILTON, 1968; KOREY and HAMILTON, 1974). (iii) There is considerable evidence that *guanidine* can increase ACh release (FENG, 1940; DESMEDT, 1956; OTSUKA and ENDO, 1960; BARZAGHI et al., 1962; HOFMANN et al., 1966; VIZI and KNOLL, 1971), though it has not been shown to increase the presynaptic spike. Its mode of action is unknown; in some ways it resembles that of calcium (DEBECKER, 1972). Guanidine induces repetitive activity in nerve terminals, but this action need not imply that it will enhance evoked ACh release, for veratrum alkaloids and related compounds also cause repetitive activity (see FLACKE et al., 1972) but they do not increase e.p.p. amplitude or duration or quantal content (KUFFLER, 1948; DETWILER, 1972). (iv) The anticurare action of *adrenaline* was discovered over 50 years ago (PANELLA, 1907) and has been confirmed repeatedly, but it cannot be elicited under all experimental conditions. It is now well established that adrenaline and other catecholamines, acting presynaptically, can either facilitate or depress neuromuscular and ganglionic transmission. Correspondingly, experiments on sympathetic ganglia have shown both increased (BIRKS and MACINTOSH, 1961) and decreased (PATON and THOMPSON, 1953) ACh output when adrenaline is added to the perfusion fluid. For a fuller account the review by BOWMAN and NOTT (1969) and the articles by DE GROAT and VOLLE (1966) and NISHI (1970) should be consulted. (v) Certain phenols which antagonize neuromuscular block due to tubocurarine (MOGEY and YOUNG, 1949) also increase ACh release (OTSUKA and NONOMURA, 1963) in an unknown way. Catechol (GALLAGHER and BLABER, 1973) acts similarly, and may promote calcium influx into nerve terminals (BLABER, 1973). A synthetic "*calcium ionophore*" studied by KITA and VAN DER KLOOT (1974) increases both spontaneous and evoked ACh release at the frog neuromuscular junction. (vi) *Caffeine* and the related purine bases might be expected to promote ACh release by mobilizing calcium from intracellular stores, as in muscle fibres, and such an effect has indeed been reported (HOFMANN, 1969). (vii) *Alcohols, anaesthetics* and *chlorpromazine*, which can accelerate the "spontaneous" release of ACh quanta at the neuromuscular junction in the almost complete absence of external calcium (QUASTEL et al., 1971; COOKE and QUASTEL, 1973a), also reinforce calcium-dependent evoked release. The reinforcement appears to be multiplicative rather than additive (COOKE and QUASTEL, 1973a). CARMODY and GAGE (1973) argue, however, that some of the effect of these drugs depends on the mobilization of intracellular calcium.

Many basic drugs that are generally supposed to act mainly on postsynaptic structures can also be shown in properly designed experiments to elicit presynaptic responses as well. The first experiments of this sort were those of MASLAND and WIGTON (1940) on anticholinesterases; the other drugs investigated have included a large number of nicotinic agonists and antagonists, including ACh itself, and a group of "facilitatory" drugs, most of which possess some anticholinesterase activity. The results obtained have been complex and often controversial. For the most part they are outside the scope of this chapter, but the data on the neuromuscular junction have been reviewed by Bowman and Webb (1972); the review by Volle (1966) and an important article by Nishi (1970) discuss the situation in sympathetic ganglia. The experimental work summarized by the above authors leaves no doubt that there are presynaptic nicotinic receptors at, or close to, the cholinergic terminals in muscles and ganglia, but it leaves much doubt about their physiological significance. One aspect of the problem, the hypothesis that ACh release at nerve endings is regenerative, was discussed on p. 137. The present writers incline to the view that the ACh receptors on cholinergic endings, like those on sensory endings and on unmyelinated axons (Brown and Gray, 1948; Douglas and Gray, 1953; Armett and Ritchie, 1960; Douglas and Ritchie, 1960), are functionally unimportant.

b) Drugs that Decrease Evoked ACh Release

These are chemically diverse and also differ greatly in their presumed modes of action. *Tubocurarine* has been asserted on the basis of electrophysiological evidence (Lille-heil and Naess, 1961; Hubbard et al., 1969; Blaber, 1970; Maeno and Nobe, 1970; Galindo, 1971) to have such an action at the neuromuscular junction, but this conclusion has been challenged by other electrophysiologists (Beranek and Vysko-čil, 1967; Chang et al., 1967; Auerbach and Betz, 1971; Bauer, 1971). Direct measurements of released ACh in muscles (Dale et al., 1936; Emmelin and MacIntosh, 1956; Krnjević and Mitchell, 1961; Cheymol et al., 1962) and in ganglia (Brown and Feldberg, 1935; Matthews, 1966) have uniformly failed to detect such an effect, although a small change could have been overlooked, and the necessary presence of an anticholinesterase might have altered the situation. At present it seems (Blaber, 1973) that most of the divergent results can be reconciled on the basis that tubocurarine has little effect on ACh release *per se*, but can interfere with replenishment of the available ACh store when stimulation frequency is elevated, especially in the somewhat unphysiological conditions that prevail in isolated muscles. *Adrenaline*, as already noted, can reduce evoked ACh release from perfused ganglia (Paton and Thompson, 1953) and from isolated gut muscle (Vizi, 1968; Paton and Vizi, 1969), and can act presynaptically to depress transmission in both muscles and ganglia, though it has opposing effects which may predominate. For further information and references the reader is referred to the work of Volle (1966), Bowman and Nott (1969) and Nishi (1970). *Morphine* is a potent inhibitor of ACh release in intestine (Paton, 1957; Lees et al., 1973), but in similar concentration it does not reduce ACh release in ganglia (Paton, 1957; Kosterlitz and Wallis, 1966) or in skeletal muscle (Frederickson and Pinsky, 1971), so morphine can hardly be regarded as a specific inhibitor of transmitter release at cholinergic synapses. The effects of morphine on ACh release in brain are outside the scope of this chapter. A number of other *central depressant drugs* have been shown to block ACh release as measured directly in ganglia (Matthews and Quilliam, 1964; Casati et al., 1973). The *antibiotics of the streptomycin-neomycin group* interfere with ACh release at the neuromuscular junction by a magnesium-like action (Vital Brazil and Corrado, 1957), competing with calcium: reduction of e.p.p. quantum content (Elmqvist and Josefsson, 1962), and of evoked ACh release measured biologically (Vital Brazil and Prado-Franceschi, 1969), have both been demonstrated. The ions of several *metals* appear to act in a generally similar fashion. This has been shown for cadmium (SMIRNOV et al., 1954), lead (KOSTIAL and VOUK, 1957; SILBERGELD et al., 1974), and manganese (KAJIMOTO and KIRPEKAR, 1972; KOSTERLITZ and WATERFIELD, 1972; MEIRI and RAHAMIMOFF, 1972; KOSTIAL et al., 1974). For completeness it may be added that agents that induce nerve-terminal depolarization can diminish the release of ACh by nerve impulses: ACh itself is such an agent (CIANI and EDWARDS, 1963; HUBBARD et al., 1965), as are metabolic inhibitors (KRAATZ and TRAUTWEIN, 1957; BEANI et al., 1966). Finally, drugs that inhibit choline uptake (p. 114—117) reduce evoked ACh output during repetitive stimulation.

8. Cyclic Nucleotides, Prostaglandins and ACh Release

The adenyl cyclase system is involved in so many physiological functions that it is not surprising to find it assigned a role in ACh release (BRECKENRIDGE et al., 1967; GOLDBERG and SINGER, 1969; SINGER and GOLDBERG, 1970; WILSON, 1974). The principal evidence for such a role is that theophylline and caffeine, which inhibit the destruction of cyclic AMP by phosphodiesterase, and dibutyryl cyclic AMP, which might mimic the actions of cyclic AMP, all increase e.p.p. quantum content (HOFMANN, 1969; WILSON, 1974). The demonstration (JOHNSON et al., 1973) that cyclic AMP and phosphodiesterase are associated with a synaptic-vesicle fraction harvested from brain is consistent with the proposed role for the nucleotide in evoked ACh release, but there are a number of difficulties. First, it is very probable that caffeine and theophylline enchance ACh release by mobilizing intracellular calcium (ELMQVIST and FELDMAN, 1965a; HOFMANN, 1969), as they do in skeletal and heart muscle when they promote excitation-contraction coupling (BIANCHI, 1961; LÜLLMANN and HOLLAND, 1962); it is as yet by no means certain that these actions are mediated by cyclic AMP. Second, neither theophylline nor dibutyryl cyclic AMP has a measurable effect on ACh release by the superior cervical ganglion during short periods of nerve stimulation (COLLIER, unpublished). Third, adenosine, which might be expected to increase intracellular cyclic AMP as it does in brain slices (SATTIN and RALL, 1970), reduces rather than increases the quantum content of the e.p.p. in rat diaphragm (GINSBORG and HIRST, 1972). Thus the case for cyclic AMP formation as a normal factor in evoked ACh release is not convincing at present.

There is even less evidence for the involvement of prostaglandins in ACh release. Nerve stimulation liberates prostaglandins, mostly E_1, from rat diaphragm (RAMWELL et al., 1965; LAITY, 1969) and from cat superior cervical ganglion (DAVIS et al., 1971), but nothing is known about the source or functional significance of these prostaglandins. Prostaglandin E_1 does not affect transmission through a sympathetic ganglion (KAYAALP and MCISAAC, 1962) or e.p.p. quantum content at the neuromuscular junction (GINSBORG and HIRST, 1971). Thus the discovery (HEDQVIST and VON EULER, 1972) that this prostaglandin controls noradrenaline release in some tissues cannot be extrapolated to ACh release. A recent report by SURIA and COSTA (1974) suggests that prostaglandins may oppose post-tetanic potentiation of ganglionic transmissions.)

9. Contractile Proteins, Microtubules and Microfilaments

It is now apparent that actomyosin-like complexes participate in many kinds of intracellular movement as well as in the sliding-filament mechanisms of the different kinds of muscle. A rise in intracellular free calcium is the usual trigger for all these movements; and it was therefore a plausible suggestion (Poisner and Trifaró, 1967), that calcium-dependent secretion and neurosecretion also involve a contractile process. Such a process is usually supposed to be responsible for the exocytosis of granular or vesicular material, but it is conceivable that it could act directly on the presynaptic membrane to create channels for the efflux of materials from the cytosol. Actomyosin-like proteins have in fact been extracted from adrenal medulla (Poisner, 1970) and from brain, where they are associated with synaptosomes (Puszkin et al., 1972; Puszkin and Berl, 1972). The brain protein, called neurostenin, can be dissociated by mild treatment into two components, neurin (actin-like) and stenin (myosin-like), and there is evidence that *in vivo* there are attached to plasma membrane and vesicles respectively (Berl et al., 1973). Wellington and his colleagues (1973) have reported that neurostenin constitutes 1 to 2% of total brain protein, and they have studied its distribution by immunofluorescence: it seems to be located in central and peripheral membranes but not within axons or perikarya. They failed to detect the claimed actomyosin-like properties of the material, whose status must therefore be regarded with reserve for the time being. There is no direct evidence yet that neurostenin is present in cholinergic terminals.

Axelrod (1972) proposed that contractile *microfilaments*, activated by calcium, might trigger transmitter release, on the grounds that cytochalasin B, which disrupts microfilaments (Carter, 1967; Wessels et al., 1971), inhibited the release of noradrenaline and of dopamine-β-hydroxylase from the vas deferens of the guinea-pig during hypogastric nerve stimulation (Thoa et al., 1972). Cytochalasin B also inhibits the release of vasopressin from the posterior pituitary, of catecholamines from the adrenal medulla, and of ACh from sympathetic ganglia (Douglas and Sorimachi, 1972a; Nakasoto and Douglas, 1973). The blocking effect of cytochalasin B on neurosecretory processes may, however, be only one more example of the nonspecificity of pharmacological agents, for Nakasoto and Douglas (1973) have shown that its blocking action on a sympathetic ganglion is partly reversed by pyruvate, as if the drug's primary effect were on energy production, possibly by inhibiting glucose uptake (Kletzien et al., 1972; Mizel and Wilson, 1972).

Microtubules have also been implicated in transmitter release, principally because of the ability of colchicine and vinblastine, drugs that cause microtubule disintegration, to decrease the release of catecholamines from the adrenal medulla by ACh (Poisner and Bernstein, 1971) and from the vas deferens in response to hypogastric nerve impulses (Thoa et al., 1972). The effect of colchicine in these experiments, however, may have been on cholinergic receptors rather than on microtubules, for in the concentrations used the drug is a cholinergic blocking agent (Spoor and Ferguson, 1965; Douglas and Sorimachi, 1972b; Trifaró et al., 1972; Turkanis, 1973). Thus colchicine would have blocked ACh-induced catecholamine release in Poisner and Bernstein's tests, and also in those of Thoa and his colleagues, because most of the fibres in the hypogastric nerve are known to be preganglionic. In any case, there is no evidence that microtubules are required for ACh release, for colchicine and vinblastine do not diminish its release from the superior cervical ganglion, at least with short exposure to the drug (Trifaró et al., 1972; Pumplin and McClure, 1974), nor do they inhibit the mobilization of ACh quanta for release at the neuromuscular junction (Katz, 1972). There is, on the other hand, excellent evidence (Section H) that microtubules are involved in axonal growth and transport, and therefore in the delivery to the terminals of materials that are important for synaptic function.

Though none of the three filamentous protein entities—neurostenin, microfilaments or microtubules—has an established role in the processes that immediately precede ACh release, it is very probable that some mechanism of the general type discussed above will eventually come to light and will help to explain the calcium-dependence of the release process. A provocative finding, so far reported only in brief, is that calcium in rather low concentration (K_m 10 µmol/l) can dissociate microtubules by a mechanism different from that of colchicine (HAGA et al., 1973).

10. Are Quanta Released by Exocytosis?

As yet this question cannot be answered with assurance. The relevant anatomical studies are reviewed in the first chapter of this volume. There are three main lines of evidence in favour of exocytosis. (a) Electron micrographs, especially of freeze-etched preparations, show vesicles fused with the presynaptic membrane and apparently open to the synaptic cleft (see for example AKERT et al., 1969; NICKEL and POTTER, 1970). (b) Vesicle counts decrease, and the presynaptic membrane area increases, during enhanced ACh release at neuromuscular junctions, as if the membrane were temporarily expanded by incorporating the membranes of vesicles (CLARK et al., 1972; HEUSER and REESE, 1973). (c) Macromolecular markers (e.g. ferritin, horseradish peroxidase) accumulate in synaptic vesicles more rapidly during repetitive stimulation (HOLTZMAN et al., 1971; CECCARELLI et al., 1973; HEUSER and REESE, 1973). None of the evidence has been expressed in sufficiently quantitative form to carry conviction.

Neurochemical evidence pertinent to the exocytosis theory is scanty in the case of cholinergic junctions. For adrenergic junctions, and especially for chromaffin cells, the evidence is much more abundant (see DOUGLAS, 1968; KIRSHNER and KIRSHNER, 1971; A. D. SMITH, 1971, 1973). It has been shown that the vesicle (granule) constituents, chromogranin A, dopamine-β-hydroxylase and ATP, are released along with noradrenaline by nerve stimulation, and usually in the same ratio as in the vesicular store. Even in this case, there are some awkward points that do not appear to fit the exocytosis theory (see BENNETT [1972] for a brief review). But at present, perhaps the strongest argument for exocytosis at cholinergic junctions is the analogy with adrenergic junctions.

Vesicle and plasma membranes from brain synaptosomes have been reported to differ in lipid (EICHBERG et al., 1964), protein (VON HUNGEN et al., 1968) and enzyme (WHITTAKER et al., 1964; HOSIE, 1965) composition, and there is some evidence (BOSMANN and HEMSWORTH, 1970; LUNT and LAPETINA, 1970) that vesicle lipids incorporate a choline label more rapidly than plasma-membrane lipids. Estimates of vesicle lifetime based on the labelling of vesicle-membrane lipids are unlikely to be of great value, because labelled phospholipids are fairly readily exchanged between the different membrane fractions in brain homogenates (MILLER and DAWSON, 1972). Similar measurements on the proteins specifically associated with vesicles might be of greater value, but apparently have not been made as yet. VON HUNGEN and his colleagues (1968) pulse-labelled brain protein with [^{3}H]leucine and followed the loss of radioactivity from the usual subcellular fractions; time constants of about 3 weeks were obtained for all the fractions, including the synaptic vesicles. The result was thought to be incompatible with the exocytosis theory of transmitter release, for all the known transmitters seem to have faster turnover rates, but this is probably too simple a view. At least some of the vesicular protein could conceivably remain bound to the vesicle membrane during exocytosis, while some of the released protein (or its constituent amino acids) could be recaptured and rerouted through the vesicle cycle. One must regretfully predict that experiments on brain are unlikely to help solve the problem of whether ACh is released by exocytosis: the synapses are too heterogeneous, and the detection and measurement of the release of macromolecules within the tissue present too formidable difficulties. In recent years, therefore, several attempts have been made to apply to peripheral cholinergic synapses the approach that has been productive in the case of peripheral adrenergic synapses, i.e. to look for the release of vesicle constituents other than the transmitter itself into a perfusing or suspending medium during nerve stimulation. In the case of skeletal muscles and ganglia, which have been used for such experiments, these other constituents have not been identified, but are supposed to be the same as in electric organs and brain; indeed the electric organ itself is now being studied in this way. As noted earlier (p. 129) its cholinergic vesicles contain a protein, vesiculin, plus nucleotide, mainly ATP (Whittaker et al., 1972a, b 1974).

Protein. Musick and Hubbard (1972) measured the release of protein from the isolated diaphragm of the mouse and showed a large spontaneous release and a small (35%) additional release during nerve stimulation. They believed that the evoked release came from nerve, not muscle, because it was dependent on calcium and was not prevented by tubocurarine in a concentration that suppressed the e.p.p.s. It was suggested (Musick and Hubbard, 1972) that the protein was similar to vesiculin, although an attempt to characterize it by polyacrylamide gel electrophoresis revealed no component specifically released by nerve stimulation. A most curious finding was that the released ACh appeared to be bound to the released protein, because only 20% of the ACh collected from the medium bathing the muscle could be removed by dialysis; nevertheless it must have been effective in transmission. It is extraordinary in the first place that ACh, a compound so water-soluble that its salts are hygroscopic, should bind strongly to any protein (even an ACh receptor protein), and secondly that the ACh so bound should be biologically active. The ACh collected from a Locke-perfused superior cervical ganglion during nerve stimulation is not attached to any macromolecule (B. Collier and M. Warner, unpublished). There is a further difficulty in supposing that the protein released by nerve stimulation in Musick and Hubbard's experiments came from synaptic vesicles. Whittaker (1971) found that the ratio of vesiculin to ACh in Torpedo vesicles was about 4:1 by weight. Even if Musick and Hubbard's mouse diaphragms had released as much ACh during stimulation at 6.25 Hz for 20 min as rat diaphragms do under similar conditions, their rate of ACh release would have been less than 2 ng/min. The corresponding amount of vesiculin, if both substances had come only from synaptic vesicles, would have been less than 10 ng/min, an increment that could not have been detected in the presence of the baseline leak of more than 400 ng/min in the experiments of Musick and Hubbard.

ATP. BOYD and FORRESTER (1968) showed that ATP is released from frog sarto-rius muscle by motor nerve stimulation. They thought that the released nucleotide came from the muscle, not the nerve; and in fact there is evidence that ATP and other adenosine esters contribute to the vasodilatation that accompanies or follows mus-cular contraction (IMAI et al., 1964; FORRESTER and LIND, 1969; DOBSON et al., 1971). SILINSKY and HUBBARD (1973) also found in experiments on rat diaphragm that motor nerve stimulation released ATP. However, since they could detect such a release when the muscle was fully paralysed by tubocurarine they believed that it originated from the nerve. SILINSKY and HUBBARD detected no release of ATP on nerve stimulation from preparations bathed in a normal medium, probably because escaping ATP was quickly destroyed by endogenous ATPases. However, after these enzymes were inhibited by removing all of the magnesium and 95% of the calcium from the bathing medium, exposure of the preparation to hyperosmotic conditions (500 mosmol/l) released ACh, as expected, along with detectable quantities of ATP (about 8 pmol in 10 min). This figure for released ATP may well be an underestimate, because ATPase activity is probably not abolished by reducing the calcium concen-tration to 0.01 mmol/l (DOUGLAS and POISNER, 1966). Supposing however that it is correct, and that the ATP came from the same source as the quanta of ACh, one can make a rough calculation of the amount of ATP per quantum, on the basis of published estimates of m.e.p.p. frequency in rat diaphragm under the same conditions: this has been recorded as about 5/sec (HUBBARD et al., 1968). Taking the number of endplates in the muscle as 10^4, the ATP discharge during hyperosmotic stimulation would be about 150000 molecules per m.e.p.p., nearly 10 times the estimated ACh content of a quantum (pp. 131, 135), whereas the molar ratio ATP/ACh in cholinergic vesicles isolated from Torpedo is about 0.1 (WHITTAKER et al., 1972b). However rough the calculation, it clearly allows one to suppose that most of the ATP collected in the experiments of SILINSKY and HUBBARD, like most of the protein collected in the experiments of MUSICK and HUBBARD, came from sources other than the nerve terminals.

Experiments on the cat's superior cervical ganglion have failed to demonstrate the release of ATP (KATO et al., 1974). In that study, ATPase activity was inhibited by removing calcium and magnesium from the perfusion medium, while the divalent cation required for transmitter release was provided by adding barium; under these conditions ATP perfused through the ganglion was not destroyed. However, when the potassium content of the medium was elevated, or when the pre-ganglionic nerve was stimulated, ACh was released without ATP. In the best of these experiments, the nucleotide would have been detected if its molar ratio to ACh had been as much as 0.02. Thus if ACh is stored together with ATP in cholinergic nerve terminals of the ganglion, either the nucleotide is not released, or it is consumed intracellularly in some reaction related to transmitter release. The latter possibility is made more attractive by some recent experiments by ZIMMERMANN and WHITTAKER (1974a). They found that synaptic vesicles prepared from electroplaques that had been stimu-lated to deplete their ACh content had lost proportionately more ATP than total nucleotide, as if the release of transmitter were accompanied by utilization of vesicu-lar ATP. The lost ATP could have been used to supply the energy for exocytosis, or for some quite different purpose inside the nerve endings.

Thus the neurochemical approach, like the electrophysiological approach and the morphological approach, or indeed all three in combination, has so far failed to produce decisive evidence for or against the vesicular-exocytosis hypothesis.

F. Acetylcholine Turnover

The term "turnover" is a convenient one, but it has a precise meaning (Sparf, 1973) only when the compartment involved is specified and is in a steady state. In the case of ACh a steady state exists when synthesis plus influx is equal to breakdown plus efflux. This ideal situation may be hard to achieve in practice, because it often takes many minutes for the nerve-ending processes to reach a new steady state after an experimental alteration, for example a change in presynaptic impulse frequency or in cholinesterase activity. Indeed it can be argued that a single nerve ending considered over any short time interval is never really in a steady state, because ACh release is quantized and ACh synthesis probably is not. For these reasons the term will be used somewhat loosely in the present context.

In all the cases so far examined, the cholinergic nerve endings of vertebrates have a significant though low rate of ACh turnover during rest and a much higher rate during synaptic activation. [In cholinergic neurones of molluscs the turnover rates during activity may be no higher than during rest (Eisenstadt et al., 1975)]. The purpose of this section is to summarize the information about ACh turnover that has been obtained from studies on whole tissues, and to relate it as far as possible to the results of experiments in which ACh turnover was measured in subcellular fractions. A principal aim of experiments of the latter sort has been to determine which subcellular store of ACh represents the ACh that is immediately available for release by nerve impulses. As already noted, this aim has not yet been achieved; however these experiments have yielded valuable information which will have to be reinterpreted when the basic processes are more fully understood.

1. Tissue ACh Turnover during Rest and Activity

a) Ganglion

ACh turnover in ganglia at rest occurs at a measurable rate. The frequency of resting quantal discharge appears to be low (Blackman et al., 1963a, c; Nishi et al., 1967; Sacchi and Perri, 1973), and in a cat's superior cervical ganglion perfused with an eserine-containing medium the maintained rate of ACh discharge amounts to no more than 0.1 to 0.2% per min of the ganglion's initial ACh store (Birks and MacIntosh, 1961). This resting discharge is thought to originate from nerve endings in the ganglion, though it is possible that some of it comes from nerve trunks and other structures adjacent to the ganglion (Brown and Feldberg, 1936b; Evans and Saunders, 1974). However, this spontaneous release accounts for only part of the ACh turnover at rest, for there is also an intracellular turnover, which is greater. This can be revealed in either of two ways. (i) The ACh of a resting ganglion that is perfused with radioactive choline is gradually replaced by radioactive ACh. The rate of replacement is about 0.4% per min in the absence of an anticholinesterase

(COLLIER and MACINTOSH, 1969; COLLIER and KATZ, 1971). (ii) Surplus ACh formation in a resting ganglion exposed to a suitable anticholinesterase drug proceeds for an hour or so at a rate of about 1.5% of initial content per min. This rate is probably the best available measure of the ACh turnover rate in the absence of the drug (BIRKS and MACINTOSH, 1961; COLLIER and KATZ, 1971).

During synaptic activity ACh turnover is considerably accelerated. In an eserine-treated superior cervical ganglion the minute output of ACh under optimal conditions (plasma perfusion, stimulation at >15 Hz) can be maintained over a long period at about 8% of initial content per minute (BIRKS and MACINTOSH, 1961; MATTHEWS, 1966). A slightly higher maintained output may be possible for the superior cervical ganglion *in situ* without eserine, for MCCANDLESS et al. (1971) calculated a minute-output of about 11% from their electrophysiological data obtained under these conditions. As these minute-output values were obtained under near steady-state conditions, they should provide a good approximation to the maximum turnover rate for the ACh store as a whole. The ACh store is in fact maintained at close to its initial concentration in a ganglion stimulated for 1 to 2 hrs at up to 20 Hz in the absence of an anticholinesterase (BIRKS and MACINTOSH, 1961; FRIESEN and KHATTER, 1971a; BIRKS and FITCH, 1974; BOURDOIS et al., 1975), though it may suffer a small transient decline during the first few minutes (MACINTOSH, 1963).

Maintenance of the overall level of stored ACh does not imply that all the ACh compartments or pools within the store are equally well maintained and make an equal contribution to ACh turnover during activity. As noted earlier, there is evidence that this is not the case. Rather, it appears that a critical part of the store becomes depleted during high-frequency synaptic activity, and that its rate of replenishment is then the limiting factor for ACh turnover. In exceptional circumstances, however, the repletion may raise the store above its initial level, with a corresponding effect on ACh turnover.

The principal evidence for this is the following. (a) Short bursts of high-frequency stimulation (e.g., 500 volleys at 16 to 64 Hz) discharge ACh at very high rates, i.e. 0.2 to 0.8% of initial ACh content per second. However such output rates cannot be maintained, and with continued stimulation the minute output falls rapidly to the 8% per min level mentioned above, and remains there (BIRKS and MACINTOSH, 1961; MATTHEWS, 1966). (b) Correspondingly, the electrically recorded postsynaptic responses from ganglia stimulated at high frequency (MCCANDLESS et al., 1971; BENNETT and MCLACHLAN, 1972b) decay initially towards a steady level at which the transmitter output is about 40% of the initial value. (c) At higher frequencies of stimulation, e.g. 50 to 60 Hz, there is an early steep fall in the ACh content of a ganglion (ROSENBLUETH et al., 1939; FRIESEN and KHATTER, 1971a); this fall is followed by a rise up to and above the initial level, especially if an interval of rest is allowed (ROSENBLUETH et al., 1939; RANGACHARI et al., 1969; BOURDOIS et al., 1970, 1975; FRIESEN and KHATTER, 1971a; BIRKS and FITCH, 1974); the rise may last for many minutes or even hours (ROSENBLUETH et al., 1939; BOURDOIS et al., 1970, 1975; BIRKS and FITCH, 1974). (d) As might be expected from the above observations, and from the ease with which post-tetanic potentiation of presynaptic origin can be elicited at ganglionic synapses (ROSENBLUETH et al., 1939; LARRABEE and BRONK, 1947; DUNANT and DOLIVO, 1968), the minute output of ACh can be increased either during (Birks and Fitch, 1974) or as a consequence of (Bourdois et al., 1970, 1975) repetitive stimulation. In ganglia perfused with choline-Locke, the minute-output of ACh rises during the first few minutes of stimulation at 4 Hz and then becomes steady (Birks and Fitch, 1974); at higher frequencies, the early fall in release is the most conspicuous feature of the ACh output curve, but when the ganglion is again tested some time after a period of conditioning high-frequency stimulation the output is found to be above the control level (Bourdois et al., 1970, 1975).

In some of the experiments just discussed, differences in ACh output rate appear to be correlated with differences in ACh content, but in other cases no such correlation is obvious. Thus with ganglia perfused with a choline-Locke medium, the maintained rate of ACh release during prolonged stimulation is only half the initial rate, although tissue ACh is not measurably depleted at the end of the experiment (Birks and MacIntosh, 1961). If however the depletion occurred mainly in a "readily releasable" pool amounting to some 25% of the original total, even a halving of that pool would be undetectable by the usual measurements, because it would be masked by the concomitant accumulation of surplus ACh in an amount that would roughly equal the initial content (Birks and MacIntosh, 1961; Collier and Katz, 1971). In ganglia exposed to HC-3 and subjected to prolonged stimulation, each nerve impulse appears to release a constant proportion of the ACh in a shrinking "readily available" pool (Birks and MacIntosh, 1961). For the sake of convenience the variations in ACh output rate discussed in the preceding paragraph may be tentatively explained in terms of changes in the level of such an ACh pool. But it must be kept in mind that a change in ACh output can also reflect a change in the probability that any ACh molecule or quantum in the readily available pool will be released by the next impulse; such changes can also be induced experimentally (see Chapter 3 in this volume).

In theory, ACh turnover in a tissue under steady-state conditions is equal to ACh synthesis, which can be measured if either of the two substrates of ChAc is isotopically labelled to known specific activity and if the rate at which the label is incorporated into ACh is measured. In practice, the use of labelled choline is likely to lead to a gross underestimate of ACh turnover, because the labelled choline is diluted by an unknown but large amount of endogenous choline, which is unlabelled. In the experiments of Collier and MacIntosh (1969), for example, preganglionic stimulation increased [^{3}H] choline incorporation into ACh by a factor of 5 or 6. However the experiments were performed in the absence of an anticholinesterase agent, so that the re-use of choline from hydrolysed ACh was not eliminated; the measured rate of choline acetylation, about 2% of ACh store per minute, was thus certainly less than half the actual rate. With good design this source of error can be kept to a minimum, even for *in vivo* experiments (Saelens et al., 1973; Sparf, 1973), but this has not yet been undertaken for ACh turnover studies in ganglia.

b) Skeletal Muscle

One major paper by Potter (1970a) presents most of the data on ACh turnover in muscle that have been obtained by measuring ACh directly. Potter, using the rat phrenic nerve-diaphragm preparation, performed biological and radiometric assays in parallel, and his results and conclusions were remarkably similar to those reported for ganglia. Thus in the absence of a cholinesterase inhibitor, tissue ACh in the resting diaphragm could be labelled from [^{14}C]choline in the medium at a rate of about 0.5% per min, and nerve stimulation could raise the rate to about 3% per min; the corresponding figures for ganglia were 0.4% and 2% per min (COLLIER and MACINTOSH, 1969; COLLIER and KATZ, 1971). In the presence of eserine, surplus ACh accumulated in the resting muscles, so that the total ACh doubled in an hour or so, as in ganglia. This suggested that intracellular turnover at rest might be as high as 1.5% per min, which is rather higher than the observed rate of spontaneous ACh release. ACh output during a 5 min period of stimulation at 20 Hz averaged 7% of the store per min, a rate within the range reported for experiments on plasma-perfused ganglia. Whether ACh turnover could have been maintained at this rate indefinitely is open to question, though the 5 min stimulation did not measurably deplete tissue ACh in POTTER's experiments; 25% depletion was reported (MACIN-TOSH, 1963) for cat leg muscles stimulated *in vivo* at 20 Hz for 30 min in the presence of gallamine. Since POTTER (1970a) found a fourfold higher rate of ACh release during bursts of stimulation lasting only 18 sec, it seems likely that stimulation for 5 min or more would have caused some depletion, at least within a small readily-releasable part of the ACh depot, as has been concluded also from comparable electrophysiological experiments (BROOKS and THIES, 1962; ELMQVIST and QUASTEL, 1965b; ČAPEK et al., 1971). On the other hand POTTER's figure of 7% for the minute-output cannot have been much in excess of the maximum rate of ACh turnover that his stimulated diaphragms could achieve, for they were able to accumulate radioactive ACh, and later to release it, at about 3% of their total ACh content per min. The true turnover rate must have been higher than this because endogenous unlabelled choline would have made some contribution. It is of interest that ČAPEK et al. (1971), who used their electrophysiological data to calculate maximum ACh turnover rates in stimulated rat diaphragms, obtained a value of 6% of store per min, while ELM-QVIST and QUASTEL (1965b) concluded from their analysis of quantum release in human intercostal muscles that the apparent rate at which quanta were made available for mobilization was about 3% per min of the quanta ultimately available.

POTTER's (1970a) experiments clearly confirmed that ACh in diaphragm preparations can be labelled from choline (SAELENS and STOLL, 1965), but other studies have failed to show this (CHANG and LEE, 1970; MCCARTY et al., 1973). It may be suggested that the negative results were due to dilution of the radioactive choline by endogenous choline. The rat diaphragm preparation contains, or forms, enough free choline to support ACh synthesis during phrenic nerve stimulation for long periods of time, even when neostigmine is present to prevent recycling of choline (STRAUGH-AN, 1960). POTTER (1970a) washed his diaphragm preparations for 4 hr with choline-free medium to remove endogenous choline before he added [^{14}C] choline, but CHANG and LEE (1970) and MCCARTY and his colleagues (1973) did not. MCCARTY et al. did find that their labelled choline was incorporated into junctional phospholipids: it seems unlikely, however, that these would turn over more rapidly than ACh, or would derive their choline from a completely different pool. A more probable explanation is that the labelling of phospholipid choline was via the calcium-dependent choline-exchange reaction described in a number of recent papers (LUNT and LAPETINA, 1970; ABDEL-LATIF and SMITH, 1972; MILLER and DAWSON, 1972; ABDEL-LATIF et al., 1973), rather than as a result of phospholipid synthesis *de novo*.

c) Brain

The turnover of brain ACh in conscious animals has been calculated from its rate of labelling after injection of isotopically labelled choline. Such calculations assume that free choline in the brain can be regarded as a single pool, with which blood-borne choline is rapidly equilibrated. Theoretically the assumption must be wrong, but in practice the errors that arise from making it are not as large as might be expected. On this basis, three separate studies have shown that the ACh of brain turns over once every 1 to 2 min on the average (Schuberth et al., 1969, 1970; Saelens et al., 1973; Jenden et al., 1974), about 10 times as fast as the most rapid rate in ganglia or muscles. Sparf (1973), who gives a valuable discussion of the validity of such measurements, points out that the calculated rates for rat brain, though possibly underestimates, are only about 25% of the maximal rate at which the ChAc of the brain can synthesise ACh *in vitro* (Schrier and Shuster, 1967). Even higher turnover rates may be possible *in vivo*: in the experiments of Richter and Crossland (1949), brain ACh recovered, after depletion by electrical stimulation, at a rate sufficient to support a turnover time of less than 30 sec, close to the theoretical maximum.

Though cholinergic nerve terminals in brain can achieve much higher ACh turn-over rates than those in ganglia or muscles, they are less efficient at maintaining their ACh stores at a nearly constant level during variations in synaptic activity. This is apparent from both *in vivo* and *in vitro* experiments, and suggests that in brain the readily releasable ACh accounts for a much larger fraction of the ACh store than in peripheral tissues. *In vivo*, the ACh content of rat brain varies inversely with the animal's functional activity: thus anaesthetics increase the content and convulsants lower it (see for example Tobias et al., 1946; Richter and Crossland, 1949; Elliott et al., 1950; Giarman and Pepeu, 1962; Szerb et al., 1970). Correspondingly, ACh release from the brain surface is lower in anaesthetized than in conscious animals (Celesia and Jasper, 1966; Collier and Mitchell, 1967; Beani et al., 1968), and labelled choline from the blood stream is incorporated more slowly into brain ACh (Schuberth et al., 1970). *In vitro*, raising the potassium content of the medium depletes the ACh content of brain slices or minces but increases both release and synthesis (Mann et al., 1938; Welsh and Hyde, 1944; Brodkin and Elliott, 1953; Bertel-Meeuws and Polak, 1968). Radiochemical measurements of ACh turnover in brain tissue support the same conclusion (Browning and Schulman, 1968; Sharkawi and Schulman, 1969; Grewaal and Quastel, 1973; Lefresne et al., 1973). In these experiments the tissue ACh was labelled on the acetyl moiety by means of radioactive glucose or pyruvate added to the medium, with the intention of bypassing the difficulties that arise when radioactive choline is used as source of the label for ACh. One puzzling feature of some of these experiments remains unexplained, however: although the specific activity of the ACh released into the medium appeared to match that of the labelled glucose or pyruvate, as if only newly-synthesized ACh had been released, the amount of radioactive ACh retained in the tissue equalled, or even exceeded, the total tissue ACh measured by bioassay (Browning and Schulman, 1968; Lefresne et al., 1973). In both cases the tissue must have contained unlabelled ACh to start with, and this should have diluted the labelled ACh that was released or retained.

d) Electric Organ

Torpedo electroplaques have been used for cell fractionation and *in vitro* ACh labelling studies for some time, but it is only recently that the intact organ has been used for the study of ACh turnover in relation to nerve stimulation. Discussion of the results obtained by DUNANT et al. (1971, 1972), ISRAËL et al. (1972) and ZIMMERMANN and WHITTAKER (1874a, b) will be deferred to a later subsection (pp. 163—165).

e) Other Tissues

There is a considerable body of work, starting with the papers of LE HEUX (1918, 1921a, b) on ACh turnover in the intestinal wall (for references see PATON and ZAR, 1968); but since most of the wall's layers contain cholinergic elements (FELDBERG and LIN, 1950), studies of ACh metabolism were rather unrewarding until a tissue preparation with a reasonably well-defined population of synapses became available. The innervated longitudinal muscle strip from the guinea-pig ileum (PATON and ZAR, 1968) is such a preparation: it contains some ganglionic synapses (PATON and ZAR, 1968; KOSTERLITZ and WATERFIELD, 1973) but most of its ACh turnover probably occurs at postganglionic terminations. So far only bioassay methods have been used. ACh output at rest, as a percentage of tissue ACh, is similar to that of a perfused ganglion, about 0.1 to 0.2% per min (PATON et al., 1971); the lower figure is the average for experiments in which hexamethonium or tetrodotoxin was used to suppress impulses in the postganglionic axons. Stimulation at 10 Hz, or contact with a solution containing a high (49 mmol/l) concentration of potassium, increases output roughly 10-fold and turnover almost as much, since tissue stores are fairly well maintained; but turnover rates comparable to the maximum rates observed with ganglia or diaphragms have not yet been reported. A remarkable feature of ACh metabolism in these terminals of AUERBACH's plexus is the steep decline of ACh output per volley as stimulation frequency increases: this holds even at frequencies of less than 1 Hz (COWIE et al., 1968; PATON and ZAR, 1968; KOSTERLITZ and WATERFIELD, 1970, 1973; KNOLL and VIZI, 1971). If the interval between stimuli is a minute or more, the ACh liberated by a single stimulus can be measured quite easily, for it is about 1% of the store (KOSTERLITZ and WATERFIELD, 1973); a second volley coming as much as 40 sec later liberates much less. This extraordinarily slow replenishment of the transmitter pool that is available for release by the next nerve impulse has no parallel elsewhere in mammalian cholinergic physiology, so far as our present knowledge goes. Radiometric studies of the phenomenon could hardly fail to give interesting results.

Other parasympathetically innervated tissues for which preliminary data on ACh turnover are available include the salivary glands of the cat (EMMELIN and MUREN, 1950) and rat (HANIN et al., 1972a, b) and the vas deferens of the rat (KNOLL et al., 1972).

2. Preferential Release of Newly Synthesized ACh

Experiments on the cat superior cervical ganglion first suggested that newly-synthesized ACh might be released preferentially (COLLIER and MACINTOSH, 1969; COLLIER, 1969). In these experiments the ACh of a perfused ganglion was initially labelled to a

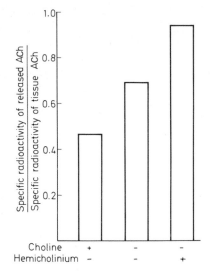

Fig. 8. The specific radioactivity of ACh released from cat superior cervical ganglia expressed as a fraction of the specific radioactivity of ganglionic ACh. Ganglia had been perfused with [³H] choline to label tissue stores of ACh (see COLLIER and MACINTOSH, 1969); released ACh was collected during preganglionic nerve stimulation (20 Hz for 20 min), in the presence or absence of choline or in the presence of HC-3

nearly constant specific activity by stimulation in the presence of [³H] choline; the perfusion medium was then replaced by one that contained unlabelled choline, to support ACh synthesis, and an anticholinesterase agent to preserve released ACh. Under these conditions, the ACh released by preganglionic stimulation was less radioactive than the ACh in the tissue; but the difference became smaller when a choline-free medium was perfused during the test stimulation, and it was almost eliminated when HC-3 was added to such a perfusion medium (Fig. 8). These results were taken to mean that most of the ACh turnover during high-frequency synaptic activity is in a rather small part of the ACh store. BIRKS and MACINTOSH (1961), noting that the ganglion's releasable ACh behaved as if it were located in two pools, suggested that the more and less readily releasable pools might be in series, with the latter replenishing the former during prolonged stimulations. However, this model is unacceptable without major modification if released ACh is replaced mainly by new synthesis rather than from a reserve store. The size of the ACh pool in which turnover is fast is not exactly known: COLLIER's (1972) estimate of it was 25 to 33% of the total ACh content of the superior cervical ganglion, about the same as BIRKS and MACINTOSH's (1961) estimate for the readily-releasable pool.

Birks and Fitch (1974) have recently suggested that such estimates were grossly in error, because they overlooked the accumulation of unlabelled ACh that must have occurred in the interval between replacement of the ganglion's endogenous ACh with radioactive ACh and the test stimulation which released ACh for measurement of its specific activity. BIRKS and FITCH found that after an hour's stimulation even at a frequency as low as 20 Hz, as in the experiments of COLLIER and MACINTOSH (1969) and COLLIER (1969), the ganglion's total store of ACh could increase by about 40% ("rebound" ACh, cf. p. 188), and this additional ACh was releasable; using this figure they calculated that the earlier results were compatible with a single-compartment model, so that there was no need to postulate preferential release of any fraction of the depot ACh. BIRKS and FITCH's criticism appears to be valid for the results published by COLLIER and MACINTOSH (1969), but not for those published by COLLIER (1969), who compared the specific radioactivity of the released ACh with that of the ACh left in the tissue at the end of the experiment. To bring COLLIER's results within range of the criticism, it would have to be supposed that the "rebound" ACh was released by the test stimulation but not replaced. The data of BIRKS and FITCH (1974) appear to show that it was both released and replenished, as if ACh turnover were proceeding normally but with an inflated total tissue content. Other experiments can be devised that would test this important point more decisively, and final judgement should perhaps be deferred until this has been done.

The preferential release of newly-synthesized ACh has also been reported for the neuromuscular junction. In POTTER's (1970a) experiments, diaphragms whose ACh had been almost completely labelled from [^{14}C] choline were then stimulated either in the presence or in the absence of unlabelled choline. With neostigmine added in both cases, almost twice as much labelled ACh was released into the choline-free medium as into the choline-containing one. While POTTER did not measure total ACh release in these experiments, it is very unlikely that the added choline reduced ACh release. A more plausible explanation is that it accelerated the turnover of a relatively small pool within the ACh store, and so caused the preferential release of the newly-made ACh that had just entered that pool.

Other cholinergic synapses may also release newly synthesized transmitter preferentially. ACh released from the electric organ of Torpedo after incomplete labelling of the store has a higher specific activity than the remaining store (DUNANT et al., 1972). Similar results have been obtained with brain slices (MOLENAAR et al., 1971, 1973a; RICHTER and MARCHBANKS, 1971a) and with brain *in vivo* (WHITTAKER, 1969). There appears also to be a selective release of newly-synthesized catecholamines from adrenergic nerve endings (KOPIN et al., 1968; STJÄRNE and WENNMALM, 1970) and from the adrenal medulla (WINKLER et al., 1971). Thus the phenomenon may be a general feature of chemically transmitting synapses.

The preferential release of newly synthesized transmitter is not in itself strong evidence for or against the hypothesis of vesicular exocytosis as the principal mechanism for quantized transmitter release. Those who support the hypothesis can suppose that the transmitter pool that turns over rapidly is in a particular subpopulation of vesicles, such as those that are closely apposed to the presynaptic membrane, while those who dislike the hypothesis can argue that the fast-turnover pool is cytoplasmic ACh, with vesicular ACh representing a highly concentrated but relatively static reserve store. There is, of course, no doubt that vesicular ACh is releasable *eventually*: this is shown by the fact that nearly all the ACh store can be released by nerve activity, and that the vesicular pool, where it can be measured, accounts for at least half the total.

3. ACh Turnover in Relation to Changes in Ultrastructure

If ACh quanta are released from synaptic vesicles by exocytosis, one might expect the immediate result of an acceleration of release to be a fall in the number of vesicles in parallel with a fall in the amount of stored ACh. If however the released quanta come from an extravesicular source, one would not expect much change in the number of vesicles, though the vesicles might become smaller if their ACh were used to replenish the releasable pool. In either case, the changes just described would be more striking if the stimulation were more intense or prolonged, and especially if synthesis of new ACh were prevented, for example by giving HC-3. The two major assumptions one has to make if one proposes to rely on the electronmicroscopic evidence are that full vesicles will look different from emptied ones, and that fixing the tissue for microscopy does not alter vesicle numbers.

In most of the earlier ultrastructural studies on cholinergic junctions (e.g. Birks et al., 1960), stimulation did not produce striking or consistent changes. Hubbard and Kwanbunbumpen (1968) however found that treatment with 20 mmol/l potassium chloride reduced the vesicle count in rat diaphragm nerve endings: the number of vesicles located opposite postsynaptic junctional folds, and presumed to be favourably placed for discharge, was also reduced. The reduction was not very great (about 25%), but it was prevented by magnesium, and so it seemed to be related to transmitter release. Jones and Kwanbunbumpen (1970a), in a limited number of experiments on the same preparation, found vesicle counts not much affected by nerve stimulation (11 Hz for 90 min), but reduced by an hour's contact with HC-3, and more strikingly reduced by 90 min of stimulation in the presence of HC-3: the reductions were by about 11% and 45% respectively. The latter figure might seem smaller than one would have expected, for on the basis of Potter's result there should have been an almost total depletion of the releasable ACh in the terminals. However, Jones and Kwanbunbumpen (1970a) also found that the individual vesicles in these tests were less than half their original size, so the agreement between ACh measurements and morphology might be regarded as acceptable.

Two important papers on ultrastructural alterations in stimulated frog muscles will be referred to only briefly, because of the absence of comparable neurochemical data for such muscles. Ceccarelli et al. (1973), who used curarized cutaneous pectoris muscles, found that vesicle counts were little changed by several hours' stimulation at 2 Hz, though transmitter stores appeared from electrophysiological findings to be severely depleted; after 20 min stimulation at 10 Hz the nerve terminals were swollen and many vesicles were lost. Heuser and Reese (1973), who used curarized sartorius muscles stimulated at 10 Hz, found that vesicle counts were reduced by 30% after stimulation for 1 min and by 60% after stimulation for 15 min; these values correlated well with the rundown of e.p.p. size and thus, perhaps, with the depletion of releasable ACh. A loss of ACh during stimulation without HC-3 would be at variance with Potter's (1970a) results on mammalian muscle, but neither Ceccarelli and his colleagues nor Heuser and Reese added choline to their media, and this deficiency may have retarded transmitter replenishment. In addition, the Ringer's solution used by Heuser and Reese was unbuffered, and stimulation might have caused serious local alterations of pH. Both the paper by Heuser and Reese and the one by Ceccarelli and his co-workers have provided valuable evidence for the recycling of vesicular membrane material after fusion with the presynaptic membrane, and for an accelerated uptake (Holtzman et al., 1971) of macromolecular labels from the extracellular space during stimulation. Such observations are compatible with vesicular exocytosis but do not prove it; vesicles could rupture and discharge their contents intracellularly before fusing with the plasma membrane, and pinocytotic uptake of macromolecules could be associated with the re-formation rather than the exocytosis of vesicles. The studies on frog sartorius muscles of LON-GENECKER et al. (1970) and CLARK et al. (1972), using black widow spider venom, were referred to earlier: they showed a clear correlation between depletion of vesicles and exhaustion of the capacity for quantal release, and it would be attractive to suppose that the venom's primary action is to interfere with the re-formation of vesicles. However this is by no means proven, and other possibilities remain open; for example, the venom might open extravesicular channels in the presynaptic membrane through which ACh quanta escape, and the loss of vesicles could then be secondary to loss of cytoplasmic ACh.

Several studies on the superior cervical ganglion have reported that preganglionic nerve stimulation reduces the number of vesicles in the axon terminals (PARDUCZ and FEHÉR, 1970; BIRKS, 1971, 1974; FRIESEN and KHATTER, 1971b; PARDUCZ et al., 1971; PERRI et al., 1972; PYSH and WILEY, 1972), but the morphological changes do not correlate particularly well with the changes in ACh content. Thus vesicle counts are depleted by stimulation at 20 Hz (BIRKS, 1971, 1974; PERRI et al., 1972; PYSH and WILEY, 1972) but there is little depletion of tissue ACh with such stimulation (BIRKS and MACINTOSH, 1961; MACINTOSH, 1963; MATTHEWS, 1966; FRIESEN and KHATTER, 1971a) unless ACh synthesis is inhibited. Prolonged stimulation in the presence of HC-3 depletes tissue ACh by 80 to 90%, but apparently is not much more effective in reducing vesicle counts than stimulation without HC-3 (PYSH and WILEY, 1972). Better agreement between vesicle counts and ACh content was reported in some of the experiments of PARDUCZ and his co-workers (1971). With stimulation at 20 Hz for 30 to 60 min the number of vesicles did not change unless HC-3 had been given, when the number fell to about 16% of the control value, which fits very well with the results of BIRKS and MACINTOSH (1961). In other experiments by PARDUCZ et al. (1971) the ultrastructural findings correlated less well with the neurochemical ones: thus stimulation during perfusion with a choline-free medium lowered vesicle counts to the same extent as when HC-3 was present, although there is much less reduction of tissue ACh in the former case than in the latter (BIRKS and MACINTOSH, 1961). PERRI and his co-workers (1972) found that stimulation altered the distribution as well as the number of the vesicles in their rat ganglia: the smallest reduction of the count was observed in the zone closest to the synaptic membrane, as if the more distant vesicles had moved towards sites of release, a result apparently the opposite of the one that HUBBARD and KWANBUNBUMPEN(1968) reported for the neuromuscular junction.

The most recent report on superior cervical ganglion ultrastructure, and in some ways the most thorough, is the one by BIRKS (1974). He used magnesium in high concentration to preserve synaptic morphology during fixation; the procedure gives better retention of tissue ACh. (Magnesium might act here as a calcium antagonist, as it does when it suppresses evoked ACh release, but whether extracellular or intracellular calcium is mainly involved is not known.) BIRKS's micrographs of magnesium-treated nerve endings are striking: a large part of each bouton profile is occupied by the outlines of vesicles packed very closely together. This had to be ascribed to better preservation of the vesicles, rather than to shrinkage of boutons or swelling of vesicles during fixation, for the areas of both boutons and vesicles were the same as in conventionally fixed tissues. In all Birks's experiments, stimulation lowered the vesicle count: the effect was significant even at physiological (e.g. 1 to 4 Hz) frequencies; with stimulation for 20 min at 20 Hz, the number of vesicles fell to about 25% of control, whether or not HC-3 was present, though in its absence the ACh content must have remained at near the resting level, while in its presence the content must have fallen by at least 50%. Under these conditions of measurement, clearly, there was no correlation between ACh content and vesicle numbers, and Birks's results suggest that previous reports on vesicle abundance may have been subject to unknown but large counting errors, which in turn resulted from loss of vesicles at the time of tissue fixation. Some of the quantitative discrepancies mentioned above may have arisen in this way, and other examples could be given: thus Pysh and Wiley (1972) and Parducz et al. (1971) obtained vesicle counts in resting ganglia that averaged 66 and 232 per μm^2 respectively, though both groups worked with the cat superior cervical ganglion left *in situ* with its blood supply intact, and their published pictures do not suggest that their tissue sections were of very different thickness. The most obvious way to account for all these findings, and especially those of Birks (1974), is to suppose, as Birks himself points out, that during repetitive activity most of the nerve ending ACh is located in the terminal cytosol and is released from it directly. To reconcile the findings with the vesicular-exocytosis hypothesis requires further postulates, for which at present there is no direct evidence. Thus, one could propose that though Birks's high-magnesium fixation preserves vesicles in resting nerve endings, it is less successful with repetitively-activated nerve endings, which would contain much more trapped calcium. Alternatively one could postulate that the number of quanta released depends more on the number of release sites activated than on the number of vesicles present, so that exocytosis might proceed at an adequate rate even with a greatly reduced vesicle population; loss of vesicles could be caused by intracellular disruption as well as by exocytosis. Still other more or less plausible schemes can be put forward, but will not be mentioned here; the main purpose of these paragraphs is to point out that the morphological evidence referred to above can be reconciled with either of the two principal hypotheses for quantal transmitter release.

Another interesting discrepancy between synaptic-vesicle numbers and ACh release comes from the study by Landmesser and Pilar (1972) of the development of transmission processes in the chick ciliary ganglion. Transmission in this structure is chemical at first, but few synaptic vesicles can be seen; later on, after hatching, transmission is 80% electrical, but there is a striking increase in the number of vesicles.

4. ACh Turnover as Studied by Cell Fractionation Techniques

In principle, information about the intracellular site of storage of releasable ACh should be obtainable by measuring the turnover of ACh in subcellular fractions prepared from a tissue rich in cholinergic endings; this information together with measurements of ACh release should also identify the sites of release.

In practice, there are difficulties about this. One approach to the problem is to label the various nerve-ending pools of ACh to different levels of specific radioactivity, then to measure the release of ACh, and try to match the specific activity of the released ACh with that of one or another of the labelled pools. The difficulty here is that the pools identified *in vivo* may not correspond to the fractions isolated *in vitro*. It is not impossible, for example, that some vesicles because of their location might release and regain ACh faster than the remaining vesicles. Thus if the conditions used to label tissue ACh are such that not all of the vesicular ACh is labelled to equilibrium, subsequent stimulation could release ACh of a higher specific activity than the ACh of the vesicle fraction; and unless there were some way of separating the "hotter" vesicles from the others, one might be tempted to conclude that the released ACh did not originate from vesicles. If on the other hand equilibrium loading is achieved, all the ACh pools will probably have the same specific activity, and the experiments will not identify the source of ACh released.

A second approach is to cause the release of ACh under conditions which prevent its replenishment, and then to measure the extent to which each of the fractions has become depleted. The main difficulty here is that of ensuring there is no exchange of ACh between the fractions in the interval between depletion and separation.

A third approach, which has not been much used, is to expand one pool selectively, see whether release is affected, and then look for a change in the distribution of ACh between the fractions. An example is the use of an anticholinesterase drug to promote the accumulation of surplus ACh.

It will be convenient to consider first the electric organ, as the only tissue so far from which cholinergic vesicles can be isolated in quantity and relative purity. Synaptosomes, harvested from whole brain or brain regions, will next be examined, then brain slices, whose behaviour is closer to that of intact brain tissue, and finally brain *in situ*. Muscles, ganglia and other peripheral tissues cannot be included, because they have not yet been studied in this way.

a) Electric Organ

The electric organ of *Torpedo* contains ACh that can be separated upon homogenization into two main fractions: "free", which is ACh lost during homogenization, and "bound", practically all of which is ACh contained in synaptic vesicles (ISRAËL et al., 1970). (Because this tissue is so rich in AChE, its free ACh cannot be satisfactorily quantitated by assaying the supernatant from a homogenate prepared in the presence of an anticholinesterase: instead, free ACh is measured as the difference between bound ACh and total ACh.) When slices of electric organ were incubated with radioactive choline, labelled ACh was synthesized, and the free ACh was labelled to higher specific activity than the bound ACh (MARCHBANKS and ISRAËL, 1971). The greater specific activity of the free ACh was especially obvious when the slices had been stimulated electrically in the presence of [^{14}C] choline (DUNANT et al., 1972). This pattern of labelling of the two ACh fractions resembles the labelling of cytoplasmic and vesicular ACh in incubated brain slices (see pp. 166—167), and it suggests that under these conditions free ACh turns over more rapidly than bound ACh. In support of this, it was shown that during intermittent stimulation the labelling of free ACh fluctuated but the labelling of bound ACh remained fairly constant. However, when slices of electric organ were incubated with [^{14}C] choline and then washed and stimulated, the specific activity of the ACh released was greater than the specific activity of either free or bound ACh in the tissue (DUNANT et al., 1972). These results indicate that the turnover of free ACh is to a large extent independent of the turnover of bound ACh, while the high specific activity of the released ACh must imply that ACh newly synthesized from residual $[^{14}C]$ choline was not fully mixed with either the free or the bound fraction before it was released.

Dunant and his colleagues made a further attempt to characterize releasable ACh in terms of the bound and free fractions by experiments in which they stimulated the nerve supplying the intact electric organ. During repetitive stimulation the electrical responses declined, so that none could be recorded after about 1500 stimuli. This failure of response could be ascribed to diminished ACh release (Feldberg and Fessard, 1942), rather than to diminished postsynaptic sensitivity to ACh, for the spontaneous junctional potentials were of normal amplitude. The decline of the electrical response during stimulation was paralleled by the depletion of free ACh, while there was little change in bound ACh. Bound ACh, however, could be reduced by continuing the stimulation after the evoked electrical response had disappeared (Dunant et al., 1972; Israël et al., 1972; Dunant et al., 1974).

These experiments on *Torpedo* by Dunant, Israël and their colleagues are noteworthy in that they are the only experiments that clearly showed that vesicular ACh, as isolated by conventional fractionation techniques, contributes little to physiological ACh release under the experimental conditions specified. But it would be premature to conclude that physiologically released ACh comes only from the cytoplasm, even in *Torpedo*.

In the first place, it has been shown (Marchbanks and Israël, 1972) that the monodisperse vesicle fraction isolated from electric-organ slices that have been exposed to radioactive choline contains two ACh compartments; one of these, the smaller and more loosely bound fraction, has about the same specific activity as the free ACh, but can apparently exchange under *in vitro* conditions with the more firmly bound ACh of the larger compartment. Marchbanks and Israël (see also Marchbanks, 1973) argue that the vesicular ACh is heterogeneous not because there are two kinds of vesicle, but because there are two kinds of vesicular ACh, namely a loosely bound surface layer and a tightly bound core. The former but not the latter might be the source of released ACh, but since the two can slowly exchange, the ACh of the core could fill the role of the reserve pool within the ACh depot, in schemes like the one proposed by Birks and MacIntosh (1961).

Secondly, reference must be made to the recent work of Zimmermann and Whittaker (1974a, b), who also fractionated the electric organ after stimulating it *in situ*. They found, as did Dunant et al. (1972), that during continuous stimulation successive electrical responses decayed steeply, but in Zimmermann and Whittaker's experiments vesicle counts and vesicle diameters also fell, and the presynaptic membrane area increased as if vesicle membranes were being recycled. Harvesting of the vesicular fraction at this stage (50% reduction of vesicle count) showed little change in protein concentration but a drastic fall (90%) in ACh and ATP concentrations, with both free and bound fractions of ACh falling sooner than ATP. Recovery from this situation was slow. The postsynaptic response to single stimuli was restored first, in 5 hrs, then the number and diameter of the vesicles (24 hrs), then ACh and last ATP (3 days); the ability to respond to repetitive excitation was correspondingly slow to recover.

It would be unwise to suppose that ACh turnover in mammalian nerve endings is governed by the same factors as in *Torpedo* nerve endings, especially in view of the latter's very slow recovery from repeated excitation. But for *Torpedo* itself, a fairly strong case can be made for the involvement of the vesicles in ACh release as well as ACh storage. If so, however, release can hardly involve the discharge of their entire internal content. Either an outer layer of ACh is removed, as MARCHBANKS and ISRAËL (1972) propose, or there is a labile subpopulation of vesicles, as ZIMMERMANN and WHITTAKER (1974a) have suggested. A third possibility is that vesicles fusing with the synaptic membrane may provide a channel of discharge for the smaller molecules (ACh, perhaps ATP, but not protein) within contiguous vesicles. This last possibility might help to account for differential depletion of substances held within the vesicles, and for the discrepancy, at present embarrassingly large, between estimates of ACh in a quantum and ACh in a vesicle. As for the slow recovery of vesicular ACh after depletion, it can be supposed that this is mainly due to the time required for the replenishment of vesicles, for there is no shortage of ChAc in the nerve endings, and it does not seem likely that the supply of either choline or acetyl-CoA would be a limiting factor.

b) Isolated Synaptosomes

When synaptosomes that have been harvested from brain are incubated with radioactive choline, they synthesize and retain labelled ACh (MARCHBANKS, 1968b, 1969; RITCHIE and GOLDBERG, 1970; HAGA, 1971; YAMAMURA and SNYDER, 1972; HAGA and NODA, 1973; KUHAR et al., 1973). By subjecting the synaptosomes to hypoosmotic shock it can be shown that most of the newly-synthesized radioactive ACh is in the cytoplasm; only 3 to 15% of it is recovered in the vesicle fraction (MARCHBANKS, 1969; RITCHIE and GOLDBERG, 1970; HAGA, 1971). This differential labelling of cytoplasmic and vesicular ACh shows that the two pools do not mix readily in this *in vitro* situation, but it does not follow that they have different turnover rates even *in vitro;* if the cytoplasm is able to retain more ACh than was present initially but the vesicles are not, the cytoplasm would be better labelled than the vesicles from the added radioactive choline. However, with synaptosomes so prepared it should be possible to distinguish between release of cytoplasmic ACh and release of vesicular ACh.

Such an experiment was undertaken by HAGA (1971), who used synaptosomes that had been exposed to [^{14}C] choline. Only about 3% of the [^{14}C] ACh synthesized by the synaptosomes was found in the vesicular fraction, but when the synaptosomes were treated with high K$^+$ they released about 25% of their labelled ACh, while the efflux of unchanged [^{14}C] choline was little affected. It is unlikely that the treatment with potassium mobilised [^{14}C] ACh from cytoplasm into vesicles as a prelude to its release, for synaptosomes that had been pre-incubated with [^{14}C] choline in a high-potassium medium released less [^{14}C] ACh than did control synaptosomes when they were subsequently challenged with potassium. The released ACh therefore came from the cytoplasm. However, whether the mechanism of its release had anything in common with the mechanism by which nerve impulses (or K$^+$ ions) release ACh from normal nerve endings may be seriously doubted, for HAGA found that the release occurred also in the absence of ionized calcium (EGTA present), whereas evoked ACh release *in vivo* is strictly calcium-dependent. The behaviour of cytoplasmic ACh could be similar to that of surplus ACh in ganglia, which might be released from nerve endings by potassium but is not released by nerve stimulation (Collier and Katz, 1971). Unfortunately Haga (1971) measured only radioactive ACh, so if his treatment of synaptosomes with potassium had released vesicular ACh together with cytoplasmic [^{14}C] ACh he would not have detected it. De Belleroche and Bradford (1972), who used bioassay techniques to measure the ACh released from isolated synaptosomes, showed that the release evoked by either raised potassium or electrical pulses was much reduced in the absence of calcium ions, so it is quite possible that potassium treatment releases vesicular ACh from synaptosomes by a calcium-dependent mechanism and cytoplasmic ACh by a second mechanism that is independent of calcium. Clearly it would be useful to combine radiochemical and bioassay (or chemical assay) techniques for experiments on ACh turnover in synaptosomes. Indeed without such experiments, preferably on synaptosomes from ACh-rich brain regions, no meaningful conclusions about the physiological mechanisms of ACh release can be drawn from studies on isolated synaptosomes.

c) Brain Slices

The incubation of brain slices with radioactive precursors labels tissue ACh, and at least part of the labelled ACh is released when the slices are transferred to a medium containing a high concentration of potassium (Browning and Schulman, 1968; Richter and Marchbanks, 1971a; Grewaal and Quastel, 1973). With [^{3}H] choline as precursor, vesicular and cytoplasmic ACh are labelled to about the same specific activity when a normal medium is used for the incubation (Richter and Marchbanks, 1971b; Collier et al., 1972). Under these conditions, therefore, the two pools either exchange readily, or turn over at the same rate while using the same source of choline for ACh synthesis. A different result is obtained when a high-potassium medium is used for the incubation: cytoplasmic ACh is then labelled to a higher specific activity than vesicular ACh (Richter and Marchbanks, 1971b), as if the two pools do not exchange readily under these conditions. Thus it appears that during stimulation by potassium cytoplasmic ACh turns over more rapidly than vesicular ACh; this is the opposite of what might be expected if the ACh that is released by potassium was vesicular.

In parallel experiments, Richter and Marchbanks (1971a) measured the specific activity of the ACh released from brain slices by potassium treatment and found it higher than the specific activity of either the vesicular or the cytoplasmic fraction; Molenaar et al. (1973a, b) subsequently obtained a similar result. Thus the vesicular and cytoplasmic fractions isolated by subcellular fractionation techniques are not identical with the store in the tissues from which newly-synthesized ACh is preferentially released.

Part of the difficulty of interpreting such experiments arises from the heterogeneity of the tissue, in which cholinergic elements form only a small part. Nevertheless it should be possible, at least in theory, to use fractionation techniques to identify the highly radioactive pool from which released ACh is derived. Richter and Marchbanks (1971b) found when they attempted to do this that such a pool was associated with their vesicle fractions, but was distinct from the rest of the vesicular ACh. This was shown when isolated vesicles from a tissue that had been incubated with [^{3}H] choline were passed through an iso-osmotic Sephadex column: most of the bioassay-able ACh, but little of the radioactive ACh, remained with the vesicles. RICHTER and MARCHBANKS (1971 b) noted that the radioactive ACh might have been in a surface layer, or in a small population of fragile vesicles, but neither they nor MOLENAAR et al. (1973 b), who also discussed this problem, could come to a firm conclusion. The experiments of MARCHBANKS and ISRAËL (1971, 1972), who worked on slices of electric organ in the hope of obtaining a clearer answer, have already been mentioned (p. 163 et seq.).

We are obliged to conclude that the experiments so far performed on brain slices do not enable us to identify the site of storage of the ACh released by nerve impulses.

d) Brain in Situ

The ACh in the intact cerebral cortex can be labelled by injecting radioactive choline systemically (SCHUBERTH et al., 1969, 1970; DIAMOND, 1971; AQUILONIUS et al., 1973; SAELENS et al., 1973; SPARF, 1973), intracortically (CHAKRIN and SHIDEMAN, 1968; CHAKRIN and WHITTAKER, 1969), or intraventricularly (BARKER et al., 1972). All these routes have been used in experiments investigated the turnover of ACh in subcellular fractions.

The results obtained depend on the experimental conditions. In early experiments on anaesthetized animals, CHAKRIN and WHITTAKER (1969) found that [^{3}H] choline infiltrated into the cortex labelled cytoplasmic ACh to a higher specific activity than vesicular ACh, as if the former were turning over faster than the latter. This was the pattern that RICHTER and MARCHBANKS (1971 b) observed in their experiments on potassium-stimulated cortical slices, and it is the opposite of what would be expected if the vesicles are the store from which ACh is released synaptically. Continuing these studies, however, and giving the labelled choline intraventricularly to unanaesthetized animals, BARKER and his associates (1970) detected a small pool of ACh with a rapid turnover. This pool was easily lost during purification of the subcellular fractions; later BARKER et al. (1972) obtained evidence that it was associated with vesicles that remained attached to ruptured nerve-ending membranes. It is attractive to suppose that such a strategically-located population of vesicles might be the subcellular counterpart of the readily-releasable pool of ACh, whose existence had been postulated on the basis of experiments on ganglia and muscles (COLLIER and MACINTOSH, 1969; COLLIER, 1969; POTTER, 1970a); however, on the basis of the evidence so far available, this supposition is at best tenuous.

CHAKRIN and his colleagues (1972) have offered some direct evidence that newly-synthesized ACh is preferentially released in the cerebral cortex in vivo, but their experiments are difficult to interpret. They placed a cylinder open at both ends on the exposed cortex of an anaesthetized rabbit, so that exchange by diffusion could take place between the cortex and a pool of saline in the cylinder. The cortex was exposed to [^{3}H] choline for 30 min, and then the efflux of ACh into an eserine-saline pool was measured either at rest or during electrical stimulation of the lateral geniculate. Stimulation was expected to enhance the activity of cholinergic afferents to the cortex, and in most cases it did increase ACh release. In such experiments, CHAKRIN and his associates found that the specific activity of the released ACh was usually higher in the resting samples than during stimulation, and they suggested that the

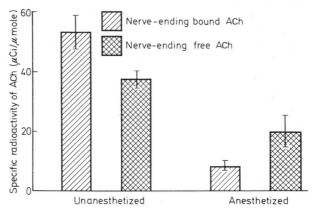

Fig. 9. Specific radioactivity of ACh in subcellular fractions prepared from mouse brain 3 min after intravenous injection of [³H] choline. Animals were either unanaesthetized or had received pentobarbitone (90 mg/kg; i.p.) 15 min before the choline. Results are expressed as mean ± s.e. (4—6 experiments). From Aquilonius et al., 1973: data from their Table 7

extra ACh released by stimulation came predominantly from an ACh pool of later origin, and therefore of lower radioactivity. In support of this idea, they found that the specific activity of the released ACh initially was higher than that of either the vesicular or the cytoplasmic ACh from synaptosomes isolated from the subjacent cortex.

The experimental situation when such techniques are used is complicated, and it is doubtful if the results can support the interpretation that has been given to them. Because the cortex has a blood flow, equilibration between the surface fluid and the more deeply situated tissue is not achieved, and it can be supposed that the ACh in surface layers will be labelled to higher specific activity than that in deeper layers. Most of the ACh released by lateral geniculate stimulation would be expected to come from synapses on cells that are excited by ACh (Collier and Mitchell, 1966, 1967), and these are found at some depth (Krnjević and Phillis, 1963; Jordan and Phillis, 1972). Spontaneous ACh release might in part represent activity at more superficial synapses, such as those that mediate cholinergic inhibition (Jordan and Phillis, 1972). If this were the case, stimulation might well increase the proportion of unlabelled ACh collected, simply because of the topographic distribution of the activated synapses. The difference in specific activity between released and tissue ACh might be explained by the thickness of the cortical slabs removed for homogenization (2 mm); the deeper layers might have contained ACh that was much less labelled than the ACh in the more superficial layers, which may have been the source of most of the released ACh.

Aquilonius and his colleagues (1973) made use of their discovery (Schuberth et al., 1969, 1970) that intravenous choline is promptly incorporated into brain ACh. Using unanaesthetized mice, they showed that within 15 sec of the injection of [³H] choline into a tail vein, about 15% of the label captured by the brain had been converted into [³H] ACh; thereafter the label disappeared slowly from the tissue. Synaptosomes from the brains were harvested, and it was found, in contrast to the results of Chakrin and Whittaker (1969), that the specific activity of the ACh in the vesicular fraction was higher than that in the cytoplasmic fraction (Fig. 9). These experiments strongly suggest that vesicles with a high turnover rate of ACh exist *in vivo* and can be harvested, and the results are thus compatible with the vesicular-exocytosis hypothesis, though they do not prove it. An incidental finding was that the newly-synthesized, labelled ACh appeared to be bound in a different way from the older, unlabelled ACh; most of the latter appeared in the crude synaptosome (P_2) fraction, while most of the former did not. This result can perhaps be interpreted in terms of the suggested heterogeneity of vesicular ACh, e.g. two kinds of vesicle (BARKER et al., 1970) or two kinds of binding within a vesicle (MARCHBANKS and ISRAËL, 1972).

The difference between the results of AQUILONIUS et al. (1973) and those of CHAKRIN and WHITTAKER (1969) is probably not wholly attributable to differences in fractionation technique or species differences (MOLENAAR and POLAK, 1973; MOLENAAR et al., 1973 b). Anaesthesia was probably the important factor (Fig. 9). Anaesthetic agents are well known to increase brain ACh, and the increase appears to be in the extravesicular store (BEANI et al., 1969); at the same time ACh release is reduced, and so presumably is ACh turnover in whatever store is releasable. On the assumption that this store is in vesicles, reduced turnover of vesicular ACh and the accumulation of cytoplasmic ACh might account for the pattern of labelling demonstrated by CHAKRIN and WHITTAKER (1969). These studies on ACh turnover in the intact brain provide valuable baseline data on the overall pattern of ACh metabolism, and they confirm that vesicular ACh turns over quite rapidly under physiological conditions, but they have not supplied much evidence for or against the vesicular exocytosis hypothesis of evoked ACh release.

5. Transfer of ACh between Pools or Compartments

a) ACh Uptake by Vesicles

If ACh upon being synthesized is at first free in the terminal cytosol and is then transferred to the vesicles, it might be expected that neurochemical experiments could demonstrate vesicular uptake of free ACh. In general, however, they have failed to do so (MARCHBANKS, 1968a). In contrast to the ease with which vesicular ACh can be labelled *in vivo*, it appears that isolated vesicles cannot take up labelled ACh from the medium in which they are suspended. Occasional positive findings may have resulted from working with a medium of low ionic strength (GUTH, 1969; see KURIYAMA et al., 1968) or with vesicles that were contaminated with intact synaptosomes (BURTON, 1964). Several possible reasons for the difference between the *in vivo* and the *in vitro* results can be considered. Vesicles might lose their ability to concentrate ACh as a result of damage during the isolation procedures; they might only be able to take up ACh when they are empty, or when they are filled with a cation (e.g. Na^+) which they can exchange for ACh (POTTER, 1972); alternatively, the suspension medium might be deficient in materials necessary for the (presumably uphill) transport process. Again, uptake of ACh may be rather tightly coupled to its synthesis at the vesicle surface; this is an idea that several authors have found attractive (RITCHIE and GOLDBERG, 1970; COLLIER and KATZ, 1971; HEBB, 1972; AQUILONIUS et al., 1973) and that has been expressed in a variant form by MARCHBANKS and

Israël (1972). No serious attempt to test these possibilities experimentally has been reported.

The experiments of Ritchie and Goldberg (1970) do not provide evidence for an obligatory linkage between the synthesis of ACh and its uptake into vesicles. Ritchie and Goldberg incubated synaptosomes with [^{14}C] choline and found that 15% of the [^{14}C] ACh formed was in the vesicles and 85% in the cytoplasm; when they repeated the experiment with [^{14}C] ACh instead of choline in the medium, they found only 1.5% of the labelled ACh in the vesicles and all the rest in the cytoplasm. At first glance this result suggests that synthesis and uptake of ACh at the vesicular surface must be closely associated, but this deduction can only be made if [^{14}C] ACh uptake from the medium into the synaptosomes involved the cholinergic synaptosomes exclusively. This is not so: ACh uptake into nervous tissue is unrelated to the presence of cholinergic neurones (Katz et al., 1973; Kuhar and Simon, 1974). On the other hand the accumulation of [^{14}C] ACh derived from [^{14}C] choline would be almost wholly in cholinergic synaptosomes, because only they would contain ChAc.

b) Mixing of Surplus ACh and Depot ACh

If surplus ACh is extravesicular though situated in the nerve endings, and the normal depot from which ACh is released is intravesicular, it might be supposed that surplus ACh would also become available for release eventually. Collier and Katz (1971) tested this in experiments on the cat superior cervical ganglion. They partly labelled the ACh in a resting ganglion, using [^{3}H] choline; in some of their tests eserine was present, and surplus [^{3}H] ACh was formed, while in others eserine was absent, and no surplus ACh was formed. In each case the preganglionic nerve was subsequently stimulated in the presence of eserine and unlabelled choline. Collier and Katz found that neither the amount nor the specific activity of the released ACh was increased by the presence of surplus ACh. These experiments confirmed that the surplus ACh of the superior cervical ganglion is not released by nerve impulses (Birks and MacIntosh, 1961) and showed in addition that it does not mix with the depot ACh, except perhaps at a slow rate. Mixing of surplus ACh and releasable ACh in phrenic nerve terminals, however, has been demonstrated by Potter (1970a). In his experiments, surplus and depot pools of ACh had been labelled simultaneously and almost completely; prolonged nerve stimulation then released more labelled ACh than could be accounted for by exhaustion of the normal depot, so in this preparation surplus ACh must eventually contribute to the release during prolonged stimulation. Whether it contributes to quantal release is unknown, and would be difficult to test. As has been pointed out earlier (pp.124—125) it is probable, though not yet certain, that the surplus ACh of peripheral tissues is located in the terminal regions of the axons and outside the vesicles. Its failure to mix with the releasable ACh depot (except to a small extent at most), even when the depot is turning over rapidly, is the strongest single piece of evidence so far available for an obligatory linkage between synthesis and storage during transmitter turnover.

c) Transfer of ACh between Pools during Stimulation in the Presence of HC-3

That ACh can be redistributed during stimulation can be inferred from the electrophysiological experiments of Elmqvist and Quastel (1965a), who measured quantum content at the neuromuscular junction in rat diaphragms subjected to exhaus-

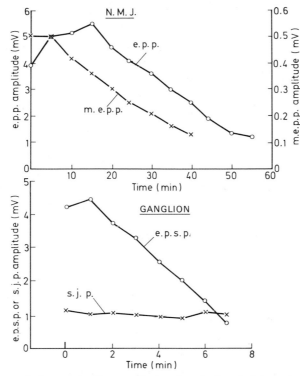

Fig. 10. Time-course of changes in the amplitude of evoked end-plate potentials (e.p.p.) and spontaneous miniature end-plate potentials (m.e.p.p.) measured from rat diaphragm (from ELMQVIST and QUASTEL, 1965a) or evoked excitatory postsynaptic potentials (e.p.s.p.) and spontaneous junctional potentials (s.j.p.) from rat superior cervical ganglion (from SACCHI and PERRI, 1973) continuously stimulated in the presence of HC-3. The diaphragm was bathed in a medium containing high magnesium concentration (15 mmol/l) to reduce transmitter release which was evoked by phrenic nerve stimulation (10.5 Hz). The ganglion was bathed in a medium containing normal magnesium concentration (1.2 mmol/l) and ACh release was evoked by stimulating a single afferent fibre (10 Hz)

tive stimulation in the presence of HC-3. They found that quantum content (the number of quanta per e.p.p.) remained unchanged under these conditions, whereas quantum size (e.g. m.e.p.p. size) steadily diminished as the preformed transmitter depot became depleted. JONES and KWANBUNBUMPEN (1970b) made similar observations. Since it can be assumed that very little new ACh was being formed in these circumstances, this finding must mean either than quanta are only formed at the moment of release, or if they are preformed, that their ACh is mutually exchangeable, so that all the individual quanta become depleted *pari passu* with the general store. This result is compatible with the cytosol-release hypothesis, for decreased quantum size would merely reflect depletion of the releasable transmitter pool; the only additional postulate needed would be a downhill leak of ACh from the reserve store in vesicles to the depleted store in the cytosol. The fall of quantum size during stimulation in the presence of HC-3 is somewhat awkward for the vesicle-exocytosis hypothesis, unless there is exchange of ACh between the vesicles. Could this kind of exchange occur, even though exchange of ACh between the vesicles and the cytosol by which they are surrounded is so difficult to demonstrate? An alternative hypothesis might be that already suggested (p.136) to help to explain why quanta seem to contain more ACh than vesicles: namely that vesicles adherent to one another might form a single compartment, functionally separate from the surrounding cytosol. It is somewhat surprising, as already noted, that ACh quanta in the rat superior cervical ganglion do not behave like quanta in the rat diaphragm during depleting stimulation in the presence of HC-3 (Fig.10). In ganglia, as Sacchi and Perri (1973) have shown, quantum size stays constant but the number of quanta released per impulse is reduced, as if only pre-formed quanta were released and there was no redistribution of ACh. These experiments offer an interesting challenge to those who favour the cytosol hypothesis of ACh release.

Cell fractionation studies to match these electrophysiological observations have not yet been made on ganglia or muscles, but have been undertaken on brain. Rodriguez de Lores Arnaiz and her colleagues (1970) injected HC-3 into the subarachnoid space of unanaesthetized rats, and measured ACh in subcellular fractions prepared from homogenates of the cortex. They found that vesicular ACh was reduced to 13% of normal, but that cytoplasmic ACh was not depleted. This result apparently conflicts with the findings discussed earlier in this section [p. 167 et seq.] which show that both cytoplasmic and vesicular fractions can be labelled from radioactive choline, and with recent experiments on rat cortex slices (S. Salehmoghaddam and B. Collier, unpublished), which showed that both fractions become depleted as potassium-evoked release of ACh falls in the presence of HC-3.

d) Differences between Tissues

As this section has shown, the data from neurochemical studies of ACh turnover in relation to its compartmentation are now rather voluminous, but only a few major facts have been established; and even these have not been established for all the tissues that have been the object of study. In brain at least, it seems clear that the vesicular and cytoplasmic stores of ACh are both relatively large, and that both can turn over rapidly during normal synaptic activity, with renewal times of the order of a minute or so in the case of cortex.

The stored ACh in ganglionic and neuromuscular terminals has renewal times that are an order of magnitude longer, and the neurochemical measures of turnover are very similar in these two peripheral tissues; however the discrepancy between quantal release patterns in HC-3 poisoned junctions (Elmqvist and Quastel, 1965a; Sacchi and Perri, 1973) suggests that the processes of ACh exchange within the terminals differ between muscles and ganglia. In both of these tissues, the phenomenon of surplus ACh formation suggests that the terminal cytoplasmic compartment normally contains little ACh, because of the activity of inwardly-directed AChE. In brain, however, surplus ACh is much less conspicuous and its existence has even been denied (Bourdois and Szerb, 1972). However, the storage capacity of cholinergic nerve terminals in brain is usually not saturated, whereas in ganglia and muscles it is. The cholinergic terminals in intestine, on which neurochemical investigation has just begun, may be different from those in either brain or ganglia and muscles. The extent of these peculiarities of individual tissues (and probably also

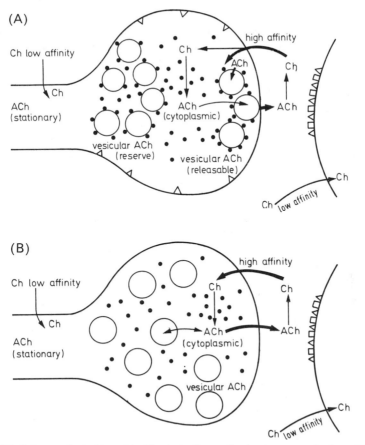

Fig. 11 A and B. Schemes that attempt to illustrate the synthesis, storage and release of ACh in a model cholinergic nerve terminal. In A, release of ACh is shown as if it were from vesicles by exocytosis, and in B, as if it were from the nerve terminal cytoplasm. Choline acetyltransferase is represented as ●, acetylcholinesterase as △ and cholinergic receptors as □. For details see the text

species) may seem depressing to investigators who would like to think that their results have a general significance and should help to explain all analogous phenomena. In fact, continued research will probably reveal that the diversity results from the varying combinations that are possible among a rather small number of basic processes at the molecular level.

6. A Tentative Model for ACh Storage and Metabolism

Tradition makes it almost obligatory to conclude a chapter of this length on this sort of topic by presenting a scheme which depicts, preferably with a diagram, the processes and compartments that the foregoing discussion has identified. Such schemes can have either positive or negative value: they are more likely to have positive value if the reader recognizes that they are inevitably distorted by the imperfect vision of those who have produced them, and if he is incited to correct them by doing further and better experiments. The scheme outlined below and illustrated in Fig. 11A may suggest that its authors cannot count past two, but it has the questionable virtue of preserving the classical vesicular-exocytosis hypothesis, which in the form stated seems to us to be marginally more plausible than the membrane-gate hypothesis. The main features of the scheme are:

a) Two Choline Uptake Mechanisms

In cholinergic nerve-endings only one of these mechanisms is important for ACh synthesis; it is a high-affinity uptake system (K_m of the order of 1 to 2 µmol/l); it serves to recapture much of the choline produced outside the terminal by the hydrolysis of released ACh, along with some of the free choline always present in the extracellular compartment, and it provides most of the choline that is used for ACh synthesis. More ubiquitous in its distribution is a low-affinity uptake system (K_m of the order of 10 to 100 µmol/l): its functions are unknown, but perhaps it is concerned with the transport of bases other than choline, or helps to provide choline for phospholipid synthesis.

Both mechanisms of uptake are inhibited by certain choline analogues such as the hemicholiniums, and by many other bases. It has not been finally proved that either of the choline uptake mechanisms is an active transport process, though each can accumulate choline against a concentration gradient. Choline can also become incorporated into pre-existing membrane phospholipids by a base-exchange process which is not blocked by hemicholiniums. In addition to these choline uptake mechanisms, it is likely that some free choline is made available within the terminal by the turnover of choline-containing phospholipids.

b) Two Sites of ACh Synthesis by Choline Acetyltransferase

The enzyme exists free in the nerve-ending cytoplasm, and also adsorbed on synaptic vesicles. The ACh that is synthesized in the cytosol does not readily enter the vesicles, while the ACh that is synthesized at the vesicular surface is much more likely to enter, and usually does so with great rapidity.

The scheme does not attempt to depict the process by which vesicles become loaded with ACh. Nothing is known about this process, except that it must be coupled directly or indirectly to a source of energy (since vesicular ACh is more concentrated than cytoplasmic ACh), is probably dependent in some way on sodium, and may involve some kind of loose binding of ACh by materials in the vesicle interior.

c) Two Compartments Containing ACh within the Nerve Ending

One of these compartments is the interior of the vesicles, and the other the cytosol; the latter is continuous with the cytosol of the cholinergic axon proximal to the terminal (or between synaptic varicosities). Cytoplasmic ACh is newly-synthesized ACh that is normally destined to become incorporated into synaptic vesicles or to be destroyed by intraterminal (membrane-bound but inward-facing) acetylcholinesterase. Inhibition of this enzyme allows cytoplasmic ACh to accumulate as surplus ACh.

Surplus ACh is a well-defined compartment at peripheral cholinergic synapses, but is probably less significant at central cholinergic synapses, from which inward-facing acetylcholinesterase may be more completely excluded. These central synapses can however increase their ACh storage capacity to well above the usual level in the absence of cholinesterase inhibition. Peripheral synapses, when excessively stimulated, also increase their ACh content (formation of "rebound" ACh: cf. pp. 188—189); it is not known whether this extra ACh, which appears to be releasable, is accommodated in vesicles or in the cytosol. In addition there is some evidence that newly-synthesized ACh can exist transiently in loose binding at the vesicular surface before passing into the vesicular core. Finally it may be noted that under abnormal conditions many kinds of cell, but especially non-cholinergic elements in brain, can take up extracellular ACh by a carrier-mediated process and hold it against a concentration gradient: this happens when ACh is in contact with brain slices in the presence of an organophosphorus inhibitor of acetylcholinesterase.

d) Two Populations of Synaptic Vesicles

One comprises the vesicles close to the presynaptic sites of release, and it turns over its ACh more rapidly than the second group which is larger, and is made up of the vesicles that are farther from release sites.

Eventually all or nearly all the vesicular ACh is releasable, so presumably the vesicles are either (i) not stationary inside the terminals, or (ii) able to exchange their stored ACh in some way.

e) Two Processes by which ACh Released from Synaptic Vesicles can be Replaced

As already noted, one is the uptake of ACh recently synthesized in close association with the membranes of the vesicles; the other is the uptake of pre-existing ACh from the cytosol, and perhaps from contiguous vesicles. The former process normally predominates, but the latter may be important when the supply of choline within the terminal is limited, as in the presence of HC-3.

Active nerve endings seem to take up choline most vigorously at or just after the instant of ACh release (p. 111), so it is conceivable that the release sites are also sites where choline is efficiently captured and acetylated. It is possible but not proven that HC-3 and related drugs block the uptake of ACh by the vesicles, as well as the uptake of choline by the nerve-endings.

As we see it the major difficulties raised by this scheme are the following:

(a) Although electronmicroscopic evidence for vesicular exocytosis has been presented, there is no evidence that such events are common or that their frequency is a linear function of the rate at which quanta are released. The accelerated uptake of macromolecular markers by active nerve endings is consistent with accelerated vesicular exocytosis but does not prove it; and so far, such uptake has not yet been shown to have been proportional to the release of either quanta or ACh. Expansion of the presynaptic membrane with depleted vesicle counts during high-frequency activity could be explained just as well by breakdown of vesicles within the terminal as by exocytosis. Moreover even the best vesicle counts made with the aid of current techniques may not be completely trustworthy.

(b) There is an appreciable difference between the estimates of the ACh content of a vesicle and the ACh content of a quantum, the latter being an order of magnitude higher in most cases. It is still possible, however, that either kind of estimate, or both, may be in error for technical reasons. It is also possible that the exocytosis of one vesicle may open a channel for the efflux of transmitter from other vesicles that are contiguous with it.

(c) The uptake of ACh into synaptic vesicles has not been demonstrated, and the concept that ACh synthesized at the vesicle membrane can readily enter the vesicle core is speculative. (It can of course be argued that no one has yet harvested vesicles that retain all their native properties, or exposed them to a medium that is identical to their natural environment in the cytoplasm.)

(d) The evidence for the existence of two kinds of synaptic vesicle, corresponding to two pools, a readily-releasable one and a reserve, of the ACh depot, is not at all convincing.

An alternative scheme (Fig. 11B) that avoids these difficulties is that ACh is released quantally from the nerve-terminal cytosol through the formation of temporary gates or pores in the presynaptic membrane, and that the vesicles function only as a high-capacity reserve store from which cytoplasmic ACh can be replenished under conditions of accelerated release. The difficulties with which this alternative scheme has to contend have been discussed, but none of them eliminates it. The most important difficulty is that the conditions that evoke the release of surplus ACh, believed to be cytoplasmic, from peripheral cholinergic terminals, are very different from the conditions that evoke the release of ACh from the regular nerve-ending depot. Reference should perhaps also be made again to the finding that in ganglia (unlike muscles) when ACh stores are depleted it is the number of quanta released by an impulse, rather than the size of the quanta, that is reduced. It is certainly not impossible to suppose that the vertebrate nervous system, which is versatile enough to employ electrical and chemical transmission at the same synapses, may on some occasions reinforce one sort of ACh release process with another sort.

G. Removal of Acetylcholine

After a neurotransmitter has been released into the synaptic cleft, its concentration rapidly declines. In general, three processes have been suggested as being responsible for the removal of transmitters: enzymatic destruction, uptake or re-uptake, and diffusion out of the synaptic cleft.

1. Enzymatic Destruction

a) Location of Acetylcholinesterase

It has been clear for many years that the presence of AChE in high concentration is characteristic of cholinergic neurones throughout their length, and indeed can serve as a useful histochemical marker for such neurones. However the enzyme occurs also in a variety of other structures, including red blood cells, afferent axons, denervated skeletal muscles, and brain regions containing little ACh, such as most of the cerebellum (BURGEN and CHIPMAN, 1952; LEWIS et al., 1967). Nevertheless it is clear that there is a particularly strong association between AChE and cholinergic junctions. This was apparent as soon as its histochemical localization became possible (KOELLE and FRIEDENWALD, 1949), and it has been confirmed both by biochemical measurements (GIACOBINI, 1959) and by radioautography (SALPETER, 1967; ROGERS et al., 1969). In skeletal muscle, where the enzyme is strongly concentrated at the end-plates, the greater part of it is located postsynaptically (COUTEAUX and TAXI, 1952; DAVIS and KOELLE, 1967, see also the review by KOELLE, 1963; and the chapter by BOWDEN and DUCHEN and also by HOBBIGER, this volume).

It has been known for many years that there is enough AChE at muscle end-plates and in sympathetic ganglia to dispose of any ACh that has been liberated by nerve impulses within less than 5 msec (GLICK, 1938; MARNAY and NACHMANSOHN, 1938). A more recent calculation by NAMBA and GROB (1968), who measured the AChE activity of membranes isolated from rat intercostal muscle, was that in 1 msec a single end-plate should be able to hydrolyse about 2.7×10^8 ACh molecules, which far exceeds the 3 to 6×10^6 molecules released there by one nerve impulse. The density of ACh-hydrolysing sites on the end-plate surface must therefore be high. By means of radioautography after labelling with [³H] DFP, using appropriate chemical devices to achieve specificity, SALPETER (1969) and BARNARD and his colleagues (1971) calculated that there are about 12000 such sites per μm^2, which means that the enzyme (one active site per half-molecule of 128000) could account for between a quarter and a half of the postsynaptic surface. The number of ACh receptor sites, as measured by α-bungarotoxin binding, is similar, and the two proteins, which are both rather firmly bound to membranes at these and other junctions, may have many structural features in common (BELLEAU and DiTULLIO, 1970). It is clear, however, that they are not identical, as has been suggested from time to time, since they can be separated from each other by appropriate chemical manipulations (e.g., HALL and KELLY, 1971; MOLINOFF and POTTER, 1972).

The location of AChE in sympathetic ganglia is less clear. Preganglionic denervation results in the loss of the enzyme (VON BRÜCKE, 1937; GLICK, 1938; COUTEAUX and NACHMANSOHN, 1940; SAWYER and HOLLINSHEAD, 1945), and histochemical studies with light microscopy showed strong specific staining in pre-ganglionic axons but only exceptionally in post-ganglionic ones (KOELLE, 1951, 1955; KOELLE and KOELLE, 1959; GROMADZKI and KOELLE, 1965). These findings were considered to prove that the AChE of a normal ganglion is associated mainly with the preganglionic terminals. An alternative explanation, however, would be that postsynaptic AChE is derived from presynaptic enzyme synthesized in the soma of the cholinergic neurone and transported down the axon (see the following section). KOELLE (1970, 1971; KOELLE et al., 1971) now favours this interpretation on the basis of histochemical studies at the electronmicroscope level on the cat's superior cervical ganglion where the enzyme seems to be located postsynaptically, though in somewhat looser binding than at the neuromuscular junction.

b) "Functional" and "Reserve" Acetylcholinesterase

This concept was proposed by KOELLE and his colleagues to take account of their finding that some of the tissue AChE behaves as if it were freely accessible to quaternary substrates and inhibitors, while some does not (KOELLE and STEINER,

1956; Koelle, 1957; Fukuda and Koelle, 1959; Koelle and Koelle, 1959; Mc-Isaac and Koelle, 1959; see also Burgen and Chipman,1952). It was suggested that "functional" AChE is oriented externally in the neuronal membrane and hydrolyses released transmitter; whereas "reserve" AChE is intracellular, is not involved in hydrolyzing released transmitter, and represents enzyme in transit from its site of synthesis in the cholinergic cell body to its site of functional activity. Inhibition of "reserve" AChE appears to correlate with the accumulation of surplus ACh in motor and preganglionic nerve terminals (Potter, 1970a; Collier and Katz, 1971): such accumulation begins promptly when an organophosphorus inhibitor or eserine (a lipid-soluble tertiary base) is employed, but only after a significant delay when neostigmine or ambenonium, both quaternary compounds, are used.

The presence of intracellular or inwardly-directed AChE in cholinergic *nerve-cell bodies* has been documented by histochemical observations at the electronmicroscope level (Lewis and Shute, 1966; Koelle et al., 1971). The histochemical evidence that the enzyme is similarly distributed in cholinergic *axons* is at least plausible, and is supported, as was noted earlier (p.125) by neurochemical evidence that nerve-trunk ACh, most of which is probably freely diffusible inside axons, slowly increases in the presence of eserine to about double its initial level (Evans and Saunders, 1974). The histochemical evidence for the existence of inwardly-directed AChE at cholinergic *nerve terminals* is weak, as would be expected in view of the formidable technical difficulty of localizing what may be a minute part of the total enzyme within structures of such small dimensions (Friedenberg and Seligman, 1972); there have, however, been occasional positive reports (e.g. Robinson and Bell, 1967; Teräväinen, 1969).

c) Subcellular Distribution of Acetylcholinesterase

When a tissue that contains AChE is homogenized, most of the enzyme activity remains associated with membranes or microsomes from which it can be removed by treatment with detergents, organic solvents or enzymes. A small fraction of the AChE is usually found in the soluble fraction of the homogenate, but since the proportion varies with the conditions of homogenization (Aldridge and Johnson, 1959; Hollunger and Niklasson, 1967, 1973; Chan et al., 1972), this does not necessarily mean that some of the enzyme was free in the cytoplasm *in vivo*. The soluble enzyme might represent the "reserve" AChE and the membrane-bound enzyme the "functional" AChE. In the case of brain homogenates, the soluble enzyme might have come mainly from cholinergic cell bodies (though in cortex at least there seem to be relatively few of these). Brain synaptosome preparations are rich in AChE, most of which is associated with membranes but not with synaptic vesicles; 5% or less is recovered with the soluble constituents (De Robertis et al., 1963; Whittaker et al., 1964; Rieger et al., 1972).

d) Effect of Anticholinesterase Agents on Synaptic Transmission

This subject will be fully discussed in other chapters of this book, and for the purpose of this section it is sufficient to mention that the effect of anticholinesterase agents on neuromuscular transmission lends support to the concept that released transmitter is hydrolysed by AChE. End-plate potentials and m.e.p.p.s recorded from skeletal muscle are increased in amplitude and in duration by drugs such as neostigmine (ECCLES et al., 1942; FATT and KATZ, 1951, 1952; MAGLEBY and STEVENS, 1972a; KATZ and MILEDI, 1973). Neostigmine, however, does not alter the magnitude or the duration of the elementary voltage change that represents the immediate consequence of the action of ACh on cholinergic receptors at the muscle end-plate (KATZ and MILEDI, 1973). This shows that acetylcholinesterase does not terminate the action of an ACh molecule on a cholinergic receptor; that action must be over before the molecule is hydrolysed by acetylcholinesterase. The potentiation of synaptic transmission by anticholinesterase presumably results from an average molecule of ACh acting more times than normal upon receptors.

The effects of anticholinesterase agents on ganglionic transmission are less dramatic (ECCLES, 1944; BLACKMAN et al., 1963a), but it is now clear that eserine increases the duration of spontaneous and evoked synaptic potentials recorded from ganglia (BORNSTEIN, 1974). That immediate hydrolysis of released ACh occurs in ganglia can also be concluded from the finding that choline formed from released ACh is recaptured by the nerve endings and used again (PERRY, 1953; COLLIER and MACINTOSH, 1969; BENNETT and MCLACHLAN, 1972b; COLLIER and KATZ, 1974). The re-utilization of choline derived from hydrolysed ACh has been shown to be a property of motor nerve terminals also (POTTER, 1970a).

2. ACh Uptake

At adrenergic and probably at other non-cholinergic synapses, the re-uptake of released transmitter helps to terminate transmitter action and conserve transmitter stores (see the reviews by WATKINS, 1972; and IVERSEN, 1973). The intense activity of AChE at many cholinergic synapses makes it unlikely that much of the released ACh will survive long enough to be recaptured. In some circumstances, however, the inactivation of AChE allows ACh uptake by neural tissue to proceed. In brain slices, as was first shown by POLAK and MEEUWS (1966) and has been repeatedly confirmed (SCHUBERTH and SUNDWALL, 1967; HEILBRONN, 1969; LIANG and QUASTEL, 1969a; POLAK, 1969), uptake of ACh in the presence of an organophosphorus inhibitor occurs against a concentration gradient and can raise the ACh content of the tissue to several times its initial value. Little or no uptake is seen when eserine is used (MANN et al., 1938; BRODKIN and ELLIOTT, 1953; POLAK and MEEUWS, 1966; LIANG and QUASTEL, 1969b). It is doubtful whether this uptake is ever a significant route for the inactivation of ACh released *in vivo*, even in the exceptional case of brain tissue in severe anticholinesterase poisoning. Certainly the accumulated ACh is not recycled in the way that choline is, for it is not available for release by potassium, and hexamethonium (which blocks ACh uptake) does not increase potassium-evoked release of endogenous ACh; moreover the uptake appears not to be specifically into cholinergic neurones (KATZ et al., 1973; KUHAR and SIMON, 1974).

At peripheral cholinergic synapses, ACh uptake seems to be neither physiologically nor pharmacologically significant. Sympathetic ganglia (COLLIER and MACINTOSH, 1969; KATZ et al., 1973) and rat diaphragms (ADAMIČ, 1970; POTTER, 1970a) accumulate very little exogenous ACh in the presence of an anticholinesterase; the amount accumulated is not increased by nerve stimulation (POTTER, 1970a; KATZ et al., 1973). Accumulated exogenous ACh is not released by nerve impulses or by potassium (Katz et al., 1973). It has been shown that the end-plate region accumulates no more ACh from a medium than the same volume of extrajunctional muscle (Adamič, 1970; Potter, 1970a), and chronically decentralized ganglia accumulate exogenous ACh just as well as acutely decentralized ganglia (Katz et al., 1973). The non-specificity of ACh uptake limits its use in experiments designed to elucidate cholinergic mechanisms.

3. Diffusion from the Synaptic Cleft

In the presence of cholinesterase inhibitors, diffusion of ACh from the synaptic cleft probably provides the mechanism by which transmitter is removed. Calculations have shown that diffusion should be able to remove ACh within the refractory period of a typical synapse (Fatt, 1954; Ogston, 1955). The binding of ACh to its receptors can apparently slow its dissipation by diffusion (Katz and Miledi, 1973), because the time for ACh removal from the neuromuscular junction in the presence of an anticholinesterase is longer than can be accounted for by unrestricted diffusion within the synaptic space (Magleby and Stevens, 1972a, b; Katz and Miledi, 1973).

H. Axonal Transport of Materials Related to Cholinergic Transmission

The viability of axons and their terminals depends on the transport of materials from their nerve-cell bodies. There is now abundant evidence that in addition to a "slow" (e.g. 1 to 10 mm/day) proximo-distal movement of certain materials along the axon (Weiss and Hiscoe, 1948), there is a "fast" (e.g. 100 to 500 mm/day) transport of the same or other materials in the same direction (for reviews see, e.g., Barondes, 1969; Dahlström, 1971; Ochs, 1972; Droz, 1973; Jeffrey and Austin, 1973). Transport towards the soma occurs simultaneously, often at an intermediate rate.

The movement of materials along axons has been studied by three main techniques. (1) Organelles have been observed under the light microscope in motion in both directions within axons of cultured neurones, and more recently in amphibian and human nerves (for references see Cooper and Smith, 1974). (2) Radioactive tracers (often amino acids) have been injected around or into nerve cell bodies, and the subsequent movement of the resulting labelled materials (often proteins) along the nerves or axons has been followed. (3) A third technique has been to interrupt the flow of materials along axons by applying ligatures to nerve trunks or by crushing or transecting them, and after a suitable interval, measuring the accumulation of specific materials near the point of obstruction. The presumed functions of axonal transport are to replace materials that have been degraded or secreted (somatofugal transport especially), and to regulate certain aspects of axonal, neuroterminal, somatal, dendritic or trans-synaptic function (both somatopetal and somatofugal transport). There is now convincing evidence that fast axonal transport depends in some way on microtubules, and that the transported materials are membrane—or particle-bound (Schmitt, 1968; Ochs, 1972); at least some of the material is glycoprotein (Karlsson and Sjöstrand, 1971; Edström and Mattson, 1972). Slow axonal transport seems to involve mainly the soluble components of the axoplasm, and its mechanism is poorly understood. The present discussion will be limited to aspects of axonal transmission that are directly pertinent to cholinergic transmission. Much of the information has come from nerve-constriction experiments.

By 1945 the presence of ACh, ChAc and AChE, in those nerve trunks that contain cholinergic fibres, was well established, and so was the early loss of these materials from the synaptic regions during Wallerian degeneration. Thus physiologists who were not attracted by the proposal that ACh was involved in axonal, rather than junctional, transmission were almost obliged to postulate axonal migration of ACh and ChAc from soma toward terminals, to account for their distribution. This idea was certainly being discussed informally by 1945, though it appears not to have been staded explicitly until some years later (DALE, 1953; BURGEN and MacINTOSH, 1955).

1. Acetylcholinesterase

That AChE moves from cholinergic cell bodies toward motor nerve terminals was suggested by SAWYER (1946), who observed that enzyme activity accumulates on the proximal side of a transected motor nerve: AChE was the first enzyme found to behave in this way. The observation has been confirmed repeatedly, for example by LUBIŃSKA and her colleagues (1961) and by FRIZELL and his colleagues (1970). That the accumulation is due to transport rather than local synthesis of the enzyme has been demonstrated by LUBIŃSKA et al. (1964), who found that in pieces of nerve isolated between two ligatures the AChE activity was redistributed with no change in the total activity, and by FRIZELL et al.(1970), who showed that the accumulation was unaffected by cyclohexamide.

The rate of axonal transport of AChE was originally calculated to be about 5 to 15 mm/day, and its transport was therefore considered to be part of the slow axoplasmic flow. It is now clear that part (10 to 15%) of the AChE moves as a component of the fast transport system, with a velocity estimated at 260 mm/day (dog peroneal nerve: LUBIŃSKA and NIEMIERKO, 1971), 430 mm/day (cat sciatic nerve: RANISH and OCHS, 1972) or 425 mm/day (rabbit vagus nerve: FONNUM et al., 1974). This rapidly-transported AChE appears to be associated with intra-axonal tubules and vesicles, which are considered to be part of the smooth endoplasmic reticulum (for references see KÁSA et al., 1973). The slowly-transported AChE is perhaps bound to the axolemma: if so, most of its active sites must be either outward-facing or masked, to permit the existence of a rather high concentration of ACh apparently free within the axon (see pp.119,122).

As yet, in spite of NACHMANSOHN's arguments (see NACHMANSOHN, 1971) AChE has no accepted role in axonal transmission. If the AChE that is transported in motor nerves is on its way to replace the functional stock of enzyme at the neuromuscular junction, it must eventually be secreted there, because most of the junctional AChE is attached to the postsynaptic membrane. There is considerable direct evidence for the trans-synaptic transfer of macromolecules (GRAFSTEIN, 1971; NEALE et al., 1972), though not yet for transfer of AChE. Two findings are consistent with, but do not prove, the idea that end-plate AChE comes at least in part from motor nerves: first, motor denervation significantly reduces end-plate AChE within two weeks (Kupfer, 1951; Snell and McIntyre, 1956; Guth et al., 1964; Eränkö and Teräväinen, 1967; Crone and Freeman, 1972):secondly, after DFP treatment, AChE recovers sooner in innervated than in denervated muscle (Filogamo and Gabella, 1967; Rose and Glow, 1967).

Retrograde movement of AChE occurs, at about half the forward velocity (Lubińska and Niemierko, 1971; Ranish and Ochs, 1972; Fonnum et al., 1974); its function is unclear. Proteins other than AChE are also transported somatopetally (Kerkut et al., 1967; Kristensson and Olsson, 1971; Watson, 1974a); these may be either exogenous (Kristensson and Olsson, 1971) or endogenous (Bisby, 1975). In the former case the movement may serve to regulate the soma's anabolic activities (Cragg, 1970), while in the latter case it may represent the recycling of worn-out protein for dismantling and rebuilding at the soma (Droz, 1973). There is some evidence of limited synthesis of proteins by nerve terminals, though they contain few if any ribosomes (Morgan and Austin, 1968; Droz and Koenig, 1971; Ramirez et al., 1972; Droz, 1973); however, it now seems unlikely that the AChE of axons or terminals arises in this fashion (Austin and James, 1970). It had been suggested (Koenig and Koelle, 1960; Koenig, 1965, 1967) that the absence of a proximo-distal gradient for AChE along the nerves of animals recovering from DFP poisoning implies that the enzyme was made or regenerated locally rather than transported, but this suggestion was made before the evidence for a fast axoplasmic flow had been completed.

2. Choline Acetyltransferase

That ChAc accumulates above a site of nerve transection or ligation was first shown by Hebb and Waites (1956) and has been confirmed repeatedly (Hebb and Silver, 1961; Frizell et al., 1970). As a cytoplasmic enzyme ChAc might be expected to be carried by the slower transport process, and rates consistent with such a process have been published (6 to 14 mm/day, Frizell et al., 1970; about 3 mm/day, Wooten and Coyle, 1973). As noted earlier, however, there is both biochemical (Fonnum, 1967) and histochemical (Kása et al., 1970a, b) evidence that a part of the enzyme may be loosely bound in vivo to subcellular organelles. ChAc so bound would be expected to migrate more rapidly, and some recent measurements by Fonnum and his colleagues (1974) support this expectation. It was found that 6% of the enzyme in vagus nerves moved at 190 mm/day, while the migration rate in hypogastric nerves, 47 mm/day, was intermediate between the fast and slow rates of transport. Fonnum et al. also observed a slower retrograde movement of the axonal enzyme, and this can be taken as further evidence that some of it is membrane- or particle-bound; it is hardly conceivable that a soluble component of the axoplasm would be moved in both directions simultaneously.

On the assumption that transported ChAc serves to replace the nerve terminal enzyme, the latter's turnover time can be calculated if the transport rate is known. Hebb et al. (1964) found that 1 mm of phrenic nerve contains about 1/50 as much ChAc as a hemidiaphragm: if 6% of the nerve enzyme were to move peripherally at 200 mm/day, the junctional enzyme could be replaced every 4 days. Fonnum et al. (1974) calculated that the half-life of ChAc in tongue muscles is 22 days. An obvious possible source of error in such estimates is that the transport rates observed experimentally may have been influenced by the nerve ligation or transection: it has been noted that axotomy reduces ChAc activity in nerve cell bodies (HEBB and SILVER, 1963; FONNUM et al., 1974). In principle, better estimates of the turnover time of specific proteins in nerve endings can be obtained from labelling experiments, provided that the protein can be isolated from extracts of the terminal region. However, such estimates have apparently not yet been attempted for any of the specific proteins of cholinergic neurones.

3. Acetylcholine

Although axonal ACh is generally assumed to be mainly in solution (see p.122), ACh accumulates along with AChE and ChAc in nerve trunks proximal to a lesion (SASTRY, 1956; DIAMOND and EVANS, 1960; EVANS and SAUNDERS, 1967; HÄGGENDAL et al., 1971). In experiments of this sort on rat sciatic nerve (HÄGGENDAL et al., 1971; DAHLSTRÖM et al., 1974), part of the ACh behaved as if it were transported at a rate of several mm/hour, which would suggest that it had migrated by the fast mechanism and was associated with some kind of particle; sequestration within particles would also account for its co-existence with the AChE that had accumulated at the same site. An accumulation of vesicular organelles above nerve lesions has in fact been observed (VAN BREEMEN et al., 1958; WEISS et al., 1962; LAMPERT and CRESSMAN, 1964), but it has not been proved that they arrived there by axonal transport or that they contain ACh. It is conceivable that they represent vesicular material in transit toward nerve endings. Though the origin of the synaptic vesicles is still debatable, a close association between them and axonal microtubules is well documented for some tissues (e.g. lamprey spinal cord: SMITH et al., 1970; SMITH, 1971). The paucity of observable vesicular profiles in axonal axoplasm could still be consistent with axonal delivery if it is remembered that the turnover time of vesicular materials in nerve endings is very long compared with the transit time from soma to synapse. A half-life of 20 to 30 days has been reported by VON HUNGEN et al. (1968) and LAPETINA et al. (1970). Thus some of the fast-moving ACh might be in vesicles, while some might be in other axonal organelles. The postulated vesicular location of some of the ACh in cholinergic axons would correspond to that of a major part of the noradrenaline in adrenergic axons, where the amine-bearing granules are believed to be in transit to the release sites (DAHLSTRÖM, 1965; KAPELLER and MAYOR, 1967; GEFFEN and RUSH, 1968; LIVETT et al., 1968; BANKS and MAYOR, 1972; but see TAXI and SOTELO, 1973). For adrenergic neurones it has been stressed repeatedly that axonal transport does not contribute significantly to the replenishment of the transmitter depots in the neuroterminals: local synthesis is the important process (DAHLSTRÖM and HÄGGENDAL, 1966; GEFFEN and RUSH, 1968). It has long been obvious, but perhaps has not been explicitly stated, that this is equally true of vertebrate cholinergic neurones. For example, the ACh content of a rat hemidiaphragm is about 220 pmol, which is about equal to the ACh content of 60 mm of phrenic nerve (HEBB et al., 1964). At the fastest recorded rate of axonal transport, 450 mm/day, it would take over 3 hrs to deliver the end-plates' store of ACh, whereas the average turnover time of the ACh in POTTER's (1970a) experiments was 10 to 20 min. A similar calculation can be made for ACh replenishment in ganglia. As TAXI and SOTELO (1973) have remarked for catecholamine transport, all these find-

ings "tend to prove that the axonal migration of [the transmitter] is only an epiphen-
omenon related to the distal migration of enzymatic and storage proteins from the
perikaryon".

Radioactive tracer techniques have not yet been used to follow the somatofugal
movement of ACh in vertebrate cholinergic neurones, but successful experiments of
this sort have been carried out on identified cholinergic neurones of *Aplysia* (Koike
et al., 1972) and in chemoreceptor axons of the wood roach (Schafer, 1973). The
estimated transport rates were 17 to 55 mm/day for the *Aplysia* axons at 15° C, and
120 to 130 mm/day for the insect axons, presumably at room temperature. Since the
Q_{10} for fast axoplasmic transport is about 2 (Grafstein et al., 1972; Koike et al.,
1972; Ochs, 1972), the observed rates in the vertebrate and invertebrate neurones are
in good agreement. At least in the case of the *Aplysia* neurones, the transported ACh
must have been particle-bound, because the axons are known to contain AChE
(Giller and Schwartz, 1971), and part of the labelled ACh could be recovered in a
particulate fraction prepared from homogenized axons (Koike et al., 1972).

4. Other Materials

Nothing is known as yet about the axonal transport of vesiculin and the other
proteins associated with synaptic vesicles, or of the (hypothetical) protein or proteins
specifically involved in choline uptake.

5. Effects of Agents that Block Axonal Transport

Colchicine and vinca alkaloids (vinblastine and vincristine) break down microtubules (Peterson and Bornstein, 1968; Wisniewski et al., 1968) and block fast, but not
slow, axonal transport (Dahlström, 1968; Karlsson and Sjöstrand, 1969; Sjöstrand et al., 1970). When applied to cholinergic axons, colchicine blocks the fast
migration of AChE (Kreutzberg, 1969; Fonnum et al., 1974), of ChAc (Sjöstrand
et al., 1970; Fonnum et al., 1974) and of ACh (Schafer, 1973). Local application of
colchicine or vinblastine to a sciatic nerve does not cause failure of neuromuscular
transmission (Albuquerque et al., 1972; Hofmann and Thesleff, 1972; Cangiano, 1973; Hofmann et al., 1973), and this demonstrates again that the nerve terminals are not immediately dependent on the rapid transport of ACh or of choline
acetyltransferase for transmitter turnover. Similarly, chronic systemic administration
of tolerated doses of colchicine does not cause neuromuscular paralysis by any
peripheral action (Ferguson, 1952; Hofmann et al., 1973), and chronic systemic
administration of vinca alkaloids does not deplete tissues of ACh (Cheney et al.,
1973). However, both chronic administration of colchicine (Ferguson, 1952), and
the direct application of colchicine or vinblastine to motor nerves (Albuquerque et
al., 1972; Hofmann and Thesleff, 1972; Cangiano, 1973), do cause important
changes in skeletal muscles: they become supersensitive to exogenous ACh, and the
ACh-sensitive region of each fibre spreads from the end-plate area to include the
entire surface. These changes are like those that follow surgical denervation (e.g.,
Brown, 1937; Axelsson and Thesleff, 1959; Miledi, 1960). In the past the effect of

denervation on ACh sensitivity has been variously attributed to the absence either of ACh release (THESLEFF, 1960), or of a "trophic" factor (see GUTH, 1968) or of muscle activity (JONES and VRBOVÁ, 1970; LØMO and ROSENTHAL, 1972). The discovery that colchicine treatment can provoke spread of sensitivity to ACh, without altering ACh release or preventing muscle activity, immediately suggested that fast axoplasmic transport might be responsible for delivering to the neuromuscular junction some material that controls the formation of ACh receptor sites in the muscle fibres. The control system must be more complex than this, however, for LØMO has recently (1974) shown that colchicine when injected into a denervated muscle that has been stimulated directly — a procedure that prevents the post-denervation spread of ACh sensitivity — reverses the inhibitory effect of the stimulation and makes the muscle fibres responsive to ACh over their whole length. In these experiments the colchicine must have acted on the muscle.

The nature of the "trophic" factor released from motor nerves is unknown, and so is the mechanism by which it affects the production or the distribution of ACh receptors in muscle. It is tempting to speculate that vesiculin (WHITTAKER, 1971) might be a trophic factor. Neurotoxins that block ACh release (botulinum toxin, tetanus toxin, β-bungarotoxin) also induce ACh sensitivity; they could act by causing muscle inactivity or by blocking the release of a trophic factor.

6. A Note on Other Trophic Influences Mediated by Cholinergic Nerves

A trophic influence of nerve on muscle might be involved in altering the speed of contraction of fast and slow skeletal muscles after denervation and cross-reinnerva- tion; e.g., after cross-union of nerves to fast and slow muscles, fast muscles develop a slower rate of contraction and slow muscles develop a faster rate of contraction (BULLER et al., 1960; BULLER and LEWIS, 1965; CLOSE, 1965). It is interesting that these changes appear not to occur in dystrophic mouse muscle (LAW and ATWOOD, 1972), and there is some evidence that a neuronal factor is involved in at least some types of muscular dystrophy (MCCOMAS and SICA, 1970; MCCOMAS et al., 1970, 1971). A particularly clear example of a neuronal defect in murine muscular dystro- phy is the recent experiment of GALLUP and DUBOWITZ (1973), in which nerve and muscle cultures were established. When axons from normal animals innervated ei- ther normal or dystrophic muscle, the muscle regenerated and functional neuromus- cular junctions were established, but when axons from dystrophic animals contacted either normal or dystrophic muscle, the muscle did not regenerate and functional neuromuscular junctions were not established. It is not yet known what factor(s) in the nerve of the dystrophic mouse may limit muscle regeneration, nor is it known whether there is a similar neuronal defect in any of the human muscular dystrophies.

Any further attempt to summarize progress in these currently active research areas would be premature at this time. It is reasonably certain that some of the mechanisms that control embryonic development in cholinergic neurones and their target cells persist into postnatal life. The embryonic development of cholinergic mechanisms is outside the scope of this chapter: for reviews see FILOGAMO and MARCHISIO (1971) and KARCZMAR et al. (1972). The related topic of plasticity as it relates to presynaptic cholinergic mechanisms is discussed in the next section.

I. Prolonged Neurochemical Changes Resulting from Synaptic Activity

1. Causes of Synaptic Plasticity

Phenomena like learning and memory are often supposed to be based on synaptic plasticity, which in turn is considered to have a biochemical basis. These topics have a voluminous and diffuse literature, which contains many references to cholinergic mechanisms; in fact not much is known about how experience can modify these mechanisms at the cellular level.

The traditional doctrine that synaptic potency is enhanced by use and diminished by disuse was severely criticized by Sharpless (1964), who pointed out that if peripheral synapses could be taken as paradigms for central ones there was at least as much evidence for an exactly contrary position. In the last decade, however, there has been a good deal of relevant experimental work, which if it has not provided the answers does allow the questions to be put in a clearer form. As a result the traditional view seems to have regained some of its plausibility. Four lines of progress can be specified:

(i) As noted in the preceding section, it has been confirmed that exchange of materials other than neurotransmitters occurs at the neuromuscular junction, and that these "trophic" materials can profoundly influence the metabolism of the cells they enter. It seems possible that such "trophic" substances can cross synapses in both directions and that their intracellular convection is dependent on microtubules. While this kind of exchange is not necessarily linked to synaptic transmission in the more usual sense, so that for example, the effects of denervation can be different from those of synaptic disuse, it is recognized that the amount of material exchanged — and therefore the magnitude of the "trophic" effect — may depend on the intensity of impulse traffic across the synapses.

(ii) It has been demonstrated that post-tetanic potentiation (the increased effectiveness of a presynaptic impulse after a period of repetitive excitation) can be brought about by more than one mechanism, and that it can last for hours.

(iii) Evidence has been obtained that under conditions of increased traffic over certain synaptic pathways there is increased synthesis and storage of enzymes specifically involved in the manufacture of the relevant neurotransmitters. (There may also be induced synthesis of the specific degradative enzymes and transport and storage proteins, but the evidence for this is less complete.)

(iv) It has been recognized that increased synaptic activity can have a striking and long-lasting effect on neighbouring glial cells, and that these in turn may alter synaptic events and processes by mechanisms that as yet are poorly understood.

The phenomena referred to above are certainly not restricted to peripheral cholinergic junctions, but examples of them have been observed there. Reference has been made in the preceding section to trophic influences at the neuromuscular junction; some of the phenomena that come under the other three headings will be mentioned below. Neurochemical studies on peripheral synapses will be emphasized; and it will be seen that while postsynaptic mechanisms may not be strengthened by use, as Sharpless (1964) noted, presynaptic potentiation may be strong and long-lasting.

2. Post-Tetanic Potentiation

Post-tetanic potentiation has been known for over a century (see HUGHES, 1958 for a historical review); as the name indicates, it was first observed in skeletal muscle. There it can have both pre-synaptic and post-synaptic (muscle fibre) components (FENG, 1938; BROWN and VON EULER, 1938), but when it is seen in the form of post-tetanic decurarization the presynaptic component is the significant one, as has been demonstrated repeatedly (HUTTER, 1952; LILEY and NORTH, 1953; BROOKS, 1956). Presynaptic post-tetanic potentiation in the superior cervical ganglion was elegantly analyzed by LARRABEE and BRONK (1947), who showed that increasing either the duration or the frequency of the conditioning stimulation can increase both the magnitude and duration of the effect. Similar results were first reported for the spinal monosynaptic reflex by LLOYD (1949), and a particularly striking example was offered by ECCLES and McINTYRE (1953) when they tested the same reflex several weeks after dorsal root section and recorded a large presynaptic post-tetanic potentiation that decayed with a half-time of 3 hrs. It is now clear that presynaptic post-tetanic potentiation is a widespread phenomenon at chemically transmitting synapses, though apparently not universal (KUNO, 1971); it is absent at some central exitatory synapses, and the evidence that it exists at muscarinic, adrenergic (cf. BENNETT, 1972) or central inhibitory synapses is rather fragmentary. Such a potentiation can last for a long time. The disused synapses examined by ECCLES and McINTYRE (1953) were no doubt a special case, but potentiations lasting an hour or several hours have been recorded from the superior cervical ganglion (DUNANT and DOLIVO, 1968); from spinal monosynaptic pathways (BESWICK and CONROY, 1965; SPENCER and WIGDOR, 1965; SPENCER and APRIL, 1970; ZABLOCKA-ESPLIN and ES-PLIN, 1971; FAREL, 1974) and from the hippocampus (BLISS and LØMO, 1970; BLISS and GARDNER-MEDWIN, 1971). Presynaptic post-tetanic potentiations lasting over an hour have not yet been recorded from the neuromuscular junction, perhaps because the conditioning stimulation was never intense enough.

All the experimenters cited above used electrophysiological methods. Their analyses have led to a fair measure of agreement about the presynaptic changes that underlie post-tetanic potentiation: for reviews see for example WALL (1970), KUNO (1971) and HUBBARD (1974). Of the various mechanisms that have been postulated two have been generally accepted. (a) Hyperpolarization developing during the tetanic stimulation may persist, increasing spike height and therefore transmitter release (LLOYD, 1949): this effect is not always seen, and it plays no part in long-lasting potentiation. (b) There is an increase in fractional release of the transmitter with no apparent change in the size of the releasable pool: this effect is the major one, and it is somehow related to the amount of calcium that can be made available to the release mechanism, perhaps from a membrane store (KATZ and MILEDI, 1965; GAGE and HUBBARD, 1966) which accumulates during the tetanus (ROSENTHAL, 1969) or becomes more readily available as a result of rising sodium concentrations within the nerve terminal (BIRKS and COHEN, 1965). It seems probable that mitochondria within the terminal are involved in calcium storage, playing a similar role to that described in other types of cell (BORLE, 1974), but direct tests are lacking.

Neurochemical studies indicate that a third mechanism may contribute to presynaptic post-tetanic potentiation, especially when the conditioning stimulation is intense and prolonged. In graphs of the time-course of ACh release by ganglia subjected to prolonged stimulation at 20 Hz, the initial fall of output, ascribed to depletion of the readily-available transmitter pool, is prominent. With plasma-perfused ganglia, however, after 5 to 10 min there is usually at least a hint of an opposing process that may correspond to presynaptic post-tetanic potentiation in its usual sense, with some tendency for the curve to show a second slow ascent after 15 to 30 min (e.g. Fig. 6 of BIRKS and MacIntosh, 1961; Fig. 1 of MATTHEWS, 1966; Fig. 1 of BIRKS and FITCH, 1974). With excitation at 5 Hz the first rise is more conspicuous (BIRKS and FITCH, 1974); with excitation at 50 Hz, the later rise appears to be dominant (BOURDOIS et al., 1975).

These findings recall the studies, long unjustly disregarded, of A. ROSENBLUETH and his colleagues during the 1930s (ROSENBLUETH and LUCO, 1939; LANARI and ROSENBLUETH, 1939). They presented evidence for two phases of potentiation of both neuromuscular and ganglionic transmission during prolonged high-frequency (60 Hz) stimulation. In the final paper of the series (ROSENBLUETH et al., 1939), they reported that the ACh content of their ganglia showed parallel changes, which they thought explained the phenomenon; the late rise in stored ACh was best seen when the ganglia were allowed a few minutes rest before being extracted. The changes in ACh content were rediscovered by FRIESEN and his colleagues about 30 years later (FRIESEN and MacCONAILL, 1967; RANGACHARI et al., 1969; FRIESEN and KHATTER, 1971a). BIRKS and FITCH (1974) have observed that the final "rebound" rise is quite evident, amounting to about 40% of the control level, even with stimulation at 20 Hz, provided that the ganglia are rested before removal; it is undetectable after stimulation at 4 Hz. BOURDOIS and his colleagues (1970, 1975), who have also studied the rebound rise, found that it averaged about 60% of the initial ACh content after 1 hr of stimulation at 50 Hz, and then decayed with a half-time of about 2 hrs. The rebound ACh must have a presynaptic location, for it disappears along with the original ACh depot during preganglionic stimulation in the presence of HC-3 and either hexamethonium or tubocurarine (BOURDOIS et al., 1975; see also BIRKS and FITCH, 1974). Rebound ACh accumulates during, as well as after, high-frequency stimulation (Fig. 12). An unexpected finding in these experiments was that the formation of rebound ACh is totally suppressed when hexamethonium or tubocurarine is present during the conditioning stimulation (BOURDOIS et al., 1970, 1975). Thus rebound ACh is one more addition to the ACh pools that have been postulated at cholinergic synapses. Its location, like that of the other pools, is uncertain: BOURDOIS et al. (1975) suggest that it is in vesicles remote from the synaptic interface. Whether it can be formed at other junctions is also uncertain, but a possibly analogous post-stimulation rise in ACh content has been observed in slices of electroplaque (ISRAËL et al., 1972; DUNANT et al., 1974).

In the ganglion, rebound ACh is something of an artefact, since in life impulses do not usually arrive there at 20 to 60 Hz (see however IGGO and VOGT, 1960), though such frequencies are common enough at the neuromuscular junction and at central synapses. If the phenomenon turns out to be a general one, and to be causally related to the very long presynaptic post-tetanic potentiations that have been observed in ganglia and elsewhere, it will be of considerable interest as the first example of a long-lasting presynaptic potentiation that apparently is elicited *only* when the presynaptic impulses have been successful in firing the postsynaptic cells. It has been

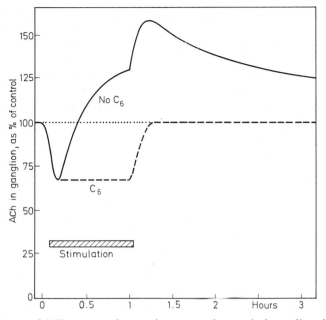

Fig. 12. Time course of ACh content changes in cat superior cervical ganglion during and after prolonged preganglionic stimulation at 50 or 60 Hz. Semi-diagrammatic representation incorporating data from FRIESEN and KHATTER (1971a, b) and BOURDOIS et al. (1975): *cf.* also ROSEN-BLUETH et al. (1939) Hexamethonium bromide (C6) given intravenously: priming dose 10 mg/kg 5 min before stimulation; followed by infusion, 0.2 mg/kg-min, until end of stimulation. Data for ACh content between 10 and 60 min in C6 experiments, by interpolation

repeatedly suggested on theoretical grounds, for example by HEBB (1949), GRIFFITH (1966) and BRINDLEY (1967), that the existence of synapses having this property could account for the main features of classical conditioning with reinforcement and extinction. At ganglia, the potentiation is a transient one, lasting only a few hours, but in other neurones, it might be more enduring.

3. Enzyme Induction

In 1969 THOENEN, MUELLER and AXELROD made the important discovery (for references see AXELROD, 1974) that the central nervous system controls the level of tyrosine hydroxylase in adrenergic neurones and cells of the adrenal medulla. The enzyme's rate of biosynthesis appears to depend on the activity of the controlling cholinergic axons; when the traffic becomes heavier the enzyme level rises in the adrenergic cell bodies and, after a lag, in the adrenergic terminals. A second enzyme in the biosynthetic pathway, dopamine-β-hydroxylase, behaves similarly, though a third, dopa-decarboxylase, does not.

These results with adrenergic neurone enzymes have naturally suggested that the enzymes peculiar to cholinergic neurones might be controlled in a similar way. Some evidence that this is so can be found in the older literature, and more has been obtained recently. For example decentralization (by preganglionic denervation) of parasympathetically innervated structures reduces their activity greatly; in the case of the parotid gland, whose ganglion cells are situated well outside the organ, decentralization reduces ACh (Chang and Gaddum, 1933), AChE (Strömblad, 1955) and ChAc (Nordenfelt, 1967; Ekström and Holmberg, 1972). In the dog, ChAc is reduced by 50—90% within 5 to 7 days. A smaller reduction of ChAc occurs in the parotid glands of rats fed on an exclusively liquid diet (Ekström, 1973), and conversely, ChAc rises by about 20% in rats fed a dry diet or treated with an atropine-like drug (Ekström, 1974b). A similar elevation occurs in the atria of rats that have been chronically exercised and can be supposed to have increased their cardiac vagal tone as a result (Ekström, 1974a). Male mice transferred from single to group cages fight viciously, and when allowed to do so for 10 to 15 min daily their adrenal ChAc increases by as much as 50% (Goldberg and Welch, 1972). For skeletal muscle, though the effects of chronically increased use or disuse on postsynaptic ACh sensitivity and on the muscle fibres themselves have been assiduously studied, not much is known about the effects on presynaptic function. Prolonged hind-limb immobilization has little effect on ACh release, measured as e.p.p. quantum content (Lømo and Rosenthal, 1972), unless the frequency of tetanic stimulation is above 10 Hz, when there is a 25% reduction (Fischbach and Robbins, 1969; Robbins and Fischbach, 1971). Perhaps disuse diminishes the ACh depot. ACh itself has not been measured in muscles subjected to increased use or disuse, but it has been reported (Diamond et al., 1974) that ChAc in rat soleus falls after tenotomy (see also Max et al., 1973), though not during cortisone-induced atrophy; and that it is not increased by work hypertrophy, though it does increase to keep pace with normal growth. The levator ani muscle of the male rat, which atrophies after castration, loses about 40% of its ChAc within 6 months, less than the percentage loss in muscle bulk (Gutmann et al., 1969). Finally, there are some significant data on ganglionic ChAc: Oesch and Thoenen (1973a, b) found that reserpine, which can cause a several-fold increase in tyrosine hydroxylase in the superior cervical ganglion and stellate ganglion of the rat, can also increase ChAc. The largest effect so far reported is a rather modest one (60%), which however may be compared with the 66% rise produced in the newborn rat superior cervical ganglion by prolonged administration of nerve growth factor (Thoenen et al., 1972). The former effect seems to be a true enzyme induction since it is blocked by cycloheximide (Oesch, 1974). It is tempting to ascribe this effect of reserpine on ChAc levels, like the drug's much bigger effect on tyrosine hydroxylase levels, to a compensatory increase in sympathetic discharge; although Iggo and Vogt (1960), who are sometimes quoted as having demonstrated such an increase, were not very positive about this. Nevertheless it has been found that severe stress mimics the effect of reserpine (Oesch and Thoenen, 1973a) and that high spinal transection blocks it (Oesch, 1974). The effect of ganglion-blocking agents has not yet been examined, so it cannot be stated whether the mechanism of enzyme induction has anything in common with the mechanism (pp. 187—188) responsible for producing increased ACh storage capacity in ganglia after repetitive activation.

Thus these results suggest that neuronal activity is probably a significant factor in controlling ChAc and the ACh storage capacity of cholinergic nerve endings, but its influence on these parameters appears to be quite limited, and may be less important than that of the trophic influences that reach the cholinergic neurone from above and below. So far as judgement can be based on the neurochemical data now available, it would seem that after early life biochemical plasticity persists in adrenergic neurones (and in some kinds of effector cell) to a much greater degree than in peripheral cholinergic neurones. However, species and local differences can be important in this context (HENDRY et al., 1973).

For embryos and neonates there is much evidence that the pre- and post-synaptic elements contribute to each other's biochemical maturation (BLACK et al., 1971, 1972a, b; THOENEN et al., 1972). Embryonic cells in tissue culture can also form functional synapses and synthesize the enzymes associated with cholinergic trans-mission. The sequence of events mimics more or less closely that of natural develop-ment. In the case of AChE, both manufacture and loss of the enzyme have been observed (JONES et al., 1956; WERNER et al., 1971). The respective roles of cessation of differentiation and cessation of cell division (BLUME et al., 1970; PRASAD and VERNA-DAKIS, 1972), and of induction by ACh as substrate (JONES et al., 1956; BURKHALTER et al., 1958; GOODWIN and SIZER, 1965), for stimulating formation of the enzyme have been debated. The appearance and rapid increase of ChAc is no doubt a more reliable index than that of AChE to the development of functional cholinergic syn-apses (WERNER et al., 1971; cf. TUČEK, 1972; PILAR et al., 1974). Neither tubocurarine, HC-3 (COHEN, 1971) nor α-bungarotoxin (GIACOBINI et al., 1973) prevents the forma-tion of normal junctions, but a number of dramatic experiments have shown that contact with some kind of non-neuronal cell — e.g. myoblasts or glia — is essential for the manufacture of ChAc by cultured neuronal elements (AMANO et al., 1973; GILLER et al., 1973; PATTERSON and CHUN, 1974). The chemical signal for induction of the enzyme has not yet been indentified; it is unlikely that it is cyclic AMP (SHAPIRO, 1973).

Some of the voluminous information that experimental psychologists and other workers have accumulated on induced changes in brain ChAc and AChE may eventually throw light on the mechanisms of cholinergic plasticity. Only a few exam-ples can be cited. ChAc levels can be altered by drug treatment (MANDELL and KRAPP, 1971; SINGER et al., 1971; LIBERTUN et al., 1973). Visual deprivation reversi-bly lowers ACh in the retina, (LIBERMAN, 1962; GLOW and ROSE, 1966), and either nutritional (ADLARD and DOBBING, 1972) or environmental (KRECH et al., 1966; MCKINNEY, 1970) impoverishment can lower AChE in brain; both enzymes are said to be more abundant in the temporal cortices of clever as compared with stupid mice (EBEL et al., 1973). Many fascinating reports, especially on the effects of cholinergic agonists and antagonists in men and animals, leave little doubt that prolonged interference with central cholinergic mechanisms can produce striking and rather specific changes in behaviour and learning capacity. Some introductory references are: CROW and GROVE-WHITE (1973), DEUTSCH (1971), DRACHMAN and LEAVITT (1974), GEORGE and MELLANBY (1974), GLICK et al., (1973), HAZRA (1970), IZQUIERDO (1972), LEHMANN and OELZNER (1971), MANDEL and EBEL (1974), VOGEL and LEAF (1972) and WIENER and MESSER (1972). The ratio of speculation to fact in these fields is still rather high, and it may be salutary to recall that in the best-studied peripheral neuroeffector system the most striking consequence of prolonged cholinergic block-ade is a striking increase in responsiveness to *adrenergic* stimulation (EMMELIN, 1965).

4. Possible Contribution by Glial Elements

A growing body of literature indicates that glial elements respond to neuronal activity (for references see Watson, 1974b). Hypertrophy and some degree of hyperplasia have been recorded. Particularly striking are the changes in autonomic ganglia following intense and prolonged preganglionic stimulation (Schwyn and Hall, 1965; Schwyn, 1967) or repeated electroshock treatment (Dropp and Sodetz, 1971); in both cases DNA synthesis is stimulated, apparently in relation to amitotic proliferation of glial nuclei (Schwyn, 1967). In the superior cervical ganglion these effects are intensified by neostigmine and abolished by atropine (Schwyn and Hall, 1965), which may suggest that they depend on the activation of dopaminergic interneurones by way of muscarinic synapses (Libet and Owman, 1974) and are unrelated to the changes that lead to the formation of rebound ACh (see pp. 187–188). Peroxidase uptake data (Krishnan and Singer, 1913) and observations on the appearance of intracellular membrane-bound inclusions (Birks, 1974) are suggestive of increased glial-neuronal exchange during activity. There is perhaps a temptation to correlate all these findings with the enduring activity-related changes that neuronal studies have shown to occur in both the adrenergic and cholinergic elements of ganglia. The temptation must be resisted, since no basis for such a correlation exists as yet: even in the case of embryonic neurones, in which contact with glia induces ChAc synthesis (Patterson and Chun, 1974), it has not been shown that the glial elements are irreplaceable in that role. The disappointingly meagre outcome of other biochemical studies on glia (Watson, 1974b) hardly encourages attempts to relate these cells to either short- or long-term alterations in specific neurotransmitter systems.

References

Abdel-Latif,A.A., Roberts,M.B., Karp,W.B., Smith,J.P.: Metabolism of phosphatidylcholine, phosphatidylinositol and palmityl carnitine in synaptosomes from rat brain. J. Neurochem. **20**, 189—202 (1973).

Abdel-Latif,A.A., Smith,J.P.: Studies on choline transport and metabolism in rat brain synaptosomes. Biochem. Pharmacol. **21**, 3005—3021 (1972).

Acara,M., Rennick,B.: Regulation of plasma choline by the renal tubule: bidirectional transport of choline. Amer. J. Physiol. **225**, 1123—1128 (1973).

Adamič,S.: Accumulation of acetylcholine by the rat diaphragm. Biochem. Pharmacol. **19**, 2445—2451 (1970).

Adlard,B.P.F., Dobbing,J.: Vulnerability of developing brain. 8. Regional acetylcholinesterase activity in early life. Brit. J. Nutr. **28**, 139—143 (1972).

Akert,K., Moor,H., Pfenninger,K., Sandri,C.: Contribution of new impregnation methods and freeze etching to the problems of synaptic fine structure. Progr. Brain Res. **31**, 223—240 (1969).

Albuquerque,E.X., Warnick,J.E., Sansone,F.M.: The pharmacology of batrachotoxin. II. Effect on electrical properties of the mammalian nerve and skeletal muscle membranes. J. Pharmacol. exp. Ther. **176**, 511—528 (1971).

Albuquerque,E.X., Warnick,J.E., Tasse,J.R., Sansone,F.M.: Effects of vinblastine and colchicine on neural regulation of the fast and slow skeletal muscles of the rat. Exp. Neurol. **37**, 607—634 (1972).

Aldridge,W.N., Johnson,M.K.: Cholinesterase, succinic dehydrogenase, nucleic acids, esterase, and glutathione reductase in sub-cellular fractions from rat brain. Biochem. J. **73**, 270—276 (1959).

Alemà,S., Calissano,P., Rusca,G., Giuditta,A.: Identification of a calcium-binding, brain-specific protein in the axoplasm of squid giant axons. J. Neurochem. **20**, 681—689 (1973).

AMANO,T., HAMPRECHT,B., KEMPER,W.: High activity of choline acetyltransferase induced in neuroblastoma x glia hybrid cells. Abstr. 4th Internat. Meet. Neurochem. 293 (1973).

ANSELL,G.B., SPANNER,S.: Studies on the origin of choline in the brain of the rat. Biochem. J. **122**, 741—750 (1971).

ANSELL,G.B., SPANNER,S.G.: The inhibition of brain choline kinase by hemicholinium-3. J. Neurochem. **22**, 1153—1155 (1974).

AQUILONIUS,S.M., FRANKENBERG,L., STENSIÖ,K.E., WINBLAD,B.: In vivo studies of two choline acetyltransferase inhibitors. Acta pharmacol. (Kbh.) **30**, 129—140 (1971).

AQUILONIUS,S.M., FLENTGE,F., SCHUBERTH,J., SPARF,B., SUNDWALL,A.: Synthesis of acetylcholine in different compartments of brain nerve terminals in vivo as studied by the incorporation of choline from plasma and the effect of pentobarbital on this process. J. Neurochem. **20**, 1509—1521 (1973).

ARMETT,C.J., RITCHIE,J.M.: The action of acetylcholine on conduction in mammalian non-myelinated fibres and its prevention by an anticholinesterase. J. Physiol. (Lond.) **152**, 141—158 (1960).

ASKARI,A.: Uptake of some quaternary ammonium ions by human erythrocytes. J. gen. Physiol. **49**, 1147—1160 (1966).

AUERBACH,A., BETZ,W.: Does curare affect transmitter release? J. Physiol. (Lond.) **213**, 691—705 (1971).

AUSTIN,L., JAMES,K.A.C.: Rates of regeneration of acetylcholinesterase in rat brain subcellular fractions following DFP inhibition. J. Neurochem. **17**, 705—707 (1970).

AXELROD,J.: Dopamine-β-hydroxylase: regulation of its synthesis and release from nerve terminals. Pharmacol. Rev. **24**, 233—243 (1972).

AXELROD,J.: Regulation of the neurotransmitter norepinephrine. In: SCHMITT,F.O., WORDEN,F.G. (EDS.): The Neurosciences Third Study Program, pp.863—876. Cambridge, Mass.: MIT Press 1974.

AXELSSON,J., THESLEFF,S.: A study of supersensitivity in denervated mammalian skeletal muscle. J. Physiol. (Lond.) **147**, 178—193 (1959).

BABEL-GUÉRIN,E.: Métabolisme du calcium et libération de l'acétylcholine dans l'organe électrique de la Torpille. J. Neurochem. **23**, 525—532 (1974).

BABEL-GUÉRIN,E., DUNANT,Y.: Entrée de calcium et libération d'acétylcholine dans l'organe électrique de la Torpille. C.R. Acad. Sci. (D) (Paris) **275**, 2961—2964 (1972).

BAKER,B.R., GIBSON,R.E.: Irreversible enzyme inhibitors. 181. Inhibition of brain choline acetyltransferase by derivatives of 4-stilbazole. J. Med. Chem. **14**, 315—322 (1971).

BANISTER,J., SCRASE,M.: Acetylcholine synthesis in normal and denervated sympathetic ganglia of the cat. J. Physiol. (Lond.) **111**, 437—444 (1950).

BANISTER,J., WHITTAKER,V.P., WIJESUNDERA,S.: The occurence of homologues of acetylcholine in ox spleen. J. Physiol. (Lond.) **121**, 55—71 (1953).

BANKS,P., MAYOR,D.: Intra-axonal transport in noradrenergic neurons in the sympathetic nervous system. Biochem. Soc. Symp. **36**, 133—149 (1972).

BARKER,L.A., DOWDALL,M.J., ESSMAN,W.B., WHITTAKER,V.P.: The compartmentation of acetylcholine in cholinergic nerve terminals. In: HEILBRONN,E., WINTER,A. (Eds.): Drugs and Cholinergic Mechanisms in the CNS, pp.193—223. Stockholm: Research Institute of National Defence 1970.

BARKER,L.A., DOWDALL,M.J., WHITTAKER,V.P.: Choline metabolism in the cerebral cortex of guinea-pigs. Biochem. J. **130**, 1063—1075 (1972).

BARKER,L.A., MITTAG,T.W.: Inhibition of synaptosomal choline uptake by naphthylvinyl-pyridiniums. FEBS Letters **35**, 141—144 (1973).

BARNARD,E.A., WIECKOWSKI,J., CHIU,T.H.: Cholinergic receptor molecules and cholinesterase molecules at mouse skeletal muscle junctions. Nature (Lond.) **234**, 207—209 (1971).

BARONDES,S.H.: Two sites of synthesis of macromolecules in neurons. Symp. Intern. Soc. Cell Biol. **8**, 351—364 (1969).

BARSOUM,G.S.: The acetylcholine equivalent of nervous tissues. J. Physiol. (Lond.) **84**, 259—262 (1935).

BARZAGHI,F., MANTEGAZZA,P., RIVA,M.: Effects of some guanidine derivatives on neuromuscular and ganglionic transmission. Brit. J. Pharmacol. **19**, 414—426 (1962).

Bauer, H.: Die Freisetzung von Acetylcholin an der motorischen Nervenendigung unter dem Einfluß von d-Tubocurarin. Pflügers Arch. ges. Physiol. **326**, 162—183 (1971).

Beani, L., Bianchi, C., Ledda, F.: The effect of 2,4-dinitrophenol on neuromuscular transmission. Brit. J. Pharmacol. **27**, 299—312 (1966).

Beani, L., Bianchi, C., Megazzini, P., Ballotti, L., Bernardi, G.: Drug induced changes in free, labile and stable acetylcholine of guinea-pig brain. Biochem. Pharmacol. **18**, 1315—1324 (1969).

Beani, L., Bianchi, C., Santinoceto, L., Marchetti, P.: The cerebral acetylcholine release in conscious rabbits with semi-permanently implanted epidural cups. Int. J. Neuropharmacol. **7**, 469—481 (1968).

Bellamy, D.: The distribution of bound acetylcholine and choline acetylase in rat and pigeon brain. Biochem. J. **72**, 165—168 (1959).

Belleau, B., DiTullio, V.: The anionic sites of acetylcholinesterase *versus* the acetylcholine receptors. In: Heilbronn, E., Winter, A. (Eds.): Drugs and Cholinergic Mechanisms in the CNS, pp. 441—453. Stockholm: Research Institute of National Defence 1970.

Belleroche, J. S. de, Bradford, H. F.: The stimulus-induced release of acetylcholine from synaptosome beds and its calcium dependence. J. Neurochem. **19**, 1817—1819 (1972).

Bennett, M. R.: Autonomic Neuromuscular Transmission. Cambridge: University Press 1972.

Bennett, M. R., McLachlan, E. M.: An electrophysiological analysis of the storage of acetylcholine in preganglionic nerve terminals. J. Physiol. (Lond.) **221**, 657—668 (1972a).

Bennett, M. R., McLachlan, E. M.: An electrophysiological analysis of the synthesis of acetylcholine in preganglionic nerve terminals. J. Physiol. (Lond.) **221**, 669—682 (1972b).

Benz, F. W., Long, J. P.: Investigations on a series of heterocyclic hemicholinium-3 analogs. J. Pharmacol. exp. Ther. **166**, 225—236 (1969a).

Benz, F. W., Long, J. P.: Structure-activity relationships of N-alkyl and heterocyclic analogs of hemicholinium-3. J. Pharmacol. exp. Ther. **168**, 315—321 (1969b).

Beranek, R., Vyskočil, F.: The action of tubocurarine and atropine on the normal and denervated rat diaphragm. J. Physiol. (Lond.) **188**, 53—66 (1967).

Berl, S., Puszkin, S., Nicklas, W. J.: Actomyosin-like protein in brain. Science **179**, 441 (1973).

Berman, R., Wilson, I. B., Nachmansohn, D.: Choline acetylase specificity in relation to biological function. Biochim. biophys. Acta (Amst.) **12**, 315—324 (1953).

Berry, J. F., Whittaker, V. P.: The acyl-group specificity of choline acetylase. Biochem. J. **73**, 447—458 (1959).

Bertel-Meeuws, M. M., Polak, R. L.: Influence of antimuscarinic substances on *in vitro* synthesis of acetylcholine by rat cerebral cortex. Brit. J. Pharmacol. **33**, 368—380 (1968).

Beswick, F. B., Conroy, R. T. W. L.: Optimal tetanic conditioning of heteronymous monosynaptic reflexes. J. Physiol. (Lond.) **180**, 134—146 (1965).

Bhatnagar, S. P., Lam, A., McColl, J. D.: Inhibition of synthesis of acetylcholine by some esters of trimethoxybenzoic acid. Nature (Lond.). **204**, 485—486 (1964).

Bhatnagar, S. P., Lam, A., McColl, J. D.: Inhibition of acetylcholine synthesis in nervous tissue by some quaternary compounds. Biochem. Pharmacol. **14**, 421—434 (1965).

Bhatnagar, S. P., MacIntosh, F. C.: Acetylcholine content of striated muscle. Proc. Canad. Fed. Biol. Soc. **3**, 12—13 (1960).

Bhatnagar, S. P., MacIntosh, F. C.: Effects of quaternary bases and inorganic cations on acetylcholine synthesis in nervous tissue. Can. J. Physiol. Pharmacol. **45**, 249—268 (1967).

Bianchi, C.: The effect of caffeine on radiocalcium movement in frog sartorius. J. gen. Physiol. **44**, 845—858 (1961).

Birks, R. I.: The role of sodium ions in the metabolism of acetylcholine. Canad. J. Biochem. Physiol. **41**, 2573—2597 (1963).

Birks, R. I.: Effects of stimulation on synaptic vesicles in sympathetic ganglia, as shown by fixation in the presence of Mg^{2+}. J. Physiol. (Lond.) **216**, 26—28 P (1971).

Birks, R. I.: The relationship of transmitter release and storage to fine structure in a sympathetic ganglion. J. Neurocytol. **3**, 133—160 (1974).

Birks, R. I., Burstyn, P. G. R., Firth, D. R.: The form of sodium-calcium competition at the frog myoneural junction. J. gen. Physiol. **52**, 887—907 (1968).

BIRKS,R.I., COHEN,M.W.: Effects of sodium on transmitter release from frog motor nerve terminals. In: PAUL,W.M., DANIEL,E.E., KAY,C.M., MONCKTON,G., (Eds.): Muscle, pp.403—420. Oxford: Pergamon Press 1965.

BIRKS,R.I., COHEN,M.W.: The action of sodium pump inhibitors on neuromuscular transmission. Proc. roy. Soc. B **170**, 381—399 (1968a).

BIRKS,R.I., COHEN,M.W.: The influence of internal sodium on the behaviour of motor nerve endings. Proc. roy. Soc. B **170**, 401—421 (1968b).

BIRKS,R.I., FITCH,S.J.G.: Storage and release of acetylcholine in a sympathetic ganglion. J. Physiol. (Lond.) **240**, 125—134 (1974).

BIRKS,R.I., HUXLEY,H.E., KATZ,B.: The fine structure of the neuromuscular junction of the frog. J. Physiol. (Lond.) **150**, 134—144 (1960)

BIRKS,R.I., MACINTOSH,F.C.: Acetylcholine metabolism at nerve endings. Brit. med. Bull. **13**, 157—161 (1957).

BIRKS,R.I., MACINTOSH,F.C.: Acetylcholine metabolism of a sympathetic ganglion. Canad. J. Biochem. Physiol. **39**, 787—827 (1961).

BISBY,M.A.: Return of axonally transported protein towards the cell body. Physiol. Canada **6**, 20 (1975).

BLABER,L.C.: The effect of facilitatory concentrations of decamethonium on the storage and release of transmitter at the neuromuscular junctions of the cat. J. Pharmacol. exp. Ther. **175**, 664—672 (1970).

BLABER,L.C.: The prejunctional actions of some non-polarizing blocking drugs. Brit. J. Pharmacol. **47**, 109—116 (1973).

BLACK,I.B., HENDRY,I.A., IVERSEN,L.L.: Trans-synaptic regulation of growth and development of adrenergic neurones in a mouse sympathetic ganglion. Brain Res. **34**, 229—240 (1971).

BLACK,I.B., HENDRY,I.A., IVERSEN,L.L.: The role of postsynaptic neurons in the biochemical maturation of presynaptic cholinergic nerves. J. Physiol. (Lond.) **221**, 149—160 (1972a).

BLACK,I.B., HENDRY,I.A., IVERSEN,L.L.: Effects of surgical decentralization and nerve growth factor on the maturation of adrenergic neurone in a mouse sympathetic ganglion. J. Neurochem. **19**, 1367—1377 (1972b).

BLACKMAN,J.G.: Stimulus frequency and neuromuscular block. Brit. J. Pharmacol. **20**, 5—16 (1963).

BLACKMAN,J.G., GINSBORG,B.L., RAY,C.: Synaptic transmission in the sympathetic ganglion of the frog. J. Physiol. (Lond.) **167**, 355—373 (1963a).

BLACKMAN,J.G., GINSBORG,B.A., RAY,C.: Some effects of changes in ionic concentration on the action potential of sympathetic ganglion cells in the frog. J. Physiol. (Lond.) **167**, 374—388 (1963b).

BLACKMAN,J.G., GINSBORG,B.L., RAY,C.: Spontaneous synaptic activity in sympathetic ganglion cells of the frog. J. Physiol. (Lond.) **167**, 389—401 (1963c).

BLACKMAN,J.G., GINSBORG,B.L., RAY,C.: On the quantal release of the transmitter at a sympathetic synapse. J. Physiol. (Lond.) **167**, 402—415 (1963d).

BLACKMAN,J.G., PURVES,R.V.: Intracellular recordings from ganglia of the thoracic sympathetic chain of the guinea-pig. J. Physiol. (Lond.) **203**, 173—198 (1969).

BLAUSTEIN,M.P.: Preganglionic stimulation increases calcium uptake by sympathetic ganglia. Science **172**, 391—393 (1971).

BLIGH,J.: The level of free choline in plasma. J. Physiol. (Lond.) **117**, 234—240 (1952).

BLIGH,J.: The role of the liver and the kidneys in the maintenance of the level of free choline in plasma. J. Physiol. (Lond.) **120**, 53—62 (1953a).

BLIGH,J.: The effect of a choline-free diet upon the level of free choline in plasma of the rat. J. Physiol. (Lond.) **120**, 440—444 (1953b).

BLIOCH,Z.L., GLAGOLEVA,I.M., LIBERMAN,E.A., NENASHEV,V.A.: A study of the mechanism of quantal transmitter release at a chemical synapse. J. Physiol. (Lond.) **199**, 11—35 (1968).

BLISS,T.V.P., GARDNER-MEDWIN,A.R.: Long-lasting increases of synaptic influence in the unanaesthetized hippocampus. J. Physiol. (Lond.) **216**, 32—33P (1971).

BLISS,T.V.P., LØMO,T.: Plasticity in a monosynaptic cortical pathway. J. Physiol. (Lond.) **207**, 61P (1970).

BLUME,A., GILBERT,F., WILSON,S., FARBER,J., ROSENBERG,R., NIRENBERG,M.: Regulation of acetylcholinesterase in neuroblastoma cells. Proc. nat. Acad. Sci. USA **67**, 786—792 (1970).

Bohan,T.P., Boyne,A.F., Guth,P.S., Narayanan,Y., Williams,T.H.: Electron-dense particle in cholinergic synaptic vesicles. Nature (Lond.) **244**, 32—34 (1973).

Borle,A.B.: Calcium and phosphate metabolism. Ann. Rev. Physiol. **36**, 361—390 (1974).

Bornstein,J.C.: The effects of physostigmine on synaptic transmission in the inferior mesenteric ganglion of guinea-pigs. J. Physiol. (Lond.) **241**, 309—325 (1974).

Boroff,D.A., del Castillo,J., Evoy,J.H., Steinhardt,R.A.: Observations on the action of type A botulinum toxin on frog neuromuscular junctions. J. Physiol. (Lond.) **240**, 227—253 (1974).

Bosmann,H.B., Hemsworth,B.A.: Synaptic vesicles — incorporation of choline by isolated synaptosomes and synaptic vesicles. Biochem. Pharmacol. **19**, 133—141 (1970).

Bourdois,P.S., McCandless,D.L., MacIntosh,F.C.: A prolonged after-effect of high frequency stimulation in a cholinergic pathway. Proc. Canad. Fed. Biol. Soc. **13**, 148 (1970).

Bourdois,P.S., McCandless,D.L., MacIntosh,F.C.: A prolonged after-effect of intense synaptic activity on acetylcholine in a sympathetic ganglion. Canad. J. Physiol. Pharmacol. **53**, 155—165 (1975).

Bourdois,P.S., Szerb,J.C.: The absence of "surplus" acetylcholine in prisms prepared from rat cerebral cortex. J. Neurochem. **19**, 1189—1193 (1972).

Bowman,W.C., Hemsworth,B.A.: Effects of triethylcholine on the output of acetylcholine from isolated diaphragm of rat. Brit. J. Pharmacol. **24**, 110—118 (1965a).

Bowman,W.C., Hemsworth,B.A.: Effects of some polymethylene-*bis*(hydroxyethyl) dimethylammonium salts on neuromuscular transmission. Brit. J. Pharmacol. **25**, 392—404 (1965b).

Bowman,W.C., Hemsworth,B.A., Rand,M.J.: Triethylcholine compared with other substances affecting ganglionic transmission. Brit. J. Pharmacol. **19**, 198—218 (1962).

Bowman,W.C., Hemsworth,B.A., Rand,M.J.: Effects of analogues of choline on neuromuscular transmission. Ann. N.Y. Acad. Sci. **144**, 471—481 (1967).

Bowman,W.C., Marshall,I.G.: Inhibitors of acetylcholine synthesis. In: Cheymol,J.,(Ed.): Neuromuscular Blocking and Stimulating Agents. International Encyclopaedia of Pharmacology and Therapeutics, Section 14, Vol.I, pp.357—390. Oxford: Pergamon Press 1972.

Bowman,W.C., Nott,M.W.: Actions of sympathomimetic amines and their antagonists on skeletal muscle. Pharmacol. Rev. **21**, 27—72 (1969).

Bowman,W.C., Rand,J.J.: Actions of triethylcholine on neuromuscular transmission. Brit. J. Pharmacol. **17**, 176—195 (1961).

Bowman,W.C., Rand,M.J.: The neuromuscular blocking action of substances related to choline. Int. J. Neuropharmacol. **1**, 129—132 (1962).

Bowman,W.C., Webb,S.N.: Acetylcholine and anticholinesterase drugs. In: Cheymol,J. (Ed.): Neuromuscular Blocking and Stimulating Agents. International Encyclopaedia of Pharmacology and Therapeutics, Section 14, Vol. II, pp.427—502. Oxford: Pergamon Press 1972.

Boyd,I.A., Forrester,T.: The release of adenosine triphosphate from frog skeletal muscle *in vitro*. J. Physiol. (Lond.) **199**, 115—135 (1968).

Boyd,I.A., Martin,A.R.: The end-plate potential in mammalian muscle. J. Physiol. (Lond.) **132**, 74—91 (1956).

Bradford,H.F.: An *in vitro* approach to the biochemistry of transmission. In: Heilbronn,E., Winter,A., (Eds.): Drugs and Cholinergic Mechanisms in the CNS, pp. 309—319. Stockholm: Research Institute of National Defence 1970.

Bragança,B.M., Quastel,J.H.: Action of snake venom on acetylcholine synthesis in brain. Nature (Lond.) **169**, 695—697 (1952).

Breckenridge,B.M.L., Burn,J.H., Matshinsky,F.M.: Theophylline, epinephrine and neostigmine facilitation of neuromuscular transmission. Proc. nat. Acad. Sci. (Wash.) **57**, 1893—1897 (1967).

Breemen,V.L. van, Andersson,E., Reger,J.F.: An attempt to determine the origin of synaptic vesicles. Exp. Cell Res., Suppl. **5**, 153—167 (1958).

Bremer,J., Greenberg,D.M.: Methyl transferring enzyme system of microsomes in the biosynthesis of lecithin (phosphatidylcholine). Biochim. biophys. Acta (Amst.) **46**, 205—216 (1961).

Brindley,G.S.: The classification of modifiable synapses and their use in models for conditioning. Proc. roy. Soc. B **168**, 361—376 (1967).

Brodkin,E., Elliott,K.A.C.: Binding of acetylcholine. Amer. J. Physiol. **173**, 437—442 (1953).

Bronk,D.W.: Synaptic mechanisms in sympathetic ganglia. J. Neurophysiol. **2**, 280—401 (1939).

BRONK,D.W., LARRABEE,M.G., GAYLOR,J.B., BRINK,F.JR.: The influence of altered chemical environment on the activity of ganglion cells. Amer. J. Physiol. **123**, 24—25 (1938).

BROOKS,V.B.: An intracellular study of the action of repetitive nerve volleys and of botulinum toxin on miniature end-plate potentials. J. Physiol. (Lond.) **134**, 264—277 (1956).

BROOKS,V.B., THIES,R.E.: Reduction of quantum content during neuromuscular transmission. J. Physiol. (Lond.) **162**, 298—310 (1962).

BROWN,D.A., JONES,K.B., HALLIWELL,J.B., QUILLIAM,J.P.: Evidence against a presynaptic action of acetylcholine during ganglionic transmission. Nature (Lond.) **226**, 958—959 (1970).

BROWN,G.L.: The actions of acetylcholine on denervated mammalian and frog's muscle. J. Physiol. (Lond.) **89**, 438—461 (1937).

BROWN,G.L., VON EULER,U.S.: The after-effects of a tetanus on mammalian muscle. J. Physiol. (Lond.) **93**, 39—60 (1938).

BROWN,G.L., FELDBERG,W.: Differential paralysis of the superior cervical ganglion. J. Physiol. (Lond.) **86**, 10—11 P (1935).

BROWN,G.L., FELDBERG,W.: The action of potassium on the superior cervical ganglion of the cat. J. Physiol. (Lond.) **86**, 290—305 (1936 a).

BROWN,G.L., FELDBERG,W.: The acetylcholine metabolism of a sympathetic ganglion. J. Physiol. (Lond.) **88**, 265—283 (1936 b).

BROWN,G.L., GRAY,J.A.B.: Some effects of nicotine-like substances and their relation to sensory nerve endings. J. Physiol. (Lond.) **107**, 306—317 (1948).

BROWN,G.L., HARVEY,A.M.: Effects of changes in dietary calcium on neuromuscular transmission. J. Physiol. (Lond.) **97**, 330—337 (1940).

BROWNING,E.T.: Free choline formation by cerebral cortical slices from rat brain. Biochem. biophys. Res. Commun. **45**, 1986—1990 (1971).

BROWNING,E.T.: Fluorometric enzyme assay for choline and acetylcholine. Analyt. Biochem. **46**, 624—638 (1972).

BROWNING,E.T., SCHULMAN,M.P.: ^{14}C-acetylcholine synthesis by cortex slices of rat brain. J. Neurochem. **15**, 1391—1405 (1968).

BRÜCKE,F.T.VON: The cholinesterase in sympathetic ganglia. J.Physiol. (Lond.) **89**, 429—437 (1937).

BULLER,A.J., LEWIS,D.M.: Further observations on mammalian cross-innervated skeletal muscle. J. Physiol. (Lond.) **178**, 343—358 (1965).

BULLER,A.J., ECCLES,J.C., ECCLES,R.M.: Differentiation of fast and slow muscles in the cat hind limb. J. Physiol. (Lond.) **150**, 399—416 (1960).

BURGEN,A.S.V., BURKE,G., DESBARATS-SCHÖNBAUM,M.L.: The specificity of brain choline acetylase. Brit. J. Pharmacol. **11**, 308—312 (1956).

BURGEN,A.S.V., CHIPMAN,L.M.: The location of cholinesterase in the central nervous system. Quart. J. exp. Physiol. **37**, 61—74 (1952).

BURGEN,A.S.V., MACINTOSH,F.C.: The physiological significance of acetylcholine. In: ELLIOTT,K.A.C., PAGE,I.H., QUASTEL,J.H., (Eds.): Neurochemistry, 1st Ed., pp.311—389. Springfield, Ill.: Thomas 1955.

BURKHALTER,A., FEATHERSTONE,R.M., SCHUELER,F.W., JONES,M.: The effects of some acetylcholine derivatives on the cholinesterases of chick embryo intestine cultured in vitro. J. Pharmacol. exp. Ther. **120**, 285—290 (1958).

BURT,A.M.: The histochemical demonstration of choline acetyltransferase activity in the spinal cord of the rat. Anat. Rec. **163**, 162 (1969).

BURT,A.M.: A histochemical procedure for the localization of choline acetyltransferase activity. J. Histochem. Cytochem. **18**, 408—415 (1970).

BURT,A.M., DETTBARN,W.-D.: A histochemical study of the distribution of choline acetyltransferase and acetylcholinesterase activity in sensory ganglia and nerve roots of the bullfrog. Histochem. J. **4**, 401—411 (1972).

BURT,A.M., SILVER,A.: Non-enzymatic imidazole catalysed acyl transfer reaction and acetylcholine synthesis. Nature (Lond.) New Biol. **243**, 157—159 (1973).

BURTON,R.M.: Gangliosides and acetylcholine of the central nervous system — the binding of radioactive acetylcholine by subcellular particles of the brain. Int. J. Neuropharmacol. **3**, 13—21 (1964).

Burton,R.M., Howard,R.E.: Gangliosides and acetylcholine in the central nervous system. VIII. Role of lipids in the binding and release of neurohormones by synaptic vesicles. Ann. N.Y. Acad. Sci. **144**, 411—430 (1967).

Burton,R.M., Howard,R.E., Baer,S., Balfour,Y.M.: Gangliosides and acetylcholine of the central nervous system. Biochim. biophys. Acta (Amst.) **84**, 441—447 (1964).

Canepa,F.G.: Acetylcholine quanta. Nature (Lond.) **201**, 184—185 (1964).

Cangiano,A.: Acetylcholine supersensitivity: the role of neurotrophic factors. Brain Res. **58**, 255—259 (1973).

Čapek,R., Esplin,D.W., Salehmoghaddam,S.: Rates of transmitter turnover at the frog neuromuscular junction estimated by electrophysiological techniques. J. Neurophysiol. **34**, 831—841 (1971).

Carlini,E.A., Green,J.P.: Acetylcholine activity in the sciatic nerve. Biochem. Pharmacol. **12**, 1367—1376 (1963).

Carlyle,R.F.: The mode of action of neostigmine and physostigmine on the guinea-pig trachealis muscle. Brit. J. Pharmacol. **21**, 137—149 (1963).

Carmody,J.J., Gage,P.W.: Lithium stimulates secretion of acetylcholine in the absence of extracellular calcium. Brain Res. **50**, 476—479 (1973).

Carter,S.B.: Effects of cytochalasins on mammalian cells. Nature (Lond.) **213**, 261—264 (1967).

Casati,C., Michalek,H., Paggi,P., Toschi,G.: Effects of triperidol on transmission and on release of acetylcholine in the rat sympathetic ganglion *in vitro*. Biochem. Pharmacol. **22**, 1165—1169 (1973).

Castillo,J.del, Engbaek,L.: Nature of the neuromuscular block produced by magnesium. J. Physiol. (Lond.) **124**, 370—384 (1954).

Castillo,J.del, Katz,B.: The effect of magnesium on motor nerve endings. J. Physiol. (Lond.) **124**, 553—559 (1954a).

Castillo,J.del, Katz,B.: Changes in end-plate activity produced by presynaptic polarization. J. Physiol. (Lond.) **124**, 586—604 (1954b).

Castillo,J.del, Stark,L.: The effect of calcium ions on the motor end-plate potentials. J. Physiol. (Lond.) **116**, 507—515 (1952).

Cavallito,G.J., Yun,H.S., Kaplan,T., Smith,J.C., Foldes,F.F.: Choline acetyltransferase inhibitors. Dimensional and substituent effects among styrylpyridine analogs. J. Med. Chem. **13**, 221—224 (1970).

Cavallito,C.J., Yun,H.S., Smith,J.C., Foldes,F.F.: Choline acetyltransferase inhibitors. Configuration and electronic features of styrylpyridine analogs. J. Med. Chem. **12**, 134—138 (1969).

Ceccarelli,B., Hurlbut,W.P., Mauro,A.: Turnover of transmitter and synaptic vesicles at the frog neuromuscular junction. J. Cell Biol. **57**, 499—524 (1973).

Celesia,G.G., Jasper,H.H.: Acetylcholine released from cerebral cortex in relation to state of activation. Neurology (Minneap.) **16**, 1053—1063 (1966).

Chakrin,L.W., Marchbanks,R.M., Mitchell,J.F., Whittaker,V.P.: Origin of acetylcholine released from the surface of the cortex. J. Neurochem. **19**, 2727—2736 (1972).

Chakrin,L.W., Shideman,F.E.: Synthesis of acetylcholine from labelled choline by brain. Int. J. Neuropharmacol. **7**, 337—349 (1968).

Chakrin,L.W., Whittaker,V.P.: The subcellular distribution of N-*Me*-^{3}H acetylcholine synthesized by brain *in vivo*. Biochem. J. **113**, 97—107 (1969).

Chan,S.L., Shirachi,D.Y., Trevor,A.J.: Purification and properties of brain acetylcholinesterase (EC 3.1.1.7). J. Neurochem. **19**, 437—447 (1972).

Chang,C.C., Chen,T.F., Lee,C.Y.: Studies of the presynaptic effect of β-bungarotoxin on neuromuscular transmission. J. Pharmacol. exp. Ther. **184**, 339—345 (1973a).

Chang,C.C., Cheng,H.C., Chen,T.F.: Does d-Tubocurarine inhibit the release of ACh from motor nerve endings? Jap. J. Physiol. **17**, 505—515 (1967).

Chang,C.C., Huang,M.C.: Comparison of the presynaptic actions of botulinum toxin and β-bungarotoxin in neuromuscular transmission. Naunyn-Schmiedebergs Arch. exp. Path. Pharmak. **282**, 129—142 (1974).

Chang,C.C., Huang,M.C., Lee,C.Y.: Mutual antagonism between botulinum toxin and β-bungarotoxin. Nature (Lond.) **243**, 166—167 (1973b).

CHANG, C. C., LEE, C. Y.: Isolation of neurotoxins from the venom of *Bungarus multicinctus* and their modes of neuromuscular blocking action. Arch. int. Pharmacodyn. **144**, 241—257 (1963).

CHANG, C. C., LEE, C.: Studies on the [^{3}H] choline uptake in rat phrenic nerve-diaphragm preparations. Neuropharmacology **9**, 223—233 (1970).

CHANG, H. C., GADDUM, J. H.: Choline esters in tissue extracts. J. Physiol. (Lond.) **79**, 255—285 (1933).

CHAO, L. P., WOLFGRAM, F.: Purification and some properties of choline acetyltransferase. J. Neurochem. **20**, 1075—1082 (1973).

CHEN, I. L., LEE, C. Y.: Ultrastructural changes in the motor nerve. Virchows Arch. Abt. B **6**, 318—325 (1970).

CHENEY, D. L., HANIN, I., MASSARELLI, R., TRABUCCHI, M., COSTA, E.: Vinblastine and vincristine: a study of their action on tissue concentration of epinephrine, norepinephrine and acetylcholine. Neuropharmacology **12**, 233—238 (1973).

CHENG, S. C., NAKAMURA, R.: A study on the tricarboxylic acid cycle and the synthesis of acetylcholine in the lobster nerve. Biochem. J. **118**, 451—455 (1970).

CHENG, S. C., NAKAMURA, R., WAELSCH, II.: Krebs cycle and acetylcholine synthesis in nervous tissue. Biochem. J. **104**, 52 P—53 P (1967).

CHEYMOL, J., BOURILLET, F., OGURA, Y.: Actions de quelques paralysants neuromusculaires sur la libération de l'acétylcholine au niveau des terminaisons nerveuses motrices. Arch. int. Pharmacodyn. **139**, 187—197 (1962).

CHIOU, C. Y.: Effects of ganglionic blocking agents on the neuromuscular junction. Europ. J. Pharmacol. **12**, 342—347 (1970).

CHIOU, C. Y.: Mechanism of acetylcholine release by drugs and its blockade. Arch. int. Pharmacodyn. **201**, 170—181 (1973).

CHIOU, C. Y., LONG, J. P.: Acetylcholine-releasing effects of some nicotinic agents on chick biventer cervicis nerve muscle preparation. Proc. Soc. exp. Biol. (N. Y.) **132**, 732—737 (1969).

CHMOULIOVSKY, M., DUNANT, Y., GRAF, J., STRAUB, R. W., RUFENER, C.: Inhibition of creatine phosphokinase activity and synaptic transmission by black widow spider venom. Brain Res. **44**, 289—293 (1972).

CIANI, S., EDWARDS, C.: The effect of acetylcholine on neuromuscular transmission in the frog. J. Pharmacol. exp. Ther. **142**, 21—23 (1963).

CLARK, A. W., HURLBUT, W. F., MAURO, A.: Changes in the fine structure of the neuromuscular junction caused by black widow spider venom. J. Cell Biol. **52**, 1—14 (1972).

CLELAND, W. W.: The kinetics of enzyme-catalyzed reactions with two or more substrates or products. I. Nomenclature and rate equations. Biochim. biophys. Acta (Amst.) **67**, 104—137 (1963).

CLOSE, R.: Effect of cross-union of motor nerves to fast and slow skeletal muscles. Nature (Lond.) **206**, 831—832 (1965).

COHEN, J. A., OOSTERBAAN, R. A.: The active site of acetylcholinesterase and related esterases and its reactivity towards substrates and inhibitors. In: KOELLE, G. B. (Ed.): Handbuch der experimentellen Pharmakologie, Ergänzungswerk XV. Cholinesterases and anticholinesterase agents, pp. 299—373. Berlin-Heidelberg-New York: Springer 1963.

COHEN, M. W.: The development of neuromuscular activity in amphibian embryonic tissue cultured *in vitro*. Proc. Intern. Union Physiol. Sci. **9**, 117 (1971).

COLLIER, B.: The preferential release of newly synthesized transmitter by a sympathetic ganglion. J. Physiol. (Lond.) **205**, 341—352 (1969).

COLLIER, B.: Preferential release of newly-synthesized acetylcholine. In: FARDEAU, M., ISRAËL, M., MANARANCHE, R. (Eds.): La Transmission Cholinergique de l'Excitation, 199—207. Paris: Inserm 1972.

COLLIER, B.: The accumulation of hemicholinium by tissues that transport choline. Canad. J. Physiol. Pharmacol. **51**, 491—495 (1973).

COLLIER, B., EXLEY, K. A.: Mechanism of the antagonism by tetraethylammonium of neuromuscular block due to *d*-tubocurarine or calcium deficiency. Nature (Lond.) **199**, 702—703 (1963).

COLLIER, B., KATZ, H. S.: The release of acetylcholine by acetylcholine in the cat's superior cervical ganglion. Brit. J. Pharmacol. **39**, 428—438 (1970).

COLLIER, B., KATZ, H. S.: The synthesis, turnover and release of surplus acetylcholine in a sympathetic ganglion. J. Physiol. (Lond.) **214**, 537—552 (1971).

Collier, B., Katz, H. S.: Acetylcholine synthesis from recaptured choline by a sympathetic ganglion. J. Physiol. (Lond.) **238**, 639—655 (1974).

Collier, B., Lang, C.: The metabolism of choline by a sympathetic ganglion. Canad. J. Physiol. Pharmacol. **47**, 119—126 (1969).

Collier, B., MacIntosh, F. C.: The source of choline for acetylcholine synthesis in a sympathetic ganglion. Canad. J. Physiol. Pharmacol. **47**, 127—135 (1969).

Collier, B., Mitchell, J. F.: The central release of acetylcholine during stimulation of the visual pathway. J. Physiol. (Lond.) **184**, 239—254 (1966).

Collier, B., Mitchell, J. F.: The central release of acetylcholine during consciousness and after brain lesions. J. Physiol. (Lond.) **188**, 83—89 (1967).

Collier, B., Poon, P., Salehmoghaddam, S.: The formation of choline and of acetylcholine by brain *in vitro*. J. Neurochem. **19**, 51—60 (1972).

Colomo, F., Rahamimoff, R.: Interaction between sodium and calcium ions in the process of transmitter release at the neuromuscular junction. J. Physiol. (Lond.) **198**, 203—218 (1968).

Comline, R. S.: Synthesis of acetylcholine by non-nervous tissue. J. Physiol. (Lond.) **105**, 6—7 P (1946).

Cooke, J. D., Quastel, D. M. J.: Cumulative and persistent effects of nerve terminal depolarization on transmitter release. J. Physiol. (Lond.) **228**, 407—434 (1973).

Cooke, W. J., Robinson, J. D.: Factors influencing choline movement in rat brain slices. Biochem. Pharmacol. **20**, 2355—2366 (1971).

Cooper, P. D., Smith, R. S.: The movement of optically detectable organelles in myelinated axons of *Xenopus laevis*. J. Physiol. (Lond.) **242**, 77—97 (1974).

Corteggiani, E., Gautrelet, J., Kaswin, A., Mentzer, C.: Sur l'existence d'un complexe libérant l'acétylcholine dans les centres nerveux sous l'influence de la chaleur. C. r. Soc. Biol. (Paris) **123**, 667—668 (1936).

Cotman, C., Herschman, H., Taylor, D.: Subcellular fractionation of cultured glial cells. J. Neurobiology **2**, 169—180 (1971).

Couteaux, R., Nachmansohn, D.: Changes of choline esterase at end-plates of voluntary muscle following section of sciatic nerve. Proc. Soc. exp. Biol. (N. Y.) **43**, 177—181 (1940).

Couteaux, R., Taxi, J.: Recherches histochimiques sur la distribution des activités cholinestérasiques au niveau de la synapse myoneurale. Arch. Anat. micr. Morph. exp. **41**, 352—392 (1952).

Cowan, S. L.: The action of eserine-like compounds upon frog's nerve-muscle preparations, and conditions in which a single shock can evoke a repetitive response. Proc. roy. Soc. B **129**, 356—391 (1940).

Cowie, A. L., Kosterlitz, H. W., Watt, A. J.: Mode of action of morphine-like drugs on autonomic neuro-effectors. Nature (Lond.) **220**, 1040—1042 (1968).

Cragg, B. G.: What is the signal for chromatolysis? Brain Res. **23**, 1—21 (1970).

Creese, R., MacLagan, J.: Autoradiography of decamethonium in rat muscle. Nature (Lond.) **215**, 988—989 (1967).

Crone, H. D., Freeman, S. E.: The acetylcholinesterase activity of the denervated rat diaphragm. J. Neurochem. **19**, 1207—1208 (1972).

Crossland, J., Slater, P.: The effect of some drugs on the "free" and "bound" acetylcholine content of rat brain. Brit. J. Pharmacol. **33**, 42—47 (1968).

Crow, T. J., Grove-White, I. G.: An analysis of the learning deficit following hyoscine administration to man. Brit. J. Pharmacol. **49**, 322—327 (1973).

Csillik, B., Haarstad, V. B., Knyihar, E.: Autoradiographic localization of ^{14}C-hemicholinium — an approach to locate sites of acetylcholine synthesis. J. Histochem. Cytochem. **18**, 58—60 (1970).

Cull-Candy, C., Neal, H., Usherwood, P. N. R.: Action of black widow spider venom on an aminergic synapse. Nature (Lond.) **241**, 353—354 (1973).

Currier, S. F., Mautner, H. G.: On the mechanism of action of choline acetyltransferase. Proc. nat. Acad. Sci. (Wash.) **71**, 3355—3358 (1974).

Dahlström, A.: Observations on the accumulation of noradrenaline in the proximal and distal parts of peripheral adrenergic nerves after compression. J. Anat. (Lond.) **99**, 677—689 (1965).

Dahlström, A.: Effect of colchicine on transport of amine storage granules in sympathetic nerves of rat. Europ. J. Pharmacol. **5**, 111—113 (1968).

DAHLSTRÖM,A.: Axoplasmic transport (with particular respect to adrenergic neurons). Phil. Trans. B **261**, 325—358 (1971).
DAHLSTRÖM,A.B., EVANS,C.A.N., HÄGGENDAL,C.J., HEIWALL,P.O., SAUNDERS,N.R.: Rapid transport of acetylcholine in rat sciatic nerve proximal and distal to a lesion. J. neural Transmission **35**, 1—11 (1974).
DAHLSTRÖM,A., HÄGGENDAL,J.: Studies on the transport and life-span of amine storage granules in a peripheral adrenergic neuron system. Acta physiol. scand. **67**, 278—288 (1966).
DALE,H.H.: Adventures in Physiology, p. 637. London: Pergamon Press 1953.
DALE,H.H., FELDBERG,W., VOGT,M.: Release of acetylcholine at voluntary motor nerve endings. J. Physiol. (Lond.) **86**, 353—380 (1936).
DAUTERMAN,W.C., MEHROTRA,K.N.: The N-alkyl group specificity of choline acetylase from brain. J. Neurochem. **10**, 113—123 (1963).
DAVIS,H.A., HORTON,E.W., JONES,K.B., QUILLIAM,J.P.: Identification of prostaglandins in prevertebral venous blood after preganglionic stimulation of the cat superior cervical ganglion. Brit. J. Pharmacol. **42**, 569—583 (1971).
DAVIS,R., KOELLE,G.B.: Electron microscopic localization of acetylcholinesterase and nonspecific cholinesterase at the neuromuscular junction by the gold-thiocholine and gold-thiolacetic acid methods. J. Cell Biol. **34**, 157—171 (1967).
DAWES,P.M., VIZI,E.S.: Acetylcholine release from the rabbit isolated superior cervical ganglion preparation. Brit. J. Pharmacol. **48**, 225—232 (1973).
DEBASSIO,W.S., SCHNITZLER,R.M., PARSONS,R.M.: Influence of lanthanum on transmitter release at the neuromuscular junction. Fed. Proc. **30**, 617 (1971).
DEBECKER,J.: Activation of neuromuscular transmission: calcium, potassium, veratrum, guanidine. In: CHEYMOL,J. (Ed.): Neuromuscular Blocking and Stimulating Agents, International Encyclopedia of Pharmacology and Therapeutics, Section 14, Vol. 11, pp. 503—513. Oxford: Pergamon Press 1972.
DEGROAT,W.C., VOLLE,R.L.: The actions of the catecholamines on transmission in the superior cervical ganglion of the cat. J. Pharmacol. exp. Ther. **154**, 1—13 (1966).
DENNIS,M.J., HARRIS,A.J., KUFFLER,S.W.: Synaptic transmission and its duplication by focally applied acetylcholine in parasympathetic neurons in the heart of the frog. Proc. roy. Soc. B **177**, 509—539 (1971).
DE ROBERTIS,E., PELLEGRINO DE IRALDI,A., RODRIGUEZ DE LORES ARNAIZ,G., GOMEZ,C.J.: On the isolation of nerve endings and synaptic vesicles. J. biophys. biochem. Cytol. **9**, 229—235 (1961).
DE ROBERTIS,E., RODRIGUEZ DE LORES ARNAIZ,G., PELLEGRINO DE IRALDI,A., SALGANICOFF,L.: Cholinergic and non-cholinergic nerve endings in rat brain. J. Neurochem. **9**, 24—35 (1962).
DE ROBERTIS,E., RODRIGUEZ DE LORES ARNAIZ,G., SALGANICOFF,L., PELLEGRINO DE IRALDI,A., ZIEHLER,L.M.: Isolation of synaptic vesicles and structural organization of the acetylcholine system within brain nerve endings. J. Neurochem. **10**, 225—235 (1963).
DESIRAJU,T.: Role of potassium and calcium in the turnover of acetylcholine. Quart. J. exp. Physiol. **51**, 177—183 (1966).
DESMEDT,J.E.: Guanidine et myasthénie grave. Rev. neurol. **94**, 154—158 (1956).
DETWILER,P.B.: The effects of germine-3-acetate on neuromuscular transmission. J. Pharmacol. exp. Ther. **180**, 244—254 (1972).
DEUTSCH,J.A.: The cholinergic synapse and the site of memory. Science **174**, 788—794 (1971).
DIAMOND,I.: Choline metabolism in brain: the role of choline transport and the effects of phenobarbital. Arch. Neurol. (Chic.) **24**, 333—339 (1971).
DIAMOND,I., FRANKLIN,G.M., MILFAY,D.: The relationship of choline acetyltransferase activity at the neuromuscular junction to changes in muscle mass and function. J. Physiol. (Lond.) **236**, 247—257 (1974).
DIAMOND,I., KENNEDY,E.P.: Carrier-mediated transport of choline into synaptic nerve endings. J. biol. Chem. **244**, 3258—3263 (1969).
DIAMOND,I., MILFAY,D.: Uptake of ^{3}H-methyl choline by microsomal, synaptosomal, mitochondrial and synaptic vesicle fractions of rat brain. The effects of hemicholinium. J. Neurochem. **19**, 1899—1909 (1972).
DIAMOND,J., EVANS,C.A.N.: Acetylcholine in regenerating motor nerves. J. Physiol. (Lond.) **154**, 69P (1960).

Di Augustine, R. P., Haarstad, V. B.: The active structure of hemicholinium inhibiting the biosynthesis of acetylcholine. Biochem. Pharmacol. **19**, 559—580 (1970).

Dobson, J. G. Jr., Rubio, R., Berne, R. M.: Role of adenine nucleotides, adenosine, and inorganic
phosphate in the regulation of skeletal muscle blood flow. Circulat. Res. **29**, 375—384 (1971).

Dodge, F. A. Jr., Miledi, R., Rahamimoff, R.: Strontium and quantal release of transmitter at the
neuromuscular junction. J. Physiol. (Lond.) **200**, 267—283 (1969).

Domino, E. F., Morhman, M. E., Wilson, A. E., Haarstadt, V. B.: Acetylsecohemicholinium-3, a
new choline acetyltransferase inhibitor, useful in neuropharmacological studies. Neuropharmacology **12**, 549—561 (1973).

Domino, E. F., Shellenberger, M. K., Frappin, J.: Inhibition of acetylcholinesterase *in vitro* by
hemicholinium. Arch. int. Pharmacodyn. **176**, 42—49 (1968).

Douglas, W. W.: Stimulus-secretion coupling: the concept and clues from chromaffin and other
cells. Brit. J. Pharmacol. **34**, 451—474 (1968).

Douglas, W. W., Gray, J. A. B.: The excitant action of acetylcholine and other substances on
cutaneous sensory pathways and its prevention by hexamethonium and D-tubocurarine. J.
Physiol. (Lond.) **119**, 118—128 (1953).

Douglas, W. W., Lywood, D. W.: The stimulant effect of tetraethylammonium on acetylcholine
output from the superior cervical ganglion: comparison with barium. Fed. Proc. **20**, 324
(1961).

Douglas, W. W., Lywood, D. W., Straub, R. W.: The stimulant effect of barium on the release of
acetylcholine from the superior cervical ganglion. J. Physiol. (Lond.) **156**, 515—522 (1961).

Douglas, W. W., Poisner, A. M.: Evidence that the secreting adrenal chromaffin cell releases
catecholamines directly from ATP-rich granules. J. Physiol. (Lond.) **183**, 236—248 (1966).

Douglas, W. W., Ritchie, J. M.: The excitatory action of acetylcholine on cutaneous non-myelinated fibres. J. Physiol. (Lond.) **150**, 501—514 (1960).

Douglas, W. W., Sorimachi, M.: Effects of cytochalasin B and colchicine on posterior pituitary
and adrenal medullary hormones. Brit. J. Pharmacol. **45**, 143—144 P (1972 a).

Douglas, W. W., Sorimachi, M.: Colchicine inhibits adrenal medullary secretion evoked by
acetylcholine without affecting that evoked by potassium. Brit. J. Pharmacol. **45**, 129—132
(1972 b).

Dowdall, M. J., Boyne, A. F., Whittaker, V. P.: Adenosine triphosphate. A constituent of cholinergic synaptic vesicles. Biochem. J. **140**, 1—12 (1974).

Dowdall, M. J., Simon, E. J.: Comparative studies on synaptosomes: uptake of [N-methyl-^{3}H]
choline by synaptosomes from squid optic lobes. J. Neurochem. **21**, 969—982 (1973).

Drachman, D. A., Leavitt, J.: Human memory and the cholinergic system. A relationship to
aging. Arch. Neurol. (Chic.) **30**, 113—121 (1974).

Dropp, J. J., Sodetz, F. J.: Changes in neuroglia and neurons of behaviourally stressed rats. Brain
Res. **33**, 419—430 (1971).

Dross, K., Kewitz, H.: Concentration and origin of choline in the rat brain. Naunyn-Schmiedeberg's Arch. exp. Path. Pharmak. **274**, 91—106 (1972).

Droz, B.: Renewal of synaptic proteins. Brain Res. **62**, 383—394 (1973).

Droz, B., Koenig, H. L.: Dynamic condition of protein in axons and axon terminals. Acta neuropath. (Berl.), Suppl. **5**, 109—118 (1971).

Duchen, L. W., Tonge, D. A.: The effects of tetanus toxin on neuromuscular transmission and on
the morphology of motor end-plates in slow and fast skeletal muscle of the mouse. J. Physiol.
(Lond.) **228**, 157—172 (1973).

Dunant, Y.: Mechanisms of synaptic transmission. Presynaptic spike and excitatory postsynaptic potential in sympathetic ganglion. Their modification by pharmacological agents. Progress in Brain Res. **31**, 131—139 (1969).

Dunant, Y.: Some properties of the presynaptic nerve terminals of a mammalian sympathetic
ganglion. J. Physiol. (Lond.) **221**, 577—588 (1972).

Dunant, Y., Dolivo, M.: Presynaptic recording in excised sympathetic ganglion of the rat. Brain
Res. **10**, 268—270 (1968).

Dunant, Y., Gautron, J., Israël, M., Lesbats, B., Manaranche, R.: Effet de la stimulation de
l'organe électrique de la Torpille sur les "compartiments libre et lié" d'acétylcholine. C. r. Acad.
Sci. (Paris) **273**, 233—236 (1971).

DUNANT,Y., GAUTRON,J., ISRAËL,M., LESBATS,B., MANARANCHE,R.: Les compartiments d'acétylcholine de l'organe électrique de la Torpille et leurs modifications par la stimulation. J. Neurochem. **19**, 1987—2002 (1972).
DUNANT,Y., GAUTRON,J., ISRAËL,M., LESBATS,B., MANARANCHE,R.: Evolution de la décharge de l'organe électrique de la Torpille et variations simultanées de l'acétylcholine au cours de la stimulation. J. Neurochem. **23**, 635—644 (1974).
EBEL,A., HERMETET,J.C., MANDEL,P.: Comparative study of acetylcholinesterase and choline acetyltransferase enzyme activity in brain of DBA and C_{57} mice. Nature (Lond.) New Biol. **242**, 56—57 (1973).
ECCLES,J.C.: The nature of synaptic transmission in a sympathetic ganglion. J. Physiol. (Lond.) **103**, 27—54 (1944).
ECCLES,J.C., KATZ,B., KUFFLER,S.W.: Nature of the "endplate potential" in curarized muscle. J. Neurophysiol. **4**, 362—387 (1941).
ECCLES,J.C., KATZ,B., KUFFLER,S.W.: Effect of eserine on neuromuscular transmission. J. Neurophysiol. **5**, 211—230 (1942).
ECCLES,J.C., MCINTYRE,A.K.: Plasticity of mammalian monosynaptic reflexes. Nature (Lond.) **167**, 466—468 (1951).
ECCLES,J.C., MCINTYRE,A.K.: The effects of disuse and of activity on mammalian spinal reflexes. J. Physiol. (Lond.) **121**, 492—516 (1953).
EDSTRÖM,A., MATTSON,H.: Fast axonal transport in the sciatic system of the frog. J. Neurochem. **19**, 205—221 (1972).
EICHBERG,J., WHITTAKER,V.P., DAWSON,R.M.C.: Distribution of lipids in subcellular particles of guinea-pig brain. Biochem. J. **92**, 91—100 (1964).
EISENSTADT,M.L., TREISTMAN,S.N., SCHWARTZ,J.H.: Metabolism of acetylcholine in the nervous system of *Aplysia californica*. II. Regional localization and characterization of choline uptake. J. gen. Physiol. **65**, 275—291 (1975).
EKSBORG,S., PERSSON,B.A.: Photometric determination of acetylcholine and choline after selective isolation by ion-pair chromatography. In: HANIN,I. (Ed.): Choline and Acetylcholine: Handbook of Chemical Assay Methods, pp.181—193. New York: Raven Press 1974.
EKSTRÖM,J.: Choline acetyltransferase and secretory responses of the rat's salivary glands after liquid diet. Quart. J. exp. Physiol. **58**, 171—179 (1973).
EKSTRÖM,J.: Choline acetyltransferase in the heart and salivary glands of the rat after physical training. Quart. J. exp. Physiol. **59**, 73—80 (1974a).
EKSTRÖM,J.: Choline acetyltransferase activity in rat salivary glands after cellulose-rich diet or treatment with an atropine-like drug. Quart. J. exp. Physiol. **59**, 191—199 (1974b).
EKSTRÖM,J., HOLMBERG,J.: Effect of decentralization on the choline acetyltransferase of the canine parotid gland. J. Physiol. (Lond.) **222**, 93—94P (1972).
ELLIOTT,K.A.C., HENDERSON,N.: Factors affecting acetylcholine found in excised rat brain. Amer. J. Physiol. **165**, 365—374 (1951).
ELLIOTT,K.A.C., SWANK,R.L., HENDERSON,N.: Effects of anaesthetics and convulsants on acetylcholine content of brain. Amer. J. Physiol. **162**, 469—474 (1950).
ELMQVIST,D., FELDMAN,D.S.: Calcium dependence of spontaneous acetylcholine release at mammalian motor nerve terminals. J. Physiol. (Lond.) **181**, 487—497 (1965a).
ELMQVIST,D., FELDMAN,D.S.: Effects of sodium pump inhibitors on spontaneous acetylcholine release at the neuromuscular junction. J. Physiol. (Lond.) **181**, 498—505 (1965b).
ELMQVIST,D., JOSEFSSON,J.O.: The nature of the neuromuscular block produced by neomycine. Acta physiol. scand. **54**, 105—110 (1962).
ELMQVIST,D., QUASTEL,D.M.J.: Presynaptic action of hemicholinium at the neuromuscular junction. J. Physiol. (Lond.) **177**, 463—482 (1965a).
ELMQVIST,D., QUASTEL,D.M.J.: A quantitative study of end-plate potentials in human muscle. J. Physiol. (Lond.) **178**, 505—529 (1965b).
EMMELIN,N.: Action of transmitters on the responsiveness of cells. Experientia (Basel) **21**, 57—65 (1965).
EMMELIN,N., MACINTOSH,F.C.: The release of acetylcholine from perfused sympathetic ganglia and skeletal muscles. J. Physiol. (Lond.) **131**, 477—496 (1956).
EMMELIN,N., MUREN,A.: Acetylcholine release at parasympathetic synapses. Acta physiol. scand. **20**, 13—32 (1950).

ENG, L. F., UYEDA, C. T., CHAO, L. P., WOLFGRAM, F.: Antibody to bovine choline acetyltransferase and immunofluorescent localization of the enzyme in neurones. Nature (Lond.) **250**, 243—245 (1974).

ERÄNKÖ, O., TERÄVÄINEN, H.: Cholinesterase and eserine-resistant carboxylic esterases in degenerating and regenerating motor end plates of the rat. J. Neurochem. **14**, 947—954 (1967).

EVANS, C. A. N., SAUNDERS, N. R.: The distribution of acetylcholine in normal and in regenerating nerves. J. Physiol. (Lond.) **192**, 79—92 (1967).

EVANS, C. A. N., SAUNDERS, N. R.: An outflow of acetylcholine from normal and regenerating ventral roots of the cat. J. Physiol. (Lond.) **240**, 15—32 (1974).

EVANS, R. H.: Some characteristics of calcium accumulation at motor end-plates of mouse diaphragm. Brit. J. Pharmacol. **49**, 168—169 P (1973).

FAREL, P. B.: Persistent increase in synaptic efficacy following a brief tetanus in isolated frog spinal cord. Brain Res. **66**, 113—120 (1974).

FATT, P.: Biophysics of junctional transmission. Physiol. Rev. **34**, 674—710 (1954).

FATT, P., KATZ, B.: An analysis of the end-plate potential recorded with an intracellular electrode. J. Physiol. (Lond.) **115**, 320—370 (1951).

FATT, P., KATZ, B.: Spontaneous subthreshold activity at motor nerve endings. J. Physiol. (Lond.) **117**, 109—128 (1952).

FEIGENSON, M. E., SAELENS, J. K.: An enzyme assay for acetylcholine. Biochem. Pharmacol. **18**, 1479—1486 (1969).

FELDBERG, W.: Present views on the mode of action of acetylcholine in the central nervous system. Physiol. Rev. **25**, 596—642 (1945).

FELDBERG, W., FESSARD, A.: The cholinergic nature of the nerves to the electric organ of the Torpedo (*Torpedo marmorata*). J. Physiol. (Lond.) **101**, 200—216 (1942).

FELDBERG, W., LIN, R. C. Y.: Synthesis of acetylcholine in the wall of the digestive tract. J. Physiol. (Lond.) **111**, 96—118 (1950).

FELLMAN, J. H.: A chemical method for the determination of acetylcholine: its application in a study of presynaptic release and choline acetyltransferase assay. J. Neurochem. **16**, 135—143 (1969).

FENG, T. P.: Studies on neuromuscular function: local potentials around neuromuscular junctions induced by single and multiple volleys. Chin. J. Physiol. **15**, 367—404 (1940).

FENG, T. P.: Studies on the neuromuscular junction. V. The succession of inhibitory and facilitatory effects of prolonged high frequency stimulation on neuromuscular transmission. Chin. J. Physiol. **11**, 451—470 (1937).

FENG, T. P., LEE, L. Y., MENG, C. W., WANG, S. C.: Studies on the neuromuscular junction. IX. The after-effects of tetanization on neuromuscular transmission in cat. Chin. J. Physiol. **13**, 79—108 (1938).

FERGUSON, F. C., JR.: Colchicine. I. General pharmacology. J. Pharmacol. exp. Ther. **106**, 261—270 (1952).

FILOGAMO, G., GABELLA, G.: Cholinesterase behavior in the denervated and reinnervated muscles. Acta anat. (Basel) **63**, 199—214 (1966).

FILOGAMO, G., GABELLA, G.: The development of neuromuscular correlations in vertebrates. Arch. Biol. (Liège) **78**, 9—60 (1967).

FILOGAMO, G., MARCHISIO, P. C.: Acetylcholine system and neural development. Neurosci. Res. **4**, 29—64 (1971).

FISCHBACH, G. D., ROBBINS, N.: Changes in contractile properties of disused soleus muscles. J. Physiol. (Lond.) **201**, 305—320 (1969).

FITZGERALD, G. G., COOPER, J. R.: Studies on ACh in the corneal epithelium. Fed. Proc. **26**, 651 (1967).

FLACKE, W. E., BLUME, R. B., SCOTT, W. R., FOLDES, F. F., OSSERMAN, K. E.: Germine mono- and diacetate in myasthenia gravis. Ann. N. Y. Acad. Sci. **183**, 316—333 (1971).

FOLKOW, B., HÄGGENDAL, J., LISANDER, B.: Extent of release and elimination of noradrenaline at peripheral adrenergic nerve terminals. Acta physiol. scand., Suppl. **307**, 5—38 (1967).

FONNUM, F.: The compartmentation of choline acetyltransferase within the synaptosome. Biochem. J. **103**, 262—270 (1967).

FONNUM, F.: Choline acetyltransferase: Binding to and release from membranes. Biochem. J. **109**, 389—398 (1968 a).

FONNUM, F.: The distribution of glutamate decarboxylase and aspartate transaminase in subcellular fractions of rat and guinea-pig brain. Biochem. J. **106**, 401—412 (1968 b).

FONNUM, F.: Isolation of choline esters from aqueous solutions by extraction with Na tetraphenylboron in organic solvents. Biochem. J. **113**, 291—298 (1969).

FONNUM, F.: Surface charge of choline acetyltransferases from different species. J. Neurochem. **17**, 1095—1100 (1970).

FONNUM, F., FRIZELL, M., SJÖSTRAND, J.: Transport, turnover and distribution of choline acetyltransferase and acetylcholinesterase in the vagal and hypoglossal nuclei of the rabbit. J. Neurochem. **21**, 1107—1120 (1974).

FONNUM, F., MALTHE-SØRENSSEN, D.: Molecular properties of choline acetyltransferase and their importance for the compartmentation of acetylcholine synthesis. Progr. Brain Res. **36**, 13—27 (1972).

FONNUM, F., MALTHE-SØRENSSEN, D.: Membrane affinities and subcellular distribution of the different molecular forms of choline acetyltransferase from rat. J. Neurochem. **20**, 1351—1359 (1973).

FORRESTER, T., LIND, A. R.: Identification of adenosine triphosphate in human plasma and the concentration in the venous effluent of forearm muscles before, during and after sustained contractions. J. Physiol. (Lond.) **204**, 347—364 (1969).

FRANKENBERG, L., HEIMBURGER, G., NILSSON, C., SÖRBO, B.: Biochemical and pharmacological studies on the sulfonium analogues of choline and acetylcholine. Europ. J. Pharmacol. **23**, 37—46 (1973).

FRAZIER, D. T., NARAHASHI, T., MOORE, J. W.: Hemicholinium-3: non-cholinergic effects on squid axons. Science **163**, 820—821 (1969).

FREDERICKSON, R. C. A., PINSKY, C.: Morphine impairs acetylcholine release but facilitates acetylcholine action at a skeletal neuromuscular junction. Nature (Lond.) New Biol. **231**, 93—94 (1971).

FRIEDENBERG, M., SELIGMAN, A. M.: Acetylcholinesterase at the myoneural junction: cytochemical ultrastructure and some biochemical considerations. J. Histochem. Cytochem. **20**, 771—792 (1972).

FRIESEN, A. J. D., KHATTER, J. C.: The effect of preganglionic stimulation on the acetylcholine and choline content of a sympathetic ganglion. Can. J. Physiol. Pharmacol. **49**, 375—381 (1971 a).

FRIESEN, A. J. D., KHATTER, J. C.: Effect of stimulation on synaptic vesicles in the superior cervical ganglion of the cat. Experientia (Basel) **27**, 285—287 (1971 b).

FRIESEN, A. J. D., MACCONAILL, M.: Choline and acetylcholine metabolism in a sympathetic ganglion. Proc. Canad. Fed. Biol. Soc. **10**, 30 (1967).

FRIESEN, A. J. D., LING, G. M., NAGAI, M.: Choline and phospholipidcholine in a sympathetic ganglion and their relationship to acetylcholine synthesis. Nature (Lond.) **214**, 722—724 (1967).

FRIZELL, M., HASSELGREN, P. O., SJÖSTRAND, J.: Axoplasmic transport of acetylcholinesterase and choline acetyltransferase in the vagus and hypoglossal nerve of the rabbit. Exp. Brain Res. **10**, 526—531 (1970).

FRONTALI, N.: Catecholamine-depleting effect of black widow spider venom on iris nerve terminals. Brain Res. **37**, 146—148 (1972).

FRONTALI, N., GRASSO, A.: Separation of three toxicologically different protein components from the venom of the spider *Latrodectus tredecimgultatus*. Arch. Biochem. **106**, 213—218 (1964).

FRONTALI, N., GRANATA, F., PARISI, P.: Effects of black widow spider venom on acetylcholine release from rat cerebral cortex slices *in vitro*. Biochem. Pharmacol. **21**, 969—974 (1972).

FUKUDA, T., KOELLE, G. B.: The cytological localization of intracellular neuronal acetylcholinesterase. J. biophys. biochem. Cytol. **5**, 433—440 (1959).

FUXE, K., GROBECKER, H., HÖKFELT, T., JONSSON, G.: Identification of dopamine, noradrenaline and 5-hydroxytryptamine varicosities in a fraction containing nerve ending particles. Brain Res. **6**, 475—480 (1967).

GAGE, P. W., HUBBARD, J. I.: An investigation of the post-tetanic potentiation of end-plate potentials at a mammalian neuromuscular junction. J. Physiol. (Lond.) **184**, 353—375 (1966).

GAGE, P. W., QUASTEL, D. M.: Competition between sodium and calcium ions in transmitter release at a mammalian neuromuscular junction. J. Physiol. (Lond.) **185**, 95—123 (1966).

Galindo, A.: Prejunctional effect of curare: its relative importance. J. Neurophysiol. **34**, 289—301 (1971).

Gallagher, J. P., Blaber, L. C.: Catechol, a facilitatory drug that demonstrates only a prejunctional site of action. J. Pharmacol. exp. Ther. **184**, 129—135 (1973).

Gallup, B., Dubowitz, V.: Failure of "dystrophic" neurones to support functional regeneration of normal or dystrophic muscle in culture. Nature (Lond.) **243**, 287—289 (1973).

Gardiner, J. E., Domer, F. R.: Movement of choline between the blood and cerebrospinal fluid in the cat. Arch. int. Pharmacodyn. **175**, 482—496 (1968).

Gardiner, J. E., Gwee, M. C. E.: The distribution in the rabbit of choline administered by injection or infusion. J. Physiol. (Lond.) **239**, 459—476 (1974).

Gardiner, J. E., Paton, W. D. M.: The control of the plasma choline concentration in the cat. J. Physiol. (Lond.) **227**, 71—86 (1972).

Gardiner, J. E., Sung, L. H.: A p-terphenyl hemicholinium compound. Brit. J. Pharmacol. **36**, 171—172P (1969).

Geffen, L. B., Rush, R. A.: Transport of noradrenaline in sympathetic nerves and the effect of nerve impulses on its contribution to transmitter stores. J. Neurochem. **15**, 925—931 (1968).

George, G., Mellanby, J.: A further study on the effect of physostigmine on memory in rats. Brain Res. **81**, 133—144 (1974).

Gerhards, K. P., Röttcher, M., Straub, R. W.: Wirkungen von Ca und Mg auf Freisetzung und Synthese von Acetylcholin am spontan aktiven Darm. Pflügers Arch. ges. Physiol. **279**, 239—250 (1964a).

Gerhards, K. P., Röttcher, M., Straub, R. W.: Wirkungen von Ca und Mg auf Freisetzung und Synthese von Acetylcholin am ruhiggestellten Darm. Pflügers Arch. ges. Physiol. **279**, 251—264 (1964b).

Gesler, R. M., Hoppe, J. O.: Pharmacology of 3,6(3-diethylaminopropoxy) pyridazine bis-methiodide, a hemicholinium-like agent. Fed. Proc. **20**, 587—593 (1961).

Gesler, R. M., Lasker, A. B., Hoppe, J. O., Steck, E. A.: Further studies on the site of action of the neuromuscular blocking agent 3, 6-bis (diethylaminopropoxy)pyridazine bis-methiodide. J. Pharmacol. exp. Ther. **125**, 323—329 (1959).

Gfeller, E. M., Kuhar, M. J., Snyder, S. H.: Neurotransmitter-specific synaptosomes in rat corpus striatum: morphological variations. Proc. nat. Acad. Sci. (Wash.) **68**, 155—159 (1971).

Giacobini, E.: The distribution and localization of cholinesterases in nerve cells. Acta physiol. scand. **45** (Suppl. 156), 1—45 (1959).

Giacobini, G., Filogamo, G., Weber, M., Boquet, P., Changeux, J.-P.: Effects of a snake α-neurotoxin on the development of innervated skeletal muscle in chick embryo. Proc. nat. Acad. Sci. (Wash.) **70**, 1708—1712 (1973).

Giarman, N. J., Pepeu, G.. Drug-induced changes in brain acetylcholine. Brit. J. Pharmacol. **19**, 226—234 (1962).

Gilbert, J. C., Hutchinson, M., Kosterlitz, H. W.: The effect of electrical stimulation of the myenteric plexus-longitudinal muscle preparation of the guinea-pig ileum on its acetylcholine content. Brit. J. Pharmacol. **49**, 166—167P (1973).

Giller, E. L. Jr., Schrier, B. K., Shainberg, A., Fisk, H. R., Nelson, P. G.: Choline acetyltransferase activity is increased in combined cultures of spinal cord and muscle cells in mice. Science **182**, 588—589 (1973).

Giller, E. L., Jr., Schwartz, J. H.: Acetylcholinesterase in identified neurons of abdominal ganglion of *Aplysia californica*. J. Neurophysiol. **34**, 108—115 (1971).

Ginsborg, B. L.: The vesicle hypothesis for the release of acetylcholine. In: Andersen, P., Jensen, J. K. S., (Eds.): Excitatory Synaptic Mechanisms, pp. 77—82. Oslo: Universitetsforlaget 1970.

Ginsborg, B. L., Hamilton, J. T.: The effect of caesium ions on neuromuscular transmission in the frog. Quart. J. exp. Physiol. **53**, 162—169 (1968).

Ginsborg, B. L., Hirst, G. D. S.: Prostaglandin E_1 and noradrenaline at the neuromuscular junction. Brit. J. Pharmacol. **42**, 153—154 (1971).

Ginsborg, B. L., Hirst, G. D. S.: The effect of adenosine on the release of the transmitter from the phrenic nerve of the rat. J. Physiol. (Lond.) **224**, 629—645 (1972).

Glick, D.: Choline esterase and the theory of chemical mediation of nerve impulses. J. gen. Physiol. **21**, 431—438 (1938).

GLICK, S. D., MITTAG, T. W., GREEN, J. P.: Central cholinergic correlates of impaired learning. Neuropharmacology **12**, 291—296 (1973).

GLOVER, V. A. S., POTTER, L. T.: Purification and properties of choline acetyltransferase from ox brain striate nuclei. J. Neurochem. **18**, 571—580 (1971).

GLOW, P. H., ROSE, S.: Activity of cholinesterase in the retina with different levels of physiological stimulation. Aust. J. exp. Biol. med. Sci. **44**, 65—72 (1966).

GOLDBERG, A. L., SINGER, J. J.: Evidence for a role of cyclic AMP in neuromuscular transmission. Proc. nat. Acad. Sci. (Wash.) **64**, 134—141 (1969).

GOLDBERG, A. M., McCAMAN, R. E.: Determination of picomole amounts of acetylcholine in brain. J. Neurochem. **20**, 1—8 (1973).

GOLDBERG, A. M., WELCH, B. L.: Adaptation of the adrenal medulla: sustained increase in choline acetyltransferase by psychosocial stimulation. Science **178**, 319—320 (1972).

GOLDBERG, M. E., SALAMA, A. I., BLUM, S. W.: Inhibition of choline acetyltransferase and hexobarbitone-metabolizing enzymes by naphthylvinyl pyridine analogues. J. Pharm. Pharmacol. **23**, 384—385 (1971).

GOLDBERG, M. E., SLEDGE, K., ROBICHAUD, R. C., DUBINSKY, B.: A comparative study of the behavioral effects of scopolamine and 4-(1-naphthylvinyl) pyridine hydrochloride (NVP), an inhibitor of choline acetyltransferase. Psychopharmacologia **23**, 34—47 (1972).

GOMEZ, M. V., DAI, M. E. M., DINIZ, C. R.: Effects of scorpion venom, tityustoxin, on the release of acetylcholine from incubated slices of rat brain. J. Neurochem. **20**, 1051—1061 (1973).

GOODWIN, B. C., SIZER, I. W.: Effects of spinal cord and substrate on acetylcholinesterase in chick embryonic skeletal muscle. Develop. Biol. **11**, 136—153 (1965).

GRAFSTEIN, B.: Transneuronal transfer of radioactivity in the central nervous system. Science **172**, 177—179 (1971).

GRAFSTEIN, B., FORMAN, D. S., McEWEN, B. S.: Effects of temperature on axonal transport and turnover of protein in goldfish optic system. Exp. Neurol. **34**, 158—170 (1972).

GRAY, E. G., WHITTAKER, V. P.: The isolation of synaptic vesicles from the central nervous system. J. Physiol. (Lond.) **153**, 35—37 P (1960).

GRAY, E. G., WHITTAKER, V. P.: The isolation of nerve endings from brain: an electron-microscopic study of cell fragments derived by homogenization and centrifugation. J. Anat. (Lond.) **96**, 79—87 (1962).

GREWAAL, D. S., QUASTEL, J. H.: Control of synthesis and release of radioactive acetylcholine in brain slices from the rat. Biochem. J. **132**, 1—14 (1973).

GRIFFITH, J. S.: A theory of the nature of memory. Nature (Lond.) **211**, 1160—1163 (1966).

GROMADZKI, C. G., KOELLE, G. B.: The effect of axotomy on the acetylcholinesterase of the superior cervical ganglion of the cat. Biochem. Pharmacol. **14**, 1745—1754 (1965).

GUTH, L.: Trophic influences of nerve on muscle. Physiol. Rev. **48**, 645—687 (1968).

GUTH, L., ALBERS, R. W., BROWN, W. C.: Quantitative changes in cholinesterase activity of denervated muscle fibres and sole plates. Exp. Neurol. **10**, 236—250 (1964).

GUTH, P. S.: Acetylcholine binding by isolated synaptic vesicles *in vitro*. Nature (Lond.) **224**, 384—385 (1969).

GUTMANN, E., TUČEK, S., HANSLIKOVA, V.: Changes in the choline acetyltransferase and cholinesterase activities in levator ani muscle of rats following castration. Physiol. bohemoslov. **18**, 195—203 (1969).

GUYENET, P., LEFRESNE, P., ROSSIER, J., BEAUJOUIN, J. C., GLOWINSKI, J.: Inhibition by hemicholinium-3 of [^{14}C] acetylcholine synthesis and [^{3}H] choline high-affinity uptake in rat striatal synaptosomes. Molec. Pharmacol. **9**, 630—639 (1973).

GWEE, M. C. E., LIM, H. S.: Hydrocortisone and the concentration of choline in the plasma of rodents. Brit. J. Pharmacol. **45**, 133—134 (1972).

HABERMANN, E.: Gewinnung und Eigenschaften von Crotactin, Phospholipase A, Crotamin und »Toxin III« aus dem Gift der brasilianischen Klapperschlange. Biochem. Z. **329**, 405—415 (1957).

HAGA, T.: Synthesis and release of ^{14}C-acetylcholine in synaptosomes. J. Neurochem. **18**, 781—789 (1971).

HAGA, T., ABE, T., KUROKAWA, M.: Formation and breakdown of microtubules *in vitro* as studied by flow birefringence. Abstr. 4th internat. Meet. Neurochem. 280 (1973).

Haga,T., Noda,H.: Choline uptake systems of rat brain synaptosomes. Biochim. biophys. Acta (Amst.) **291**, 564—575 (1973).
Häggendäl,C.J., Saunders,N.R., Dahlström,A.B.: Rapid accumulation of acetylcholine in nerve above a crush. J. Pharm. Pharmacol. **23**, 552—555 (1971).
Häggendäl,C.J., Dahlström A.B., Saunders,N.R.: Axonal transport and acetylcholine in rat preganglionic neurones. Brain Res. **58**, 494—499 (1973).
Hall,Z.W., Kelly,R.B.: Enzymatic detachment of endplate acetylcholinesterase from muscle. Nature (Lond.) New Biol. **232**, 62—63 (1971).
Hanin,I.: Ed., Choline and Acetylcholine: Handbook of Chemical Assay Methods. New York: Raven Press 1974.
Hanin,I., Jenden,D.J.: Estimation of choline esters in brain by a new gas chromatographic procedure. Biochem. Pharmacol. **18**, 837—845 (1969).
Hanin,I., Massarelli,R., Costa,E.: Environmental and technical preconditions influencing choline and acetylcholine concentrations in rat brain. In: Heilbronn,E., Winter,A. (Eds.): Drugs and Cholinergic Mechanisms in the CNS, pp.33—54. Stockholm: Research Institute of National Defence 1970.
Hanin,I., Massarelli,R., Costa,E.: An approach to the *in vivo* study of acetylcholine turnover in rat salivary glands by radio gas chromatography. J. Pharmacol. exp. Ther. **181**, 10—18 (1972a).
Hanin,I., Massarelli,R., Costa,E.: An approach to the study of biochemical pharmacology of cholinergic function. Advanc. biochem. Psychopharmacol. **6**, 181—202 (1972b).
Harris,A.J., Miledi,R.: The effect of type D botulinum toxin on frog neuromuscular junctions. J. Physiol. (Lond.) **217**, 497—515 (1971).
Harry,J.: The action of drugs on the circular muscle strip from the guinea-pig isolated ileum. Brit. J. Pharmacol. **20**, 397—417 (1963).
Hart,L.G., Dixon,R.L., Long,J.P., MacKay,B.: Studies using Clostridium botulinum toxin — type A. Toxicol. appl. Pharmacol. **7**, 84—89 (1965).
Harvey,A.M., MacIntosh,F.C.: Calcium and synaptic transmission in a sympathetic ganglion. J. Physiol. (Lond.) **97**, 408—416 (1940).
Hazra,J.: Effect of hemicholinium-3 on slow wave and paradoxical sleep of cat. Europ. J. Pharmacol. **11**, 395—397 (1970).
Hebb,C.: Cholinergic neurons in vertebrates. Nature (Lond.) **192**, 527—529 (1961).
Hebb,C.: Biosynthesis of acetylcholine in nervous tissue. Physiol. Rev. **52**, 918—957 (1972).
Hebb,C.: Formation, storage and liberation of acetylcholine. In: Koelle,G.B. (Ed.): Handbuch der experimentellen Pharmakologie, Ergänzungswerk XV. Cholinesterases and Anticholinesterase Agents, pp. 55—88. Berlin-Heidelberg-New York: Springer 1963.
Hebb,C.O., Krnjević,K., Silver,A.: Acetylcholine and choline acetyltransferase in the diaphragm of the rat. J. Physiol. (Lond.) **171**, 504—513 (1964).
Hebb,C., Morris,D.: Identification of acetylcholine and its metabolism in nervous tissue. In: Bourne,G.H. (Ed.): The Structure and Function of Nervous Tissue, Vol.3, Biochemistry and Disease, pp.25—60. New York: Academic Press 1969.
Hebb,C.O., Silver,A.: Gradient of choline acetylase activity. Nature (Lond.) **189**, 123—125 (1961).
Hebb,C.O., Silver,A.: The effect of transection on the level of choline acetylase in the goat's sciatic nerve. J. Physiol. (Lond.) **169**, 41—42P (1963).
Hebb,C.O., Waites,G.M.H.: Choline acetylase in antero- and retrograde degeneration of a cholinergic nerve. J. Physiol. (Lond.) **132**, 667—671 (1956).
Hebb,C.O., Whittaker,V.P.: Intracellular distributions of acetylcholine and choline acetylase. J. Physiol. (Lond.) **142**, 187—196 (1958).
Hebb,D.O.: The Organization of Behavior. p. 62—66. New York: Wiley 1949.
Hedqvist,P., von Euler,U.S.: Prostaglandin controls neuromuscular transmission in guinea-pig vas deferens. Nature (Lond.) New Biol. **236**, 113—115 (1972).
Heilbronn,E.: The effect of phospholipases on the uptake of atropine and acetylcholine by slices of mouse brain cortex. J. Neurochem. **16**, 627—635 (1969).
Heilbronn,E.: Further experiments on the uptake of acetylcholine and atropine and the release of acetylcholine from mouse brain cortex slices after treatment with phospholipases. J. Neurochem. **17**, 381—389 (1970).

HEILBRONN, E., CEDERGREN, E.: Chemically induced changes in the acetylcholine uptake and storage capacity of brain tissue. In: HEILBRONN, E., WINTER, A. (EDS.): Drugs and Cholinergic Mechanisms in the CNS, pp. 245—265. Stockholm: Research Institute of National Defence 1970.

HEMSWORTH, B. A., DARMER, K. I., JR., BOSMANN, H. B.: The incorporation of choline into isolated synaptosomal and synaptic vesicle fractions in the presence of quaternary ammonium compounds. Neuropharmacology **10**, 109—120 (1971).

HEMSWORTH, B. A., FOLDES, F. F.: Preliminary pharmacological screening of styrylpyridine choline acetyltransferase inhibitors. Europ. J. Pharmacol. **11**, 187—194 (1970).

HEMSWORTH, B. A., MORRIS, D.: A comparison of the N-alkyl group specificity of choline acetyltransferase from different species. J. Neurochem. **11**, 793—803 (1964).

HEMSWORTH, B. A., SMITH, J. C.: The enzymic acetylation of choline analogues. J. Neurochem. **17**, 171—177 (1970a).

HEMSWORTH, B. A., SMITH, J. C.: Enzymic acetylation of the stereoisomers of alpha- and beta-methyl choline. Biochem. Pharmacol. **19**, 2925—2927 (1970b).

HENDERSON, G. I., SASTRY, B. V. R.: Kinetic studies of the reaction mechanism of human placental choline acetyltransferase. Fed. Proc. **30**, 621 (1971).

HENDRY, I. A., IVERSEN, L. L., BLACK, I. B.: A comparison of the neural regulation of tyrosine hydroxylase activity in sympathetic ganglia of adult mice and rats. J. Neurochem. **20**, 1683—1689 (1973).

HESTRIN, S.: The reaction of acetylcholine and other carboxylic acid derivatives with hydroxylamine and its analytical application. J. biol. Chem. **180**, 249—261 (1949).

HEUSER, J., MILEDI, R.: Effect of lanthanum ions on function and structure of frog neuromuscular junction. Proc. roy. Soc. B **179**, 247—260 (1971).

HEUSER, J., REESE, T. S.: Evidence for recycling of synaptic vesicle membrane during transmitter release at the frog neuromuscular junction. J. Cell Biol. **57**, 315—344 (1973).

HODGKIN, A. L., KEYNES, R. D.: Movements of labelled calcium in squid giant axons. J. Physiol. (Lond.) **138**, 253—281 (1957).

HODGKIN, A. L., MARTIN, K.: Choline uptake by giant axons of *Loligo*. J. Physiol. (Lond.) **179**, 26—27 P (1965).

HOEZL, J., FRANCK, H. P.: Proceedings of the Second International Meeting of the International Society of Neurochemistry, 219. Tamburini Editore (1969).

HOFMANN, W. W.: Caffeine effects on transmitter depletion and mobilization at motor nerve terminals. Amer. J. Physiol. **216**, 621—629 (1969).

HOFMANN, W. W., PARSONS, R. L., FEIGEN, G. A.: Effects of temperature and drugs on mammalian motor nerve terminals. Amer. J. Physiol. **211**, 135—140 (1966).

HOFMANN, W. W., STRUPPLER, A., WEINDL, A., VELHO, F.: Neuromuscular transmission with colchicine-treated nerves. Brain Res. **49**, 208—213 (1973).

HOFMANN, W. W., THESLEFF, S.: Studies on the trophic influence of nerve on skeletal muscle. Europ. J. Pharmacol. **20**, 256—260 (1972).

HOLLUNGER, G., NIKLASSON, B.: The occurence of soluble acetylcholinesterases in mammalian brain. Acta pharmacol. (Kbh.) **25**, Suppl. 4, 78 (1967).

HOLLUNGER, E. G., NIKLASSON, B. H.: The release and molecular state of mammalian brain acetylcholinesterase. J. Neurochem. **20**, 821—836 (1973).

HOLTZMAN, E., FREEMAN, A. R., KASHNER, L. A.: Stimulation-dependent alterations in peroxidase uptake at lobster neuromuscular junctions. Science **173**, 733—736 (1971).

HOSIE, R. J. A.: The localization of adenosine triphosphatases in morphologically characterized subcellular fractions of guinea-pig brain. Biochem. J. **96**, 404—412 (1965).

HRDINA, P. D., MANECKJEE, A.: "Free" and "bound" acetylcholine concentrations in rat brain: variability in determination of "free" acetylcholine fraction. J. Pharm. Pharmacol. **23**, 540—541 (1971).

HUBBARD, J. I.: Mechanism of transmitter release. Progr. Biophys. **21**, 33—124 (1970).

HUBBARD, J. I.: Neuromuscular transmission — presynaptic factors. In: HUBBARD, J. I. (ED.): The Peripheral Nervous System, pp. 151—180. New York: Plenum Press 1974.

HUBBARD, J. I., JONES, S. F., LANDAU, E. M.: An examination of the effects of osmotic pressure changes upon transmitter release from mammalian motor nerve terminals. J. Physiol. (Lond.) **197**, 639—657 (1968).

Hubbard, J. I., Kwanbunbumpen, S.: Evidence for the vesicle hypothesis. J. Physiol. (Lond.) **194**, 407—420 (1968).

Hubbard, J. I., Quastel, D. M. J.: Micropharmacology of vertebrate neuromuscular transmission. Ann. Rev. Pharmacol. **13**, 199—216 (1973).

Hubbard, J. I., Schmidt, R. F., Yokota, T.: The effect of acetylcholine upon mammalian motor nerve terminals. J. Physiol. (Lond.) **181**, 810—829 (1965).

Hubbard, J. I., Wilson, D. F.: Neuromuscular transmission in a mammalian preparation in the absence of blocking drugs and the effect of D-tubocurarine. J. Physiol. (Lond.) **228**, 307—325 (1973).

Hubbard, J. I., Wilson, D. F., Miyamoto, M.: Reduction of transmitter release by tubocurarine. Nature (Lond.) **223**, 531—533 (1969).

Hughes, J. R.: Post-tetanic potentiation. Physiol. Rev. **38**, 91—113 (1958).

Hughes, R., Whaler, B. C.: Influence of nerve ending activity and of drugs on the rate of paralysis of rat diaphragm preparations by *Cl. botulinum* type A toxin. J. Physiol. (Lond.) **160**, 221—233 (1962).

Hunt, R.: A physiological test for choline and some of its applications. J. Pharmacol. exp. Ther. **7**, 301—337 (1915).

Hurlbut, W. P., Longenecker, H. E., Jr., Mauro, A.: Effects of calcium and magnesium on the frequency of miniature end-plate potentials during prolonged tetanization. J. Physiol. (Lond.) **219**, 17—38 (1971).

Hutter, O. F.: Post-tetanic restoration of neuromuscular transmission blocked by D-tubocurarine. J. Physiol. (Lond.) **118**, 216—222 (1952).

Hutter, O. F., Kostial, K.: Effect of magnesium and calcium ions on the release of acetylcholine. J. Physiol. (Lond.) **124**, 234—241 (1954).

Hutter, O. F., Kostial, K.: Relationship of sodium ions to release of acetylcholine. J. Physiol. (Lond.) **129**, 159—166 (1955).

Iggo, A., Vogt, M.: Preganglionic activity in normal and in reserpine-treated cats. J. Physiol. (Lond.) **150**, 114—133 (1960).

Imai, S., Riley, A. L., Berne, R. M.: Effect of ischemia on adenine nucleotides in cardiac and skeletal muscle. Circulat. Res. **15**, 443—450 (1964).

Israël, M., Gautron, J., Lesbats, B.: Fractionnement de l'organe électrique de la torpille: localisation subcellulaire de l'acétylcholine. J. Neurochem. **17**, 1441—1450 (1970).

Israël, M., Lesbats, B., Manaranche, R.: Variations d'acétylcholine en relation avec l'évolution de la décharge, pendant la stimulation de l'organe électrique de la Torpille. C. r. Acad. Sci. (Paris) **275**, 2957—2960 (1972).

Israël, M., Tuček, S.: Utilization of acetate and pyruvate for the synthesis of "total", "bound" and "free" acetylcholine in the electric organ of Torpedo. J. Neurochem. **22**, 487—491 (1974).

Iversen, L. L.: Catecholamine uptake processes. Brit. med. Bull. **29**, 130—135 (1973).

Izquierdo, J. A.: Cholinergic mechanism-monoamines relation in certain brain structures. Progr. Drug Res. **16**, 334—363 (1972).

Jeffrey, P. L., Austin, L.: Axoplasmic transport. Progr. Neurobiol. **2**, 207—255 (1973).

Jenden, D. J., Choi, L., Silverman, R. W., Steinborn, J. A., Roch, M., Booth, R. A.: Acetylcholine turnover estimation in brain by gas chromatography / mass spectrometry. Life Sci. **14**, 55—63 (1974).

Johnson, G. A., Boukma, S. J., Lahti, R. A., Mathews, J.: Cyclic AMP and phosphodiesterase in synaptic vesicles from mouse brain. J. Neurochem. **20**, 1387—1392 (1973).

Jones, J. J., Laity, J. L. H.: A note on an unusual effect of gallamine and tubocurarine. Brit. J. Pharmacol. **24**, 360—364 (1965).

Jones, M., Featherstone, R. M., Bonting, S. L.: The effect of acetylcholine on the cholinesterases of chick embryo intestine cultured *in vitro*. J. Pharmacol. exp. Ther. **116**, 114—118 (1956).

Jones, R., Vrbová, G.: Effect of muscle activity on denervation hypersensitivity. J. Physiol. (Lond.) **210**, 144—145 P (1970).

Jones, S. F., Kwanbunbumpen, S.: The effects of nerve stimulation and hemicholinium on synaptic vesicles at the mammalian neuromuscular junction. J. Physiol. (Lond.) **207**, 31—50 (1970a).

Jones, S. F., Kwanbunbumpen, S.: Some effects of nerve stimulation and hemicholinium on quantal transmitter release at the mammalian neuromuscular junction. J. Physiol. (Lond.) **207**, 51—61 (1970b).

JORDAN, L. M., PHILLIS, J. W.: Acetylcholine inhibition in the intact and chronically isolated cerebral cortex. Brit. J. Pharmacol. **45**, 584—595 (1972).

KAHANE, E., LÉVY, J.: Sort de la choline. Administration au rat et à la souris. Arch. Sci. physiol. **4**, 173—183 (1950).

KAHLSON, G., MACINTOSH, F. C.: Acetylcholine synthesis in a sympathetic ganglion. J. Physiol. (Lond.) **96**, 277—292 (1939).

KAITA, A. A., GOLDBERG, A. M.: Control of acetylcholine synthesis — the inhibition of choline acetyltransferase by acetylcholine. J. Neurochem. **16**, 1185—1191 (1969).

KAJIMOTO, N., KIRPEKAR, S. M.: Effect of manganese and lanthanum on spontaneous release of acetylcholine at frog motor nerve terminals. Nature (Lond.) New Biology **235**, 29—30 (1972).

KAPELLER, H., MAYOR, D.: The accumulation of noradrenaline in constricted sympathetic nerves as studied by fluorescence and electron microscopy. Proc. roy. Soc. B **167**, 282—292 (1967).

KARCZMAR, A. G., SRINAVASAN, R., BERNSOHN, J.: Cholinergic function in the developing fetus. In: BOREUS, L. O. (ED.): Fetal Pharmacology, pp. 127—176. New York: Raven Press 1972.

KARLSSON, J. O., SJÖSTRAND, J.: The effect of colchicine on the axonal transport of protein in the optic nerve and tract of the rabbit. Brain Res. **13**, 612—616 (1969).

KARLSSON, J. O., SJÖSTRAND, J.: Transport of microtubular proteins in axons of retinal ganglion cells. J. Neurochem. **18**, 975—982 (1971).

KASA, P.: Identification of cholinergic neurones in the spinal cord: an electron histochemical study of choline acetyltransferase. J. Physiol. (Lond.) **210**, 89—90 P (1970).

KÁSA, P., MANN, S. P., HEBB, C.: Localization of choline acetylase: histochemistry at the light microscope level. Nature (Lond.) **226**, 812—814 (1970a).

KÁSA, P., MANN, S. P., HEBB, C.: Localization of choline acetylase: ultrastructural localization in spinal neurons. Nature (Lond.) **226**, 814—816 (1970b).

KÁSA, P., MANN, S. P., KARCSU, S., TOTH, L., JORDAN, S.: Transport of choline acetyltransferase and acetylcholinesterase in the rat sciatic nerve: a biochemical and histochemical study. J. Neurochem. **21**, 431—436 (1973).

KATO, A. C., KATZ, H. S., COLLIER, B.: Absence of adenine nucleotide release from autonomic ganglion. Nature (Lond.) **249**, 576—577 (1974).

KATZ, B., MILEDI, R.: The effect of calcium on acetylcholine release from motor nerve terminals. Proc. roy. Soc. B **161**, 496—503 (1965).

KATZ, B., MILEDI, R.: The release of acetylcholine from nerve endings by graded electrical pulses. Proc. roy. Soc. B **167**, 23—38 (1967).

KATZ, B., MILEDI, R.: The binding of acetylcholine to receptors and its removal from the synaptic cleft. J. Physiol. (Lond.) **231**, 549—574 (1973).

KATZ, H. S., SALEHMOGHADDAM, S., COLLIER, B.: The accumulation of radioactive acetylcholine by a sympathetic ganglion and by brain: failure to label endogenous stores. J. Neurochem. **20**, 569—579 (1973).

KATZ, N. L.: The effects on frog neuromuscular transmission of agents which act upon microtubules and microfilaments. Europ. J. Pharmacol. **19**, 88—93 (1972).

KATZ, N. L., EDWARDS, C.: Effects of metabolic inhibitors in spontaneous and neurally evoked transmitter release from frog motor nerve terminals. J. gen. Physiol. **61**, 259—260 (1973).

KAYAALP, S. O., MCISAAC, R. J.: Absence of effects of prostaglandins E_1 and E_2 on ganglionic transmission. Europ. J. Pharmacol. **4**, 283—288 (1968).

KELLY, J. S.: The antagonism of Ca^{++} by Na^+ and other monovalent ions at the frog neuromuscular junction. Quart. J. exp. Physiol. **53**, 239—249 (1968).

KERKUT, G. A., SHAPIRA, A., WALKER, R. J.: The transport of ^{14}C-labelled material from CNS to and from muscle along a nerve trunk. Comp. Biochem. Physiol. **23**, 729—748 (1967).

KESTON, A. S., WORTIS, S. B.: The antagonistic action of choline and its triethyl analogue. Proc. Soc. exp. Biol. (N. Y.) **61**, 439—440 (1946).

KIRSHNER, N., KIRSHNER, A. G.: Chromogranin A, dopamine β-hydroxylase and secretion from the adrenal medulla. Phil. Trans. B **261**, 279—288 (1971).

KITA, H., VAN DER KLOOT, W.: Calcium ionophore X-537A increases spontaneous and phasic quantal release of acetylcholine at frog neuromuscular junction. Nature (Lond.) **250**, 658—660 (1974).

KLETZIEN, R. F., PERDUE, J. F., SPRINGER, A.: Cytochalasin A and B. Inhibition of sugar uptake in cultured cells. J. biol. Chem. **247**, 2964—2966 (1972).

Knoll, J., Somogyi, G. T., Illes, P., Vizi, E. S.: Acetylcholine release from isolated vas deferens of the rat. Naunyn-Schmiedeberg's Arch. exp. Path. Pharmak. 274, 198—202 (1972).

Knoll, J., Vizi, E. S.: Effect of frequency of stimulation on the inhibition by noradrenaline of the acetylcholine output from parasympathetic nerve terminals. Brit. J. Pharmacol. 42, 263—272 (1971).

Knyihár, E., Csillik, B.: Localizations of inhibitors of the acetylcholine- and GABA-synthesizing systems in the rat brain. Exp. Brain Res. 11, 1—16 (1970).

Koelle, G. B.: The elimination of enzymatic diffusion artefacts in the histochemical localization of cholinesterases and a survey of their cellular distributions. J. Pharmacol. exp. Ther. 103, 153—171 (1951).

Koelle, G. B.: The histochemical identification of acetylcholinesterase in cholinergic, adrenergic and sensory neurons. J. Pharmacol. exp. Ther. 114, 167—184 (1955).

Koelle, G. B.: Histochemical demonstration of reversible anticholinesterase action at selective cellular sites in vivo. J. Pharmacol. exp. Ther. 120, 488—503 (1957).

Koelle, G. B.: A proposed dual neurohumoral role of acetylcholine: its function at the pre- and post-synaptic sites. Nature (Lond.) 190, 208—211 (1961).

Koelle, G. B.: A new general concept of the neurohumoral function of acetylcholine and acetylcholinesterase. J. Pharm. Pharmacol. 14, 65—90 (1962).

Koelle, G. B.: Cytological distributions and physiological functions of cholinesterases. In: Koelle, G. B. (Ed.): Handbuch der experimentellen Pharmakologie. Ergänzungswerk XV, Cholinesterases and Anticholinesterase Agents, pp. 187—298. Berlin-Heidelberg-New York: Springer 1963.

Koelle, G. B.: Improvement in the accuracy of histochemical localization of acetylcholinesterase: facts and artifacts. In: Heilbronn, E., Winter, A. (Eds.): Drugs and Cholinergic Mechanisms in the CNS. Stockholm: Research Institute of National Defence (1970).

Koelle, G. B.: Current concepts of synaptic structure and function. Ann. N. Y. Acad. Sci. 183, 5—20 (1971).

Koelle, G. B., Davis, R., Smyrl, E. G.: New findings concerning the localization by electronmicroscopy of acetylcholinesterase in autonomic ganglia. Progr. Brain Res. 34, 371—375 (1971).

Koelle, G. B., Friedenwald, J. S.: A histochemical method for localizing cholinesterase activity. Proc. Soc. exp. Biol. (N. Y.) 70, 617—622 (1949).

Koelle, G. B., Steiner, E. C.: The cerebral distributions of a tertiary and a quaternary anticholinesterase agent following intravenous and intraventricular injection. J. Pharmacol. exp. Ther. 118, 420—434 (1956).

Koelle, W. A., Koelle, G. B.: The localization of external or functional acetylcholinesterase at the synapses of autonomic ganglia. J. Pharmacol. exp. Ther. 126, 1—8 (1959).

Koenig, E.: Synthetic mechanisms in the axon. I. Local axonal synthesis of acetylcholinesterase. J. Neurochem. 12, 343—355 (1965).

Koenig, E.: Synthetic mechanisms in the axon. III. Stimulation of acetylcholinesterase synthesis by actinomycin-D in the hypoglossal nerve. J. Neurochem. 14, 429—435 (1967).

Koenig, E., Koelle, G. B.: Acetylcholinesterase regeneration in peripheral nerve after irreversible inactivation. Science 132, 1249—1250 (1960).

Koike, H., Eisenstadt, M., Schwartz, J. H.: Axonal transport of newly synthesized acetylcholine in an identified neuron of Aplysia. Brain Res. 37, 152—159 (1972).

Koketsu, K.: Action of tetraethylammonium chloride on neuromuscular transmission. Amer. J. Physiol. 193, 213—218 (1958).

Koketsu, K., Nishi, S.: Cholinergic receptors at sympathetic preganglionic nerve terminals. J. Physiol. (Lond.) 196, 293—310 (1968).

Kopin, I. J., Breese, G. R., Krauss, K. R., Weisse, V. K.: Selective release of newly synthesized noradrenaline from cat spleen during sympathetic nerve stimulation. J. Pharmacol. exp. Ther. 161, 271—278 (1968).

Korey, A., Hamilton, J. T.: The effect of replacement of potassium by cesium ions on neuromuscular blockade of the rat phrenic nerve-diaphragm preparation in vitro. Canad. J. Physiol. Pharmacol. 52, 61—69 (1974).

KOSTERLITZ, H. W., WALLIS, D. I.: The effects of hexamethonium and morphine on transmission in the superior cervical ganglion of the rabbit. Brit. J. Pharmacol. **26**, 334—344 (1966).

KOSTERLITZ, H. W., WATERFIELD, A. A.: The effect of the interval between electrical stimuli on the acetylcholine output of the myenteric plexus-longitudinal muscle preparation of the guinea-pig ileum. Brit. J. Pharmacol. **40**, 162—163 P (1970).

KOSTERLITZ, H. W., WATERFIELD, A. A.: Effect of calcium and manganese on acetylcholine release from the myenteric plexus of guinea-pig and rabbit ileum. Brit. J. Pharmacol. **45**, 157—158 P (1972).

KOSTERLITZ, H. W., WATERFIELD, A. A.: Characteristics of the morphine receptor in the myenteric plexus of the guinea-pig ileum. Abstr. 4th int. Meet. Neurochem. 34,(1973).

KOSTIAL, D., LANDEKA, M., ŠLAT, B.: Manganese ions and synaptic transmission in the superior cervical ganglion of the rat. Brit. J. Pharmacol. **51**, 231—236 (1974).

KOSTIAL, K., VOUK, V. B.: Lead ions and synaptic transmission in the superior cervical ganglion of the cat. Brit. J. Pharmacol. **12**, 219—222 (1957).

KRAATZ, H. G., TRAUTWEIN, W.: Die Wirkung von 2,4-Dinitrophenol auf die neuromuskulare Erregungsübertragung. Naunyn-Schmiedeberg's Arch. exp. Path. Pharmak. **231**, 419—439 (1957).

KRECH, D., ROSENZWEIG, M. R., BENNETT, E. L.: Environmental impoverishment, social isolation and changes in brain chemistry and anatomy. Physiol. Behav. **1**, 99—104 (1966).

KREUTZBERG, G. W.: Neuronal dynamics and axonal flow. IV. Blockage of intra-axonal enzyme transport by colchicine. Proc. nat. Acad. Sci. (Wash.) **62**, 722—728 (1969).

KRISHNAN, N., SINGER, M.: Penetration of peroxidase into peripheral nerve fibres. Amer. J. Anat. **136**, 1—13 (1973).

KRISTENSSON, K., OLSSON, Y.: Uptake and retrograde axonal transport of peroxidase in hypoglossal neurons. Electron microscopical localization in the neuronal perikaryon. Acta Neuropath. (Berl.) **19**, 1—9 (1971).

KRNJEVIĆ, K., MILEDI, R.: Acetylcholine in mammalian neuromuscular transmission. Nature (Lond.) **182**, 805—806 (1958).

KRNJEVIĆ, K., MITCHELL, J. F.: The release of acetylcholine in the isolated diaphragm. J. Physiol. (Lond.) **155**, 246—262 (1961).

KRNJEVIĆ, K., PHILLIS, J. W.: Acetylcholine-sensitive cells in the cerebral cortex. J. Physiol. (Lond.) **166**, 296—326 (1963).

KRNJEVIĆ, K., STRAUGHAN, D. W.: The release of acetylcholine from the denervated rat diaphragm. J. Physiol. (Lond.) **170**, 371—378 (1964).

KUFFLER, S. W.: Physiology of neuromuscular junctions: electrical aspects. Fed. Proc. **7**, 437—446 (1948).

KUHAR, M. J., SETHY, V. H., ROTH, R. H., AGHAJANIAN, G. K.: Choline: selective accumulation by central cholinergic neurons. J. Neurochem. **20**, 581—593 (1973).

KUHAR, M. J., SIMON, J. R.: Acetylcholine uptake: lack of association with cholinergic neurons. J. Neurochem. **22**, 1135—1137 (1974).

KUNO, M.: Quantum aspects of central and ganglionic synaptic transmission in vertebrates. Physiol. Rev. **51**, 647—678 (1971).

KUPERMAN, A. S., OKAMOTO, M.: A comparison of the effects of some ethonium ions and their structural analogues on neuromuscular transmission in the cat. Brit. J. Pharmacol. **24**, 223—239 (1965).

KUPFER, C.: Histochemistry of muscle cholinesterase after motor nerve section. J. cell. comp. Physiol. **38**, 469—473 (1951).

KURIYAMA, K., ROBERTS, E., VOS, J.: Some characteristics of binding of γ-amino butyric acid and acetylcholine to a synaptic vesicle fraction from mouse brain. Brain Res. **9**, 231—252 (1968).

LAITY, J. L. H.: The release of prostaglandin E_1 from the rat phrenic nerve-diaphragm preparation. Brit. J. Pharmacol. **37**, 698—704 (1969).

LAM, D. M. K.: Biosynthesis of acetylcholine in turtle photoreceptors. Proc. nat. Acad. Sci. (Wash.) **69**, 1987—1991 (1972).

LAMPERT, P., CRESSMAN, M.: Axonal regeneration in the dorsal columns of the spinal cord of adult rats. Lab. Invest. **13**, 825—839 (1964).

LANARI, A., ROSENBLUETH, A.: The fifth stage of transmission in autonomic ganglia. Amer. J. Physiol. **127**, 347—355 (1939).

Landmesser, L., Pilar, G.: The outset and development of transmission in the chick ciliary ganglion. J. Physiol. (Lond.) **222**, 691—713 (1972).

Lapetina, E.G., Lunt, G.G., De Robertis, E.: The turnover of phosphatidyl choline in rat cerebral cortex membranes *in vivo*. J. Neurobiol. **1**, 295—302 (1969).

Larrabee, M.G., Bronk, D.W.: Prolonged facilitation of synaptic excitation in sympathetic ganglia. J. Neurophysiol. **10**, 139—154 (1947).

Laskowski, M.B., Thies, R.: Interaction between calcium and barium on the spontaneous release of transmitter from mammalian motor nerve terminals. Inter. J. Neurosci. **4**, 11—16 (1972).

Law, P.K., Atwood, H.L.: Cross-reinnervation of dystrophic mouse muscle. Nature (Lond.) **238**, 287—288 (1972).

Lees, G.M., Kosterlitz, H.W., Waterfield, A.A.: Characteristics of morphine-sensitive release of neuro-transmitter substances. In: Kosterlitz, H.W., Collier, H.O.J., Villareal, J.E. (Eds.): Agonist and Antagonist Actions of Narcotic Analgesic Drugs, pp. 142—152. Baltimore: University Park Press 1973.

Lefresne, P., Guyenet, P., Glowinski, J.:. Acetylcholine synthesis from [2-^{14}C] pyruvate in rat striatal slices. J. Neurochem. **20**, 1083—1098 (1973).

Le Heux, J.W.: Cholin als Hormon der Darmbewegung. Pflügers Arch. ges. Physiol. **173**, 8—27 (1918).

Le Heux, J.W.: Cholin als Hormon der Darmbewegung. III. Die Beteiligung des Cholins an der Wirkung verschiedener organischer Säuren auf den Darm. Pflügers Arch. ges. Physiol. **190**, 280—300 (1921).

Le Heux, J.W.: Cholin als Hormon der Darmbewegung. IV. Über den Einfluß des Cholins auf die normale Darmbewegung. Pflügers Arch. ges. Physiol. **190**, 301—310 (1921 b).

Lehmann, K., Oelszner, W.: Die Beteiligungen zentral-cholinergischer Mechanismen an Ausbildung und Hemmung bedingter Reaktionen bei Ratten. Acta biol. med. germ. **26**, 559—566 (1971).

Lewartowski, B., Bielecki, K.: The influence of hemicholinium no.3 and vagal stimulation on acetylcholine content of rabbit atria. J. Pharmacol. exp. Ther. **142**, 24—30 (1963).

Lewis, P.R., Shute, C.C.D.: The distribution of cholinesterase in cholinergic neurones demonstrated with the electron microscope. J. Cell. Sci. **1**, 381—390 (1966).

Lewis, P.R., Shute, C.C.D., Silver, A.: Confirmation from choline acetylase analyses of massive cholinergic innervation to the rat hippocampus. J. Physiol. (Lond.) **191**, 215—224 (1967).

Li, T.H.: Study of neuromuscular junction; N-M transmission in rats on choline-deficient diets. Chin. J. Physiol. **16**, 9—12 (1941).

Liang, C.C., Quastel, J.H.: Uptake of acetylcholine in rat brain cortex slices. Biochem. Pharmacol. **18**, 1169—1185 (1969 a).

Liang, C.C., Quastel, J.H.: Effect of drugs on the uptake of acetylcholine in rat brain cortex slices. Biochem. Pharmacol. **18**, 1187—1194 (1969 b).

Liberman, R.: Retinal cholinesterase in rats raised in darkness. Science **135**, 372—373 (1962).

Libertun, C., Timiras, P.S., Kragt, C.L.: Sexual differences in the hypothalamic cholinergic system before and after puberty: inductory effect of testosterone. Neuroendocrinology **12**, 73—85 (1973).

Libet, B., Owman, C.H.: Concomitant changes in formaldehyde-induced fluorescence of dopamine interneurones and in slow inhibitory postsynaptic potentials of the rabbit superior cervical ganglion, induced by stimulation of the preganglionic nerve or by a muscarinic agent. J. Physiol. (Lond.) **237**, 635—662 (1974).

Ièvremont, M., Czajka, M., Tazieff-Depierre, F.: Cycle du calcium à la jonction neuromusculaire, C. r. Acad. Sci. (Paris) **268**, 379—382 (1969).

Liley, A.W.: An investigation of spontaneous activity at the neuromuscular junction of the rat. J. Physiol. (Lond.) **132**, 650—666 (1956 a).

Liley, A.W.: The effects of presynaptic polarization on the spontaneous activity at the mammalian neuromuscular junction. J. Physiol. (Lond.) **134**, 427—443 (1956 b).

Liley, A.W., North, K.A.K.: An electrical investigation of effects of repetitive stimulation on mammalian neuromuscular junction. J. Neurophysiol. **16**, 509—527 (1953).

Lilleheil, G., Naess, K.: A presynaptic effect of d-tubocurarine in the neuromuscular junction. Acta physiol. scand. **52**, 120—136 (1961).

LIPICKY,R.J., HERTZ,L., SHANES,A.M.: Ca^{45} transfer and acetylcholine release in the rabbit superior cervical ganglion. J. cell. comp. Physiol. **62**, 233—241 (1963).

LISSÁK,K.: Effect of extracts of adrenergic fibers on the frog heart. Amer. J. Physiol. **125**, 778—785 (1939).

LIVETT,B.G., GEFFEN,L.B., AUSTIN,L.: Proximo-distal transport of [^{14}C] noradrenaline and protein in sympathetic nerves. J. Neurochem. **15**, 931—939 (1968).

LLOYD,D.P.C.: Post-tetanic potentiation of response in monosynaptic reflex pathways of the spinal cord. J. gen. Physiol. **33**, 147—170 (1949).

LOEWI,O., HELLAUER,H.: Über das Acetylcholin in peripheren Nerven. Pflügers Arch. ges. Physiol. **240**, 769—775 (1939).

LØMO,T.: Neurotrophic control of colchicine effects on muscle? Nature (Lond.) **249**, 473—474 (1974).

LØMO,T., ROSENTHAL,J.: Control of acetylcholine sensivity by muscle activity in the rat. J. Physiol. (Lond.) **221**, 493—513 (1972).

LONG,J.P., EVANS,C.T., WONG,S.: A pharmacological evaluation of hemicholinium analogs. J. Pharmacol. exp. Ther. **155**, 223—230 (1967).

LONG,J.P., SCHUELER,F.W.: A new series of cholinesterase inhibitors. J. Amer. pharm. Ass. **43**, 79—86 (1954).

LONGENECKER,H.E.Jr., HURLBUT,W.P., MAURO,A., CLARK,A.W.: Effects of black widow spider venom on the frog neuromuscular junction. Nature (Lond.) **225**, 701—703 (1970).

LORENTE DE NÓ,R.: On the effect of certain quaternary ions upon frog nerve. J. cell. comp. Physiol. **33**, Suppl. 1—291 (1949).

LUBIŃSKA,L., NIEMIERKO,S.: Velocity and intensity of bidirectional migration of acetylcholinesterase in transected nerves. Brain Res. **27**, 329—342 (1971).

LUBIŃSKA,L., NIEMIERKO,S., OBERFELD,B.: Gradient of cholinesterase activity. Nature (Lond.) **189**, 122—123 (1961).

LUBINSKA,L., NIEMIERKO,S., ODERFELD-NOWAK,B., SZWARC,L.: Behaviour of acetylcholinesterase in isolated nerve segments. J. Neurochem. **11**, 493—503 (1964).

LÜLLMANN,H., HOLLAND,W.: Influence of ouabain on an exchangeable calcium fraction, contractile force, and resting tension of guinea-pig atria. J. Pharmacol. exp. Ther. **137**, 186—192 (1962).

LUNT,G.G., LAPETINA,E.G.: Incorporation of [Me^{14}C] choline into phosphatidyl choline of rat cerebral cortex membranes *in vitro*. Brain Res. **18**, 451—459 (1970).

MACINTOSH,F.C.: The distribution of acetylcholine in the peripheral and the central nervous system. J. Physiol. (Lond.) **99**, 436—442 (1941).

MACINTOSH,F.C.: Formation, storage and release of acetylcholine at nerve endings. Canad. J. Biochem. Physiol. **37**, 343—356 (1959).

MACINTOSH,F.C.: Effect of HC-3 on acetylcholine turnover. Fed. Proc. **20**, 562—568 (1961).

MACINTOSH,F.C.: Synthesis and storage of acetylcholine in nervous tissue. Canad. J. Biochem. Physiol. **41**, 2555—2571 (1963).

MACINTOSH,F.C., BIRKS,R.I., SASTRY,P.B.: Pharmacological inhibition of acetylcholine synthesis. Nature (Lond.) **178**, 1181 (1956).

MACINTOSH,F.C., BIRKS,R.I., SASTRY,P.B.: Mode of action of an inhibitor of acetylcholine synthesis. Neurology (Minneap.) **8** (Suppl. 1), 90—91 (1958).

MACINTOSH,F.C., PERRY,W.L.M.: Biological estimation of acetylcholine. Meth. med. Res. **3**, 78—92 (1950).

MAENO,T., NOBE,S.: Analysis of presynaptic effect of d-tubocurarine on the neuromuscular transmission. Proc. Japan Acad. **46**, 750—754 (1970).

MAGLEBY,K.L., STEVENS,C.F.: The effect of voltage on the time course of end-plate currents. J. Physiol. (Lond.) **223**, 151—171 (1972a).

MAGLEBY,K.L., STEVENS,C.F.: A quantitative description of end-plate currents. J. Physiol. (Lond.) **223**, 173—197 (1972b).

MAGNAN,J.L., WHITTAKER,V.P.: Distribution of free amino acids in subcellular fractions of guinea-pig brain. Biochem. J. **98**, 128—137 (1966).

MANDEL,P., EBEL,E.: Correlations between alterations in cholinergic system and behavior. In: DEROBERTIS,E.,SCHACHT,J. (Eds.): Neurochemistry of Cholinergic Receptors, pp.131—139. New York: Raven Press 1974.

Mandell, A. J., Krapp, S.: The effects of chronic administration of some cholinergic and adrenergic drugs on the activity of choline acetyltransferase in the optic lobes of the chick brain. Neuropharmacology **10**, 513—516 (1971).

Mann, P. J. G., Tennenbaum, M., Quastel, J. H.: On the mechanism of acetylcholine formation in brain *in vitro*. Biochem. J. **32**, 243—261 (1938).

Mannervik, B., Sörbo, B.: Inhibition of choline acetyltransferase from bovine caudate nucleus by sulfhydryl reagents and reactivation of the inhibited enzyme. Biochem. Pharmacol. **19**, 2509—2516 (1970).

Marchbanks, R. M.: Exchangeability of radioactive acetylcholine with the bound acetylcholine of synaptosomes and synaptic vesicles. Biochem. J. **106**, 87—95 (1968a).

Marchbanks, R. M.: The uptake of [^{14}C] choline into synaptosomes *in vitro*. Biochem. J. **110**, 533—541 (1968b).

Marchbanks, R. M.: The conversion of ^{14}C-choline to ^{14}C-acetylcholine in synaptosomes *in vitro*. Biochem. Pharmacol. **18**, 1763—1766 (1969).

Marchbanks, R. M.: Problems concerning the compartmentation of acetylcholine in the synaptic region. In: Balazs, R., Cremer, J. E. (Eds.): Molecular Compartmentation in the Brain, pp. 21—33. New York: Wiley 1973.

Marchbanks, R. M., Israël, M.: Aspects of acetylcholine metabolism in the electric organ of *Torpedo marmorata*. J. Neurochem. **18**, 439—448 (1971).

Marchbanks, R. M., Israël, M.: The heterogeneity of bound acetylcholine and synaptic vesicles. Biochem. J. **129**, 1049—1061 (1972).

Marnay, A., Nachmansohn, D.: Choline esterase in voluntary muscle. J. Physiol. (Lond.) **92**, 37—47 (1938).

Marshall, F. N., Long, J. P.: Pharmacologic studies on some compounds structurally related to the hemicholinium HC-3. J. Pharmacol. exp. Ther. **127**, 236—240 (1959).

Martin, A. R.: Quantal nature of synaptic transmission. Physiol. Rev. **46**, 51 (1966).

Martin, A. R., Orkand, R. K.: Postsynaptic effects of HC-3 on the neuromuscular junction of the frog. Canad. J. Biochem. **39**, 343—349 (1961).

Martin, A. R., Pilar, G.: Dual mode of synaptic transmission in the avian ciliary ganglion. J. Physiol. (Lond.) **168**, 443—463 (1963a).

Martin, A. R., Pilar, G.: Transmission through the ciliary ganglion of the chick. J. Physiol. (Lond.) **68**, 464—475 (1963b).

Martin, A. R., Pilar, G.: Quantal components of the synaptic potential in the ciliary ganglion of the chick. J. Physiol. (Lond.) **175**, 1—16 (1964).

Martin, K.: Concentrative accumulation of choline by human erythrocytes. J. gen. Physiol. **51**, 497—516 (1968).

Martin, K.: Effects of quaternary ammonium compounds on choline transport in red cells. Brit. J. Pharmacol. **36**, 458—469 (1969).

Martin, K.: Extracellular cations and the movement of choline across the erythrocyte membrane. J. Physiol. (Lond.) **224**, 207—230 (1972).

Masland, R. L., Wigton, R. S.: Nerve activity accompanying fasciculation produced by prostigmin. J. Neurophysiol. **3**, 269—275 (1940).

Masuoka, D.: Monoamines in isolated nerve ending particles. Biochem. Pharmacol. **14**, 1688—1689 (1968).

Matthews, E. K.: The effects of choline and other factors on the release of acetylcholine from the stimulated perfused superior cervical ganglion of the cat. Brit. J. Pharmacol. **21**, 244—249 (1963).

Matthews, E. K.: The presynaptic effects of quaternary ammonium compounds on the acetylcholine metabolism of a sympathetic ganglion. Brit. J. Pharmacol. **26**, 552—566 (1966).

Matthews, E. L., Quilliam, J. P.: Effect of central depressant drugs on acetylcholine release. Brit. J. Pharmacol. **22**, 415—440 (1964).

Max, S. R., Snyder, S. H., Rifenberick, D. H.: Effect of neuromuscular activity on choline acetyltransferase and acetylcholinesterase. Abstr. 4th int. Meet. Neurochem. 409 (1973).

McCaman, R. E., Hunt, J. M.: Microdetermination of choline acetylase in nervous tissue. J. Neurochem. **12**, 253—260 (1965).

McCaman, R. E., Weinreich, D., Borys, H.: Endogenous levels of acetylcholine and choline in individual neurons of *Aplysia*. J. Neurochem. **21**, 473—476 (1973).

McCandless, D. L., Zablocka-Esplin, B., Esplin, D. W.: Rates of transmitter turnover in the cat superior cervical ganglion estimated by electrophysiological techniques. J. Neurophysiol. **34**, 817—830 (1971).

McCarty, L. P., Knight, A. S., Chenoweth, M. B.: Incorporation of ^{14}C-choline into phospholipids in the isolated phrenic nerve-diaphragm of the rat. J. Neurochem. **20**, 487—494 (1973).

McComas, A. J., Sica, R. E. P.: Muscular dystrophy: myopathy or neuropathy? Lancet 1970 I 1119.

McComas, A. J., Sica, R. E. P., Currie, S.: Muscular dystrophy: evidence for a neural factor. Nature (Lond.) **226**, 1263—1264 (1970).

McComas, A. J., Sica, R. E. P., Currie, S.: An electrophysiological study of Duchenne dystrophy. J. Neurol. Neurosurg. Psychiat. **34**, 461—468 (1971).

McGeer, P. L., McGeer, E. G., Singh, J. K., Chase, W. H.: Choline acetyltransferase localization in the control nervous system by immunohistochemistry. Brain Res. **81**, 373—379 (1974).

McGovern, S., Maguire, M. E., Gurd, R. S., Mahler, H. R., Moore, W. J.: Separation of adrenergic and cholinergic synaptosomes from immature rat brain. FEBS Letters **31**, 193—198 (1973).

McIsaac, R. J., Koelle, G. B.: Comparison of the effects of inhibition of external, internal and total acetylcholinesterase upon ganglionic transmission. J. Pharmacol. exp. Ther. **126**, 9—20 (1959).

McKinney, T. D.: Brain cholinesterase in grouped and singly caged adrenal-demedullated rats. Amer. J. Physiol. **219**, 331—334 (1970).

McKinstry, D. N., Koelle, G. B.: Acetylcholine release from the cat superior cervical ganglion by carbachol. J. Pharmacol. exp. Ther. **157**, 319—327 (1967a).

McKinstry, D. N., Koelle, G. B.: Effects of drugs on acetylcholine release from the cat superior cervical ganglion by carbachol. J. Pharmacol. exp. Ther. **157**, 328—336 (1967b).

McLennan, H., Elliott, K. A. C.: Factors affecting the synthesis of acetylcholine by brain slices. Amer. J. Physiol. **163**, 605—613 (1950).

Meiri, V., Rahamimoff, R.: Activation of transmitter release by strontium and calcium ions at the neuromuscular junction. J. Physiol. (Lond.) **215**, 709—726 (1971).

Meiri, V., Rahamimoff, R.: Neuromuscular transmission: inhibition by manganese ions. Science **154**, 266—267 (1972).

Mellanby, J., Thompson, P. A.: The effect of tetanus toxin at the neuromuscular junction in the goldfish. J. Physiol. (Lond.) **224**, 407—419 (1972).

Michaelson, I. A., Whittaker, V. P.: The subcellular localization of 5-hydroxytryptamine in guinea pig brain. Biochem. Pharmacol. **12**, 203—211 (1963).

Miledi, R.: The acetylcholine sensitivity of frog muscle fibres before and after complete or partial denervation. J. Physiol. (Lond.) **151**, 1—23 (1960).

Miledi, R.: Transmitter release induced by the injection of calcium ions into nerve terminals. Proc. roy. Soc. B **183**, 421—425 (1973).

Miledi, R., Slater, C. R.: Electrophysiology and electron microscopy of rat neuromuscular junctions after denervation. Proc. roy. Soc. B **169**, 289—306 (1968).

Miledi, R., Thies, R. E.: Post-tetanic increase in frequency of miniature end-plate potentials in calcium-free solutions. J. Physiol. (Lond.) **192**, 54—55 P (1967).

Miledi, R., Thies, R.: Tetanic and post-tetanic rise in frequency of miniature end-plate potentials in low-calcium solutions. J. Physiol. (Lond.) **212**, 245—257 (1971).

Miller, E. K., Dawson, R. M. C.: Can mitochondria and synaptosomes of guinea-pig brain synthesize phospholipids? Biochem. J. **126**, 805—821 (1972).

Minz, B.: Pharmakologische Untersuchungen am Blutegelpräparat, zugleich eine Methode zum biologischen Nachweis von Azetylcholin bei Anwesenheit anderer pharmakologisch wirksamer körpereigener Stoffe. Naunyn-Schmiedebergs Arch. exp. Path. Pharmak. **168**, 292—304 (1932).

Mitchell, J. F., Silver, A.: The spontaneous release of acetylcholine from the denervated hemidiaphragm of the rat. J. Physiol. (Lond.) **165**, 117—129 (1963).

Mizel, S. V., Wilson, L.: Inhibition of the transport of several hexoses in mammalian cells by cytochalasin B. J. biol. Chem. **247**, 4102—4105 (1972).

Mogey, G. A., Young, P. A.: The antagonism of curarizing activity by phenolic substances. Brit. J. Pharmacol. **4**, 359—365 (1949).

Molenaar,P.C., Nickolson,V.J., Polak,R.L.: Preferential release of newly synthesized acetyl-choline from cerebral cortex. J. Physiol. (Lond.) **213**, 64—65P (1971).

Molenaar,P.C., Nickolson,V.J., Polak,R.L.: Preferential release of newly synthesized ^{3}H-acetylcholine from rat cerebral cortex slices *in vitro*. Brit. J. Pharmacol. **47**, 97—108 (1973a).

Molenaar,P.C., Polak,R.L.: Newly formed acetylcholine in synaptic vesicles in brain tissue. Brain Res. **62**, 537—542 (1973).

Molenaar,P.C., Polak,R.L., Nickolson,V.J.: Subcellular localization of newly-formed [^{3}H] acetylcholine in rat cerebral cortex *in vitro*. J. Neurochem. **21**, 667—678 (1973b).

Molinoff,P.B., Potter,L.T.: Isolation of the cholinergic receptor protein of *Torpedo* electric tissue. Advanc. biochem. Psychopharmacology **6**, 111—134 (1972).

Morgan,I.G., Austin,L.: Synaptosomal protein synthesis in a cell-free system. J. Neurochem. **15**, 41—51 (1968).

Morris,D.: The choline acetyltransferase of human placenta. Biochem. J. **98**, 754—763 (1966).

Morris,D., Grewaal,D.S.: Halogen substituted derviatives of acetylcholine as inhibitors of choline acetyltransferase. Life Sci. **8**, II, 511—516 (1969).

Morris,D., Maneckjee,A., Hebb,C.: The kinetic properties of human placental choline acetyl-transferase. Biochem. J. **125**, 857—863 (1971).

Morris,S.J.: Removal of residual amounts of acetylcholinesterase and membrane contamina-tion from synaptic vesicles isolated from the electric organ of Torpedo. J. Neurochem. **21**, 713—715 (1973).

Moss,J., Colburn,R.W., Kopin,I.J.: Scorpion toxin-induced catecholamine release from synap-tosomes. J. Neurochem. **22**, 217—221 (1974).

Mulder,A.H., Yamamura,K.I., Kuhar,M.J., Snyder,S.H.: Release of acetylcholine from hip-pocampal slices by potassium depolarization: dependence on high affinity choline uptake. Brain Res. **70**, 372—376 (1974).

Musick,J., Hubbard,J.I.: Release of protein from mouse motor nerve terminals. Nature (Lond.) **237**, 279—281 (1972).

Nachmansohn,D., Machado,A.L.: The formation of acetylcholine. A new enzyme, "choline acetylase". J. Neurophysiol. **6**, 397—403 (1943).

Nachmansohn,D.: Chemical events in conducting and synaptic membranes during electrical activity. Proc. nat. Acad. Sci. (Wash.) **68**, 3170—3174 (1971).

Nakamura,R., Cheng,S.C.: Evidence for the compartmentalization of acetyl-coenzyme A in rat brain slices and its relation to the synthesis of acetylcholine and glutamate. Life Sci. **8**, 657—662 (1969).

Nakamura,R., Cheng,S.C., Naruse,H.: A study on the precursors of the acetyl moiety of acetylcholine in brain slices. Biochem. J. **118**, 443—450 (1970).

Nakasoto,Y., Douglas,W.W.: Cytochalasin blocks sympathetic ganglion transmission — a presynaptic effect antagonized by pyruvate. Proc. nat. Acad. Sci. (Wash.) **70**, 1730—1733 (1973).

Namba,T., Grob,D.: Cholinesterase activity of the motor endplate in isolated muscle membrane. J. Neurochem. **15**, 1445—1454 (1968).

Neale,J.H., Neale,E.A., Agranoff,B.W.: Radioautography of the optic tectum of the goldfish after intraocular injection of [^{3}H] proline. Science **176**, 407—410 (1972).

Nickel,E., Potter,L.T.. Synaptic vesicles in freeze-etched electric tissue of Torpedo. Brain Res. **23**, 95—100 (1970).

Nishi,S.: Cholinergic and adrenergic receptors at sympathetic preganglionic nerve terminals. Fed. Proc. **29**, 1957—1965 (1970).

Nishi,S., Soeda,H., Koketsu,K.: Release of acetylcholine from sympathetic preganglionic nerve terminals. J. Neurophysiol. **30**, 114—134 (1967).

Nordenfelt,I.: Choline acetylase in normal and denervated salivary glands. Quart. J. exp. Physiol. **48**, 67—79 (1963).

Nordenfelt,I.: Metabolism of transmitter substances in salivary glands. In: Schneyer,L.H., Schneyer,G.A. (Eds.): Secretory Mechanisms of Salivary Glands, pp. 142—154. New York: Academic Press 1967.

Ochs,S.: Fast transport of materials in mammalian nerve fibers. Science **176**, 252—260 (1972).

Oesch,F.: Trans-synaptic induction of choline acetyltransferase in the preganglionic neurone of the peripheral sympathetic nervous system. J. Pharmacol. exp. Ther. **188**, 439—446 (1974).

OESCH, F., THOENEN, H.: Increased activity of the peripheral nervous system: induction of choline acetyltransferase in the preganglionic cholinergic neuron. Nature (Lond.) **242**, 536—537 (1973a).

OESCH, F., THOENEN, H.: Induction of choline acetyltransferase in the preganglionic sympathetic neuron. Experientia (Basel) **29**, 765 (1973b).

OGSTON, A. G.: Removal of acetylcholine from a limited volume by diffusion. J. Physiol. (Lond.) **128**, 222—223 (1955).

O'NEILL, J. J., SAKAMOTO, T.: Enzymatic fluorometric determination of acetylcholine in biological extracts. J. Neurochem. **17**, 1451—1460 (1970).

OTSUKA, M., ENDO, M.: The effect of guanidine on neuromuscular transmission. J. Pharmacol. exp. Ther. **128**, 273—282 (1960).

OTSUKA, M., NONOMURA, Y.: The action of phenolic substances on motor nerve endings. J. Pharmacol. exp. Ther. **140**, 41—45 (1963).

PAGGI, P., ROSSI, A.: Effect of *Latrodectus mactans tredecimgultatus* venom on sympathetic ganglion isolated *in vitro*. Toxicon **9**, 265—269 (1971).

PANELLA, A.: Action du principe actif surrénal sur la fatigue musculaire. Arch. ital. Biol. **48**, 430—463 (1907).

PARDUCZ, A., FEHÉR, O.: Fine structural alterations of presynaptic endings in the superior cervical ganglion of the cat after exhausting preganglionic stimulation. Experientia (Basel) **26**, 629—630 (1970).

PARDUCZ, A., FEHÉR, O., JOÓ, F.: Effects of stimulation and hemicholinium (HC-3) on the fine structure of the nerve endings in the superior cervical ganglion of the cat. Brain Res. **34**, 61—72 (1971).

PATON, W. D. M.: The action of morphine and related substances on contraction and on acetylcholine output of coaxially stimulated guinea-pig ileum. Brit. J. Pharmacol. **12**, 119—127 (1957).

PATON, W. D. M.: Cholinergic transmission and acetylcholine output. Canad. J. Biochem. Physiol. **41**, 2637—2653 (1963).

PATON, W. D. M., THOMPSON, J. W.: The mechanism of action of adrenaline on the superior cervical ganglion of the cat. Abstr. Commun. *XIX* International Physiological Congress 664—665 (1953).

PATON, W. D. M., VIZI, E. S.: The inhibitory action of noradrenaline and adrenaline on acetylcholine output by guinea-pig ileum longitudinal muscle strip. Brit. J. Pharmacol. **35**, 10—28 (1969).

PATON, W. D. M., VIZI, E. S., ZAR, M. A.: The mechanism of acetylcholine release from parasympathetic nerves. J. Physiol. (Lond.) **215**, 819—848 (1971).

PATON, W. D. M., ZAR, M. A.: The origin of acetylcholine released from guinea-pig intestine and longitudinal muscle strips. J. Physiol. (Lond.) **194**, 13—33 (1968).

PATTERSON, P. H., CHUN, L. L. Y.: The influence of non-neuronal cells on catecholamine and acetylcholine synthesis and accumulation in cultures of dissociated neurons. Proc. nat. Acad. Sci. (Wash.) **71**, 3607—3610 (1974).

PERRI, V., SACCHI, O., RAVIOLA, E., RAVIOLA, G.: Evaluation of the number and distribution of synaptic vesicles at cholinergic nerve endings after sustained stimulation. Brain Res. **39**, 526—529 (1972).

PERRY, W. L. M.: Acetylcholine release in the cat's superior cervical ganglion. J. Physiol. (Lond.) **119**, 439—454 (1953).

PERSSON, B. O., LARSSON, L., SCHUBERTH, J., SÖRBO, B.: 3-bromoacetonyltrimethylammonium bromide, a choline acetyltransferase inhibitor. Acta chem. scand. **21**, 2283—2284 (1967).

PETERSON, E. R., BORNSTEIN, M. B.: The neurotoxic effects of colchicine on tissue cultures of cord-ganglia. J. Neuropath. exp. Neurol. **27**, 121—122 (1968).

PILAR, G.: Effect of acetylcholine on pre- and postsynaptic elements of avian ciliary ganglion synapses. Fed. Proc. **28**, 670 (1969).

PILAR, G., CHIAPPINELLI, V., UCHIMURA, H., GIACOBINI, E.: Changes of acetylcholinesterase (AChE) and choline acetyltransferase (ChAc) correlated with the formation of cholinergic synapses in chick embryo. Physiologist **17**, 307 (1974).

PILAR, G., JENDEN, D., CAMPBELL, B.: Change in acetylcholine content in postganglionic cells of adult pigeon ciliary ganglion after denervation. Physiologist **13**, 284 (1970).

Pilar, G., Jenden, D. J., Campbell, B.: Distribution of acetylcholine in the normal and denervated pigeon ciliary ganglion. Brain Res. **49**, 245—256 (1973).

Poisner, A. M.: Actomyosin-like protein from the adrenal medulla. Fed. Proc. **29**, 545 (1970).

Poisner, A. M., Bernstein, J. C.: A possible role of microtubules in catecholamine release from the adrenal medulla: effect of colchicine, vinca alkaloids and deuterium oxide. J. Pharmacol. exp. Ther. **177**, 102—108 (1971).

Poisner, A. M., Trifaró, J. M.: The role of ATP and ATPase in the release of catecholamines from the adrenal medulla. ATP-evoked release of catecholamines, ATP, and protein from isolated chromaffin granules. Molec. Pharmacol. **3**, 561—571 (1967).

Polak, R. L.: The influence of drugs on the uptake of acetylcholine by slices of rat cerebral cortex. Brit. J. Pharmacol. **36**, 144—152 (1969).

Polak, R. L., Meeuws, M. M.: The influence of atropine on the release and uptake of acetylcholine by the isolated cerebral cortex of the rat. Biochem. Pharmacol. **15**, 989—992 (1966).

Politoff, A. L., Rose, S., Pappas, G. D.: The calcium-binding sites of synaptic vesicles of the frog sartorius neuromuscular junction. J. Cell Biol. **61**, 818—823 (1974).

Potter, L. T.: Uptake of choline by nerve endings isolated from the rat cerebral cortex. In: Campbell, P. N. (Ed.): The Interaction of Drugs and Subcellular Components of Animal Cells, pp. 293—303. London: Churchill 1968.

Potter, L. T.: Synthesis, storage and release of [^{14}C] acetylcholine in isolated rat diaphragm muscles. J. Physiol. (Lond.) **206**, 145—166 (1970a).

Potter, L. T.: Acetylcholine, choline acetyltransferase and acetylcholinesterase. Handbook of Neurochemistry, Vol. *IV*, pp. 263—284 (1970b).

Potter, L. T.: Acetylcholine metabolism at vertebrate neuromuscular junctions. Advanc. biochem. Psychopharmacol. **2**, 163—168 (1970c).

Potter, L. T.: Synthesis, storage and release of acetylcholine from nerve terminals. In: Bourne, G. H. (Ed.): The Structure and Function of the Nervous System, Vol. IV, pp. 105—128. New York: Academic Press 1972.

Potter, L. T., Glover, V. A. S., Saelens, J. K.: Choline acetyltransferase from rat brain. J. biol. Chem. **243**, 3864—3870 (1968).

Powers, M. F., Krueger, S., Schueler, F. W.: Synthesis and pharmacological studies of some aliphatic hemicholinium analogs. J. pharm. Sci. **51**, 27—31 (1962).

Prasad, K. N., Vernadakis, A.: Morphological and biochemical study in X-ray- and dibutyryl cyclic AMP-induced differentiated neuroblastoma cells. Exp. Cell. Res. **70**, 27—32 (1972).

Pumplin, D. W., McClure, W. O.: Effects of cytochalasin B and vinblastine on the release of acetylcholine from a sympathetic ganglion. Europ. J. Pharmacol. **28**, 316—325 (1974).

Puszkin, S., Berl, S.: Actomyosin-like protein from brain: separation and characterization of the actin-like component. Biochim. biophys. Acta (Amst.) **256**, 695—709 (1972).

Puszkin, S., Nicklas, W. J., Berl, S.: Actomyosin-like protein in brain: subcellular distribution. J. Neurochem. **19**, 1319—1333 (1972).

Pysh, J. J., Wiley, R. G.: Morphologic alterations of synapses in electrically stimulated superior cervical ganglion of the cat. Science **176**, 191—193 (1972).

Quarles, R., Folch-Pi, J.: Some effects of physiological cations on the behaviour of gangliosides in a chloroform-methanol-water biphasic system. J. Neurochem. **12**, 543—553 (1965).

Quastel, D. M. J.: The role of sodium ions in acetylcholine metabolism in sympathetic ganglia. Ph. D. thesis, McGill University, Montreal (1962).

Quastel, D. M. J., Hackett, J. T., Cooke, J. D.: Calcium: is it required for transmitter secretion? Science **172**, 1034—1036 (1971).

Quastel, J. H., Tennenbaum, M., Wheatley, A. H. M.: Choline ester formation in, and choline esterase activities of, tissues *in vitro*. Biochem. J. **30**, 1668—1681 (1936).

Ramirez, G., Levitan, I. B., Mushynski, W. E.: Highly purified synaptosomal membranes from rat brain: incorporation of amino acids into membrane proteins *in vitro*. J. biol. Chem. **247**, 5382—5390 (1972).

Ramwell, P. W., Shaw, J. E., Kucharski, J.: Prostaglandin: release from the rat phrenic nerve diaphragm preparation. Science **149**, 1390—1391 (1965).

Rangachari, P. K., Khatter, J. C., Friesen, A. J. D.: Effect of stimulation on acetylcholine content of a sympathetic ganglion. Proc. Canad. Fed. Biol. Soc. **12**, 5 (1969).

RANISH, N., OCHS, S.: Fast axoplasmic transport of acetylcholinesterase in mammalian nerve fibres. J. Neurochem. **19**, 2641—2649 (1972).

RASSIN, D. K.: Amino acids as putative transmitters: failure to bind in synaptic vesicles of guinea-pig cerebral cortex. J. Neurochem. **19**, 139—148 (1972).

REID, W. D., HAUBRICH, D. R., KRISHNA, G.: Enzymic radioassay for acetylcholine and choline in brain. Analyt. Biochem. **42**, 390—397 (1971).

REISBERG, R. B.: Properties and biological significance of choline acetylase. Yale J. Biol. Med. **29**, 403—435 (1957).

REITZEL, N. L., LONG, J. P.: The neuromuscular blocking properties of α,α'-dimethylami-noethanol-4,4'-biacetophenone (hemicholinium). Arch. int. Pharmacodyn. **119**, 20—30 (1959).

RENKIN, E. M.: Permability of frog skeletal muscle cells to choline. J. gen. Physiol. **44**, 1159—1164 (1961).

RENNICK, B. R.: The renal tubular excretion of choline and thiamine in the chicken. J. Pharmacol. exp. Ther. **122**, 448—456 (1958).

RICHTER, D., CROSSLAND, J.: Variation in acetylcholine content of the brain with physiological state. Amer. J. Physiol. **159**, 247—255 (1949).

RICHTER, J. A., GOLDSTEIN, A.: Effects of morphine and levorphanol on brain acetylcholine content in mice. J. Pharmacol. exp. Ther. **175**, 685—691 (1970).

RICHTER, J. A., MARCHBANKS, R. M.: Synthesis of radioactive acetylcholine from [^{3}H]choline and its release from cerebral cortex slices *in vitro*. J. Neurochem. **18**, 691—703 (1971a).

RICHTER, J. A., MARCHBANKS, R. M.: Isolation of [^{3}H]acetylcholine pools by subcellular fractionation of cerebral cortex slices incubated with [^{3}H]choline. J. Neurochem. **18**, 705—712 (1971b).

RIEGER, F., TSUJI, S., MASSOULIE, J.: Formes natives et globulaires de l'acétylcholinesterase dans la moëlle épinière et le cerveau de gymnote, *Electrophorus electricus*. Europ. J. Biochem. **30**, 73—80 (1972).

RIKER, W. F., Jr.: Pharmacologic considerations in a re-evaluation of the neuromuscular synapse, Arch. Neurol. Psychiat. (Chic.) **3**, 488—499 (1960).

RIKER, W. F., JR., ROBERTS, J., STANDAERT, F. G., FUJIMORI, H.: The motor nerve terminal as the primary focus for drug-induced facilitation of neuromuscular transmission. J. Pharmacol. exp. Ther. **121**, 286—312 (1957).

RIKER, W. F., JR., WERNER, G., ROBERTS, J., KUPERMAN, A.: Pharmacologic evidence for the existence of a presynaptic event in neuromuscular transmission. J. Pharmacol. exp. Ther. **125**, 150—158 (1959).

RITCHIE, J. A., GOLDBERG, A. M.: Vesicular and synaptoplasmic synthesis of acetylcholine. Science **169**, 489—490 (1970).

ROBBINS, N., FISCHBACH, G. D.: Effects of chronic disuse of rat soleus neuromuscular junctions on presynaptic function. J. Neurophysiol. **34**, 570—578 (1971).

ROBERTS, D. V.: Neuromuscular activity of the triethyl analogue of choline in the frog. J. Physiol. (Lond.) **160**, 94—105 (1962).

ROBINSON, P. M., BELL, C.: The localization of acetylcholinesterase at the autonomic neuromuscular junction. J. Cell Biol. **33**, 93—102 (1967).

RODRIGUEZ DE LORES ARNAIZ, G., ZIEHER, L. M., DE ROBERTIS, E.: Neurochemical and structural studies on the mechanism of action of hemicholinium-3 in central cholinergic synapses. J. Neurochem. **17**, 221—229 (1970).

ROGERS, A. W., SALPETER, M. M., OSTROWSKI, K., DARZYNKIEWICZ, Z.: Quantative studies on enzymes in structures in striated muscles by labeled inhibitor methods. I. The number of acetylcholinesterase molecules and of other DFP reactive sites at motor endplates, measured by radioautography. J. Cell Biol. **41**, 665—685 (1969).

ROSE, S., GLOW, P. H.: Denervation effects on the presumed de novo synthesis of muscle cholinesterase and the effects of acetylcholine availability on retinal cholinesterase. Exp. Neurol. **18**, 267—275 (1967).

ROSENBERG, P., KREMZNER, L. T., MCCREERY, D., WILLETTE, R. E.: Inhibition of choline acetyltransferase activity in squid giant axon. Biochim. biophys. Acta (Amst.) **268**, 49—60 (1972).

ROSENBLUETH, A., LISSÁK, K., LANARI, A.: An explanation of the five stages of neuromuscular and ganglionic synaptic transmission. Amer. J. Physiol. **128**, 31—44 (1939).

Rosenblueth, A., Luco, J. V.: The fifth stage of neuromuscular transmission. Amer. J. Physiol. **126**, 39—57 (1939).

Rosenthal, J.: Post-tetanic potentiation at the neuromuscular junction of the frog. J. Physiol. (Lond.) **203**, 121—134 (1969).

Roskoski, R.: Choline acetyltransferase. Inhibition by thiol reagents. J. biol. Chem. **249**, 2156—2159 (1974).

Ross, S. B., Florvall, L., Frödén, O.: Inhibiton of choline acetyltransferase by 2-dimethyl-aminoethyl chloroacetate and related compounds. Acta pharmacol. (Kbh.) **30**, 396—402 (1971).

Ross, S. B., Jenden, D. J.: Failure of hemicholinium-3 to inhibit the uptake of ^{3}H-choline in mouse brain *in vivo*. Experientia (Basel) **29**, 689—690 (1973).

Rubin, R. P.: The role of calcium in the release of neurotransmitter substances and hormones. Pharmacol. Rev. **22**, 389—428 (1970).

Ryan, K. J., Kalant, H., Thomas, E. L.: Free-flow electrophoretic separation and electrical surface properties of subcellular particles from guinea-pig brain. J. Cell Biol. **49**, 235—246 (1971).

Sacchi, O., Perri, V.: Quantal mechanism of transmitter release during progressive depletion of the presynaptic stores at a ganglionic synapse. J. gen. Physiol. **61**, 342—360 (1973).

Saelens, J. K., Simke, J. P., Allen, M. P., Conroy, C. A.: Some of the dynamics of choline and acetylcholine metabolism in rat brain. Arch. int. Pharmacodyn. **203**, 305—312 (1973).

Saelens, J. K., Simke, J. P., Schuman, J., Allen, M. P.: Studies with agents which influence acetylcholine metabolism in mouse brain. Arch. int. Pharmacodyn. **209**, 250—255 (1974).

Saelens, J. K., Stoll, W. R.: Radiochemical determination of choline and acetylcholine flux from isolated tissue. J. Pharmacol. exp. Ther. **147**, 336—342 (1965).

Salpeter, M. M.: Electron microscopic radioautography as a quantitative tool in enzyme cytochemistry. The distribution of acetylcholinesterase at motor and plates of a vertebrate twitch muscle. J. Cell Biol. **32**, 379—389 (1967).

Salpeter, M. M.: Electron microscopic radioautography as a quantitative tool in enzyme cytochemistry. The distribution of DFP-reactive sites at motor endplates of a vertebrate twitch muscle. J. Cell Biol. **42**, 122—134 (1969).

Sastry, B. V. R., Henderson, G. I.: Kinetic mechanisms of human placental choline acetyltransferase. Biochem. Pharmacol. **21**, 787—802 (1972).

Sastry, P. B.: Ph. D. thesis, McGill University, Montreal (1956).

Sattin, A., Rall, T. W.: The effect of adenosine and adenine nucleotides on the cyclic adenosine 3′-5′-phosphate content of guinea pig cerebral cortex slices. Molec. Pharmacol. **6**, 13—23 (1970).

Sawyer, C. H.: Cholinesterases in degenerating and regenerating peripheral nerves. Amer. J. Physiol. **146**, 246—253 (1946).

Sawyer, C. H., Hollinshead, W. H.: Cholinesterases in sympathetic fibers and ganglia. J. Neurophysiol. **8**, 137—153 (1945).

Schafer, R.: Acetylcholine: fast axoplasmic transport in insect chemoreceptor fibers. Science **180**, 315—317 (1973).

Schmidt, D. E., Szilagyi, P. I. A., Alkon, D. A., Green, J. P.: A method for measuring nanogram quantities of acetylcholine by pyrolysis-gas chromatography: the demonstration of acetylcholine in effluents from the rat phrenic nerve-diaphragm preparation. J. Pharmacol. exp. Ther. **174**, 337—345 (1970).

Schmitt, F. O.: Fibrous proteins — neuronal organelles. Proc. nat. Acad. Sci. (Wash.) **60**, 1092—1101 (1968).

Schrier, B. K., Shuster, L.: A simplified radiochemical assay for choline acetyltransferase. J. Neurochem. **14**, 977—985 (1967).

Schuberth, J.: Choline acetylase purification and effect of salts on the mechanism of the enzyme-catalyzed reaction. Biochim. biophys. Acta (Amst.) **122**, 470—481 (1966).

Schuberth, J., Sparf, B., Sundwall, A.: A technique for the study of acetylcholine turnover in mouse brain *in vivo*. J. Neurochem. **16**, 695—700 (1969).

Schuberth, J., Sparf, B., Sundwall, A.: On the turnover of acetylcholine in nerve endings of mouse brain *in vivo*. J. Neurochem. **17**, 461—468 (1970).

Schuberth, J., Sundwall, A.: Effect of some drugs on the uptake of acetylcholine in′ cortex slices of mouse brain. J. Neurochem. **14**, 807—812 (1967).

SCHUBERTH,J., SUNDWALL,A.: Differences in the subcellular localization of choline, acetylcholine and atropine taken up by mouse brain slices *in vitro*. Acta physiol. scand. **72**, 65—71 (1968).

SCHUBERTH,J., SUNDWALL,A., SÖRBO,B.: Relation between Na^+-K^+ transport and the uptake of choline by brain slices. Life Sci. **6**, 293—296 (1967).

SCHUBERTH,J., SUNDWALL,A., SÖRBO,B., LINDELL,J.O.: Uptake of choline by rat brain slices. J. Neurochem. **13**, 347—352 (1966).

SCHUELER,F.W.: A new group of respiratory paralyzants. J. Pharmacol. exp. Ther. **115**, 127—143 (1955).

SCHUELER,F.W.: The mechanism of action of the hemicholiniums. Int. Rev. Neurobiol. **2**, 77—97 (1960).

SCHWYN,R.C.: An autoradiographic study of satellite cells in autonomic ganglia. Amer. J. Anat. **121**, 727—740 (1967).

SCHWYN,R.C., HALL,J.L.: Studies of neurological activity in autonomic ganglia during electrical stimulation and drug administration. Anat. Rec. **151**, 414 (1965).

SELLINGER,O.Z., DOMINO,E.F., HAARSTAD,V.B., MOHRMAN,M.E.: Intracellular distribution of $[C^{14}]$-hemicholinium-3 in the canine caudate nucleus and hippocampus. J. Pharmacol. exp. Ther. **167**, 63—76 (1969).

SEVERIN,S.E., ARTENIE,V.: The isolation, partial purification and some properties of cholineacetyl transferase from rabbit brain. Biokhimiya **32**, 125—132 (1967). (Russian.)

SHAPIRO,D.L.: Morphological and biochemical alterations in foetal rat brain cells cultivated in the presence of monobutyryl cyclic AMP. Nature (Lond.) **241**, 203—204 (1973).

SHARKAWI,M.: Effects of some centrally acting drugs on acetylcholine synthesis by rat cerebral cortex slices. Brit. J. Pharmacol. **46**, 473—479 (1972).

SHARKAWI,M., SCHULMAN,M.P.: Relationship between acetylcholine synthesis and its concentration in rat cerebral cortex. Brit. J. Pharmacol. **36**, 373—379 (1969).

SHARPLESS,S.K.: Reorganization of function in the nervous system — use and disuse. Ann. Rev. Physiol. **26**, 357—388 (1964).

SHEA,P.A., APRISON,M.H.: An enzymatic method for measuring picomole quantities of acetylcholine and choline in CNS tissue. Analyt. Biochem. **56**, 165—177 (1973).

SHERIDAN,M.N., WHITTAKER,V.P., ISRAËL,M.: The subcellular fractionation of the electric organ of Torpedo. Z. Zellforsch. **74**, 291—307 (1966).

SIEGEL,F., BROOKS,J., CHILDERS,S., CAMPBELL,J.: Calcium binding proteins from adrenergic and cholinergic tissue. Abstr. 4th Int. Meet. Neurochem. 72 (1973).

SILBERGELD,E.K., FALER,J.T., GOLDBERG,A.M.: Evidence for a junctional effect of lead in neuromuscular function. Nature (Lond.) **247**, 49—50 (1974).

SILINSKY,E.M., HUBBARD,J.I.: Release of ATP from rat motor nerve terminals. Nature (Lond.) **243**, 404—405 (1973).

SIMPSON,L.L.: The role of calcium in neurohumoral and neurohormonal extrusion processes. J. Pharm. Pharmacol. **20**, 889—910 (1968).

SIMPSON,L.L.: Ionic requirements for the neuromuscular blocking action of botulinum toxin: implications with regard to synaptic transmission. Neuropharmacology **10**, 673—684 (1971).

SIMPSON,L.L.: The interaction between divalent cations and botulinum toxin type A in the paralysis of the rat phrenic nerve-hemidiaphragm preparation. Neuropharmacology **12**, 165—176 (1973).

SIMPSON,L.L., RAPPORT,M.M.: Ganglioside inactivation of botulinum toxin. J. Neurochem. **18**, 1341—1343 (1971a).

SIMPSON,L.L., RAPPORT,M.M.: The binding of botulinum toxin to membrane lipids: sphingolipids, steroids and fatty acids. J. Neurochem. **18**, 1751—1759 (1971b).

SINGER,J.J., GOLDBERG,A.L.: Cyclic AMP and transmission at the neuromuscular junction. Advances in Biochemical Psychopharmacology **3**, 335—348 (1970).

SINGER,S., HO,A., GERSHON,S.: Changes in activity of choline acetylase in central nervous system of rat after intraventricular administration of noradrenaline. Nature (Lond.) New Biology **230**, 152—153 (1971).

SJÖSTRAND,J., FRIZELL,M., HASSELGREN,P.O.: Effects of colchicine on axonal transport in peripheral nerves. J. Neurochem. **17**, 1563—1570 (1970).

Slater, P.: Effect of triethylcholine and hemicholinium-3 on acetylcholine content of rat brain. Int. J. Neuropharmacol. **7**, 421—427 (1968).

Slater, P.: The estimation of the "free" and "bound" acetylcholine content of rat brain. J. Pharm. Pharmacol. **23**, 514—518 (1971).

Slater, P., Stonier, P. D.: The uptake of hemicholinium-3 by rat brain cortex slices. J. Neurochem. **20**, 637—639 (1973 a).

Slater, P., Stonier, P. D.: The uptake of hemicholinium-3 by rat diaphragm and isolated perfused heart. Arch. int. Pharmacodyn. **204**, 407—414 (1973 b).

Smirnov, G. D., Byzov, A. L., Rampan, Yu. I.: Effects of some thiol poisons on the synaptic conduction of excitation in a sympathetic ganglion. Fiziol. Zh. (Mosk.) **40**, 424—430 (1954).

Smith, A. D.: Secretion of proteins (chromogranin A and dopamine β-hydroxylase) from a sympathetic neuron. Phil Trans. B **261**, 363—370 (1971).

Smith, A. D.: Release of noradrenaline from sympathetic nerves. Brit. med. Bull **29**, 123—129 (1973).

Smith, D. S.: On the significance of cross-bridges between microtubules and synaptic vesicles. Phil. Trans. B **261**, 395—405 (1971).

Smith, D. S., Järlfors, U., Beránek, R.: The organization of synaptic axoplasm in the lamprey (*Petromyzon marinus*) central nervous system. J. Cell Biol. **46**, 199—219 (1970).

Smith, J. C., Cavallito, C. J., Foldes, F. F.: Choline acetyltransferase inhibitors: a group of styryl-pyridine analogs. Biochem. Pharmacol. **16**, 2438—2441 (1961).

Snell, R. S., McIntyre, N.: Changes in the histochemical appearances of cholinesterase at the motor end plate following denervation. Brit. J. exp. Path. **37**, 44—48 (1956).

Sollenberg, J., Sörbo, B.: On the origins of the acetyl moiety of acetylcholine in brain studied with a differential labelling technique using ^{3}H-^{14}C-mixed labelled glucose and acetate. J. Neurochem. **17**, 201—207 (1970).

Sorimachi, M., Kataoka, K.: Choline uptake by nerve terminals: a sensitive and specific marker of cholinergic innervation. Brain Res. **72**, 350—353 (1974).

Sparf, B.: On the turnover of acetylcholine in the brain: an experimental study using intravenously injected radioactive choline. Acta physiol. scand., Suppl. **397**, 7—47 (1973).

Spencer, W. A., April, R. S.: Plastic properties of monosynaptic pathways in mammals. In: Horn, G., Hinde, R. A. (Eds.): Short-term Changes in Neural Activity and Behaviour, pp. 433—474. Cambridge: University Press 1970.

Spencer, W. A., Wigdor, R.: Ultra-late PTP of monosynaptic reflex responses in the cat. Physiologist **8**, 278 (1965).

Spoor, R. P., Ferguson, F. C., Jr.: Colchicine *IV*. Neuromuscular transmission in isolated frog and rat tissues. J. pharm. Sci. **54**, 779—780 (1965).

Stavinoha, W. B., Weintraub, S. T., Modak, A. T.: The use of microwave heating to inactivate cholinesterase in the rat brain prior to analysis for acetylcholine. J. Neurochem. **20**, 361—371 (1973).

Stevenson, R. W., Wilson, W. S.: Drug-induced depletion of acetylcholine in the rabbit corneal epithelium. Biochem. Pharmacol. **23**, 3449—3457 (1974).

Stjärne, L., Wennmalm, A.: Preferential secretion of newly formed noradrenaline in the perfused rabbit heart. Acta physiol. scand. **80**, 428—430 (1970).

Stone, W. E.: Acetylcholine in the brain. I. "Free", "bound" and total acetylcholine. Arch. Biochem. **59**, 181—192 (1955).

Stovner, J.: The effect of low calcium and of tetraethylammonium (TEA) on the rat diaphragm. Acta physiol. scand. **40**, 285—296 (1957).

Straughan, D. W.: The release of acetylcholine from mammalian motor nerve endings. Brit. J. Pharmacol. **15**, 417—422 (1960).

Strömblad, R.: Acetylcholine inactivation and acetylcholine sensitivity in denervated salivary glands. Acta physiol. scand. **34**, 38—58 (1955).

Suria, A., Costa, E.: Diazepam inhibition of post-tetanic potentiation in bullfrog sympathetic ganglia: possible role of prostaglandins. J. Pharmacol. exp. Ther. **180**, 690—696 (1974).

Szerb, J. C.: The estimation of acetylcholine, using leech muscle in a microbath. J. Physiol. (Lond.) **158**, 8—9 P (1961).

Szerb, J. C., Malik, H., Hunter, E. G.: Relationship between acetylcholine content and release in the cat's cerebral cortex. Canad. J. Physiol. Pharmacol. **48**, 780—790 (1970).

SZERB, J. C., SOMOGYI, G. T.: Variation in the release of newly synthesized acetylcholine from the longitudinal muscle of the guinea-pig ileum stimulated at low and high frequencies. Proc. Canad. Fed. Biol. Soc. **16**, 8 (1973).

SZILAGYI, P. I. A., SCHMIDT, D. E., GREEN, J. P.: Microanalytical determination of acetylcholine, other choline esters and choline by pyrolysis-gas chromatography. Analyt. Chem. **40**, 2009—2013 (1968).

TAKAHASHI, R., APRISON, M. H.: Acetylcholine content of discrete areas of the brain obtained by a near-freezing method. J. Neurochem. **11**, 887—898 (1964).

TAKENO, K., NISHIO, A., YANAGIYA, I.: Bound acetylcholine in the nerve ending particles. J. Neurochem. **16**, 47—52 (1969).

TAUC, L., HOFFMANN, A., TSUJI, S., HINZEN, D. H., FAILLE, L.: Transmission abolished on a cholinergic synapse after injection of acetylcholinesterase into the presynaptic neurone. Nature (Lond.) **250**, 496—498 (1974).

TAXI, J., SOTELO, C.: Cytological aspects of the axonal migration of catecholamines and of their storage material. Brain Res. **62**, 431—437 (1973).

TAYLOR, D. B., NEDERGAARD, O. Z., CREESE, R., CASE, R.: Labelled depolarizing drugs in normal and denervated muscle. Nature (Lond.) **208**, 901—902 (1965).

TERÄVÄINEN, H.: Histochemical localization of acetylcholinesterase in isolated brain synaptosomes. Histochemie **18**, 191—194 (1969).

THAMPI, S. N., DOMER, F. R., HAARSTAD, V. B., SCHUELER, F. W.: Pharmacological studies of nor-phenyl hemicholinium 3. J. pharm. Sci. **55**, 381—386 (1966).

THESLEFF, S.: Supersensitivity of skeletal muscle produced by botulinum toxin. J. Physiol. (Lond.) **151**, 598—607 (1960).

THIES, R. E.: Neuromuscular depression and the apparent depletion of transmitter in mammalian muscle. J. Neurophysiol. **28**, 427—442 (1965).

THIES, R. E., BROOKS, V. B.: Postsynaptic neuromuscular block produced by hemicholinium no. 3. Fed. Proc. **20**, 569—578 (1961).

THOA, N. B., WOOTEN, G. F., AXELROD, J., KOPIN, I. J.: Inhibition of release of dopamine-β-hydroxylase and noradrenaline from sympathetic nerves by colchicine, vinblastine, or cytochalasin-B. Proc. nat. Acad. Sci. (Wash.) **69**, 520—522 (1972).

THOENEN, H., KETTLER, R., SANER, A.: Time course of the development of enzymes involved in the synthesis of norepinephrine in the superior cervical ganglion of the rat from birth to adult life. Brain Res. **40**, 459—468 (1972).

THOENEN, H., MUELLER, R. A., AXELROD, J:: Increased tyrosine hydroxylase activity after drug-induced alteration of sympathetic transmission. Nature (Lond.) **221**, 1264 (1969).

THOENEN, H., MUELLER, R. A., AXELROD, J.: Phase difference in the induction of tyrosine hydroxylase in cell body and nerve terminals of sympathetic neurones. Proc. nat. Acad. Sci. (Wash.) **65**, 58—62 (1970).

TOBIAS, J. M., LIPTON, M. A., LEPINAT, A.: Effect of anaesthetics and convulsants on brain acetylcholine content. Proc. Soc. exp. Biol. (N.Y.) **61**, 51—54 (1946).

TORU, M., APRISON, M. H.: Brain acetylcholine studies: a new extraction procedure. J. Neurochem. **13**, 1533—1544 (1966).

TRETHEWIE, E. R.: Experiments on the problem of "free" and "bound" histamine and acetylcholine. Aust. J. exp. Biol. med. Sci. **16**, 225—232 (1938).

TRIFARÓ, J. M., COLLIER, B., LASTOWECKA, A., STERN, D.: Inhibition by colchicine and by vinblastine of acetylcholine-induced catecholamine release from the adrenal gland: an anticholinergic action, not an effect upon microtubules. Molec. Pharmacol. **8**, 264—267 (1972).

TRIMBLE, M. E., ACARA, M., RENNICK, B.: Effect of hemicholinium-3 on tubular transport and metabolism of choline in the perfused rat kidney. J. Pharmacol. exp. Ther. **189**, 570—576 (1974).

TROTTER, J. L., BURTON, R. M.: Acetylcholinesterase activity of synaptic vesicle fractions and membrane fractions prepared from rat brain tissue. J. Neurochem. **16**, 805—812 (1969).

TUČEK, S.: On subcellular localization and binding of choline acetyltransferase in the cholinergic nerve endings of the brain. J. Neurochem. **13**, 1317—1327 (1966 a).

TUČEK, S.: On the question of the localization of choline acetyltransferase in synaptic vesicles. J. Neurochem. **13**, 1329—1332 (1966 b).

Tuček,S.: Subcellular localization of enzymes generating acetyl-CoA and their possible relation to the biosynthesis of acetylcholine. In: Heilbronn,E., Winter,A. (Eds.): Drugs and Cholinergic Mechanisms in the CNS, pp.117—131. Stockholm: Research Institute of National Defence 1970.

Tuček,S.: Choline acetyltransferase activity in rat skeletal muscles during postnatal development. Exp. Neurol. **36**, 378—388 (1972).

Tuček,S., Cheng,S.-C.: Precursors of acetyl groups in acetylcholine in the brain *in vivo*. Biochim. biophys. Acta (Amst.) **208**, 538—540 (1970).

Tuček,S., Cheng,S.-C.: Provenance of the acetyl group of acetylcholine and compartmentalization of acetyl-CoA and Krebs cycle intermediates in the brain *in vivo*. J. Neurochem. **22**, 893—914 (1974).

Turkanis,S.A.: Some effects of vinblastine and colchicine on neuromuscular transmission. Brain Res. **54**, 324—329 (1973).

Ulmar,G., Whittaker,V.P.: Immunological approach to the characterization of cholinergic vesicular protein. J. Neurochem. **22**, 451—454 (1974).

Üvnäs,B.: An attempt to explain nervous transmitter release as due to nerve impulse-induced cation exchange. Acta physiol. scand. **87**, 168—175 (1973).

Vander,A.J.: Renal excretion of choline in the dog. Amer. J. Physiol. **202**, 319—324 (1962).

Vincenzi,F.F., West,T.C.: Effects of hemicholinium on the release of autonomic mediators in the sinoatrial node. Brit. J. Pharmacol. **24**, 773—780 (1965).

Vital Brazil,O., Corrado,A.P.: The curariform action of streptomycin. J. Pharmacol. exp. Ther. **120**, 452—459 (1957).

Vital Brazil,O., Excell,B.F.: Action of crotoxin and crotactin from the venom of *Crotalus durissus terrificus* (South American rattlesnake) on the frog neuromuscular junction. J. Physiol. (Lond.) **212**, 34—35P (1971).

Vital Brazil,O., Prado-Franceschi,J.: The nature of neuromuscular block produced by neomycin and gentamycin. Arch. int. Pharmacodyn. **179**, 78—85 (1969).

Vizi,E.S.: The inhibitory action of noradrenaline and adrenaline on release of acetylcholine from guinea-pig ileum longitudinal strips. Naunyn-Schmiedebergs Arch. exp. Path. Pharmak. **259**, 199—200 (1968).

Vizi,E.S.: Stimulation, by inhibition of $(Na^+-K^+-Mg^{2+})$-activated ATP-ase, of acetylcholine release in cortical slices from rat brain. J. Physiol. (Lond.) **226**, 95—118 (1972).

Vizi,E.S., Knoll,J.: The effects of sympathetic nerve stimulation and guanethidine on parasympathetic neuroeffector transmission; the inhibition of acetylcholine release. J. Physiol. (Lond.) **23**, 918—925 (1971).

Vogel,J.R., Leaf,R.C.: Initiation of mouse killing in non-killer rats by repeated pilocarpine treatment. Physiol. Behav. **8**, 421—424 (1972).

Volle,R.L.: Modification by drugs of synpatic mechanisms in autonomic ganglia. Pharmacol. Rev. **18**, 839—869 (1966).

Von Hungen,K., Mahler,H.R., Moore,W.J.: Turnover of protein and ribonucleic acid in synaptic subcellular fractions from rat brain. J. biol. Chem. **243**, 1415—1423 (1968).

Vos,J., Kuriyama,K., Roberts,E.: Electrophoretic mobilities of brain subcellular particles and binding of γ-aminobutyric acid, acetylcholine, norepinephrine and 5-hydroxytryptamine. Brain Res. **9**, 224—230 (1968).

Wall,P.D.: Habituation and post-tetanic potentiation in the spinal cord. In: Horn,G., Hinde,R.A. (Eds.): Short-term Changes in Neural Activity and Behaviour, pp.181—210. Cambridge: University Press 1970.

Waser,P.G., Lüthi,V.: Autoradiographische Lokalisation von ^{14}C-Calebassen-Curarin I und ^{14}C-Decamethonium in der motorischen Endplatte. Arch. int. Pharmacodyn. **112**, 272—296 (1957).

Watkins,J.C.: Metabolic regulation in the release and action of excitatory and inhibitory amino acids in the central nervous system. Biochem. Soc. Symp. **36**, 33—47 (1972).

Watson,W.E.: Cellular responses to axotomy and to related procedures. Brit. med. Bull. **30**, 112—115 (1974a).

Watson,W.E.: Physiology of neuroglia. Physiol. Rev. **54**, 245—271 (1974b).

Weiss,P., Hiscoe,H.B.: Experiments on the mechanism of nerve growth. J. exp. Zool. **107**, 315—396 (1948).

WEISS, P., TAYLOR, A. C., PILLAI, P. A.: The nerve fiber as a system in continuous low microcinematographic and electronmicroscopic demonstration. Science 136, 330 (1962).

WELLINGTON, B. S., LIVETT, B. G., JEFFREY, P. L., AUSTIN, L.: Neurostenin: isolation, biochemical characterization and histochemical localization in chick brain. Abstr. 4th int. Meet. Neurochem. 170 (1973).

WELSH, J. H., HYDE, J. E.: The distribution of acetylcholine in brains of rats of different ages. J. Neurophysiol. 7, 41—49 (1944).

WELSH, J. H., TAUB, R.: The action of choline and related compounds on the heart of *Venus mercenaria*. Biol. Bull. Marine Biol. Lab. Woods Hole 95, 346—353 (1948).

WERNER, I., PETERSON, G. R., SHUSTER, L.: Choline acetyltransferase and acetylcholinesterase in cultured brain cells from chick embryos. J. Neurochem. 18, 141—151 (1971).

WESSELLS, N. K., SPOONER, B. S., ASH, J. F., BRADLEY, M. O., LUDUENA, M. A., TAYLOR, E. L., WRENN, J. T., YAMADA, K. M.: Microfilaments in cellular and developmental processes. Science 171, 135—143 (1971).

WHITE, H. L., CAVALLITO, C. J.: Inhibition of bacterial and mammalian choline acetyltransferases by styrylpyridine analogues. J. Neurochem. 17, 1579—1589 (1970a).

WHITE, H. L., CAVALLITO, C. J.: Choline acetyltransferase. Enzyme mechanism and mode of inhibition by a styrylpyridine analogue. Biochim. biophys. Acta (Amst.) 206, 343—358 (1970b).

WHITE, H. L., WU, J. C.: Kinetics of choline acetyltransferases (E.C. 2.3.1.6) from human and other mammalian central and peripheral nervous tissues. J. Neurochem. 20, 297—307 (1973a).

WHITE, H. L., WU, J. C.: Separation of apparent multiple forms of human brain choline acetyltransferase by isoelectric focussing. J. Neurochem. 21, 939—948 (1973b).

WHITTAKER, V. P.: The isolation and characterization of acetylcholine containing particles from brain. Biochem. J. 72, 694—706 (1959).

WHITTAKER, V. P.: Identification of acetylcholine and related esters of biological origin. In: KOELLE, G. B. (Ed.): Handbuch der experimentellen Pharmakologie, Ergänzungswerk XV, Cholinesterase and Anticholinesterase Agents, pp. 1—39. Berlin-Heidelberg-New York: Springer 1963.

WHITTAKER, V. P.: The application of subcellular fractionation techniques to the study of brain function. Progr. Biophys. molec. Biol. 15, 39—96 (1965).

WHITTAKER, V. P.: Some properties of synaptic membranes isolated from the central nervous system. Ann. N. Y. Acad. Sci. 137, 982—998 (1966).

WHITTAKER, V. P.: The nature of the acetylcholine pools in tissue. Progr. Brain Res. 31, 211—222 (1969).

WHITTAKER, V. P.: The vesicle hypothesis. In: ANDERSEN, P., JANSEN, J. K. S. (Eds.): Excitatory Synaptic Mechanisms, pp. 67—76. Oslo: Universitets Forlaget 1970.

WHITTAKER, V. P.: Origin and function of synaptic vesicles. Ann. N. Y. Acad. Sci. 183, 21—32 (1971).

WHITTAKER, V. P., SHERIDAN, M. N.: The morphology and acetylcholine content of isolated cerebral cortical synaptic vesicles. J. Neurochem. 12, 363—372 (1965).

WHITTAKTER, V. P., DOWDALL, M. J., BOYNE, A. F.: The storage and release of acetylcholine by cholinergic nerve terminals: recent results with non-mammalian preparations. Biochem. Soc. Symp. 36, 49—68 (1972b).

WHITTAKER, V. P., DOWDALL, M. J., DOWE, G. H. C., FACINO, R. M., SCOTTO, J.: Proteins of cholinergic synaptic vesicles from the electric organ of Torpedo: characterization of a low molecular weight acidic protein. Brain Res. 75, 115—131 (1974).

WHITTAKER, V. P., ESSMAN, W. B., DOWE, G. H. C.: The isolation of pure cholinergic synaptic vesicles from the electric organs of elasmobranch fish of the family *Torpedinidae*. Biochem. J. 128, 833—846 (1972a).

WHITTAKER, V. P., MICHAELSON, I. A., KIRKLAND, R. J.: The separation of synaptic vesicles from nerve-endings particles ("synaptosomes"). Biochem. J. 90, 293—303 (1964).

WIEGANDT, H.: The subcellular localization of gangliosides in the brain. J. Neurochem. 14, 671—674 (1967).

WIENER, N. I., MESSER, J.: Hemicholinium-3 induced amnesia: some temporal properties. Psychonomic Sci. 26, 129—130 (1972).

Wilson, H., Long, J. P.: The effect of hemicholinium (HC-3) at various peripheral cholinergic transmitting sites. Arch. int. Pharmacodyn. **120**, 343—352 (1959).

Wilson, P. F.: The effects of dibutyryl-3′, 5′-cyclic adenosine monophosphate, theophylline and aminophylline on neuromuscular transmission in the rat. J. Pharmacol. exp. Ther. **188**, 447—452 (1974).

Wilson, W. S., Cooper, J. R.: The preparation of cholinergic synaptosomes from brain superior cervical ganglia. J. Neurochem. **19**, 2779—2790 (1972).

Wilson, W. S., Schulz, R. A., Cooper, J. R.: The isolation of cholinergic synaptic vesicles from brain superior cervical ganglion and estimation of their acetylcholine content. J. Neurochem. **20**, 659—667 (1973).

Winkler, H., Hörtnagl, H., Schöpf, J. A. L., Hörtnagl, H., zur Nedden, G.: Bovine adrenal medulla: synthesis and secretion of radioactively labelled catecholamines and chromogranins. Naunyn-Schmiedebergs Arch. exp. Path. Pharmak. **271**, 193—203 (1971).

Wisniewski, H., Shelanski, M. L., Terry, R. D.: Effects of mitotic spindle inhibitors on neurotubules and neurofilaments in anterior horn cells. J. Cell Biol. **38**, 224 (1968).

Wolff, D. J., Siegel, F. L.: Purification of a calcium-binding phosphoprotein from pig brain. J. biol. Chem. **247**, 4180—4185 (1972).

Wooten, G. F., Coyle, J. T.: Axonal transport of catecholamine synthesizing and metabolizing enzymes. J. Neurochem. **20**, 1361—1371 (1973).

Yamamura, H. I., Snyder, S. H.: Choline: high-affinity uptake by rat brain synaptosomes. Science **178**, 626—628 (1972).

Yamamura, H. I., Snyder, S. H.: Affinity transport of choline into synaptosomes of rat brain. J. Neurochem. **21**, 1355—1374 (1973).

Zablocka-Esplin, B., Esplin, D. W.: Persistent changes in transmission in spinal monosynaptic pathway after prolonged tetanization. J. Neurophysiol. **34**, 860—867 (1971).

Zacks, S. I., Metzger, J. F., Smith, C. W., Blumberg, J. M.: Localization of ferritin-labelled botulinum toxin in the neuromuscular junction of the mouse. J. Neuropath. exp. Neurol. **21**, 610—633 (1962).

Zimmermann, H., Whittaker, V. P.: Effect of electrical stimulation on the yield and composition of synaptic vesicle from the cholinergic synapses of the electric organ of Torpedo: a combined biochemical, electrophysiological and morphological study. J. Neurochem. **22**, 435—450 (1974a).

Zimmermann, H., Whittaker, V. P.: Different recovery rates of the electrophysiological, biochemical and morphological parameters in the cholinergic synapses of the Torpedo electric organ after stimulation. J. Neurochem. **22**, 1109—1114 (1974b).

CHAPTER 3

Transmission of Impulses from Nerve to Muscle

B. L. GINSBORG and D. H. JENKINSON

A. Introduction

In this chapter neuromuscular transmission will be discussed mainly from an electro-physiological standpoint although some specifically pharmacological topics, in particular the properties of the acetylcholine receptors, will also be considered. Since most of what is known about pre-synaptic mechanisms is based on electrical recordings of the muscle response, we have thought it best to discuss the relevant properties of muscle, as well as post-synaptic events during transmission, before considering the details of transmitter release. The main emphasis throughout will be on results obtained from experiments on isolated tissues; information on corresponding *in vivo* work, and a more broadly based account of the pharmacology of neuromuscular transmission, may be found in Chapter IV.

Much of what is known about the electrical events during transmission stems from discoveries by BERNARD KATZ and his coworkers. In addition to the papers and reviews mentioned in the following pages, two books, "Nerve, muscle and synapse" (KATZ, 1966) and "The release of neural transmitter substances" (KATZ, 1969), are especially recommended.

B. The Muscle Fibre and the Action of Acetylcholine

I. Some Relevant Properties of Muscle Fibres

1. The Membrane Potential and its Measurement

a) Intracellular Recording

The most direct way of determining the membrane potential (the potential of the myoplasm with respect to the exterior) is by inserting a fine-tipped electrolyte-filled micropipette into the fibre (LING and GERARD, 1949; NASTUK and HODGKIN, 1950; FATT and KATZ, 1951). Detailed accounts of the technique have been provided by FRANK and BECKER (1964), HUBBARD et al. (1969), LAVALLÉE et al. (1969) and GEDDES (1972), and a brief description of some factors which may affect the accuracy of the measurements is all that is needed here.

1. A potential difference often exists between the microelectrode tip and the surrounding medium, and this is likely to change as the tip passes from the extracellular fluid into the myoplasm. Consequently the membrane potential may be underestimated. Another complication is that this "tip potential" occasionally alters while the microelectrode is in the fibre, giving

rise to a spurious change in "membrane potential". Accounts of the origin, characteristics and consequences of the tip potential can be found in articles by del Castillo and Katz (1955b), Adrian (1956), Agin and Holtzman (1966), Niedergerke and Orkand (1966), and in the books by Lavalée et al. (1969) and Geddes (1972).

2. Insertion of a microelectrode into a cell inevitably causes some damage to the membrane. In electrical terms this is equivalent to the introduction of an unspecific leak conductance which will cause the resting potential to fall. Although the depolarization is usually small, this may not be the case when the input conductance of the cell is low. As noted on page 18, input conductance decreases with fibre diameter. It is accordingly much more difficult to record from frog "slow" muscle fibres, which are relatively small, and in addition have a low specific membrane conductance (Burke and Ginsborg, 1956a; Stefani and Steinbach, 1969) than from the twitch fibres of the same species. Similarly, it has so far proved impracticable to obtain reliable intracellular recordings from the motor nerve terminals in skeletal muscle.

b) Extracellular Recording

Changes in membrane potential can also be followed, though less directly, with extracellular recording. In one procedure often used *in vivo* a narrow electrode (which may be a platinum or a chloride-coated silver wire, or a wick soaked in agar) is placed on the surface of the muscle, and the potential between this electrode and a reference electrode at an inactive region (e.g. at or near the tendon) is recorded. At rest, since the membrane potential is the same throughout each fibre, there should be no voltage gradient along the muscle. When the nerve is stimulated, or a depolarizing agent applied, current will flow through the extracellular fluid to enter the fibres at the end-plate region which therefore becomes more negative than elsewhere. Thus by moving the active electrode to the point of maximum negativity, it is possible to locate the end-plate region (Burns and Paton, 1951; Maclagan and Vrbová, 1966; Paton and Waud, 1967).

The same technique can be applied to isolated preparations although it is often better to mount the muscle vertically in a bath in which the fluid level can be altered so that the tissue is only partly immersed during recordings; the meniscus then serves as an easily adjustable extracellular electrode. The method was introduced in 1950 by Fatt (see also Niedergerke, 1956).

Extracellular recording is often convenient, and is sometimes the only suitable method of measuring changes in membrane potential, but several possible complications must be borne in mind:

1. The proportionality factor between the surface and the transmembrane potential depends on the values of the extracellular and intracellular resistances, and these (particularly the former) may alter during long experiments.

2. The extracellular potential may sometimes give only a poor indication of a change in membrane potential as when, for example, a denervated mammalian muscle is exposed to a large concentration of acetylcholine. Since chronic denervation causes the entire fibre surface to become sensitive to acetylcholine (p. 261), depolarization will extend over the length of the muscle. In the extreme instance of a uniform fall in membrane potential, there would be no longitudinal current flow, and thus no extracellular potential difference.

3. The potential recorded from a whole muscle may reflect the contribution of many fibres, the number depending on the size of the electrode, the extracellular resistance, and the thickness of the preparation. This can be important in kinetic studies with isolated tissues. Thus the time course of the extracellularly-recorded response to a depolarizing agent will be influenced by the rate at which the drug diffuses through the tissue, as well as by the sequence of events in individual fibres.

2. Factors Influencing the Membrane Potential

a) General Considerations

Although much remains to be learnt about the membrane potential of muscle fibres, its existence can be explained in general terms as a consequence of the differences between (1) the concentrations of ions in the myoplasm and the external medium and (2) the permeability of the membrane to these ions. These factors will be discussed in turn. We may first note that although cell membranes do not show absolute ionic selectivity, it is useful (especially when discussing the actions of neurotransmitters) to consider what the membrane potential would be if the membrane allowed the passage of only one ion species, X.

This potential is given by

$$E_X = 2.3 \, \frac{RT}{ZF} \log_{10} \frac{[X]_0}{[X]_i}. \tag{1}$$

Here $[X]_0$ and $[X]_i$ are the concentrations of X in the extracellular fluid and in the myoplasm respectively, Z is the valency, R the gas constant, T the absolute temperature and F the Faraday. At 37° C the value of 2.3 RT/ZF is 61.5 mV for a univalent cation (cf. 58.2 mV at 20° C). E_X is often referred to as the *equilibrium potential* for the ion in question, since it indicates the value of the membrane potential at which there would be no net movement of the ion across the membrane.

b) The Ionic Composition of Muscle

The ionic composition of skeletal muscle has been studied under several experimental conditions. Rat and frog muscles have received particular attention, and Table 1 lists values for fresh samples of rat leg muscles. It may also be noted that the ionic composition of "slow" and "fast" twitch muscles of mammals differ slightly; for example, the latter contain a higher concentration of potassium (SRÉTER and WOO, 1963; HOH and SALAFSKY, 1971). The information available for other species, including man, has been comprehensively reviewed by ZACHAR (1971). A study of human muscle by CUNNINGHAM et al. (1971) also deserves mention. These authors reported values of 149, 26.5 and 4.1 mmol/l for the intracellular concentrations of potassium, sodium and chloride respectively in biopsy samples from healthy adults. The corresponding membrane potential was − 88 mV. In severe systemic illness the respective concentrations change to 151, 37.7 and 8.8 mmol/l, and the membrane potential to − 66 mV.

The conditions required for mammalian muscle to maintain a stable ionic content *in vitro* have been closely examined, particularly by CREESE and his co-workers. Oxygenation has been shown to be critical, so that the best results can be obtained with thin muscles, other factors being equal. It has also been shown that the addition of insulin and of a globulin fraction from human plasma to the bathing fluid allows the intracellular sodium in isolated rat diaphragm to be maintained at the same low level (about 6 mmol/l) as *in vivo* (CREESE and NORTHOVER, 1961; CREESE, 1968; ARMSTRONG and KNOEBEL, 1966; ZIERLER et al., 1966; MOORE, 1973).

Without such supplements to the bathing fluid, the intracellular concentrations of potassium and sodium in the isolated rat diaphragm *in vitro* are 168 and 13 mmol/

Table 1. Composition of rat skeletal muscle and plasma. (After CONWAY and HINGERTY, 1946; reproduced from KERNAN, 1972)

	Muscle		Plasma	
	mmol/kg	mmol/l fibre water	mmol/kg	mmol/l plasma water
Potassium	101 ± 1.9	152	5.9 ± 0.2	6.4
Sodium	27.1 ± 1.1	16	138 ± 1.8	150
Calcium	1.6 ± 0.04	(1.9)	3.1 ± 0.1	3.4
Magnesium	11.0 ± 0.3	(16.1)	1.5 ± 0.1	1.6
Chloride	16.2 ± 1.5	5.0	110 ± 0.9	119
Bicarbonate	2.5 ± 0.6	1.2	22.4 ± 0.5	24.3
Total phosphorus	82.9 ± 0.9	—	—	—
Total acid soluble phosphate	61.1 ± 0.8	—	—	—
Phosphocreatine	24.4 ± 0.4	36.9	—	—
Adenosinetriphosphate	6.5 ± 0.8	9.8	—	—
Total hexose monophosphate	10.0 ± 0.9	15.1	—	—
Triosephosphate and phospho- glycerate	3.5	5.3	—	—
Fructose diphosphate	0.2 ± 0.06	0.3	—	—
Remaining acid-soluble phosphate (incl. inorganic P)	(3.5)	5.3	2.2 ± 0.5	2.3
Phospholipids	(10.0)	(15.0)	—	—
Carnosine	1.4 ± 0.1	2.1	—	—
Anserine	20.3 ± 4.9	30.7	—	—
Urea	5.2 ± 0.6	7.0	6.7 ± 0.8	7.0
Amino acids	(20)	(30)	3	3
Lactate	(2)	(3)	1	1
Glucose	—	—	5	5
Acid-labile CO_2 (Ba-soluble)	(10)	(15)	—	—
Protein	3	4	1	1
Water (g kg^{-1})	768	—	923	—

kg fibre water respectively when the corresponding outside levels are 5.0 and 145 mmol/kg water (CREESE and NORTHOVER, 1961; CREESE, 1968). The equilibrium potentials, E_K and E_{Na}, are therefore -94 and $+64$ mV respectively [from Eq. (1)], the difference in sign arising because there is less sodium inside the fibre. The membrane potential is found to be -78 mV under similar experimental conditions (KERNAN, 1963) i.e. between E_K and E_{Na}, though very much closer to E_K. This is consistent with the membrane being considerably more permeable to potassium than to sodium, as suggested by much other evidence (e.g. BOYLE and CONWAY, 1941; HODGKIN and HOROWICZ, 1959 a, b; CREESE, 1968; see also below).

c) The Dependence of Membrane Potential on Ionic Permeabilities

The idea that each of the different ion species present in the extracellular fluid influences the membrane potential to an extent determined mainly by the permeability to the ion in question and by the corresponding transmembrane concentration gradient can be formulated in quantitative terms. Several assumptions about the properties of the membrane must be made, however, since direct information is lacking. The usual approach is to suppose that the membrane, and the electric field within it, are uniform in the transverse direction. Using this "constant field" assumption it can be shown that the membrane potential should be given by the following expression (GOLDMAN, 1943; HODGKIN and KATZ, 1949):

$$E_m = \frac{RT}{F} \ln \frac{P_K[K]_0 + P_{Na}[Na]_0 + P_{Cl}[Cl]_i}{P_K[K]_i + P_{Na}[Na]_i + P_{Cl}[Cl]_0}. \qquad (2)$$

Here the permeability to an ion X is denoted by P_X; the other symbols have been defined on p. 231. It has also been assumed that the contribution of ions other than sodium, potassium and chloride can be ignored.

Because the membrane potential normally lies between E_K and E_{Na}, there is a tendency for the cell to gain sodium at the expense of potassium (even in the absence of action potentials). Thus steady intracellular concentrations of these ions can only be maintained by the active transport of both ions in the opposite direction to their electrochemical gradients. In a resting muscle the active uptake of potassium is exactly matched by the extrusion of sodium so that there is no net transfer of charge to make a contribution to the membrane potential. If a muscle is made to gain sodium and to lose potassium (a common experimental procedure being to soak an isolated preparation in a potassium deficient solution at low temperature) it is found that when normal conditions are restored sodium extrusion may exceed the uptake of potassium. The active transport mechanism now brings about a net ionic current in such a direction as to increase the membrane potential, i.e., it becomes "electrogenic". This was first demonstrated in the frog (KERNAN, 1962) but can also occur in mammalian skeletal muscle (DOCKRY et al., 1966; KERNAN, 1968, 1972; for additional references, and a detailed account of electrogenic transport, see THOMAS, 1972).

It seems unlikely that chloride ions are actively transported in skeletal muscle since the concentration of chloride within the fibres is about what would be expected if chloride ions were distributed passively according to the membrane potential, so that E_{Cl} is close to E_m (HODGKIN, 1958; HODGKIN and HOROWICZ, 1959b; ADRIAN, 1961). This being so Eq.(2) can be replaced by the simpler expression

$$E_m = \frac{RT}{F} \ln \frac{[K]_0 + \alpha[Na]_0}{[K]_i + \alpha[Na]_i} \qquad (3)$$

where α is the ratio of the sodium to the potassium permeability of the membrane. This equation has been extensively tested (e.g. HODGKIN and HOROWICZ, 1959b) and is found to hold over a considerable range of concentrations, breaking down (in the sense that α can no longer be regarded as a constant) only when the external potassium concentration is low, or when there is a strong outwardly-directed electrochemical gradient for potassium ions. Under resting conditions α is found to be about 0.01 for frog twitch fibres, i.e. the membrane is only about one hundredth as permeable to sodium as to potassium. In contrast, the permeability to chloride, which depends on pH (see below, p. 241), is two to three times greater than that to potassium (HUTTER and PADSHA, 1959; HODGKIN and HOROWICZ, 1959b). Mammalian muscle is also considerably more permeable to chloride than to potassium (BRYANT and MORALES-AGUILERA, 1971; RÜDEL and SENGES, 1972; HEAD, 1975), whereas the reverse may hold for the multiply-innervated slow muscles of amphibians (STEFANI and STEINBACH, 1969).

II. The End-Plate Potential

1. Introduction

The development of present ideas about the electrical events occurring during neuro-muscular transmission effectively began with the discovery by GÖPFERT and SCHAE-FER (1938) that stimulation of the motor nerve to curarized frog skeletal muscle caused a transient electronegativity of that part of the muscle surface at which the axons were known to end. A similar potential change was observed by ECCLES and O'CONNOR (1939) in experiments with cat skeletal muscle *in vivo*. With an appropri-ate interval between two motor nerve stimuli the second nerve impulse could be made to reach the axon endings whilst the muscle fibres were refractory. The impulse then caused a relatively slow monophasic potential change (similar to that observed by GÖPFERT and SCHAEFER) at the end-plate region but not elsewhere. The response was accordingly named the end-plate potential.

These findings, following as they did the demonstration by DALE and his cowork-ers that acetylcholine was released from the nerve endings during activity (see Chap-ter 2), and COWAN's observation (1936) that acetylcholine added to the bathing fluid caused end-plate electronegativity similar to that seen on nerve stimulation, led to the recognition of the main steps in neuromuscular transmission. A further impor-tant advance was the demonstration by ECCLES et al. (1941) that the time course of the end-plate potential could be accounted for by supposing that the depolarizing action of acetylcholine lasted only a few msec; when this 'active phase' was complete, repolarization occured at a rate determined by the passive electrical properties of the membrane (see also p.245).

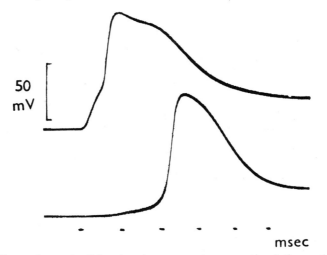

50
mV

msec

Fig. 1. Muscle fibre action potentials set up in response to nerve stimulation and recorded with an intracellular microelectrode placed at the end-plate region (upper) and 2.5 mm away (lower). Frog sartorius preparation. (From FATT and KATZ, 1951; records reproduced from FATT, 1959)

In 1951 FATT and KATZ described the use of micro-electrodes to investigate the responses of individual muscle fibres to nerve stimulation. Figure 1 compares the membrane potential changes occurring at the end-plate region with those recorded some mm away in the same fibre. The action potential set up at the end-plate differs in three main respects: (1) there is a marked "step" on the rising phase; (2) the peak amplitude is less and (3) there is a transient delay ("hump") during the early phase of repolarization.

The initial step clearly corresponds to the point at which the depolarization caused by nerve-released acetylcholine had become large enough to reach the threshold of the muscle fibre. FATT and KATZ suggested that not only this initial depolarization but also the other characteristic features of the action potential could be explained by supposing that acetylcholine acted by increasing the ionic permeability of the end-plate region of the muscle in such a way as to, in effect, "short-circuit" the resting membrane potential (see also p.239). This proposal was in keeping with the earlier finding that the membrane resistance of the muscle fell during the end-plate potential (KATZ, 1942).

As discussed in greater detail in a later section (p.280), the neuromuscular blocking action of the curare alkaloids is readily understood in these terms, since a sufficient reduction in post-synaptic sensitivity to acetylcholine will reduce the permeability increase, and hence the depolarization, to a level at which a muscle action potential is no longer set up. Only the end-plate potential can then be recorded, as originally described by GÖPFERT and SCHAEFER. Unlike the action potential, the end-plate potential is not, of course, propagated and its decline with time and distance from the end-plate is illustrated in Fig.2 (see also Fig.2 in BOYD and MARTIN, 1956b).

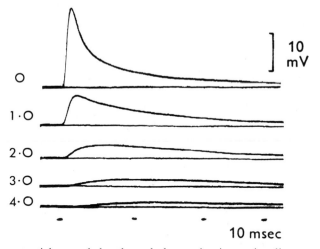

Fig. 2. End-plate potentials recorded at the end-plate and at increasing distances (left, mm) away in the same frog sartorius muscle fibre. Neuromuscular transmission blocked by tubocurarine. (From FATT and KATZ, 1951; records reproduced from FATT, 1959)

2. General Characteristics of the Permeability Change Caused by the Transmitter

As already noted (p.230), the equilibrium potentials for potassium and sodium ions are very different, being about −95 and +65 mV respectively in the mammal, and −100 and +50 mV in the frog. If acetylcholine acted by increasing the permeability of

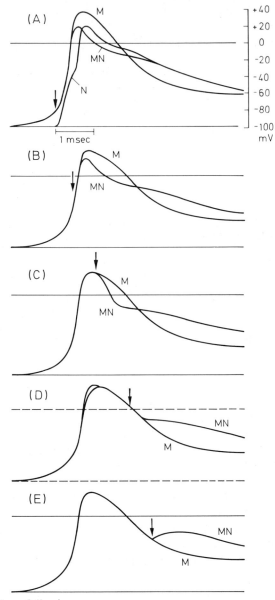

Fig. 3A—E. Legend see following page

the membrane to sodium ions alone, the membrane potential would be displaced towards E_{Na}. If, however, the rise in permeability was less selective the membrane
potential would tend to a value between E_{Na} and the equilibrium potential(s) for the
additional ion(s) involved. Del Castillo and Katz (1954e) distinguished between
these alternatives by examining the response to a nerve stimulus at various times
during an action potential set up in a frog sartorius muscle fibre by a direct stimulus
to the muscle. With appropriate intervals between the shocks to the nerve and to the

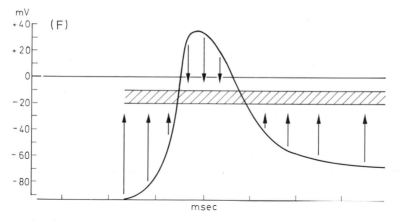

Fig. 3 A—E. The effect of the transmitter on an action potential propagating through the end-plate region of a muscle fibre. *M* in each section shows the control action potential set up by direct stimulation of the muscle fibre. *MN* illustrates the modifications (commencing at the arrows) produced when transmitter is released in response to a nerve stimulus. The action potential set up by nerve stimulation alone is also shown *(N)* in A. The records in D were considered technically less satisfactory than the others.

F summarises the effect of transmitter action on the muscle fibre membrane potential at the different levels attained during an action potential. The arrows indicate the direction and relative magnitude of the potential changes caused by the transmitter. The shaded band shows the approximate level at which the effect of transmitter on membrane potential reverses in direction. (From DEL CASTILLO and KATZ, 1954 e)

muscle, the effect of nerve-released acetylcholine on the muscle fibre membrane potential at values of the latter ranging from –90 mV (the resting potential) to + 35 mV (at the peak of the action potential) could be determined (Fig. 3). It was found that when the membrane potential was more negative than about –15 mV, acetylcholine release caused a *decline* in electronegativity, whereas an *increase* occurred when the potential was more positive than this value. Thus acetylcholine displaced the membrane potential towards a "null point" of about –15 mV. This is often referred to as the *reversal potential*, since it is the point at which the effect of the transmitter on membrane potential changes sign. The term "acetylcholine equilibrium potential", sometimes abbreviated to E_{ACh}, is also used [1].

The existence of a reversal potential for acetylcholine has been confirmed in other kinds of experiments.

a) Frog slow muscle fibres do not generate action potentials so that their response to nerve-released acetylcholine could be explored over a wide range of membrane potentials (BURKE and GINSBORG, 1956 a, b), allowing a direct demonstration of reversal, as illustrated in Fig. 4 A.

---

[1] The term "equilibrium potential" is employed here in a rather different sense from that generally used in relation to tissue electrolytes. E_{ACh} is the one value of the membrane potential at which acetylcholine causes neither hyper- nor depolarization since the sums of the currents carried by the ions affected by acetylcholine becomes zero. In contrast, the equilibrium potential for an inorganic ion, e.g. potassium, is the membrane potential at which there would be no net movement of the ion in question across the membrane.

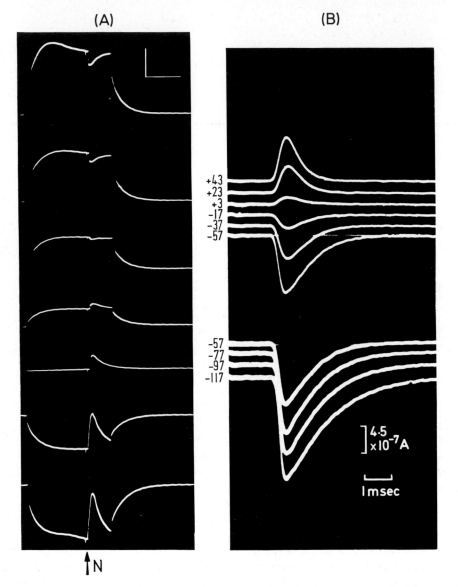

Fig. 4 A.   The effect of changing the membrane potential of a frog slow muscle fibre on the response to nerve stimulation (at *N*). Depolarization upwards. Note that the potential change which the transmitter causes reverses in direction when the membrane is depolarized beyond a certain value. Intracellular recording: a second microelectrode was used to displace the membrane potential. Calibrations (upper right): horizontal, 100 msec; vertical, 10 mV. (From Burke and Ginsborg, 1956 b.)

B. End-plate currents (see also Fig. 8) set up by nerve stimulation and recorded at different membrane potentials (indicated on left for each trace). Again note reversal as the membrane is depolarized. Glycerol-treated frog sartorius preparation. (From Kordaš, 1969)

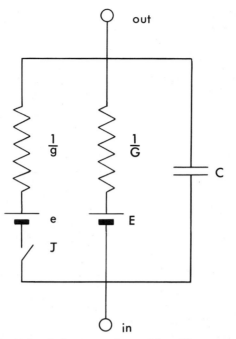

Fig. 5. A simple equivalent circuit for transmitter action. The properties of the part of the membrane that is not chemosensitive are represented by a battery, E, (with an *e.m.f.* equal to the resting potential), a conductance of value G (the reciprocal of the membrane resistance) and a capacitance C. The circuit elements on the left indicate the additional ion channels opened by the transmitter, and comprise another battery, e, (of *e.m.f.* equal to the equilibrium potential for transmitter action) in series with a conductance of value g, and a switch, J, which closes transiently to mimic transmitter action. See text for further details

    b) Axelsson and Thesleff (1959) applied acetylcholine ionophoretically to chronically denervated cat tenuissimus muscle and found that the response changed sign when the membrane potential was more positive than about -10 mV.

    c) By measuring the current needed to "voltage clamp" the end-plate membrane at different potentials during nerve activity (see p. 244 and Fig. 8), Takeuchi and Takeuchi (1959, 1960) confirmed that the "null point" lay at about -15 mV. Even more direct evidence was obtained by applying the voltage clamp technique to detubulated fibres (see p. 244) which do not contract even when strongly depolarized. Records obtained in this way by Kordaš (1969) are shown in Fig. 4B.

3. The Representation of Transmitter Action in Electrical Terms

As discussed by Fatt and Katz (1951), the hypothesis that acetylcholine acts by increasing the ionic permeability of the muscle fibre can be usefully formulated in terms of an electrical model of the kind shown in Fig. 5. Acetylcholine is considered to introduce an additional pathway for current flow, so that a fall in potential results. The time course is given by

$$(\Delta V)_t = \frac{g}{g + G} \cdot V_0 \{1 - \exp(-t/\theta)\} \qquad (4)$$

where $V_0 = e - E$, $\theta = C/(g+G)$, t is the time after switch J is closed, and the other symbols are as defined in the legend to Fig. 5. In a muscle fibre with a resting potential of -90 mV, V_0 would be $-15 - (-90) = 75$ mV.

When t is large with respect to θ, the depolarization would reach a steady value

$$\Delta V = \frac{g}{g+G} \cdot V_0. \tag{5}$$

If the action of acetylcholine ends abruptly, as represented by reopening the switch, the depolarization declines from its initial value $(\Delta V)_0$ with a time course given by

$$(\Delta V)_t = (\Delta V)_0 \exp(-t/\phi). \tag{6}$$

Here t is the time after the switch opens, and ϕ represents C/G. (For derivations of these expressions, and for further discussion, see Hubbard et al. (1969, p. 62 *et seq*) and Ginsborg (1967, 1973)).

The electrical properties of skeletal muscle fibres are of course more complicated than indicated in Fig. 5. Thus both the conductance and the capacitance of the membrane are uniform along the fibre, whereas the conductance, g, introduced by acetylcholine is localised. A more realistic model is therefore to represent transmitter action in terms of the insertion of an additional conductance at the centre point of an extended cable made up of elements to represent the conductance and capacitance of the rest of the membrane. It can be shown that the potential changes which result have a more complex time course than the simple exponentials predicted by Eq. (4) and (6). This has been discussed by Fatt and Katz (1951) whose paper should be consulted for the solution of the corresponding cable equations. One result which may be mentioned here is that the steady state depolarization will be related to g by the expression

$$\Delta V = \frac{g}{g+G_0} \cdot V_0, \tag{7}$$

where G_0 is the input conductance of the fibre, given by $2\sqrt{g_m/r_i}$. Here g_m represents the membrane conductance of the fibre and r_i the longitudinal resistance of the fibre interior, both expressed per unit length (see also p. 242).

Equations (5) and (7) are of the same form, and imply that the depolarization, ΔV, does not increase linearly with the conductance change except when $g \ll G_0$. The divergence from linearity becomes important under several circumstances, if for example the amplitude of the end-plate potential is to be used as a measure of transmitter release. The problem was first discussed in detail by Martin (1955).

Rearrangement of Eq. (7) gives

$$g = \frac{\Delta V}{V_0 - \Delta V} \cdot G_0, \tag{8}$$

which can be used either to calculate g from the observed depolarization, ΔV, if V_0 and G_0 are known, or, if G_0 is uncertain, to provide a "correction factor" (often referred to as "Martin's correction") for the non-linearity. Thus the product, $\Delta V'$, of the observed depolarization, ΔV, and the dimensionless quantity $(1 - \Delta V/V_0)^{-1}$ provides a measure which should be directly proportional to g.

The situation is somewhat complicated, however, by two further factors. First, account may have to be taken of the potential differences set up by extracellular current flow. Second, Eqs.(5), (7), and (8), and the derived "correction factor", apply only to the steady state condition. When transients are considered (as when the end-plate potential is to be analysed) the effect of the membrane capacitance must also be considered. For a valuable discussion of these complications, see HUBBARD et al. (1969, pp. 66—68). It is to be noted that G has been taken to remain constant as the membrane potential falls; this is likely to hold only when ΔV is relatively small. Also, when the amplitude of the end-plate potential is to be used as a measure of transmitter release, it is important that the recording electrode should be as close to the end-plate as possible. If this is not ensured attenuation of the response will mean that the correction factor for non-linear summation will be underestimated (see discussion by AUERBACH and BETZ, 1971).

4. The Influence of the Non-Synaptic Membrane on the Response to Acetylcholine

An important feature illustrated by the model of Fig. 5 is that the amplitude of the depolarization which results from a given increase in permeability at the end-plate region will be influenced by the conductance and capacitance of the rest of the membrane. Some consequences of this will now be considered.

a) Factors which Alter Membrane Conductance

A change in external pH will affect conductance by altering the chloride permeability of the membrane (HUTTER and WARNER, 1967a, b; WOODBURY and MILES, 1973). The effect can be substantial, since chloride contributes as much as 70% of the resting conductance of frog twitch muscle, and 85% of that of goat intercostal fibres (BRYANT and MORALES-AGUILERA, 1971). Is was shown by DEL CASTILLO et al. (1962) that lowering the external pH to 4.0 caused a more than twofold increase in the depolarizing action of acetylcholine on toad muscle, and that this effect could be attributed to a reduction in membrane conductance. HUTTER and WARNERS' findings make it likely that a decline in chloride permeability underlies this action, and also suggest that a less drastic reduction in pH (to about 5.3) should suffice to give a comparable effect.

Other procedures which effect chloride conductance include the application of some other inorganic anions (e.g. nitrate; HUTTER and PADSHA, 1959; HARRIS 1958; ADRIAN, 1961) and cations (e.g. copper and zinc; HUTTER and WARNER, 1967c); the administration of monocarboxylic acids (e.g. anthracene-9-carboxylic acid; BRYANT and MORALES-AGUILERA, 1971) and also, of course, the replacement of chloride by impermeant anions such as methylsulphate and isethionate.

Potassium ion conductance can be selectively reduced by tetraethyl ammonium salts (e.g., STANFIELD, 1970) as well as by prolonged application of local anaesthetics (ADRIAN and FREYGANG, 1962; HARRIS and OCHS, 1966).

Membrane conductance may change in certain pathological conditions. Thus studies of myotonic human (LIPICKY et al., 1971) and goat skeletal muscle (BRYANT and MORALES-ANGUILERA, 1971; ADRIAN and BRYANT, 1974) have shown that the membrane conductance is less than half of the normal value, mainly because the chloride conductance is much lower.

Chronic denervation also causes the membrane conductance to fall, as first shown by NICHOLLS (1956), though see also NASLEDOV and THESLEFF (1974), and analysed by HARRIS and NICHOLLS (1956), KLAUS et al. (1960a) and S.J.HUBBARD (1963). This is mainly because of a decline in potassium conductance, and contributes to the increased sensitivity of denervated muscle to acetylcholine, although quantitatively it is less important than the spread in the acetylcholine-sensitive area (see p. 261).

b) Influence of Muscle Fibre Dimensions

As discussed on p. 299, the amplitude of the miniature end-plate potentials (see p. 295) can vary greatly from fibre to fibre in the same muscle, being largest in the smallest fibres. An analysis of this variation by KATZ and THESLEFF (1957a) has shown that it is largely attributable to differences in the effective membrane conductance of the muscle fibres, rather than to presynaptic factors.

The input conductance, G_0(mho), of a long "cable" made up of elements comprising a conductance and a capacitance in parallel (see p. 240) is $2\sqrt{g_m/r_i}$. Since $g_m = G_m \times \pi d$, and $r_i = 4R_i/\pi d^2$, then $G_0 = 2\sqrt{\dfrac{G_m \cdot \pi d \cdot \pi d^2}{4R_i}} = \pi \cdot d^{\frac{3}{2}} \cdot \sqrt{G_m/R_i}$, where G_m is the membrane conductance per unit area (mho/cm^2) and R_i is the specific resistance of the sarcoplasm (ohm $\cdot$ cm). Thus smaller fibres will have lower input conductances, because of the $d^{\frac{3}{2}}$ term. In addition the specific membrane conductance is less in such fibres, at least in the frog (HODGKIN and NAKAJIMA, 1972a). The response to a steady application of acetylcholine can therefore be expected to be correspondingly greater, other factors remaining equal.

The same general considerations apply to the response to nerve released acetylcholine although it is then necessary to take into account membrane capacitance as well as conductance (because of the transient nature of the conductance increase). This has been discussed by GAGE and MCBURNEY (1972b) whose calculations show that the maximum depolarization to be expected from a brief localized rise in conductance in a detubulated fibre is relatively insensitive to changes in the specific membrane conductance. Nevertheless, the response to a quantum of transmitter is greater in smaller fibres because of their larger effective input impedance. It is interesting that this factor is to some extent offset (so far as the end-plate potential is concerned) by a greater release of acetylcholine from motor nerves terminating on larger muscle fibres (see p. 329).

c) The Influence of the Internal Structure of the Muscle Fibre

An important limitation of the models so far discussed is that they do not take into account the existence of the network of sarcoplasmic tubules which extend from the surface into the interior of the fibre. It is now clear, largely from the work of FALK and FATT (1964, 1965) that this "transverse tubular system", together with its associated lateral elements, contributes substantially to the electrical characteristics of muscle and provides a convincing explanation of the previously puzzling discrepancy between different estimates of the membrane capacity. Thus impedance measurements with low frequency alternating current provide values of from about 5 to more than $8 \mu F/cm^2$, depending on the fibre diameter (see HODGKIN and NAKAJIMA, 1972a) whereas much lower values ($2 \mu F/cm^2$) are observed at relatively high frequencies (FATT, 1964, see also GAGE and EISENBERG, 1969; SCHNEIDER, 1970; HODGKIN and NAKAJIMA, 1972a, b). FALK and FATT (1964) noted that this and certain other aspects of the electrical behaviour of the fibre could be accounted for more accurately by adding two further circuit elements, a capacitance (C_e) and a resistance (R_e) in series (Fig.6, upper right), to the simple model hitherto considered (Figs.5, 6,

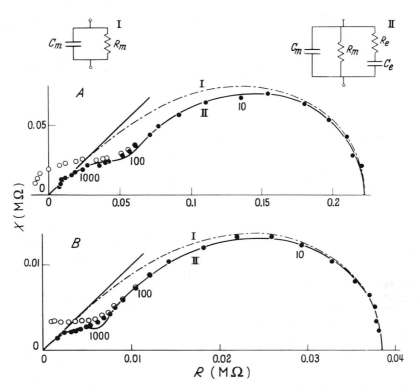

Fig. 6 A and B. Evidence that the electrical properties of a muscle fibre are reproduced more accurately by a model (upper right, II) containing additional elements (C_e and R_e) to represent the tubular system than by the simple equivalent circuit hitherto considered (upper left, I; see also Fig. 5). A and B show impedance-locus plots (see. e.g. Schwan, 1957) obtained on passing alternating current of different frequencies, indicated by numbers (Hz) for some of the points, across the membranes of frog sartorius and crayfish muscle fibres respectively. The filled circles were obtained from the open ones after allowing for stray capacitances around the microelectrodes. The broken and continuous lines show theoretical impedance loci for models I and II respectively. (From FALK and FATT, 1965, based on results obtained by FALK and FATT, 1964)

upper left). FALK and FATT suggested that the elements R_m and C_m reflected the properties of the surface membrane, whereas R_e and C_e represented a separate pathway contributed by the tubular membranes.

On this basis, a more complete model for transmitter action is illustrated in Fig. 7. Since the additional conductance generated by the action of the transmitter does not rise to, or fall from, a final value in an abrupt way, it has been represented by a variable resistance. However, even in the simple model of Fig. 5, the changes in membrane potential are considerably slower than the changes in conductance. The effect of the new elements G_e and C_e is to exaggerate the difference (see also FALK and FATT, 1965). Thus the very large increase in the duration of the end-plate potential caused by certain local anaesthetics may be explained by a relatively small increase in the duration of transmitter action. A striking example has been given by STEINBACH, 1967, 1968 a, b) for the effect of some quaternary derivatives of lignocaine.

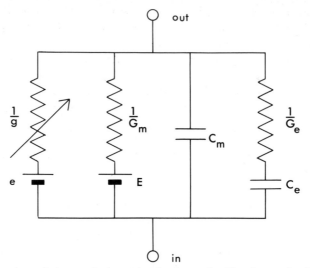

Fig. 7. A modification of the equivalent circuit shown in Fig. 5 to take into account the tubular system which is represented by a conductance, G_e, and a capacitance, C_e (cf. Fig. 6). G_m and C_m are the conductance and capacitance respectively of the surface membrane. Other circuit elements are as defined in Fig. 5. Transmitter action is considered to be equivalent to a rapid increase in g from zero and back. The circuit would require expansion to take into account the cable properties of the muscle fibre

It is possible to simplify the situation by "detubulating" muscle fibres, by a process first used by HOWELL and JENDEN (1967). It was found that immersion of a muscle in Ringer's fluid made strongly hypertonic with glycerol, followed by restoration of a normal medium, effectively disconnected the sarcoplasmic tubules from the surface membrane. Fibres detubulated in this way often had rather low membrane potentials but a modification of the procedure by EISENBERG et al. (1971) has proved more satisfactory (see also SEVCIK and NARAHASHI, 1971).

An advantage of such preparations for experimental purposes is that the muscle fibres, though electrically excitable, do not contract. An analysis of transmitter action in detubulated muscle has been made by GAGE and McBURNEY (1972a, b; see also KORDAŠ, 1969, 1972a; MAGLEBY and STEVENS, 1972a, and ANDERSON and STEVENS, 1973).

III. The Ion Selectivity of the Permeability Change Produced by the Transmitter

1. The Voltage Clamp Technique

The finding (p. 237) that the reversal potential for the action of acetylcholine is, at -15 mV, more negative than E_{Na} implied that the conductance increase must extend to other ions in addition to sodium. The subsequent demonstration (DEL CASTILLO and KATZ, 1955b) that ionophoretically-applied acetylcholine still increased membrane conductance when the muscle was bathed in a fluid containing only potassium sulphate strongly suggested that potassium permeability was also affected. Further evidence on this point, and on the general question of the relative contributions of the main environmental ions to the overall conductance increase, came from an important series of experiments by TAKEUCHI and TAKEUCHI (1959, 1960) using the voltage clamp technique.

In this procedure, two microelectrodes are inserted at the end-plate region, one to monitor membrane potential, and the other to pass current from an external source. By using a negative feedback arrangment whereby the flow of current is controlled by the potential measured it is possible to "clamp" the membrane potential at a pre-determined steady level. The additional current required to maintain the clamp during transmitter action can then provide a more accurate measure of the conductance increase than the depolarization which would otherwise occur; because the potential is held constant throughout, the complication of current flow through the surface membrane capacitance should not arise.

Considering again the circuit diagram in Fig. 5, it is evident that when the switch J is open a current $(V − E)G$ will be needed to change the membrane potential from E to a new value V. If J is now closed (to represent the onset of transmitter action) an additional current (the "end-plate current"), given by $(V − e)g$, will be needed to maintain the potential at V. Thus the end-plate current should be proportional both to g and to $(V − e)$, and should reverse when $V = e$. Before discussing the results of experiments to test these predictions, some details of the application of the method deserve brief mention.

1. The phase changes introduced by stray capacitances set an upper limit to the usable gain of the feed-back amplifier. Thus some residual change in membrane potential is unavoidable.

2. The nerve terminals in a frog twitch muscle fibre may extend for as much as $600 \mu m$ in the longitudinal plane so that some of the end-plate membrane will "escape" a clamp applied from a single microelectrode, effectively a point source of current (see also RANG, 1975, p. 323). "Escape" may also occur if the microelectrodes are not positioned focally, and this may complicate the study of pre- as well as of post-synaptic events (see discussion by AUERBACH and BETZ, 1971).

3. The current needed to clamp the end-plate region during normal transmitter action is likely to exceed the limit which can be passed through a microelectrode. Further, stimulation of the nerve trunk will generally cause contraction of other parts of the muscle so that one or both electrodes may be displaced. Accordingly, clamping experiments are usually made with blocked or detubulated preparations. A more drastic procedure is to transect the muscle on either side of the end-plate region (see also p. 231).

2. The End-Plate Current

Figure 8 illustrates the time course of the end-plate current as measured by the voltage clamping technique (see also Fig. 4 B). The peak amplitude is reached in less than a msec and thereafter the current falls almost exponentially, with a half-time of 1.1 msec in frog muscle at 17° C (TAKEUCHI and TAKEUCHI, 1959; see also KORDAŠ, 1972 a, b, and MAGLEBY and STEVENS, 1972 a, b). Thus current flow is almost complete after 5 msec, confirming earlier conclusions based on analysing the time course of the end-plate potential.

TAKEUCHI and TAKEUCHI (1959, 1960) also examined the dependence of the end-plate current on membrane potential over the range $− 50$ to $− 100 \, mV$, finding an approximately linear relationship (see Fig. 9) which on extrapolation suggested a reversal potential of between $− 10$ to $− 20 \, mV$, in good agreement with the value obtained in experiments of the kind discussed on pp. 237 and 239. Figure 9 also

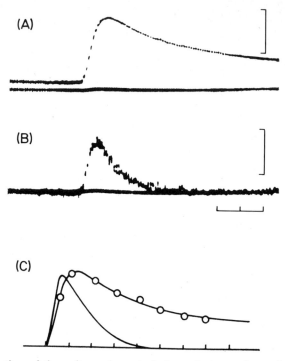

Fig. 8 A—C. Application of the voltage clamp technique. A shows the end-plate potential recorded intracellularly from a superficial fibre in a curarized frog nerve-sartorius preparation. In
B the clamp had been applied in the same fibre so that the transmitter now caused a transient
flow of current (upper trace) rather than a fall in potential (monitored in the lower trace).
Calibrations: voltage, 5 mV (A); current, 10^{-7} A (B); time, msec. In C records of the end-plate
potential and current have been superimposed. The circles indicate the potential changes calculated from the end-plate current, assuming appropriate values for the conductance and capacitance of the fibre membrane. (From TAKEUCHI and TAKEUCHI, 1959)

shows that the reversal potential is not affected by a change in the concentration of
tubocurarine in the bathing fluid.

Application of the clamping technique to muscles which have been detubulated
(p. 244) allows the voltage dependence of the end-plate current to be explored over a
wider range than would otherwise be practicable. It is then found (KORDAŠ, 1969,
1972 a, b; MAGLEBY and STEVENS, 1972 a, b) that the rate of decay of the current
varies with the membrane potential, becoming greater as the membrane is depolarized. It is also observed that the relationship between end-plate current and membrane potential deviates somewhat from linearity. Several explanations can be suggested. One possibility raised by KORDAŠ (1969, 1972 a, b) is that the membrane
potential influences the stability of the transmitter-receptor complex, and MAGLEBY
and STEVENS (1972 a, b) have outlined a model (based on the idea that conformational changes in the receptor alter the dipole moment of the transmitter-receptor
complex) which could explain how this might occur (see also ANDERSON and STEV-
ENS, 1973).

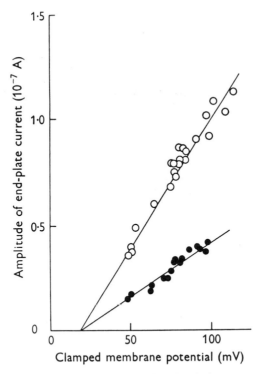

Fig. 9. The relationship between membrane potential and end-plate current as determined by the voltage clamp method. The open and closed circles indicate values measured before and after raising the concentration of tubocurarine from 3 to 4 µg/ml. (From TAKEUCHI and TAKEUCHI, 1960)

3. Relative Contribution of Different Ions to the Conductance Increase

As TAKEUCHI and TAKEUCHI (1959) showed, the voltage-clamp technique provided direct means of finding the equilibrium potential for transmitter action, and so could be applied to the problem of determining the contributions of different ions to the net increase in conductance. If the equilibrium potential for a given ion is altered (e.g. by adjusting the external concentration), the null point for transmitter action should change only if the conductance change involves the ion in question. Using this criterion, TAKEUCHI and TAKEUCHI were able to confirm that the effect of acetylcholine on membrane permeability extended to sodium and potassium; chloride ions, however, were found not to be involved to any substantial extent (contrast C with A and B in Fig. 10).

In a later study, TAKEUCHI (1963 b) showed that acetylcholine still produced de-polarization when applied in a fluid in which sodium had been completely replaced by calcium. Indeed miniature end-plate potentials (although reduced in amplitude) can be recorded from muscles bathed in isotonic calcium or magnesium chloride (80 mM), plus 2 mM potassium chloride (KATZ and MILEDI, 1969 b). These observations (see also PARSONS and NASTUK, 1969, and p. 251) show that acetylcholine increases both

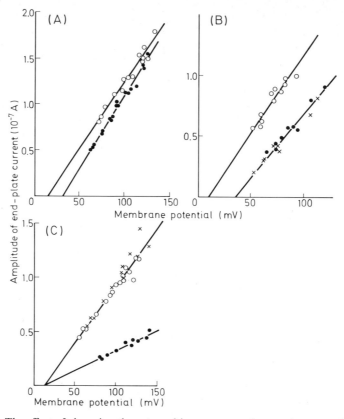

Fig. 10 A—C. The effect of changing the external ion concentration on the reversal potential for transmitter action. Each panel shows the relationship between the end-plate current and membrane potential, as in Fig. 9. In A the open and closed circles indicate values obtained with bathing fluids containing 113.6 and 33.6 mmol/l sodium respectively. Reducing the sodium concentration makes the sodium equilibrium potential less positive, and it can be seen that the transmitter reversal potential (the membrane potential at which the end-plate current would be zero) then becomes more negative. This is consistent with the idea that the transmitter increases sodium permeability. B shows the effect of changing potassium from 0.5 mmol/l (filled circles) to 4.5 mmol/l (open circles) and back (crosses). Raising the external potassium concentration makes the reversal potential less negative, as is to be expected if the transmitter increases potassium permeability. C Effect of changing external chloride. The filled circles were obtained in normal solution. The open circles and crosses show values measured 2 to 3 and 15 min respectively after replacing all the chloride by glutamate; the concentrations of calcium and tubocurarine were also adjusted. Note that the reversal potential remains unchanged. (From TAKEUCHI and TAKEUCHI, 1960)

calcium and magnesium conductance, although under normal circumstances only a small part of the total end-plate current is carried by divalent ions.

There is also evidence that acetylcholine enhances the permeability to certain organic cations, including ammonium and tetramethylammonium (NASTUK, 1959), methyl- and ethylammonium (FURUKAWA and FURUKAWA, 1959) hydrazinium (KOKETSU and NISHI, 1959) and probably also decamethonium (CREESE and ENGLAND, 1970; CREESE and MACLAGAN, 1970).

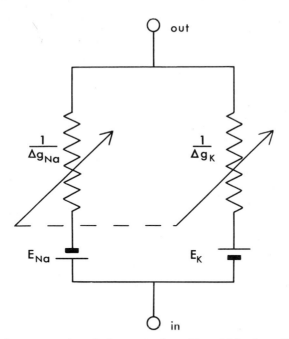

Fig. 11. An electrical representation of a "separate channel" model for the action of acetylcholine (see text). The circuit can be regarded as one of several possible expansions of the circuit elements shown on the left of Fig. 5. (After TAKEUCHI and TAKEUCHI, 1960)

4. Characteristics of the Additional Ion Channels

The finding that the transmitter affects only cation permeability raises the additional questions of whether the resulting net movements of sodium and potassium ions are comparable, and occur through common or separate channels. If distinct pathways exist, it might be possible to represent them by separate conductances Δg_{Na} and Δg_K, each in series with an E.M.F. equivalent to the corresponding equilibrium potential (see TAKEUCHI and TAKEUCHI, 1960 and ECCLES, 1972). In such a model (Fig. 11), the total current, I, which flows through the synaptic channels during transmitter action is the sum of the sodium and potassium currents, i_{Na} and i_K. If the conductances Δg_{Na} and Δg_K behave ohmically, I can be written as

$$(V - E_{Na})\, \Delta g_{Na} + (V - E_K)\, \Delta g_K,$$

where V is the membrane potential.

Rearranging, $I = (\Delta g_{Na} + \Delta g_K)\, V - (\Delta g_{Na} \cdot E_{Na} + \Delta g_K \cdot E_K)$.

Thus I should be linearly related to V, becoming zero when V is at the equilibrium potential, e. In that condition

$$(\Delta g_{Na} + \Delta g_K)\, e - (\Delta g_{Na} E_{Na} + \Delta g_K E_K) = 0.$$

Hence

$$e = \frac{\Delta g_K E_K + \Delta g_{Na} E_{Na}}{\Delta g_K + \Delta g_{Na}},$$

or

$$e = \frac{E_K + \theta E_{Na}}{1+\theta}, \tag{9}$$

where $\theta = \Delta g_{Na}/\Delta g_K$. Taking e, E_K and E_{Na} for frog muscle as -15, -99 and $+50$ mV respectively, θ is calculated to be 1.29.

TAKEUCHI and TAKEUCHI (1960) also examined the dependence of e on E_K and E_{Na} which were varied independently by adjusting the composition of the bathing fluid. The results were consistent with Eq.(9), although the range of values which could be explored was limited by the need to preserve conduction in the nerve endings. In a later study, TAKEUCHI (1963a) investigated the response to iono-phoretically-applied rather than nerve-released acetylcholine, thereby allowing a wider range of sodium and potassium concentrations to be tested. It was found that when the external potassium was considerably increased, the value of θ fell (from 1.29 to 0.66 on raising $[K]_0$ from 2.5 to 50 mmol/l). However, θ did not alter when the external sodium was varied over a wide range.

The implications of these results are still somewhat uncertain and it may be mentioned that the finding of an approximately linear relationship between end-plate current and membrane potential does not necessarily imply the existence of two separate "linear" ion channels for sodium and potassium (see GINSBORG, 1973, and RANG, 1975, for discussions of this point). If there are separate channels, it might be feasible to block either of them by pharmacological means. Indeed it has been suggested (MAENO, 1966; MAENO et al., 1971) that procaine may reduce Δg_{Na} in relation to Δg_K during the early phase of the end-plate current (see also DEGUCHI and NARAHASHI, 1971) although this interpretation has not been universally accepted (see STEINBACH, 1968b, KORDAŠ, 1970, 1972b). A decline in the ratio of Δg_{Na} to Δg_K may also underlie the increase in the negativity of the reversal potential seen on raising external calcium (TAKEUCHI, 1963b). Large concentrations of atropine, in contrast, cause the reversal potential to become less negative, and it has been suggested that this is because of a rise in $\Delta g_{Na}/\Delta g_K$ (MAGAZANIK and VYSKOČIL, 1969).

There is much evidence to show that the ion channels controlled by the transmitter are not those concerned either in the action potential or in the passive passage of ions across the resting membrane. Thus the action of acetylcholine is little affected by tetrodotoxin (FURUKAWA et al., 1959; ELMQVIST and FELDMAN, 1965a; KATZ and MILEDI, 1967b) even at concentrations many times greater than those needed to suppress the action potential. Further, the additional potassium conductance which results from the action of acetylcholine shows little rectification, in marked contrast to the potassium conductance of the rest of the membrane (see DEL CASTILLO and KATZ, 1955b).

5. Evidence on Ion Selectivity from the Use of Radio-Isotopes

Strictly speaking, electrophysiological experiments can provide direct information only about ion *conductances*. Since radioisotopes of the main ions of physiological interest are available, it should, in principle, be possible to detect whether acetylcholine or some related substance increases the *permeability* of the membrane to a given ion simply by testing the effect of the agent on the rate of exchange of a suitable isotope. Such experiments have been undertaken, but encountered several difficulties.

In the first place, the acetylcholine-sensitive region normally forms only a small part of the total surface area of a skeletal muscle fibre, so that any increase in flux due to the direct effect of acetylcholine at the motor end-plate may be masked by the flux across the rest of the membrane. It is not surprising therefore that bath-applied depolarizing agents have generally been found to cause little change in the overall movement of labelled potassium and sodium ions in normally innervated muscles (e.g. KLAUS et al., 1960b; HENDERSON and HANCOCK, 1971). Although AHMAD and LEWIS (1962) reported large effects of suxamethonium, carbachol, decamethonium and nicotine on ion flux in normal muscle, the concentrations tested were so great (e.g. suxamethonium, 12 mmol/l, carbachol, 27.3 mmol/l) that the possibility of unspecific effects involving the whole membrane cannot be ruled out.

The problem raised by the spatially-restricted sensitivity to acetylcholine is less important (at least for influx measurements) when changes in end-plate permeability to cations such as calcium and decamethonium (p. 258) are to be examined. This is because these ions on entering the myoplasm become bound to intracellular components and hence, in effect, immobilised. Thus the additional entry of decamethonium at the end-plate can be measured by autoradiography (CREESE and MACLAGAN, 1970), and LIÈVREMONT et al. (1968), NASTUK (1971) and EVANS (1971, 1974) have used a histochemical method to demonstrate accumulation of calcium at the end-plate region of muscles exposed to acetylcholine and carbachol.

A second general difficulty with the isotope technique is that the changes in membrane potential (i.e. depolarization and possibly also propagated action potentials) which result from the action of a depolarizing agent such as acetylcholine can be expected to alter ion flux, so that it may not be easy to distinguish between primary and secondary effects of the agent on tracer movement. One way of simplifying the situation (although at the cost of departing from physiological conditions) is to keep the muscle depolarized throughout the experiment by applying a potassium-rich bathing solution. Acetylcholine then causes little change in membrane potential (DEL CASTILLO and KATZ, 1955b; JENKINSON and NICHOLLS, 1961) so that alterations in ion flux should provide a more reliable indication of changes in permeability. This has been examined in chronically denervated mammalian skeletal muscle in which the whole fibre surface has become sensitive to acetylcholine (see p. 261). Under these conditions large increases in the exchange of sodium, potassium and calcium are observed in response to acetylcholine while there is no comparable effect on chloride flux, in keeping with the conclusions about the selectivity of the permeability change reached from electrophysiological experiments on muscles with intact innervation (see KLAUS et al., 1960b, 1961; JENKINSON and NICHOLLS, 1961; ADAMIČ, 1965).

The effect of depolarizing agents on ion flux in denervated frog and mammalian muscles bathed in more physiological fluids has also been examined (see KLAUS et al., 1961; HENDERSON and HANCOCK, 1971). As would be expected, large increases in ^{42}K efflux and ^{24}Na uptake (associated with a net loss of tissue potassium, and a net gain of sodium) are readily observed.

IV. Localization of Acetylcholine Receptors

1. Introduction

The "receptor concept" was introduced and developed equally by EHRLICH, LAN-
GLEY and MICHAELIS. LANGLEY's contribution is of special interest here since his
conclusions were based for the most part on experiments with skeletal muscle. An
early finding was that nicotine caused contraction of skeletal muscle even after the
motor nerve had been cut and allowed to degenerate. Noting that the response could
still be abolished by curare, LANGLEY wrote in 1905:

"Since there is evidence that the axon-endings in skeletal muscle degenerate after section of
the nerves supplying the muscle, I conclude that nicotine and curari do not act on the axon-
endings but on the muscle itself ... Since in the normal state both nicotine and curari abolish the
effect of nerve stimulation, but do not prevent contraction from being obtained by direct stimulations of the muscle or by a further adequate injection of nicotine, it may be inferred that neither
the poison nor the nervous impulse act directly on the contractile substance of the muscle but on
some accessory substance. Since this accessory substance is the recipient of stimuli which it
transfers to the contractile material, we may speak of it as the *receptive substance* of the muscle."

Evidence on the localization of the "receptive substance" was obtained by the
simple expedient of using a fine brush to apply droplets of a dilute solution of
nicotine from point to point along the length of the fibres. It was found that twitching was readily elicited at the region of the nerve endings but rarely, if ever, elsewhere
(LANGLEY, 1907).

LANGLEY also showed that the antagonism between curare and nicotine was
reversible as well as dose-dependent, and he put forward the view, still widely held
(see also pp. 280) that

"such antagonistic poisons formed chemical compounds with the same constituent in the
tissues, that the compounds were reversible and that the amount of each compound formed
depended on the relative masses (i.e. on the relative concentrations) of the two poisons" (LAN-
GLEY, 1914).

2. The Ionophoretic Method of Drug Application

More precise information about the spatial distribution of acetylcholine sensitivity
was not obtained until some 40 years later with the development of the micro-
ionophoretic technique. This was introduced by NASTUK (1953), and refined by
DEL CASTILLO and KATZ (1955a) and by PEPER and MACMAHAN (1972).

A fine-tipped glass micropipette is filled with a strong solution of the substance to
be applied, which preferably should be mainly or wholly ionized. Leakage from the
tip (if fine enough) can largely be prevented by passing a "braking" current through
the pipette. When the drug is to be applied the current is reduced or reversed for a
brief period so that a pulse of the substance is released. The method has been
described in detail by CURTIS (1964). It should also be mentioned that some neutral
substances can be released from micropipettes by electro-osmosis, by high frequency
vibration of the whole pipette (CHOWDHURY, 1969), or by diffusion. In the latter case
the release rate may be controlled by an electrically operated micro-tap, which can
be made very rapid in action (BRYANT et al., 1967).

The relationship between the amount of a charged molecule delivered and the current passed
through an ionophoretic micropipette has been much studied. Unfortunately it appears to depend to some extent on the particular micropipette and current duration tested. Direct proportionality is generally assumed, and ionophoretic doses are usually expressed in terms of the total

charge passed, from which the quantity released could be calculated if the transport number for the ion in question were known under the particular experimental circumstances. For acetylcholine the transport number appears to be about 0.4 when release is from a micropipette filled with 3 M acetylcholine chloride; there is little electro-osmosis (see KRNJEVIĆ et al., 1963, and BRADLEY and CANDY, 1970).

However, when brief pulses of drug are ejected at relatively low frequencies (less than 1 Hz), as in most ionophoretic experiments with skeletal muscle, the concentration of the drug in the tip will not be the same as when the releasing current in passed continuously or in trains of pulses, and the appropriate transport number is even less certain (CLARKE et al., 1973).

Even if the amount released were accurately known, the concentration attained at the receptor would still be uncertain; it is however clear that high values may be reached directly under the tip of a focally-placed micropipette. Thus the end-plate depolarization produced by a low concentration of acetylcholine (e.g. 1 µM) applied in the bathing fluid in the presence of an anticholinesterase (and so presumably reaching all the available receptors) can be matched without difficulty by ionophoretic application to a small fraction (perhaps no more than a percent or so) of the total sensitive area. Several factors rule out exact computations, however. These include: (1) the difficulty of determining the distance between the pipette tip and the receptors; (2) the uptake of some of the drug by the receptors (and possibly other tissue components) and, (3) the likely non-uniformity of the sensitive area. As a first approximation, taking the tip as a point source in an infinite volume can account for the general features of the time course of the end-plate response to ionophoretically applied acetycholine, although a detailed examination reveals some discrepancies (DEL CASTILLO and KATZ, 1955a, see also KAHN and LE YAOUANC, 1971).

Against the limitations of the ionophoretic method can be set the advantage that drugs can be applied within milliseconds to specified minute areas of the end-plate membrane. This is illustrated by the records shown in Figs. 12 and 13. In both experiments the micro-pipette had been placed at a highly sensitive spot, and it may be seen that the responses began without appreciable latency, and reached their peak within a few milliseconds.

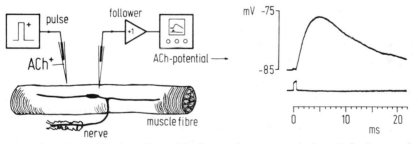

Fig. 12. Ionophoretic application of acetylcholine to the motor end-plate. Left, the experimental arrangement. Right, the depolarization produced by a brief pulse of acetylcholine (releasing current, 1.5×10^{-8} A for 0.5 msec). The coulomb potency (see text) was 1260 mV/nC. Frog cutaneous pectoris preparation. (From PEPER and MCMAHAN, 1972)

It has become usual to express the sensitivity to ionophoretically-applied drugs in units of the potential change (mV) produced per nanocoulomb (nC) of charge passed. Very high values, up to 5000 mV/nC (KUFFLER and YOSHIKAMI, 1975) have been described. Thus for the responses illustrated in Figs. 12 and 13, the quantities of acetylcholine released were only about 3×10^{-17} and 1.5×10^{-16} mol respectively (taking the transport number to be 0.4). These amounts are, however, greater than the quantities of nerve-released acetylcholine which would produce a

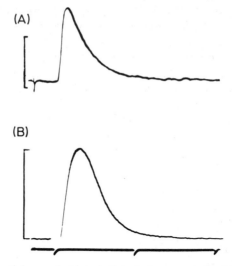

Fig. 13 A. End-plate potential recorded intracellularly from a rat diaphragm muscle fibre: transmission blocked by magnesium. B The end-plate response to ionophoretically-applied acetylcholine in another rat diaphragm under similar conditions; releasing pulse 3.5×10^{-8} A for 1 msec. Voltage calibrations: A, 5 mV; B, 10 mV. Time scale, 10 msec. Temperature 24—25°C. (From Krnjević and Miledi, 1958b)

similar depolarization. Thus each nerve impulse has been estimated to release at most 7×10^{-18} mol (i.e. about 4×10^6 molecules) per rat diaphragm end-plate (see Potter, 1970, and Chapter 2). The discrepancy presumably arises because of the different geometrical situations, and of the limitations of the ionophoretic method. Thus the receptors under the pipette may be saturated, and it is possible that some become desensitized (p. 275).

The relationship between ionophoretic sensitivity (mV/nC) and receptor density (as assessed by the bungarotoxin method; p. 258) has been studied by Hartzell and Fambrough (1972; see also Barnard et al., 1975, and Dreyer and Peper, 1975).

3. Evidence on Receptor Distribution from Ionophoretic Experiments

Much information about the distribution of acetylcholine sensitivity in both normally innervated and denervated muscle has been obtained using the ionophoretic method. The main findings with normal muscles can be summarized as follows:

(1) As the earlier experiments of Langley (1907) and of Ginetzinksy and Shamarina (1942) (see p. 261), had indicated, the sensitivity to acetylcholine is greatest in the vicinity of the nerve endings (Axelsson and Thesleff, 1959; Miledi, 1960 a, b; Katz and Miledi, 1964 a; Feltz and Mallart, 1971 a). The possibility that even higher sensitivities might be found under the nerve terminals has been tested by Peper and McMahan (1972) who were able to "peel off" the terminals (after the preparations had been exposed to collagenase) and thus expose the surface immediately under the nerve ending. The procedure did not cause any appreciable change in the responsiveness to ionophoretically-applied acetylcholine (see also Kuffler and Yoshikami, 1975).

(2) The sensitivity extends beyond the nerve endings but falls away steeply with increasing distance along the fibre (MILEDI, 1960b; see also (4) and (5) below). In the frog, experiments by PEPER and MCMAHAN (1972), DREYER and PEPER (1974a) and KUFFLER and YOSHIKAMI (1975) suggest that the spatial decrement can be even greater than had been indicated by earlier work, and is subject to seasonal variation. These authors used an optical system which enabled the nerve-endings to be visualised at high magnifications without the need for vital staining (Fig. 14 A), thus allowing the experiments illustrated in Figs. 14 B and C to be performed. It was found that the sensitivity could decline as much as ten-fold when the pipette tip was moved only 5 to 10 μm from the edge of a nerve terminal.

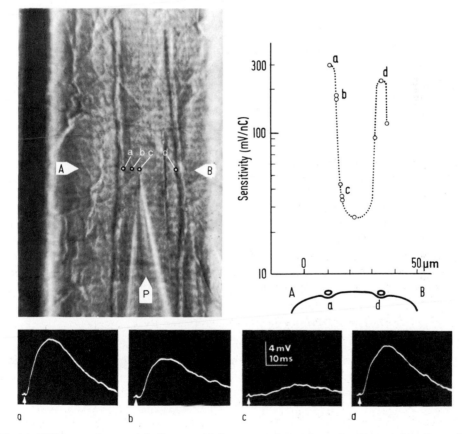

Fig. 14. Differences in acetylcholine sensitivity across the surface of a frog muscle fibre with closely spaced nerve terminals. *Photomicrograph.* Cutaneous pectoris muscle fibre viewed under Nomarski optics. Acetylcholine was applied at a series of points along a line running perpendicularly to two parallel terminals about 22 μm apart. P = acetylcholine pipette. *Records.* Acetylcholine potentials at each of the spots marked with a white dot on the photomicrograph. Moving the pipette as little as 3 μm from the edge of the terminal caused a 34% drop in sensitivity. Pulse duration 1 msec; amplitude 3.2×10^{-8} A. Resting potential of fibre, — 72 mV. *Graph.* Profile of sensitivity between the two terminals. (From PEPER and MCMAHAN, 1972)

(3) Katz and Miledi (1964 a) observed that in frog muscle the sensitivity of the non-junctional region to acetylcholine varied greatly from fibre to fibre, ranging from less than $^1/_{500\,000}$ to as much as $^1/_{100}$ of the maximum at the end-plate.

(4) In the same series of experiments, Katz and Miledi made the surprising discovery that the response to ionophoretically-applied acetycholine often increased again as the exploring micro-pipette was moved to the end of frog muscle fibres. Although the sensitivity at the end was never more than a small fraction of that at the end-plate, it was often as much as 1000 times greater than at intermediate points. Interestingly, this response to acetylcholine (unlike that at the end-plate) was not potentiated by the anti-cholinesterases edrophonium and neostigmine even though histochemical techniques show cholinesterase localization at the extreme tips of the fibres, (e.g. Lubinska and Zelená, 1967, though see Hall, 1973, and Chapter 1). The response was, however, reduced by tubocurarine to much the same extent as that at the end-plate.

(5) The spatial distribution of acetylcholine sensitivity in slow and fast mammalian twitch muscle has been examined by Miledi and Zelená (1966), Miledi et al. (1968) and Albuquerque and Thesleff (1968). In the rat soleus (a slow-contracting muscle) there is a low but clearly detectable responsiveness along the entire length of the fibre (although with areas of increased sensitivity at the muscle-tendon junctions as well as at the end-plate) whereas in the extensor digitorum longus (a fast-contracting muscle) the sensitivity is restricted to the neuromuscular junction and the immediately surrounding area (see also Lømo and Rosenthal, 1972).

4. Other Electrophysiological Evidence on the Distribution of Receptors

Receptor localization has also been studied by applying agonists (usually either acetylcholine, carbachol or suxamethonium) to the entire muscle, and measuring the changes in membrane potential at different points along the fibres by either intracellular or extracellular recording. This may be done *in vivo*, when the drug is given by intravenous infusion, or *in vitro* when it can be added to the bathing fluid.

The method, while convenient, has the limitation that because of the cable properties of the fibres the depolarization will extend away from the chemosensitive region. However, the decline with distance is such that there should be little change in membrane potential at the ends of any but the shortest fibres. (Although the muscle-tendon junctions are responsive to acetylcholine, the sensitivity is much lower than that at the end-plate, as already noted.) Nevertheless, there have been several reports of a generalized depolarization in response to bath applied agonists (Thesleff, 1955b; Ochs and Mukherjee, 1959; Ras et al., 1972; Ras and Mooij, 1973). While it has not been possible to repeat some of these observations (see e.g. the reassessments by Katz and Miledi, 1961, and by Ochs, 1966), others remain and require explanation. One factor which may be concerned is the gradual change in intracellular ionic concentrations brought about by the continued action of the depolarizing agent. Not only will sodium and potassium levels be affected, but also chloride (since the membrane potential becomes less negative than E_{Cl}), and the gradual rise in chloride content along the fibre can be expected to contribute to the spread of depolarization (see Jenkinson and Terrar, 1973; Feltz and Jaoul, 1974).

Nevertheless, some authors (e.g. PORTELA et al., 1970) have attributed the generalised depolarization which they have observed to the existence of substantial numbers of "cholinoceptive" sites along the whole length of the fibre. This is in disagreement with the general conclusions from ionophoretic experiments, as well as with observations with labelled antagonists. One factor which could contribute to the discrepancy is the variability of the acetylcholine sensitivity of the non-junctional regions of individual muscle fibres (see p. 255). In view of work on the causes of denervation supersensitivity (p.261), it seems possible that the density of extrajunctional receptors may depend on the activity of the animal which, certainly in the frog, will vary seasonally and with storage temperature (OCHS, 1966; FELTZ and MALLART, 1971a; DREYER and PEPER, 1974a; for the effect of hibernation in the mammal, see MORAVEC et al., 1973).

5. Evidence on Receptor Distribution from Experiments with Labelled Antagonists

The location of receptors has also been studied using isotopically-labelled substances (usually neuromuscular blocking drugs) which are thought to combine with either the receptor or a closely related site. The amounts taken up by different parts of the muscle, and hence, (provided that certain assumptions hold) the relative number of receptors can be assessed by quantitative autoradiography, or by counting serial sections.

a) Studies with Reversible Antagonists

This approach was introduced by WASER and his co-workers (WASER and LÜTHI, 1957; TRUOG and WASER, 1970; WASER, 1970, 1973) who have studied the distribution of labelled toxiferine, C-curarine, dimethyl-tubocurarine, pancuronium and decamethonium in the diaphragm of the mouse. A problem with such agents is that their combination with the receptors is readily reversible[2] so that after a muscle has been exposed to the labelled drug, it is difficult to wash away unbound material from the extracellular spaces without at the same time losing some of the label from the receptors. Nevertheless, subsequent work suggests that the error involved does not invalidate the main conclusions reached[3].

Using this technique, WASER and his co-workers were able to show that the endplate region of the muscle fibres took up much more of the antagonist drug than elsewhere. The magnitude of the extra uptake was measured by quantitative autoradiography, and was found to be similar when equiactive doses of toxiferine, curarine and dimethytubocurarine were injected intravenously in mice. Thus about 3.3×10^6 molecules were found per endplate at doses of each drug just sufficient to kill all the animals. This was about 80% of the maximum binding capacity ($4-5 \times 10^6$ molecules/end plate), as determined by S. MEILI (quoted by WASER, 1970). A comparable value was observed with pancuronium (WASER, 1973).

[2] This has been examined in most detail with tubocurarine, using the ionophoretic method (p.252). It has been found that after a "pulse" of tubocurarine the blocking action subsides with a half-time which may be no more than a second or two (DEL CASTILLO and KATZ, 1957a), and possibly even less (WAUD, 1967).
[3] For a critical discussion of the underlying assumptions, the reader is referred to "The Molecular Properties of Drug Receptors", ed. R. PORTER and M. O'CONNOR (1970) PP. 69—75.

Similar experiments with decamethonium also showed increased binding at the end-plate region, although the uptake was much greater than with the curare alkaloids, and extended for more than a mm along the fibres. This was taken as evidence that the binding sites for decamethonium and curare may be different. However, other explanations can be envisaged, and the problem has been re-examined by Creese and his co-workers (Creese et al., 1963; Taylor et al., 1965; Creese and England, 1970; Creese and Maclagan, 1970). Waser's finding that decamethonium fixation extended well beyond the confines of the end-plate was confirmed. However, it was also shown that the uptake could be blocked by tubocurarine. While more complicated explanations were not ruled out, a simple interpretation of the greater uptake of decamethonium was therefore that the drug, by activating the receptors, had brought about a permeability increase which facilitated the passage of drug molecules into the myoplasm (see p. 250). The mobility of decamethonium in myoplasm has been found to be very low (Taylor et al., 1967), and Creese and Maclagan (1970) consider this to rule out the otherwise attractive possibility that the presence of substantial amounts of the drug in the fibres at a distance from the end-plate was due to longitudinal diffusion of material which had entered at the end-plate. Creese and Maclagan suggested instead that the additional uptake may be a consequence of the presence of extrajunctional receptors (see p. 255).

b) Irreversible Antagonists; Counting and Isolation of Receptors

An important modification of the technique described above has been made possible by the discovery and purification of snake venom toxins which selectively block neuromuscular transmission by irreversibly inactivating the receptors, probably by becoming attached to them (Chang and Lee, 1963). The general properties of these toxins have been reviewed by Meldrum (1965) and Lee (1972); see also Simpson (1974). Two agents which have been studied in particular detail are α-bungarotoxin, from the venom of the Formosan snake *Bungarus multicinctus*, and cobra toxin, from the venom of the cobra *Naja naja* (*siamensis* or *nigricollis*). Both are very long acting, many hours at least being required for the response to acetylcholine to recover after an isolated preparation is returned to toxin-free solution (see Lee, 1972; Lee et al., 1972 and Lester, 1972 a, b).

These substances can be labelled with radioisotopes (Lee et al., 1967; Miledi and Potter, 1971; Barnard et al., 1971; Berg et al., 1972; Fambrough and Hartzell, 1972; Vogel et al., 1972; Chang et al., 1973 a) and this not only provides another means of studying the location and density of receptors, but also, because of the stability of the receptor-toxin complex, may allow the receptors to be isolated and characterised[4]. (Early attempts at receptor isolation using labelled gallamine (see Chagas, 1959) had been vitiated by the rapidity with which the drug dissociates from the receptors when the tissue is restored to gallamine-free solution). Although many interesting results have already been obtained, it is too early for a detailed evaluation, particularly since only preliminary reports have appeared in several instances, and also because the homogeneity and stability of some labelled toxin

---

[4] It is also possible to label α-bungarotoxin with a fluorescent dye so that the distribution of receptors *in situ* can be visualized by fluorescence microscopy (Anderson and Cohen, 1974; see Fig. 20, p. 54 in Chapter 1).

Table 2. Binding of labelled antagonists at the end-plate region of skeletal muscle

Tissue	Antagonist	Molecules of antagonist bound per end-plate[a]	Density of binding (molecules/μm^2)	Reference
Mouse diaphragm	C-curarine toxiferine pancuronium }	4—5×10^6		1
Mouse diaphragm	α-bungarotoxin	2—3×10^7		2, 3
Mouse diaphragm	α-bungarotoxin	1.4—2.1×10^7	8.5×10^3	3,8
Mouse sternomastoid	α-bungarotoxin	8.7×10^7	8.8×10^3	3,8
Rat diaphragm	α-bungarotoxin	4×10^7	1.3×10^4	4, 7
Rat diaphragm	α-bungarotoxin	$2 \times 10^{7\ b}$		5
Rat diaphragm	α-bungarotoxin	4.7×10^7		6
Frog sartorius	α-bungarotoxin	10^9		6
Frog sartorius	α-bungarotoxin	3×10^7		2
Normal human deltoid	α-bungarotoxin	3.8×10^7		7
Myasthenic human deltoid	α-bungarotoxin	see [c] below		7
Bat diaphragm	α-bungarotoxin	—	8.8×10^3	8

References: (1) WASER (1970, 1973); (2) PORTER et al. (1973b); (3) PORTER et al. (1973a); (4) FAMBROUGH and HARTZELL (1972); (5) CHANG et al. (1973a); (6) MILEDI and POTTER (1971); (7) FAMBROUGH et al. (1973); (8) PORTER and BARNARD (1975). See also SALPETER and ELDEFRAWI (1973) and FERTUCK and SALPETER (1974) for evidence on variations in receptor density along the sub-synaptic folds.

[a] Varies with fibre size [see Ref. (3)]. May correspond to number of functional receptors (see p. 260).
[b] Decreases in response to chronic administration of neostigmine (CHANG et al., 1973b; see also FAMBROUGH et al., 1973).
[c] From 11 to 30% of the value in normal muscle.

preparations, while adequate for qualitative work, may fall short of the attainable limits (see discussion by CHANG et al., 1973a). It seems best, therefore, merely to summarize the main findings to date and to provide references where further details may be sought.

1. LEE et al. (1967; see also MILEDI and POTTER, 1971; BARNARD et al., 1971; BERG et al., 1972; PORTER et al., 1973b, as well as individual papers in the symposium volume edited by RANG, 1973) have shown that toxin binding is much greater at the end-plate region than elsewhere. The number of additional toxin molecules taken up under saturation conditions has been estimated by several groups, and the figures obtained are summarized in Table 2. Although these values could well correspond to the number of functional receptors, the point is not yet certain and some authors have suggested that there may be more than one binding site on the receptive mechanism [see (3) and (4) below]. The possibility that the toxins may also combine with cholinesterase has been raised by STALC and ŽUPANČIČ (1972) but is made unlikely by the finding that α-bungarotoxin does not reduce the catalytic activity of the acetylcholinesterases found in the rat diaphragm (CHANG and SU, 1974) and in Electrophorus electricus (CHANGEUX et al., 1970; see also MILEDI et al., 1971a).

2. Following chronic denervation of skeletal muscle, toxin binding is no longer restricted mainly to the end-plate region so that the total amount taken up by the whole muscle increases greatly, up to 30 fold for α-bungarotoxin (LEE et al., 1967; MILEDI and POTTER, 1971; BERG et al., 1972; HARTZELL and FAMBROUGH, 1972; CHANG et al., 1973a; COLQUHOUN et al., 1974). This is discussed further on p. 261.

3. The inhibitory actions as well as the binding of α-bungarotoxin and cobra venom have been shown to be reduced by simultaneous exposure of the tissue to tubocurarine (Miledi and Potter, 1971; Berg et al., 1972; Lester, 1972b; Vogel et al., 1972). While the simplest explanation is that these substances share a common binding site, there have been reports that tubocurarine even at high concentration does not reduce the amount of toxin bound after a given time by more than about half (Miledi and Potter, 1971; Porter et al., 1973b; Albuquerque et al., 1973). The explanation is uncertain, and must await more detailed studies of the kinetics of toxin binding in the presence and absence of curare alkaloids (see Colquhoun et al., 1974). One way of accounting for the apparent failure of curare to "protect" is to suppose that α-bungarotoxin becomes attached to other end-plate structures as well as to the receptor proper. Alternatively there may be two toxin-binding sites on the receptor, only one of which can combine with curare (see 4. below). However, tubocurarine can almost completely inhibit toxin binding by chick embryo muscle (Vogel et al., 1972), as well as by rat diaphragm, provided that a relatively low concentration (3.75×10^{-8} M) of bungarotoxin is used (Chang et al., 1973a; see also Anderson and Cohen, 1974; Colquhoun et al., 1974; Porter and Barnard, 1974).

4. The conclusion that there may be two binding sites for α-bungarotoxin is supported by studies with the perhydro derivative of histrionicotoxin, a toxic substance isolated from the Colombian arrow-poison frog *Dendrobates histrionicus* (Albuquerque et al., 1973). This toxin also blocks neuromuscular transmission, and reduces the rate of binding of α-bungarotoxin (though, as with tubocurarine, not to zero). When, however, perhydrohistrionicotoxin and tubocurarine were given together, α-bungarotoxin binding was almost completely blocked. Albuquerque et al. in discussing these results, propose that α-bungarotoxin might combine with two separate sites. One, the acetylcholine receptor proper, is curare-sensitive, and the other, it is proposed, is part of the structure (the "ionic conductance modulator" or "ionophore") that mediates the permeability change which follows receptor activation. This latter site is thought to be blocked by perhydrohistrionicotoxin.

The idea that the entity with which the transmitter combines and the "conductance modulator" are distinct structures, and therefore susceptible to selective blockade, is also suggested by the work of Kasai and Changeux (1971) on microsac preparations from the electroplax of *Electrophorus electricus*. The same concept appears in the suggestion by Magazanik and Vyskočil (1973) that desensitization may involve not the receptors but a later stage in the transduction process (see p. 278).

5. Simultaneous exposure of a muscle to acetylcholine or carbachol reduces the inhibitory effects of both α-bungarotoxin (Miledi and Potter, 1971) and cobra toxin (Lester, 1972b). The binding of labelled α-bungarotoxin is also reduced (Miledi and Potter, 1971; Berg et al., 1972; Vogel et al., 1972). This does not seem to be a consequence of simple competition for the receptor, since the inhibition of toxin binding develops slowly, and can be observed several minutes after the agonist has been washed out of the tissue. It has been suggested instead that desensitized receptors may have a lower affinity for such toxins (see also p. 280).

6. As noted, the stability of the bungarotoxin-receptor complex suggests a means of isolating the receptors for acetylcholine. While some preliminary work with skeletal muscle has already been reported (Miledi and Potter, 1971; Berg et al., 1972), greater effort has been directed towards the electric organs of *Electrophorus electricus* and *Torpedo marmorata*. These tissues are much more densely innervated than skeletal muscle, and are correspondingly richer sources of nicotinic receptors. There is already some evidence to suggest that the receptor from *Torpedo* is a protein made up of about six sub-units each with a molecular weight in the order of 40000. A detailed account of this work can be found in the reviews by O'Brien et al. (1972), Landowne et al. (1975) and Rang (1975). It is likely that the isolation procedures now being developed for fish electric organ tissue will also prove applicable to muscle. An intriguing finding which suggests a close relationship between the structures of *Electrophorus* and mammalian nicotinic receptors is that repeated injections of *Electrophorus* receptor extracts in rabbits causes an immune response associated with muscle weakness and eventual paralysis (Patrick and Lindstrom, 1973; Patrick et al., 1973; Sugiyama et al., 1973; Heilbronn and Mattson, 1974).

7. The complex between α-bungarotoxin and the receptor dissociates so slowly that the disappearance of labelled toxin from the end-plate region of a muscle may give an indication of the rate of turnover of receptors. Preliminary studies of this kind suggest that receptor half-life may be about a week in the rat. References and further details may be found in the article by Vincent (1975).

6. Denervated Muscle

The control of the acetylcholine sensitivity of skeletal muscle is still only partly understood. One of the main pieces of evidence comes from studies of the consequences of interfering with the motor nerve supply. Chronic denervation has long been known to cause skeletal muscle to become many times more sensitive to diffusely-applied acetylcholine. Several factors contribute to this, including a fall in membrane conductance (see p. 241, and a reduction in the cholinesterase content of the tissue. Much more important, however, is an increase in the area of the muscle which responds to acetylcholine. This was first shown by GINETZINSKY and SHAMARINA (1942) using a technique similar to LANGLEY's in which they examined the response of different regions of the muscle fibres to droplets of acetylcholine solution applied from a fine pipette. It was found that chronically denervated rabbit muscle became responsive over the entire length of the fibres. Regrettably, this work did not become widely known outside Russia until much later (see DIAMOND and MILEDI, 1962) and the spread of sensitivity was in effect independently rediscovered by AXELSSON and THESLEFF (1959) and MILEDI (1960a).

An important consequence of the increase in the sensitive area is that diffuse application of agonists will cause a generalised depolarization. This can account for the maintained contractures unaccompanied by action potentials (except at the outset) observed when acetylcholine is injected into the arterial supply to a denervated muscle *in situ*, or even into the general circulation (BROWN, 1937; ROSENBLUETH and LUCO, 1937). Since both the depolarization and the increase in permeability which underlies it occur over the whole fibre, the associated ionic movements (e.g. potassium loss) are greater than in normal muscle (PERRY and ZAIMIS, quoted in ZAIMIS, 1954; see also p. 251, and Chapter 4A).

Some further aspects of receptor control will now be briefly mentioned, with emphasis on findings which could throw light on the mechanism of the spread of sensitivity.

(1) Although the entire fibre surface becomes responsive after denervation, a gradient in acetylcholine sensitivity remains with a peak at the site of the original end-plate. This is particularly marked in the frog (MILEDI, 1960a), but even in mammals the original end-plate region is probably more responsive (MILEDI, 1962) and, as illustrated in Fig. 15, binds much more α-bungarotoxin than elsewhere (LEE et al., 1967; HARTZELL and FAMBROUGH, 1972; CHANG et al., 1973a; see also VINCENT, 1975). Thus HARTZELL and FAMBROUGH found that the non-junctional part of normally innervated adult rat diaphragm muscle took up less than 5 toxin molecules per μm^2; after denervation this rose to $1700/\mu m^2$, as compared with $10^4/\mu m^2$ at the end-plate. A consequence of the differential sensitivity is that the response of a denervated muscle to a small dose of diffusely-applied depolarizing agent is likely to be greater at the original end-plate region than elsewhere.

(2) The spread of sensitivity which follows denervation develops much more slowly in the frog (MILEDI, 1960a; DREYER and PEPER, 1974b) than in mammals (AXELSSON and THESLEFF, 1959; ELMQVIST and THESLEFF, 1960; MILEDI and SLATER, 1968; ALBUQUERQUE and MCISAAC, 1970; JONES and VRBOVÁ, 1974). It can also be shown to occur in muscles maintained *in vitro* under organ culture conditions (MILEDI and TROWELL, 1962; FAMBROUGH, 1970).

(3) Many muscle fibres in foetal and newborn rats and rabbits are sensitive to acetylcholine over their entire length, the adult distribution only being attained several weeks after birth (GINETZINSKY and SHAMARINA, 1942; DIAMOND and MILEDI, 1962). Sensitivity may still be widespread even after the nerve has made contact with the muscle, as indicated by the presence of miniature end-plate potentials.

It is interesting that cultured embryonic chick and rat muscle cells bind labelled α-bungarotoxin over their whole surface although discrete areas with a higher binding capacity are also observed (VOGEL et al., 1972).

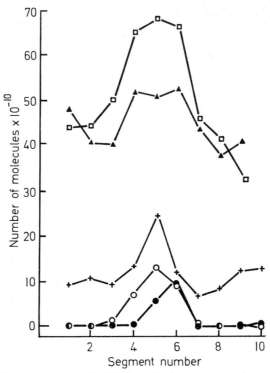

Fig. 15. The effect of denervation on the binding of α-bungarotoxin by rat diaphragm muscle. The diaphragms were first incubated with labelled N, O-diacetyl α-bungarotoxin (125 nmol/l) for 2 hr at 32° C. After repeated washings for 5 hrs, they were then dried and cut into segments 1·5 mm wide, parallel to the end-plate zone. The radioactivity of each segment was expressed in terms of the number of toxin molecules bound and has been plotted (ordinate) against segment number (abscissa) counted from the central tendon.
The closed circles ● refer to normally innervated diaphragms: there is little binding away from segments 5 and 6 (the presumed end-plate region). The symbols O, +, ▲ and □ show the results for diaphragms denervated 2, 4, 8, and 18 days beforehand, respectively. Uptake away from the end-plate increases greatly after denervation although note that the original end-plate region still binds more toxin than elsewhere. (From Chang et al., 1973a)

(4) Complete transection ("myotomy") of skeletal muscle at a point between the nearest end-plate region and the tendon (so as to create a separate nerve-free portion) is followed, after a short recovery period, by the development of acetylcholine sensitivity over the whole aneural portion. The sensitivity is greatest near the region of the cut. The healed end of the innervated part also becomes more responsive, though not to the same degree (Katz and Miledi, 1964b).

(5) Individual muscle fibres in the frog sartorius have at least two end-plates, and the distribution of the nerve branches is such that it is possible to cut the supply to one of the end-plate regions so that individual fibres can be partially denervated. The denervated end-plates are found to become more sensitive to diffusely-applied acetylcholine than those which still receive an axon (Miledi, 1960a). Further, the membrane conductance of the denervated region of the fibre declines, as in fully denervated muscle. These changes occur despite the continued mechanical and electrical activity of the muscle.

(6) Acetylcholine sensitivity spreads following prolonged application of agents which block neuromuscular transmission either by reducing acetylcholine release, e.g. botulinum toxin (Thesleff, 1960) and β-bungarotoxin (Hofmann and Thesleff, 1972) or by a post-synaptic action, e.g., tubocurarine, suxamethonium and α-bungarotoxin (Berg and Hall, 1975).

(7) Chronic application of vinblastine or colchicine to a motor nerve also causes an increase in extrajunctional sensitivity (ALBUQUERQUE 1972; HOFMANN and THESLEFF, 1972). These substances are thought to interfere with axoplasmic transport but not with the conduction of action potentials; neither the mechanical response of the muscle to nerve stimulation nor the spontaneous release of transmitter are affected. However, there is some evidence that colchicine may have acted directly on the muscle membrane (for further discussion see BERG and HALL, 1975).

(8) Blockade of conduction in motor nerves *in situ* either by application of a silicone rubber cuff which slowly released a local anaesthetic [bupivacaine (Marcaine) or lignocaine], or by injection of diptheria toxin into the nerve trunk, caused the fibres in the soleus and extensor digitorum longus muscles of the rat to become sensitive over their entire length; neither the miniature end-plate potentials nor the response to nerve stimulation distal to the blocked region were affected (LØMO and ROSENTHAL, 1972). ROBERT and OESTER (1970) however, found no comparable change in sensitivity in similar experiments with rabbit muscle.

LØMO and ROSENTHAL also showed that the spread in sensitivity produced by nerve block could be prevented by chronic nerve stimulation distal to the block. Furthermore, chronic direct stimulation of denervated soleus or extensor digitorum longus muscles could prevent the development of the usual denervation supersensitivity, or cause it to decline once present. A similar result was obtained by DRACHMAN and WITZKE (1972) who found the acetylcholine sensitivity of denervated rat diaphragms which had been directly stimulated *in situ* to be much less than that of unstimulated controls. This can also be demonstrated *in vitro* with previously-denervated rat diaphragm preparations maintained under organ culture conditions (PURVES and SAKMANN, 1974). There is evidence that direct electrical stimulation is most effective in preventing the development of extrajunctional sensitivity if begun within 2 to 3 days of nerve section (JONES and VRBOVÁ, 1974).

(9) Muscles from mice with hereditary "motor end-plate disease" are exceptionally sensitive to acetylcholine, and this is associated with an increase in the responsive area (DUCHEN and STEFANI, 1971).

(10) Placing either a segment of a severed peripheral nerve or a piece of thread on the surface of a muscle has been found to cause a localised increase in the acetylcholine sensitivity of the underlying fibres (VRBOVÁ, 1967; JONES and VRBOVÁ, 1974).

As yet no single hypothesis seems able to account for all these observations (see LØMO and ROSENTHAL, 1972; ALBUQUERQUE et al., 1972; HOFMANN and THESLEFF, 1972; JONES and VRBOVÁ, 1974; PURVES and SAKMANN, 1974; BERG and HALL, 1975).

One possibility is that both denervation and "nerve-block" supersensitivity are consequences of the quiescence of the muscle (JONES and VRBOVÁ, 1970, 1974; DRACHMANN and WITZKE, 1972; LØMO and ROSENTHAL, 1972). However, as these authors note, it might be objected that "supersensitive" muscles fibres are often observed to fibrillate, i.e. show spontaneous, unsynchronised contractions (see LI et al., 1957; JOSEFSSON and THESLEFF, 1961; BELMAR and EYZAGUIRRE, 1966; SALAFSKY et al., 1968). The objection is not conclusive since PURVES and SAKMANN (1974) who studied the pattern of fibrillation in denervated rat diaphragm maintained *in vitro* under organ culture conditions found that activity in individual fibres was cyclical, lasting for about 20 hours followed by a somewhat longer quiescent period. Direct electrical stimulation for 24 hours (to mimic a period of spontaneous activity) caused little change in acetylcholine sensitivity; however, more prolonged stimulation (for 7 to 8 days, applied in a pattern comparable to that during breathing) caused a marked fall in sensitivity. PURVES and SAKMANN therefore concluded that the mechanical and electrical activity associated with fibrillation in denervated muscle was not sufficiently sustained to interfere with supersensitivity.

Another possibility is that the nerve exerts a "trophic" influence (see GUTH, 1968) which in some way restricts the acetylcholine sensitivity of the muscle to the end-plate region. This is compatible with several of the findings mentioned above (see in particular sub-sections 5 and 7) but it would not explain how direct stimulation of a previously-denervated muscle reduces its extrajunctional sensitivity.

The origin and integrity of the nerve supply also influences other characteristics of the membrane, including both the resting conductance and the action potential. Thus frog slow muscle fibres, which are normally inexcitable, become capable of propagating action potentials, following either denervation or replacement of the original innervation by a "fast" motor nerve supply (MILEDI et al., 1971 b; see also SCHMIDT and TONG, 1973, and the following section).

A further question raised by the phenomenon of denervation supersensitivity is whether the spread of the sensitive area reflects the making of new receptors, or the activation or uncovering of entities already present in the membrane. The latter possibility has been examined by subjecting normally-innervated muscles to treatments (e.g. application of phospholipase, collagenase, detergents) which might be expected to unmask any such hidden structures. So far only negative results have been obtained (KATZ and MILEDI, 1964 b). The development of extra-junctional sensitivity in denervated muscle can however be inhibited by substances such as cycloheximide, actinomycin D and puromycin which interfere with protein synthesis (FAMBROUGH, 1970; GRAMPP et al., 1972).

As already noted, the characteristics of the action potential also alter when a skeletal muscle is denervated; in mammals the rate of depolarization decreases, and, surprisingly, the mechanism becomes relatively resistant to the action of tetrodotoxin (REDFERN and THESLEFF, 1971). These changes are again sensitive to inhibitors of protein synthesis (GRAMPP et al., 1972; see also SCHMIDT and TONG, 1973).

A possible link between the two phenomena could be that the voltage-dependent sodium channels concerned in the initial phase of the action potential in normal muscle become responsive to acetylcholine after denervation, and insentitive to tetrodotoxin. It is even conceivable that they could be converted to the usual acetylcholine receptors although evidence against this has been obtained by COLQUHOUN et al. (1974). Labelled tetrodotoxin and α-bungarotoxin were used to estimate the number of normal sodium channels and receptors respectively, and it was found that the additional α-bungarotoxin binding sites which appeared after denervation considerably outnumbered the sodium channels in normal muscle. A direct, one-to-one, conversion of channels into receptors thus seems unlikely (see also THESLEFF, 1973).

7. Characteristics of Acetylcholine Receptors in Denervated Muscle

The evidence presently available, though clearly not decisive (see LUNT et al., 1971), would suggest that new receptors are formed when acetylcholine sensitivity spreads. This raises the further question of whether these receptors are the same as those normally present. If they are not, the difference could lie in their pharmacological characteristics, or in the properties of the ion channels they control. The first possibility could best be tested by comparing the affinity constants for the binding of a range of agonists and antagonists by the receptors in intact normal and denervated muscles. However, as discussed on pp. 267 and 281 at present this is only practicable for antagonists, and the methods available are indirect. Thus, although the results of an early study of this kind (JENKINSON, 1960) might suggest that the affinity for tubocurarine increases by a small amount after denervation, the evidence is by no means decisive, especially since the extracellular recording technique used (see p. 230) was such that the responses to agonists were measured at the most sensitive region of the muscle, i.e. at the original end-plate. It would be of greater interest to study the action of tubocurarine at other parts of the fibre, so as to ensure that "new" receptors were involved.

Other evidence on the question has been provided by BERÁNEK and VYSKOČIL (1967) who compared the effectiveness of tubocurarine and atropine in blocking (1) the end-plate potential in normal rat diaphragm, and (2) the depolarizations caused by ionophoretic application of acetylcholine to non-endplate regions of denervated diaphragms. The latter response was found to be less sensitive to the action of tubocurarine, and this was taken to reflect differences in the properties of the receptors involved. Atropine had no such differential effect, so that the curare/atropine coefficient (the ratio of the antagonist concentrations causing equal reductions in response) was greater for denervated than for normal muscle, the actual values being 0.003 and 0.0005 respectively. This coefficient has also been used as a measure of the "differentiation" of acetylcholine receptors in the muscles of species at different points on the evolutionary scale, an interesting field which has been reviewed by KHROMOV-BORISOV and MICHELSON (1966).

It is worth noting that the assessment of differences in receptors by comparison of the effectiveness of a given antagonist in reducing the response to an agonist is in general less satisfactory (although sometimes the only course open) than measuring agonist dose ratios, i.e. the factors by which the agonist concentration must be increased to restore the original response when an antagonist has been applied. This is because the former measure is influenced by the form of the stimulus-response relationship (which will differ between tissues, and may not be the same for nerve-released as for externally-applied acetylcholine), as well as by the affinity of the receptor for the antagonist. The latter factor alone should determine the agonist dose ratio, provided that certain conditions hold (p. 281).

Further evidence on the identity or otherwise of receptors in normal and denervated muscle can be expected to result from progress in receptor isolation and characterisation (see VINCENT, 1975).

Finally we may consider the possibility that the characteristics of the ion channels controlled by "denervated" receptors may not be the same as those in normal muscle. Different equilibrium potentials (p. 237) might then be expected. The only detailed studies of this point have been made by FELTZ and MALLART (1971b) and by MALLART and TRAUTMANN (1973). It was found that the equilibrium potential for the action of acetylcholine was $-42\,\text{mV}$[5] in denervated frog muscle, as compared with the normal value of –15 mV. (However, it may be noted that AXELSSON and THESLEFF (1959) observed no appreciable change in equilibrium potential on denervating the tenuissimus muscle of the cat, nor did MAGAZANIK and POTAPOVA (1969) in similar experiments with the rat diaphragm. A species difference may exist, or the time course of the change in the receptors may not be the same). Other experiments by FELTZ and MALLART suggested that receptors near, but not at, the nerve endings in a normal muscle also had an equilibrium potential of $-42\,\text{mV}$[5]. Interestingly, a similar value[5] was found for junctional receptors, again in normally innervated muscle, when the external pH was increased to 9.0 (MALLART and TRAUTMANN, 1973).

---

[5] Note added in Proof. MALLART, DREYER and PEPER (Pflügers Archiv, 1976, in Press) have provided grounds for revising this conclusion, and they suggest that the equilibrium potential has the standard value under these conditions.

V. The Interaction between Acetylcholine and its Receptors

There is as yet no direct means of measuring the rate at which acetylcholine combines with the receptors, nor is there any simple way of finding the proportion of receptors occupied by acetylcholine (or indeed any comparable agonist) under equilibrium conditions. An indirect approach which has been explored in some detail attempts to deduce receptor occupancy from the response of the tissue. The validity of the conclusions reached clearly depends on the correctness of the assumptions which have to be made about the connection between these quantities. This will now be discussed briefly in relation to various models which have been proposed to account for receptor action.

1. Classical Models of Receptor Action

It has been usual to suppose that the response to acetylcholine or a similar agonist will be determined by (1), the proportion, p_A, of the receptors which are occupied by the agonist, and (2), the quantitative relationship between p_A and the events which ensue in the tissue. With regard to (1) it is usually assumed, following HILL (1909) and CLARK (1926 a, b), that the law of mass action can be applied to the combination of the agonist with the receptor. The value of p_A at equilibrium should then be related to the agonist concentration, $[A]$, by

$$p_A = \frac{K_A [A]}{1 + K_A [A]}, \tag{10}$$

where K_A is the affinity constant, i.e. the reciprocal of the "dissociation" or "equilibrium" constant for the agonist-receptor interaction.

This also supposes (1) that only one molecule of agonist combines with each binding site, (2) that the total number of sites can be regarded as constant, (3) that the sites do not interact (i.e., occupation of a site by agonist does not change the affinity of others nearby), (4) that the concentration of the drug at the receptors is the same as that in the external fluid, and (5) that the relevant activity coefficients are close to unity.

We may now consider the relationship between receptor occupancy and the ensuing increase in conductance. It has often been assumed that this is one of direct proportionality. The additional membrane conductance introduced by the action of an agonist, A, could then be written

$$g = g_{max} p_A \tag{11}$$

or

$$\frac{g}{g_{max}} = \frac{K_A [A]}{1 + K_A [A]}. \tag{12}$$

Substitution into Eq. (7) gives an expression for the relationship between agonist concentration and depolarization:

$$\Delta V = \frac{g_{max} K_A [A]}{G_0 + (g_{max} + G_0) K_A [A]} \cdot V_0. \tag{13}$$

On such a scheme, variations in the maximum response attainable with different agonists could perhaps be expressed in terms of differences in the proportionality factor, g_{max}. However, the underlying assumption of direct proportionality between p_A and g is highly questionable (see p. 268).

A more flexible way of formulating the relation between agonist concentration and response was developed by STEPHENSON (1956). Following his line of argument and nomenclature, one may write in place of Eq.(11)

$$g = f(e\,p_A) = f\left(e\,\frac{K_A[A]}{1 + K_A[A]}\right).$$

Here g is regarded as a function (not necessarily linear) of the product of receptor occupancy and the "efficacy", e, of the depolarizing agent in question. Efficacy is a measure of the activation of the receptors at a given occupancy, and is defined in relative terms: if two agents, A and B, elicit the same response, it is supposed that

$$e_A\,p_A = e_B\,p_B\,.$$

Hence, from (10):

$$\frac{e_A\,K_A[A]}{1 + K_A[A]} = \frac{e_B\,K_B[B]}{1 + K_B[B]}\,. \tag{14}$$

It is interesting to consider the relation which holds when the two agonists differ considerably in efficacy. Let us suppose that substance A has a high efficacy, that is, it can produce a substantial response when $K_A[A] \ll 1$, so that few receptors are occupied, whereas e_B is relatively small. (Substances which even at high concentrations fail to elicit the maximum response obtainable with a 'full' agonist such as acetylcholine are often termed *partial agonists* (see e.g. STEPHENSON, 1956; ÄRIENS, 1964, pp. 137—139). For submaximal responses, Eq.(14) can then be simplified to

$$e_A\,K_A[A] = \frac{e_B\,K_B[B]}{1 + K_B[B]}\,,$$

so that:

$$\frac{1}{[A]} = \frac{e_A\,K_A}{e_B\,K_B} \cdot \frac{1}{[B]} + \frac{e_A}{e_B} \cdot K_A\,. \tag{15}$$

Hence it should be possible to estimate the affinity constant, K_B, for the agonist with the lower efficacy from the ratio of the intercept to the slope of a double reciprocal plot of the concentrations of A and B which produce the same levels of response. This argument has been developed by MACKAY (1966) and by BARLOW, SCOTT and STEPHENSON (1967; see also BARLOW et al., 1969; WAUD, 1969; COLQUHOUN, 1973, and RANG, 1973b) and has been used to compare affinities and relative efficacies of several substances which activate nicotinic receptors.

The method does not, however, allow the affinity constant for a "full" agonist to be determined. It has often been thought that K_A might be obtainable from a double reciprocal plot of agonist concentration against response (by analogy with the Lineweaver-Burk plot of enzyme chemistry) or, even more simply, from the reciprocal of the concentration of agonist producing a half maximal response. This assumption was made in the past for the effect of nicotine and acetylcholine in causing contraction of the isolated frog rectus abdominis muscle (HILL, 1909; CLARK, 1926a, b;

Kirschner and Stone, 1951; Cavanaugh and Hearon, 1954). It is now generally accepted, however, that the complexity of the events which link receptor activation to contraction make it quite unlikely that a linear relationship should hold. A somewhat better procedure is to measure electrical changes, preferably in single fibres, since this should provide a rather more direct index of events at the receptor. Nevertheless, difficulties in interpretation remain. Thus Eqs.(12) and (13) predict that both the conductance increase and the resulting depolarization should be directly proportional to the agonist concentration when this is small. However, it is generally found that linear plots of dose-response relationships for the action of depolarizing agents on skeletal muscle begin with a region of increasing slope. This has been shown for depolarizations elicited by agonists applied either ionophoretically (Katz and Thesleff, 1957b; Dreyer and Peper, 1975; Hartzell et al., 1975) or in the bathing fluid (Jenkinson, 1960; Jenkinson and Terrar, 1973), and for end-plate conductance increases measured either directly (Johnson and Parsons, 1972) or by the voltage clamp technique (Rang, 1971, 1973c). When the response is small, it is generally proportional to the agonist concentration raised to a power which is commonly about 1.5 and rarely more than 2. If the whole dose-response relationship is accessible, as it may be for partial agonists, the Hill plot (Brown and Hill, 1923) in which $\log(y/y_{max}-y)$ is plotted against $\log[A]$, where y is the response, also gives a slope of about 1.5 rather than unity. A possible explanation is that more than one molecule of acetylcholine combines with each binding site, although this does not seem likely. Alternatively the sites may interact in the sense that either the overall affinity may increase as more agonist becomes bound (as in the "allosteric" model outlined on p. 269), or two or more neighbouring sites might need to be occupied for an ion channel to be opened. This remains to be settled; for further discussion see Werman (1969), Johnson and Parsons (1972), Colquhoun (1973, 1975) and Rang (1975).

The interpretation of differences in efficacy in terms of events at the receptors is still far from clear. Since the first event to be detected is an increase in membrane conductance, perhaps the simplest model of receptor action would be to suppose that the additional ion channels are formed as a direct consequence of the combination of the agonist with the receptor. One might imagine, for example, that a cation such as acetylcholine could enter the membrane and alter the separation between two adjacent negatively charged structures, and in this way create access to pre-existing channels through the membrane. If such a simple arrangement operated, the extent to which various agonists could open the channels might differ. It is further conceivable that the ionic selectivity of the channels could depend on the degree of opening, in which case the equilibrium potential (p. 237) would vary between agonists. This possibility has been tested by several workers. The weight of the evidence suggests that the agents so far examined, which include carbachol, decamethonium, phenyltrimethylammonium and suberyldicholine, have the same equilibrium potential as acetylcholine, at least when applied in a solution containing the normal amount of potassium (Dunin-Barkovskii et al., 1969; see also Werman and Manalis, 1970; Koester and Nastuk, 1970, and Feltz and Mallart, 1971 b). Interestingly, when the external potassium is lowered, suberyldicholine gives a different value to the other substances (Dunin-Barkovskii et al., 1969). Possible explanations have been discussed by Rang (1975, pp. 292, 319).

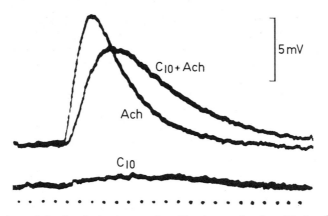

Fig. 16. Comparison of the depolarization produced by decamethonium (C_{10}) and acetylcholine (Ach) separately and together (C_{10} + Ach). In the upper two records, a brief acetylcholine pulse (13 msec, 4.4×10^{-10} C) was applied, first by itself, and then immediately preceded by a longer decamethonium pulse (84 msec, 1.7×10^{-9} C). Frog sartorius preparation. Time marks, 50 Hz. (From DEL CASTILLO and KATZ, 1957c)

Another interpretation of efficacy was suggested by a comparison of the time course of action of different agonists (DEL CASTILLO and KATZ, 1957c). It was found that the depolarization produced by ionophoretically-applied decamethonium developed more slowly than a comparable response to carbachol or acetylcholine. The possibility that this was simply because decamethonium combined less rapidly with the receptors was examined by applying a pulse of acetylcholine or carbachol just after one of decamethonium. The experiment is illustrated in Fig. 16. It can be seen that decamethonium reduced the rate of rise of the response to added acetylcholine at a time when the same dose of decamethonium given alone produced little depolarization. A possible explanation is that the agonist-receptor complex, AR, is inactive when first formed, but changes to an active configuration, AR_A:

$$A + R \underset{k_{-1}}{\overset{k_1}{\rightleftharpoons}} AR \underset{k_{-2}}{\overset{k_2}{\rightleftharpoons}} AR_A \qquad (16)$$

At equilibrium,

$$[AR_A] = K_2 [AR], \qquad (17)$$

where K_2 is an equilibrium constant equal to k_2/k_{-2}. Clearly, K_2 could be regarded as a measure of efficacy, being small for a weak agonist, and negligible for a competitive antagonist (see KATZ and MILEDI, 1972, p. 693, and 1973a, p. 717).

2. The "Allosteric" Model of the Receptor

The concept that the agonist-receptor complex can exist in two forms, one active and the other not, bears a close relationship to another model. Here the underlying idea is that the receptor is analogous to a special class of "allosteric" enzymes which in addition to catalysing single reactions in the usual way also regulate the overall rate of the sequence of reactions in which they participate. This control is exerted because the rate at which the substrate is transformed can be changed in either direction by specific molecules which are sometimes products of the reaction chain, but need not closely resemble the substrate (for further details the reader is referred to MAHLER and CORDES, 1971, pp. 299—311). Such enzymes have several common features. One of the most striking is that the usual Michaelis-Menten kinetics are not obeyed: in particular, the substrate concentration—velocity curve begins with a region of increasing slope so that its shape becomes that of an elongated S rather than part of a rectangular hyperbola.

MONOD et al. (1965) have shown that this and the other characteristic features can be explained by supposing, first, that an enzyme of this kind has several identical binding sites for the substrate, second, that it exists in two forms which are in equilibrium and, third, that the affinity between the substrate and its binding sites is the same for all the sites on one form of the enzyme, but is in general different between the forms. Thus, on adding substrate, the equilibrium will be displaced towards the form with the higher substrate affinity, and this will facilitate further binding. Other ligands which combine with either the same or a different site on the enzyme may also influence the equilibrium in a similar way, and hence alter the rate of substrate transformation.

As first discussed by KARLIN (1967), these ideas may be applicable to the acetylcholine receptor which could also be imagined to exist in two forms, one active or "open" (bearing in mind the ion channel concept) and the other "closed". The equilibrium between them would be such that the closed form predominates in the resting tissue. It is also supposed, however, that the "open" receptors have a much higher affinity for acetylcholine, so that in the presence of acetylcholine the equilibrium between the two configurations is displaced towards the active form.

Correspondingly, substances which have an equal or greater affinity for the binding sites on the closed as compared with the open form will antagonise the action of a "strong" agonist such as acetylcholine. The interaction between agonists and antagonists to be expected on this basis has been examined by COLQUHOUN (1973) and THRON (1973) who have shown that if certain conditions hold the allosteric model can demonstrate the characteristics of "classical" competitive antagonism, i.e. parallel displacement of dose-response curves, and adherence to the Schild equation (see p. 281).

The same authors have also discussed the concept of efficacy in terms of the allosteric model. It was shown that variations in efficacy between agonists could be explained in terms of differences in the ratio of the affinities of the particular agonists for the open and closed forms of the receptor. This ratio also determines the maximum activation attainable with a large concentration of a given agent.

A further prediction of the allosteric model is that under some circumstances the proportion of active receptors should increase more than linearly with small values of the agonist concentration. The finding that the dose-response relationship in skeletal muscle often begins with a region of increasing slope (p. 268) has accordingly been taken as evidence in favour of this model of the receptor, although it is clearly not decisive. The reader is referred to discussions by KARLIN (1967), RANG (1971, 1973 b, 1975), COLQUHOUN (1973, 1975) and THRON (1973).

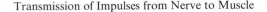
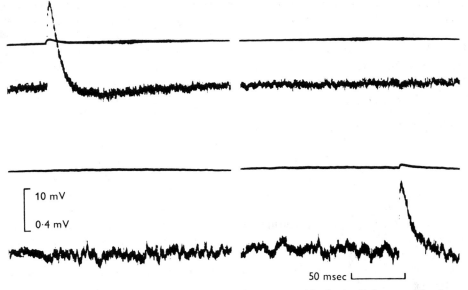

Fig. 17. The "acetylcholine noise" phenomenon, demonstrated by intracellular recording from a frog sartorius end-plate. 21° C. The two traces in each block were simultaneously recorded on a low-gain direct coupled channel (upper trace, voltage scale, 10 mV) and on a high gain condenser coupled channel (lower trace, voltage scale 0.4 mV). The upper blocks are controls (no acetylcholine): the lower ones were taken during the application of acetylcholine from a micropipette. The upward displacement of the low gain d.c. traces indicates a net depolarization during the action of acetylcholine; note the increased "noise" of the corresponding high gain records. Two spontaneous miniature end-plate potentials are also seen. (From KATZ and MILEDI, 1972)

3. New Evidence on Receptor Action: Acetylcholine "Noise"

An important development has been the analysis of the fluctuations in the "steady" depolarization which occurs when acetylcholine (or an analogue) is added to the bathing solution. The acetylcholine "noise" was first described by KATZ and MILEDI (1970, 1972, 1973a, b, c) and is illustrated in Fig. 17. Qualitatively, it can be explained on the assumption that the seemingly steady depolarization is in fact made up of an enormous number of components each resulting from the transient opening of an "elementary" ion channel; the noise thus results from the fluctuations in the number of channels open from moment to moment.

KATZ and MILEDI (1972; see also STEVENS, 1972; ANDERSON and STEVENS, 1973, and the review by VERVEEN and DE FELICE, 1974) have based their quantitative analysis on Campbell's theorem: if the overall response is made up of components $f(t)$ occurring at a frequency of n per sec, the mean value V of the depolarization will be given by

$$V = n \int f(t)\, dt, \tag{17}$$

and its variance $\overline{E^2}$ by

$$\overline{E^2} = \overline{(V_t - V)^2} = n \int f^2(t)\, dt, \tag{18}$$

where V_t is the value at time t. To integrate the equations, the function $f(t)$ is required explicitly but in fact the main conclusions are not greatly affected by its exact form. If $f(t)$ is taken to be a "blip" which rises instantaneously to a value a and then declines exponentially with a time constant τ, i.e. $f(t) = a \exp(-t/\tau)$, the integrations give

$$V = na\tau \tag{19}$$

and

$$\overline{E^2} = \frac{na^2\tau}{2}$$

from which

$$\overline{E^2} = \frac{aV}{2}$$

or

$$a = 2\overline{E^2}/V, \tag{20}$$

which it may be noted is independent of τ. Substituting the experimental values from frog muscle fibres into (20), KATZ and MILEDI obtained a value of about $0.25\,\mu V$ for a. If τ is taken to be the membrane time constant, 10 msec, it can be estimated from Eq. (19) that the number of elementary events needed to produce a mean depolarization of 10 mV is in the order of 4×10^6 per sec. During a maintained depolarization of this magnitude, the current flowing through the synaptic channels of a typical sartorius fibre with an input conductance, G, of $4 \times 10^{-6}\,\Omega^{-1}$ will be V times G, i.e., about 4×10^{-8} A. This corresponds to a net flow of charge of 4×10^{-8} coulombs per sec. Thus each elementary event would cause the transfer of 10^{-14} C, equivalent to 6×10^4 univalent ions. ANDERSON and STEVENS (1973) have suggested a rather higher figure (2×10^5 ions) on the basis of their analysis of the fluctuations in the end-plate current recorded from voltage-clamped frog muscle at 8° C.

A value of the same order is obtained by considering the relative magnitudes of the elementary events and the normal end-plate potential for which the total transfer of charge was measured by FATT and KATZ (1951). This came to the equivalent of 5×10^9 univalent ions for a depolarization of 25 mV, so that the corresponding value for a $0.25\,\mu V$ elementary potential of similar time course would be 5×10^4 ions (KATZ and MILEDI, 1972).

The falling phase of the elementary potential change is effectively determined by the time constant of the fibre membrane (as with miniature and normal end-plate potentials) and does not therefore provide information about the duration of the elementary events. This question can, however, be approached by recording acetylcholine noise extracellularly using a focally placed microelectrode. The potential differences detected in this way are set up by the flow of current into the immediately adjacent muscle fibre and so should reflect the conductance increase rather than the ensuing membrane potential change (see e.g. DEL CASTILLO and KATZ, 1956). Records of this kind obtained during the action of acetylcholine and carbachol are shown in Fig. 18. It may be seen that the carbachol noise is much "faster" than that produced by acetylcholine. Such records can be analysed by the procedure of power

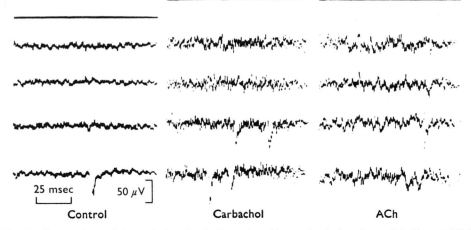

Fig. 18. Comparison of the end-plate "noise" produced by carbachol and acetylcholine at 21°C in a frog sartorius preparation. The upper trace in each block was recorded intracellularly at low gain, as in Fig. 17; the upward displacement during the release of carbachol (centre) or acetylcholine (right) from a double-barrel micropipette indicates a depolarization of about 5 mV. The four other traces in each block were recorded extracellularly at high gain from a focally-placed microelectrode. Note that the additional noise during carbachol action is much "faster" than that caused by acetylcholine. (Magnetic tape playback: the very large deflections (e.g. in the bottom traces of control and carbachol records) arose from external miniature end-plate potentials which saturated the tape amplifier). (From KATZ and MILEDI, 1972)

density spectrum analysis (BENDAT and PIERSOL, 1971). This allows an estimate to be made of the "duration" of the elementary conductance changes or, in other words, of the life time of the ion channels. Once again, although a precise estimate would require a knowledge of the exact form of their time course, the main results are relatively insensitive to this. If an exponential decline is assumed, analysis of the power spectrum suggests that the time constant for decay is about 1 msec for acetylcholine and about 0.35 msec for carbachol. Decamethonium, acetylthiocholine and suberyldicholine have also been studied in this way (KATZ and MILEDI, 1973a). The decay times were found to cover a ten-fold range, from about 0.12 msec for acetylthiocholine to 1.65 msec for suberyldicholine.

Whether or not these values reflect the lifetime of the drug-receptor complex is an open question which has an interesting bearing on the interpretation of efficacy. If they do not, a possible explanation for efficacy in elementary terms is that it is a measure of the ratio of the lifetime of the channel to that of the complex, since by definition efficacy is the parameter which distinguishes between the effects of different drugs at the same level of occupancy.

4. The Response to Prolonged Application of Depolarizing Agents

a) Desensitization

Under physiological conditions the receptors are exposed to acetylcholine for no more than a msec or so after each nerve impulse. The response to longer applications of depolarizing agents is nevertheless of interest, not only because such exposures are often used in experimental work but also because of the need to understand the mechanism of action of depolarizing neuromuscular blocking drugs such as decamethonium and suxamethonium.

The simplest expectation is that the membrane should remain depolarized as long as the agonist concentration is maintained. This is often not the case, certainly in *in vitro* experiments; rather, the response falls away to reach a steady level which may be only a small fraction of the original (FATT, 1950; THESLEFF, 1955a, b; KATZ and THESLEFF, 1957b; GISSEN and NASTUK, 1966; RANG and RITTER, 1970a). The

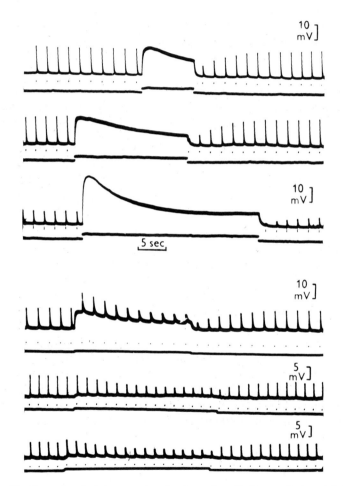

Fig. 19. Desensitization of end-plate receptors by ionophoretically-applied acetylcholine. *Upper panel*: single pipette technique. As the records begin, brief test doses of acetylcholine were applied at regular intervals, producing transient depolarizations which appear as "spikes" on the records. The pulses were then stopped and a steady conditioning dose of acetylcholine applied by reducing the braking current (p.252) which was monitored on the lower of each pair of recordings. Note the spontaneous fall in the depolarization. The response to the test pulses rapidly recovered when the braking current was restored. *Lower panel*: as above, but using twin pipettes. One barrel was used to apply test pulses throughout, and the other to administer the conditioning dose. (From KATZ and THESLEFF, 1957b)

phenomenon is referred to as *inactivation* or *desensitization* and has been the object of much study and some dispute in recent years. Controversy centres primarily on the extent to which desensitization occurs *in vivo*. This is discussed in Chapter 4A and will not be considered further here other than by mentioning some problems that complicate the assessment of desensitization *in vivo* or *in vitro*.

The first quantitative study of the phenomenon was made by KATZ and THESLEFF (1957b). As illustrated in Fig. 19, the depolarization produced by a maintained ionophoretic application of acetylcholine declined spontaneously and this was associated with a fall in the response to acetylcholine released as brief test pulses from a second micropipette. Normal sensitivity was rapidly regained when the "conditioning" application was stopped. The phenomenon could still be observed when the tissue was bathed in either isotonic potassium sulphate solution (see also ADAMIČ, 1965) or strongly hypertonic Ringers fluid, i.e., under conditions where the contractile response is much reduced or absent.

KATZ and THESLEFF also found that the rate of onset of desensitization could be equal to or slower than the subsequent recovery, and they concluded (see also RANG and RITTER, 1970a) that this together with other kinetic findings could best be explained in terms of a model of the following kind:

$$A + R \underset{\text{(fast)}}{\rightleftharpoons} AR \quad \text{(active)}$$

$$\text{(slow)} \updownarrow \qquad\qquad \updownarrow \text{(slow)}$$

$$A + R_D \underset{\text{(fast)}}{\rightleftharpoons} AR_D \quad \text{(inactive)}$$

Here A is the agonist and R the receptor which it is supposed can exist in two forms, one of which (R_D) is inactive in the sense that it cannot influence membrane permeability, though still able to combine with A. Under resting conditions, the proportion of the receptors in the inactive form is small. However, prolonged application of an agonist causes R_D and AR_D to rise at the expense of R and AR so that the response declines.

For completeness, another step could be added to this scheme to allow for the possibility that the active receptor is formed from an initially inactive agonist-receptor complex, as mentioned on p. 269. A variant of this idea was considered by RANG and RITTER (1970a) who speculated that the active form of the receptor could be a transitional state in the passage of the initial complex to the inactive configuration, AR_D. This is now thought unlikely on thermodynamic grounds (RANG, 1973b).

b) The Assessment of Desensitization

The extent of desensitization is sometimes gauged from the decline in the depolarization produced by a maintained application of an agonist. While this is satisfactory for many purposes, complications arise if the depolarization is large and lasts for more than a minute or so. One possibility is that the gradients of sodium and potassium across the membrane may change as a direct consequence of the increase in permeability to these ions. In addition, chloride will enter the fibre (p. 256). This will tend to cause the membrane potential to fall further (as E_{Cl} becomes less negative) and so may mask the onset of desensitization (JENKINSON and TERRAR, 1973).

It is also conceivable that the rise in intracellular sodium could initiate electrogenic transport (p. 233) which might then contribute to the "spontaneous" recovery of the membrane potential in the presence of the agonist. However, this does not seem to occur in frog muscle under the conditions so far examined (TERRAR, 1974).

These complications are likely to be less important when desensitization is studied using the ionophoretic technique since the total exposure to agonist need then be no more than a few seconds (see Fig. 19). The fact that desensitization is much more rapid when examined with this technique than when depolarizing agents are applied in the bathing fluid seems likely to be a consequence of the greater agonist concentrations attained with the ionophoretic method (p. 253).

This raises the question of the possible occurence of desensitization during neurotransmission since the concentration of acetylcholine reached at the receptors may again be high, albeit for a very short period. The point has been examined by OTSUKA et al. (1962) who compared the response to ionophoretically-applied acetylcholine before and after nerve stimulation. No appreciable change was seen, suggesting that there had been little desensitization (certainly of those receptors most accessible to external application). The same general conclusion is suggested by the finding that there is no obvious reduction in the amplitude of miniature end-plate potentials during and after repetitive nerve stimulation (see p. 310). This is not unexpected since each quantum of transmitter is shortlived and acts over a limited area. Thus a particular receptor is likely to experience a high concentration of acetylcholine for no more than a small fraction of the total duration of the tetanus.

A more direct index of desensitization can be obtained by measuring the decline in the effect of an agonist on the conductance rather than the potential of the membrane. This approach has been used by NASTUK, MANTHEY, PARSONS and their coworkers. While the main results are summarised later, we may note that MANTHEY (1966) has shown that during maintained application of carbachol to frog muscle the depolarization subsides less rapidly than the increase in membrane conductance. As discussed by NASTUK and PARSONS (1970), this is probably a consequence of (1) the increased chloride content of the fibre, and (2) the non-linearity of the relationship between membrane potential and conductance. Clearly both factors have to be borne in mind when potential changes are to be used as a measure of desensitization.

It is also possible to monitor desensitization by following changes in the current needed to voltage-clamp the end-plate during the action of depolarizing agents (COCHRANE et al., 1972; HARRINGTON, 1973; JENKINSON and TERRAR, 1973; ADAMS, 1974a). However, the difficulty of achieving a steady and uniform clamp is not to be underestimated (see p. 245).

An indirect procedure sometimes used in *in vivo* studies on the mechanism of action of depolarizing neuromuscular blocking agents is to assess the polarization of the end-plate membrane (and hence the occurrence or otherwise of desensitization) by monitoring the pharmacological characteristics of the neuromuscular block produced by the agent in question. If transmission cannot be restored by an anticholinesterase such as neostigmine, one such argument runs, the membrane is still depolarized and little desensitization can have occurred. While this could well be so, care is needed in the interpretation of such findings because of the complexity of depolarization blockade.

At least four interacting post-synaptic factors contribute:

(1) The depolarization which results from activation of the receptors by the drug will cause inactivation of the potential-dependent sodium carrier mechanism which underlies the rising phase of the action potential. Hence the electrical threshold of the fibre will rise, although this may be offset to a limited extent by the fall in the membrane potential on which the end-plate potential is superimposed.

(2) Fewer receptors will be capable of activation by nerve-released acetylcholine; some will already be occupied by the applied depolarizing agent, whereas others may be in an inactive form.

(3) The depolarizing action of the acetylcholine will be reduced because the conductance of the end-plate is higher than normal due to the action of the depolarizing agent.

(4) The depolarized and electrically less excitable area around the end-plate gradually extends along the fibre, probably because of changes in intracellular ion concentrations, as well as in membrane conductance (see BURNS and PATON, 1951).

Other aspects of depolarization blockade are considered in Chapter IV A (see also COOKSON and PATON, 1969).

These difficulties notwithstanding, there is some evidence that desensitization may be less marked *in vivo* than *in vitro* (MACLAGAN, 1962; ZAIMIS, 1962). One possibility is that the simple bathing solutions used in experiments with isolated tissues lack an important factor normally present in plasma. This has yet to be studied in detail, although it has been shown that the addition to Ringer's fluid of materials (e.g. foetal calf serum, and the constituents of Wolf and Quimby's "amphibian culture medium") which help to preserve isolated cells or tissues has no appreciable effect on the decline of the response of frog skeletal muscle to bath-applied carbachol (TERRAR, 1974).

c) Factors which Influence the Rate of Desensitization

1. The Nature of the Agonist. Some depolarizing agents (e.g. phenyltrimethylammonium and C_{13} bis-trimethylammonium) cause more rapid desensitization than others (e.g. carbachol and suxamethonium), as shown by GISSEN and NASTUK (1966) and by RANG and RITTER (1970a).

2. The Preparation. Desensitization differs in the fast and slow muscles of the frog (MAGAZANIK and SHEKHIREV, 1970) and between mammalian species (AXELSSON and THESLEFF, 1958).

3. Temperature. Desensitization in frog muscle becomes much slower as the temperature is lowered (MAGAZANIK and VYSKOČIL,1973, 1975).

4. External Calcium Concentration. This has been studied by MANTHEY (1966, 1970, 1972) and by NASTUK and PARSONS (1970) using as a test object the changes in membrane conductance produced by carbachol applied from a pipette with a tip diameter of 50 to 75 μm. It was found that desensitization became slower in nominally calcium-free solution and considerably faster when the external calcium was raised to 10 mmol/l (see also MAGAZANIK, 1968 and MAGAZANIK and SHEKHIREV, 1970). It has been proposed on the basis of these and other observations (NASTUK and PARSONS, 1970) that desensitization may be influenced by the amount of calcium at a specific site at the inner surface of the membrane. Other ions, e.g. lanthanum (MAGAZANIK and VYSKOČIL, 1970; LAMBERT and PARSONS, 1970; PARSONS et al., 1971) which affect the rate of desensitization could perhaps act at the same point.

Curiously, a reduction in the concentration of carbachol from 2.7 to 0.14 mmol/l causes the calcium sensitivity of desensitization (as assessed by Manthey's technique) to disappear (MANTHEY, 1970). A further complication is that the initial conductance increase produced by carbachol is influenced by the external calcium concentration (p. 289).

5. Application of SKF 525 A and Related Compounds. MAGAZANIK 1970; 1971a; VYSKOČIL and MAGAZANIK, 1972) and his co-workers have shown that SKF 525 A and several allied compounds cause a large increase in the rate of desensitization to ionophoretically-applied acetylcholine. As illustrated in Fig. 20, SKF 525 A is also active when applied intracellularly, and the effect can be observed when both the agonist and the desentitization-enhancing agent are

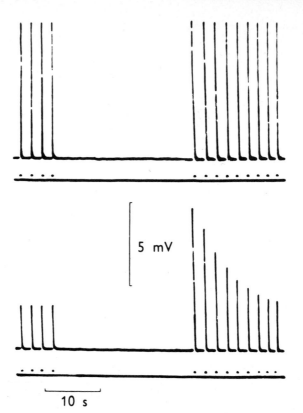

Fig. 20. The effect of intracellularly-applied SKF-525A on desensitization. The upper trace of each pair shows transient depolarizations produced by ionophoretically applied pulses of acetylcholine. The lower trace monitors the current through the pipette. The response scarcely changed after a rest period of 26 sec, suggesting that there had been little desensitization during the train. The lower pair of traces were taken 10 min after the intracellular injection of SKF-525A at a distance of about 50 μm from the acetylcholine pipette. The response to acetylcholine is reduced (left) but recovers during a rest period. When pulses were resumed, the amplitude of the response declined, presumably as desensitization was re-established. (From Vyskočil and Magazanik, 1972)

added to the bathing fluid (Fig. 21). The mechanism is unclear; Magazanik and Vyskočil (1972, 1973) consider that a step beyond the agonist binding site may be implicated, perhaps involving the ionophore (see p. 260). A similar proposal was made by Nastuk and Karis (1964) for the blocking action of hexafluorenium.

Such a desensitization-enhancing action might be expected to alter the nature of the neuromuscular block caused by depolarizing blocking agents, and it is interesting that Suarez-Kurtz et al. (1969) have reported that in chicks, hens, and toads SKF 525 A changed the "typical depolarizing blockade" caused by suxamethonium and decamethonium to what was described as a "competitive-like" or "dual" block.

6. Other Drugs and Toxins. The response to bath or ionophoretically-applied agonists has been reported to decline more rapdly in the presence of several agents, including chlorpromazine, promethazine, diphenhydramine, procaine, lignocaine, methylpentynol, mephenesin, pentobarbitone (Payton, 1966; Magazanik, 1971b) caffeine (Cochrane and Parsons, 1972, though see also Magazanik and Vyskočil, 1970) and α-bungarotoxin, even when the last mentioned is

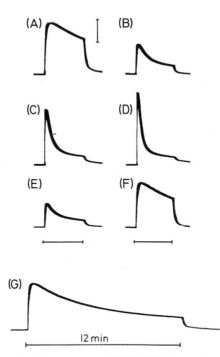

Fig. 21 A—G. Effect of pipenzolate (a congener of SKF-525A) on carbachol-induced depolarizations recorded in sequence from the end-plate region of a frog sartorius fibre (resting potential, −97 mV). Room temperature, chloride-free bathing fluid throughout. Pen recorder traces A, F and G show the responses to carbachol alone (10 µmol/l for 3 min in A and F, 12 min in G). B to E were recorded in the presence of pipenzolate (10 µmol/l); the carbachol concentrations were 10 µmol/l for B and E, 20 µmol/l for C and 30 µmol/l for D. Pipenzolate is seen to accelerate the spontaneous decline in the carbachol depolarization. Voltage calibration 10 mV. (From TERRAR, 1974)

applied intracellularly (MAGAZANIK and VYSKOČIL, 1972, 1973). In contrast, desensitization has been reported to be reduced by nystatin (MAGAZANIK, 1968), catecholamines (STAMENOVIĆ, 1968; MAGAZANIK, 1969) and by methoxyambenonium (KIM and KARCZMAR, 1967). The mechanism of these actions is unknown.

7. **Membrane Potential.** MAGAZANIK and VYSKOČIL (1970) have shown that desensitization becomes more rapid when the membrane is hyperpolarized. The mechanism is unclear, although the inference that receptor function may be influenced by the transmembrane potential difference is in keeping with the general conclusions of KORDAŠ (1969) and of MAGLEBY and STEVENS (1972a, b) as mentioned on p. 246.

d) Have Desensitized Receptors Different Pharmacological Properties?

Most models which have been put forward to explain desensitization suppose that the receptor can exist in an inactive as well as an active form. This raises the possibility that these forms may have different pharmacological properties, and recent evidence suggests that this is indeed so. (1) RANG and RITTER (1969) have shown that certain antagonists related to decamethonium become much more effective when applied in the presence of a depolarizing agent such as carbachol. Further work (RANG and RITTER, 1970a, b) indicated that this could best be explained by supposing desensitized receptors to have a greater affinity for "metaphilic" antagonists of this kind. (2) As mentioned on p. 260, MILEDI and POTTER (1971) found that the binding of α-bungarotoxin by the end-plate region of frog muscle is greatly reduced by prior exposure of the tissue to acetylcholine. A possible interpretation is that the affinity for α-bungarotoxin falls when receptors become desensitized. LESTER (1972b) has obtained evidence that the same may hold for cobra toxin.

VI. Modification of Transmitter Action

1. Competitive Antagonism

Although considered in greater detail in other chapters, competitive antagonists such as the curare alkaloids must also be mentioned here because of their continuing importance in the development of ideas about neuromuscular transmission. Most work has been done with tubocurarine which has long been known to reduce the responsiveness of the end-plate to both nerve-released and externally-applied acetylcholine (see pp. 235 and 246). This action is usually ascribed to competitive antagonism. It is worth noting that the term "competitive" is often used in two rather different senses. One is to convey the idea that a substance reduces the proportion of receptors occupied by another by becoming attached to the same site, or to a point so close that the binding of the two agents is mutually hindered. The other is to indicate merely that the inhibitory effect of an antagonist can be overcome by increasing the dose of the agonist, and that this can be done over a wide range of concentrations. While the second meaning is included in the first (provided that the drug-receptor complexes are readily reversible), the converse need not apply.

These usages can be illustrated in relation to the mechanism of action of depolarizing neuromuscular blocking agents such as suxamethonium. As already mentioned, it is likely that these substances combine with the same receptors as acetylcholine, with which they could be said to compete, using the first sense considered above. However, this is not the main cause of the block which is attributable rather to the relatively maintained depolarization which such agents bring about (see p. 277). It is also observed that under particular conditions discussed in greater detail in Chapter 4A, the characteristics of the block may change with time; in particular it may become possible to restore transmission by inhibiting cholinesterase, and so raising the local concentration of acetylcholine. This alteration in the nature of the block is sometimes described by saying that the blocking agent is now acting competitively; here the term is being used in the second sense above. No confusion need arise if this distinction is kept in mind. In the following pages "competitive" will be used in the first sense discussed.

2. Evidence for Competition between Curare Alkaloids and Acetylcholine

a) In vitro Studies under Equilibrium Conditions

The last few years have seen the development of methods which should allow a direct test of the idea that antagonists such as tubocurarine combine with the same site as acetylcholine. Radio-isotopes offer the most promising approach since it should, in principle, be possible to demonstrate displacement of labelled agonists by antagonists, and vice versa (although even this might not be decisive since it is possible to envisage allosteric models in which combination of an antagonist with a separate "inhibitory" site could reduce the binding of the agonist). So far, however, this method has not provided a clear-cut answer (see below), and other approaches have had to be examined. Some of these will now be discussed.

If it is assumed tentatively that the agonist, A, and the antagonist, I, compete for the receptor in a reversible and one-to-one manner, application of the law of mass action to the simultaneous equilibria

$$A + R \rightleftharpoons AR \quad \text{(affinity constant } K_A)$$

$$I + R \rightleftharpoons IR \quad \text{(affinity constant } K_I)$$

shows that the proportion of the receptors occupied by agonist and antagonist respectively should be given by

$$p_A = \frac{K_A[A]}{1 + K_A[A] + K_I[I]}, \qquad (21) \quad \text{(cf. 10)}$$

$$p_I = \frac{K_I[I]}{1 + K_A[A] + K_I[I]}. \qquad (22)$$

Clearly the best way of testing these expressions would be to measure p_A and p_I for a range of values of $[A]$ and $[I]$. However, as mentioned, this is not yet practicable. For example, attempts to estimate p_A directly by using labelled agonists are likely to be complicated by the passage of the agents into the muscle fibres (see p. 258). Nor is it at all straightforward to estimate p_A from the relationship between dose and response (p. 267).

A more fruitful approach, although applicable only to antagonists, was developed by GADDUM (1937; GADDUM et al., 1955) and SCHILD (1949; ARUNLAKSHANA and SCHILD, 1959). The underlying assumption is that the same proportion of receptors is occupied by an agonist when a standard response is evoked first by the agonist acting alone, and then by an x-fold greater concentration of agonist applied in the presence of the antagonist at concentration $[I]$. We may then write, from Eqs. (10) and (21),

$$p_A = \frac{K_A[A]}{1 + K_A[A]} = \frac{K_A x[A]}{1 + K_A x[A] + K_I[I]} \qquad (23)$$

from which

$$x - 1 = K_I[I]. \qquad (24)$$

Since only the dose *ratio*, x appears in (24), the value of x for a given concentration of antagonist should be the same regardless of the magnitude of $[A]$, and hence of the level of the response. This implies that log dose-response curves determined in the presence and absence of the antagonist will be parallel (a constant ratio of concentrations being equivalent to a constant separation on a logarithmic plot).

Table 3. "Affinity constants" for the action of tubocurarine on skeletal muscle

Animal	Muscle	Temperature °C	"Affinity constant" μM^{-1}	Notes	Ref.
Frog	rectus abdominis	room	1—4	2	a
Frog	rectus abdominis	19—23	3.1		b
Frog	m. ext. dig. long. IV.	19—23	2.3	3	b
Frog	semitendinosus	19—23	1.7		c
Frog	sartorius	25	2.9	4	d
Chick	biventer cervicis	37	2.6	5	e
Guinea-pig	diaphragm	38	9.2	6	f
Guinea-pig	latissimus dorsi	38	10.5		f
Guinea-pig	serratus anterior	38	10.4		f
Guinea-pig	lumbrical	36	9.9	7	g
Hamster	diaphragm	30	2.6	8	h

References: (a) van Maanen (1950); (b) Jenkinson (1960); (c) Waud (1971); (d) Bowen (1972a); (e) Rang and Ritter (1969); (f) Lu (1970); (g) Waud et al. (1973); (h) Kruckenberg and Bauer (1971).

1. Although the point is rather academic, values reported in molar units before 1971 should be reduced by 1.8%; the molecular weight of tubocurarine chloride pentahydrate (the form most often used) is known to be 772, not 786, following the demonstration that tubocurarine is a mono-rather than a bis-quaternary alkaloid (Everett et al., 1970).
2. C-toxiferine II, C-curarine I and β-erythroidine were also studied. Changes in temperature and external potassium shown to have little effect.
3. Changes in external Na^+, K^+, Ca^{2+}, and Mg^{2+} also examined (for a more comprehensive study with mammalian muscle, see Goldfine, 1973). Temperature shown to have little influence.
4. Non-equilibrium dose ratio method used; see text.
5. Gallamine also examined.
6. Gallamine, dimethyltubocurarine and C-toxiferine also studied.
7. Pancuronium, and the effects of halothane on the antagonism, also studied.
8. Method based on depression of quantal response; see text.

Equation (24) (the "Schild equation") has been found to apply to the action of tubocurarine and several other neuromuscular blocking agents (see Table 3 for references), although some deviation occurs with large concentrations (Jenkinson, 1960; Lu, 1970). The usual test is to plot $\log(x-1)$ against $\log[I]$ when a straight line with a slope of unity and an intercept of $\log K_I$ should be observed (the "Schild plot": see Fig. 22). Values for K_I obtained in this way have been listed in Table 3.

A more general form of Eq. (24) is

$$x^m - 1 = K_I [I]^n.$$

This might be expected to apply were m molecules of agonist and n molecules of antagonist to combine with each receptor. Parker and Goldfine (1973) concluded that the dependence of x on $[I]$ for a range of agonists and antagonists acting on guinea-pig lumbrical muscle was best accounted for by supposing both m and n to be unity. However Rang and Ritter (1969) have found the slope of the Schild plot to be significantly less than one (though only by a small amount) for the action of tubocurarine and gallamine on chick muscle.

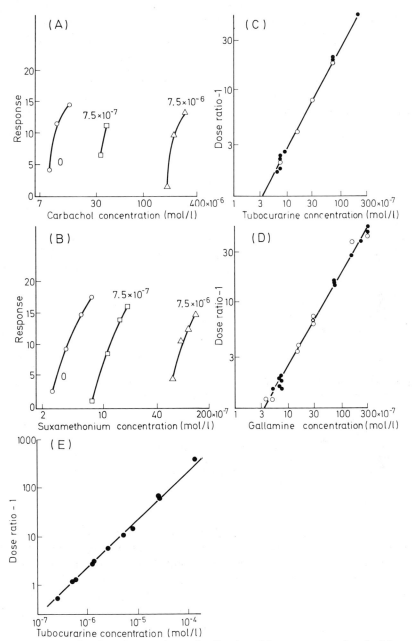

Fig. 22 A—E. Antagonism by tubocurarine and gallamine of the response to depolarizing agents. A and B illustrate the effect of two concentrations of tubocurarine on the contractile response (ordinates, arbitrary units) of the isolated chick biventer cervicis muscle to various concentrations (abscissae, log scale) of carbachol and suxamethonium. 38° C. C and D show double log plots of (dose ratio — 1) against the concentration of tubocurarine and gallamine respectively (see Text). Each point represents a single measurement; filled circles were obtained with carbachol as agonist, and open ones with suxamethonium. (From RANG and RITTER, 1969.) E Result of similar experiments on the effectiveness of tubocurarine in blocking acetylcholine depolarizations in isolated frog ext. dig. long IV muscles at room temperature. (From JENKINSON, 1960)

It should be recognized that the demonstration that Eq. (24) holds cannot be taken as decisive proof that the antagonism is competitive in the sense defined on p. 280 (see discussion by Stephenson, 1956; Arunlakshana and Schild, 1959; Rang, 1966, and Hubbard et al., 1969, pp. 176—186). All that can be said is that the results of such tests as have been applied are consistent with the idea that acetylcholine and tubocurarine compete on a one-to-one basis for the receptors. Other models which make the same predictions can be devised, however. For example, if the antagonist acts non-competitively (in the sense that it combines with a second independent site on the receptor, and by so doing renders the receptor inactive, even when combined with agonist) the following relationship should hold in place of Eq. (24):

$$x - 1 = K_I[I](1 + x K_A[A]). \tag{25}$$

This becomes identical to equation 24 if $x K_A[A] \ll 1$. This condition (which implies that few receptors need be occupied by the agonist) can only be evaluated when reliable estimates for K_A become available.

*b) The Effect of Competitive Antagonists on Transmitter Action:
Studies with Isolated Tissues*

We turn now to the more difficult problem of the influence of competitive antagonists on the response to acetylcholine released from the nerve endings rather than applied in the bathing fluid under equilibrium conditions. If a resting muscle is exposed to a steady concentration, $[I]$, of a competitive antagonist, the proportion of receptors occupied will be given by an expression analogous to Eq. (10), namely,

$$p_I = \frac{K_I[I]}{1 + K_I[I]}. \tag{26}$$

The extent to which p_I will fall as a consequence of transmitter release will depend on the concentration of acetylcholine attained at the receptor, as well as on the values of the association and dissociation rate constants for the combination of acetylcholine and antagonist with the receptor. These quantities are as yet unknown, although it is evident from the time course of the end-plate current and of the response to ionophoretically-applied acetylcholine (Katz and Miledi, 1965b) that the rates can be very high (see also Katz and Miledi, 1973b). Another problem is that the concentration of acetylcholine at the receptors will not be uniform. It seems likely, however, that the maximum levels attained during transmission will be much greater than the concentrations commonly used in experiments in which agonists and antagonists are applied in the bathing fluid. This suggestion is made on grounds similar to those outlined on p. 253 where it was noted that ionophoretic application of e.g. acetylcholine to a small fraction of the end-plate could match the response to a uniform concentration of the same agonist. The action of a quantum of acetylcholine is likely to be even more restricted, and the local concentration correspondingly higher (see also Salpeter and Eldefrawi, 1973).

Despite these uncertainties, it is clear that the transmitter is present for only a millisecond or so after each nerve impulse, and it seems unlikely that a new equilibrium between acetylcholine, the antagonist and the receptor can be reached within so short a time. Indeed it is possible that the proportion of receptors occupied by an antagonist such as tubocurarine does not fall appreciably during the brief presence of the transmitter. If so, the response will be determined by the proportion of receptors which are free (p_f). This is given by $1 - p_I$, from which

$$p_f = \frac{1}{1 + K_I[I]}. \tag{27}$$

If it is further assumed (though this may well be an over simplification—see p. 268) that the response to the transmitter is directly proportional to p_f, we may write

$$\frac{R_I}{R_0} = \frac{1}{1 + K_I[I]} \tag{28}$$

where R_0 is the control response (e.g. the increase in end-plate conductance, or the end-plate potential corrected for non-linear summation), and R_I is the value in the presence of the antagonist. This has been tested in several recent studies.

(1) CECCARELLI, HURLBUT and MAURO (1973) observed that the effect of tubocurarine in reducing the end-plate potential in frog cutancous pectoris nerve-muscle preparations could be fitted by Eq.(28), K_I being found to be 2.4 μM^{-1}, i.e., close to the values observed using the equilibrium dose-ratio method (Table 3),

(2) KRUCKENBERG and BAUER (1971) similarly found that Eq.(28) (with K_I equal to 2.6 μM^{-1}) described the effect of small concentrations of tubocurarine on the amplitude of both the miniature end-plate potential and the unit potential of the end-plate potential (as estimated by the variance method discussed on p. 318) in the hamster diaphragm. However, with concentrations greater than about 2 $\mu mol/l$ the degree of antagonism was less than predicted. This may have reflected the displacement of tubocurarine from some of the receptors during transmitter action, although other explanations were not excluded.

(3) A further test was made by BOWEN (1972a) who measured the increase in transmitter release (again assessed by the variance method) needed to counteract the effect of different concentrations of tubocurarine on the end-plate potential recorded from frog muscle. The necessary changes in release were produced by raising the external calcium, by varying the rate of stimulation, or by making use of pre-synaptic facilitation (p. 335). It was found that the dose-ratios obtained could be fitted by Eq.(24) with K_I equal to 2.9 μM^{-1}. Since this is again similar to the values obtained in equilibrium dose-ratio studies in which the agonist was applied in the bathing solution, it was concluded that "d-tubocurarine antagonises endogenously and exogenously applied agonists to a similar extent" (see also DEL CASTILLO and KATZ, 1957b).

An interesting situation will arise if a "fast" antagonist which can dissociate appreciably from the receptors during the presence of the transmitter is applied to a preparation already exposed to a "slow" antagonist which cannot dissociate rapidly. A paradoxical increase in response may then occur. This is because the transmitter can displace some of the fast antagonist from the receptors whereas there can be no corresponding fall in the proportion of receptors blocked when the slow antagonist alone is present. The phenomenon was first demonstrated in smooth muscle by STEPHENSON (1956; see also STEPHENSON and GINSBORG, 1969) and has been analysed by RANG (1966) and by GINSBORG and STEPHENSON (1974). An explanation of this kind was invoked by FERRY and MARSHALL (1973) to account for the paradoxical "decurarising" effect of hexamethonium on the rat diaphragm.

c) Quantitative Studies of Competitive Antagonism in vivo

It might by thought that the difficulty of measuring the concentration of free drug in the extracellular spaces, let alone in the immediate vicinity of the receptors, would rule out quantitative studies of antagonism *in vivo*. However, the dose-ratio method discussed in the preceding section requires only a knowledge of the factor by which the agonist concentration has to be raised to maintain a given response in the presence of the antagonist; absolute concentrations are not required provided that proportionality to the amounts administered can be assumed. This approach has been examined by PATON and WAUD (1967) in experiments with anaesthetised cats, dogs and rabbits. The doses of tubocurarine, gallamine and DF-596 (N,N′-4,9-dioxo-3,10-dioxodecamethylenebis(3-phenylacetoxy-tropanium bromide) needed to produce various degrees of neuromuscular block were first determined. The effects of these doses on the end-plate depolarizations produced by several depolarizing agents (including suxamethonium and decamethonium) were next assessed by the dose-ratio method (p. 281). The dose-ratios (x) observed could then be used to calculate the proportion of receptors occupied by the antagonist at the doses tested by means of the equation

$$p_I = \frac{x-1}{x}. \tag{29}$$

Two models will be considered in deriving this expression. First, if the antagonism is competitive, and if dynamic equilibrium between the agonist, the antagonist and the receptor is reached during the dose-ratio measurement (model I), Eq. (24) and the following expression for antagonist occupancy in the presence of A and I at concentrations $x[A]$ and $[I]$ respectively

$$p_I = \frac{K_I[I]}{1 + K_I[I] + K_A x[A]} \tag{30}$$

can then be combined to give

$$p_I = \frac{x-1}{x(1 + K_A[A])}. \tag{31}$$

This reduces to Eq. (29) if $K_A[A] \ll 1$, as may well be the case. Of equal or greater interest is the occupancy by antagonist *in the absence of agonist*. This can also be estimated using Eq. (29) which in this instance can be simply derived by combining Eq. (24) and (26).

If however the equilibrium between the antagonist and the receptor remains unaltered during the brief application of agonist (model II), p_I will be given throughout by Eq. (26). If it is also assumed (1) that the agonist can equilibrate very rapidly with those receptors which are free of antagonist and (2), as before, that equal responses correspond to equal receptor occupation by agonist, we may write from Eqs. (10) and (27)

$$\frac{K_A[A]}{1 + K_A[A]} = \frac{K_A x[A]}{1 + K_A x[A]} \cdot \frac{1}{1 + K_I[I]}$$

from which

$$x - 1 = K_I[I](1 + x K_A[A])$$

and

$$p_I = \frac{x - 1}{x(1 + K_A[A])}.$$

This is identical to Eq.(31) and approximates to Eq.(29) if $K_A[A] \ll 1$. If the latter condition does not hold, the log dose-response curves in the absence and presence of antagonist will not be parallel, and a deviation in the direction expected on this basis was noted by PATON and WAUD. This was taken as evidence that "Model II" conditions may have obtained, i.e., that the antagonist occupancy did not fall appreciably during the presence of agonist either because of slow dissociation from the receptor proper, or as a consequence of limitations to free diffusion in the immediate vicinity of the receptor (see also discussion by COLQUHOUN, 1975). In any case, PATON and WAUD were able to conclude that estimates of p_I based on the use of Eq.(29) rather than Eq.(31) would not be greatly in error under the particular conditions of their work.

The main conclusion from these experiments was that a large proportion (in the order of 75%) of the receptors had to be occluded before there was any impairment in neuromuscular transmission when the nerve was stimulated at a low rate (once every 10 sec). The corresponding value for complete block was about 90%. This is illustrated in Fig.23 and is in accord with electrophysiological evidence which shows that under normal conditions the end-plate potential would reach a value up to four times greater than the threshold of the fibre, were not an action potential to be set up

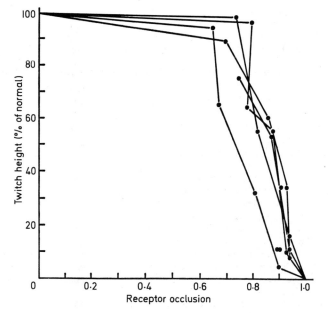

Fig. 23. Relation between twitch amplitude (in response to nerve stimulation) and the proportion of receptors occupied by a competitive blocking agent. Cat tibialis preparation: lines connect points from the same animal. (From PATON and WAUD, 1967)

(FATT and KATZ, 1951;BOYD and MARTIN, 1956b). Clearly either the release or the action of the transmitter has to be considerably reduced before the end-plate potential falls below the threshold value, and this is the main factor contributing to the striking non-linearity of the relationship plotted in Fig. 23. A similar conclusion was reached by BARNARD et al. (1971) who correlated the proportion of receptors occupied by α-bungarotoxin with the extent of the neuromuscular block produced.

The existence of a "safety margin" of this order has implications for the study of transmission under circumstances in which changes in muscle twitch are to be used as a measure of the release or activity of the transmitter (see PATON and WAUD, 1967; COOKSON and PATON, 1969, and LU, 1970). Thus, as already noted, the twitch may be normal even when as many as 70% of the receptors are occupied by an antagonist; beyond this point, however, the response will become a steep function of occupancy. As demonstrated by WAUD and WAUD (1971, 1972), the exact relationship will depend on the frequency of motor nerve impulses since this strongly influences the amount of acetylcholine released (see p. 339).

3. Other Agents which Influence Transmitter Action

a) Inorganic Ions

1. Monovalent Cations. Changes in the concentrations of sodium and potassium on either side of the muscle fibre membrane can be expected to alter the response to the transmitter, not only because both ions are involved in the increase in permeability which underlies the end-plate potential, but also by virtue of their contribution to the conductance of the non-synaptic membrane. From time to time the possibility has been considered that these cations might affect the receptor mechanism more directly, for example, by occupying the negatively-charged sites with which the transmitter combines.[An account of the evidence which has led to the formulation of tentative models of the surface configuration and charge distribution of the acetylcholine receptor would be beyond the scope of this article but can be found in, e.g., Chapters 5 and 6 in "Introduction to Chemical Pharmacology" by BARLOW (1964), and Chapters 4 and 5 in "Acetylcholine" by MICHELSON and ZEIMAL (1973)].

The possibility of a direct action of cations on the receptor sites was first suggested by ING and WRIGHT (1932), and the early finding that the blocking action of curare could be reversed by increasing the external potassium over a narrow range of concentrations was taken as evidence that potassium and curare alkaloids compete for the same binding site (for references see TAYLOR and NEDERGAARD, 1965). However, increased understanding of the details of neuromuscular transmission has made it clear that many other factors could be involved, for example, the effect of changes in potassium concentration on membrane potential. Indeed, such evidence as there is suggests that potassium has no specific action on the receptor. Thus alterations in external potassium cause little change in the affinity constant, K_I, for tubocurarine (see Table 3 for references). K_I does, however, increase when external sodium is partly replaced by sucrose although the concomitant fall in the ionic strength of the bathing fluid makes interpretation difficult.

Finally, it may be noted that the action of the transmitter in increasing the influx of sodium and the efflux of potassium at the end-plate will bring about a transient change in the ionic environment of the receptors, and of the immediately adjacent nerve endings. While this does not seem to have been studied in any detail, TAKEU-CHI and TAKEUCHI (1961) have examined the related problem of the effect of externally applied current on the concentration of potassium near the muscle membrane, and on neurotransmission.

2. Divalent Cations. Increases in external calcium and magnesium reduce the depolarization caused either by the transmitter or by carbachol or acetylcholine added to the bathing fluid (DEL CASTILLO and ENGBAEK, 1954; TAKEUCHI, 1963b; MAMBRINI and BENOIT (1964); NASTUK and LIU, 1966; HUBBARD et al., 1968a; TAYLOR et al., 1970; NASTUK, 1971; TAYLOR, 1973; see also ENGBAEK's comprehensive review, 1972, of the effects of magnesium on synaptic transmission). It has been suggested (e.g. NASTUK and LIU, 1966; TAYLOR, 1973) that this is because the receptor is normally occupied by calcium or magnesium, so that the combination of quaternary ammonium compounds such as acetylcholine or tubocurarine is in effect an ion exchange reaction of the kind originally envisaged for potassium by ING and WRIGHT. While magnesium has been found to affect the affinity constant for tubocurarine in the way which might be expected on this basis (JENKINSON, 1960; GOLD-FINE, 1973), more direct evidence is needed before such an explanation can be accepted for the partial inhibition of the action of acetylcholine by divalent ions. Thus calcium and magnesium may influence the equilibrium potential for acetylcholine (see TAKEUCHI, 1963b) and possible changes in the conductance of the nonsynaptic membrane must also be considered (p. 241). It is also conceivable that alterations in divalent ion concentration may affect the properties of the binding sites by an allosteric mechanism, and there could be changes in the characteristics of the "elementary events" discussed on p. 271. The general question of the criteria by which an "ion-exchange" model of the reaction between drug and receptor could be distinguished from the "classical" schemes considered in earlier sections has been examined by WAUD (1974).

Several heavy metal ions (e.g. lead, uranyl) also reduce post-synaptic sensitivity although it is generally found that the pre-synaptic actions are more important (Tables 6 and 9). The mechanisms have not been established.

3. Anions. Although acetylcholine does not increase anion permeability in skeletal muscle, the post-synaptic response will be influenced by the high chloride conductance of the muscle fibre, as already discussed (pp. 241, 256).

b) Drugs

Neuromuscular transmission can be blocked by agents as diverse as local and general anaesthetics, antibiotics, anticholinesterases and cholinesterase reactivators, ganglion blockers, and atropine and its congeners (Table 4). This has practical consequences which are discussed in detail in following chapters. Several of these substances are also of interest in the present context because of the light which their action may shed on post-synaptic mechanisms.

1. Effects of Anticholinesterases on the Time Course of Transmitter Action; Interactions with Tubocurarine. It has long been known that the amplitude and duration of miniature end-plate potentials are enhanced in the presence of anticholinesterases

Table 4. Some agents which alter post-junctional sensitivity to the transmitter, and which have been studied by electrophysiological techniques[a]

Agent	Reference	Species	Method of acetylcholine application (N: release from nerve, I: ionophoretic, M: microperfusion, B: in bathing fluid)	Response to acetylcholine measured[b]	Concentration of agent tested	Main conclusions, and notes; reduction in post-junctional sensitivity denoted by ↓; rise by ↑
General anaesthetics						
Ether	KARIS et al. (1966a)	frog	N, B(carb)	e.p.p., m.e.p.p., ΔV	0.5—5.0%	↓: see also KARIS et al.(1967)
Halothane	KARIS et al. (1967)	frog	N, I(carb,ACH) B(carb)	m.e.p.p., ΔV	0.1—4.0%	↓: see also GALINDO (1971)
	WAUD et al. (1973)	guinea pig	B(carb)	ΔV	1.0—4.0%	↓: effectiveness of tubocurarine and pancuronium unaffected
Ketamine	CRONELLY et al.(1973)	frog	N, I	m.e.p.p., ΔV	1—32 µg/ml	→
Methohexitone	WESTMORELAND et al. (1971)	rat	N	m.e.p.p.	0.1—3.0 mmol/l	→
Other centrally active drugs						
Barbiturates[c]						
Phenobarbitone	THOMSON and TURKANIS (1973)	frog	N	m.e.p.p.	200 µmol/l	→
CHEB[d]	THOMSON and TURKANIS (1973)	frog	N	m.e.p.p.	200 µmol/l	→
Alcohols[c]						
Ethyl	GAGE (1965)	rat	N	e.p.p., m.e.p.p.	8—1250 mmol/l	↑ e.p.p. prolonged; input conductance reduced
Ethyl	OKADA (1967,1970)	frog/toad	N, I	e.p.p., m.e.p.p.	2—8%	↑, then ↓ with increasing concentration; e.p.p. and m.e.p.p. prolonged
Methyl, propyl C_2—C_6	GAGE (1965)	rat	N	e.p.p., m.e.p.p. m.e.p.c., ACh "noise"	0.13 mol/l	↑ m.e.p.c. duration increased
	GAGE et al. (1975)	toad	N		up to 1 mol/l	

Table 4 (continued)

Drug	Reference	Species	Type	Measures	Concentration	Effect / Notes
Chlorpromazine[c]	MUCHNIK and YARYURA (1969)	frog	N. B (carb)	e.p.p., m.e.p.p., ΔV	100—500 µmol/l	↓ irreversible; see also QUASTEL et al. (1971)
Mephenesin	PAYTON (1966)	frog	N, B (carb)	e.p.p., ΔV	<2.9 mmol/l	→ desensitization increased
Methylpentynol	PAYTON (1966)	frog	N, B (carb)	e.p.p., ΔV	<19 mmol/l	→ desensitization increased
Paraldehyde	PAYTON (1966)	frog	N, B (carb)	e.p.p., ΔV	<17 mmol/l	→ desensitization increased
Adrenergic neurone blockers						
Bretylium	FERRY and NORRIS (1971)	rat	N, I	e.p.p., m.e.p.p., ΔV	0.2—2.4 mmol/l	little change, because of balance between curare-like and anticholinesterase activity
Bretylium	CHANG et al. (1967)	rat, frog	N	e.p.p., m.e.p.p.	50—300 µg/ml	→
Guanethidine	CHANG et al. (1967)	rat, frog	N	e.p.p., m.e.p.p.	150—400 µg/ml	→
Adrenaline receptor blockers						
Propranolol	WERMAN and WISLICKI (1971)	frog	N, I	e.p.p., m.e.p.p., ΔV	5—300 µg/ml	↓; high concentrations depolarize
Anti-mitotic agents						
Colchicine	TURKANIS (1973b)	frog	N	e.p.p., m.e.p.p.	500—750 µmol/l	↓; 50% reduction with 500 µmol/l
Vinblastine	TURKANIS (1973b)	frog	N	e.p.p., m.e.p.p.	20—180 µmol/l	↓; 50% reduction with 60 µmol/l
Disulphide bond reagents						
Dithiothreitol	del CASTILLO et al. (1970)	frog	I (ACH, carb)	ΔV		↓; heavy metal ions also examined
Dithiothreitol	BEN-HAIM et al. (1973, 1975)	frog	N	e.p.p., m.e.p.p.	0.1—2.0 mmol/l	↓; could be restored by 5,5'-dithiobis-(2-nitrobenzoic acid) — see also ALBUQUERQUE et al. (1968), and RANG and RITTER (1971)
Miscellaneous						
AMPMT[e]	NASTUK and POPPERS (1966)	frog	N, M	e.p.p., ΔV	0.1—1 mmol/l	→

Table 4 (continued)

Agent	Reference	Species	Method of acetylcholine application (N: release from nerve, I: ionophoretic, M: microperfusion, B: in bathing fluid)	Response to acetylcholine measured[b]	Concentration of agent tested	Main conclusions, and notes; reduction in post-junctional sensitivity denoted by ↓; rise by ↑
Acetone	Okada (1967)	frog, toad	N, I	e.p.p., m.e.p.p., ΔV	0.2—0.5%	↑; then ↓ with increasing concentration. E.p.p. and m.e.p.p. prolonged
1-fluoro-2,4-dinitrobenzene	Edelson and Nastuk (1973)	frog	N, I(carb)	e.p.p., ΔV	0.4—2.0 mmol/l	↑
Hexafluorenium	Nastuk and Karis (1964)	frog	M(carb)	A.P., ΔV	5—30 µmol/l	↓; possibly because of post-receptor block (see p. 278)
Hexafluorenium	Johnson and Parsons (1972)	frog	B(carb), M(carb)	ΔV	10—40 µmol/l	↓; non-competitive
Hexamethonium	Ferry and Marshall (1973)	rat	N	e.p.p.	300 µmol/l	has anti-curare action—see p. 286
Histamine	Scuka (1973)	frog	N	e.p.p., m.e.p.p.	100—500 µmol/l	↓; e.p.c. decays more quickly
5-hydroxytryptamine	Colomo et al. (1968)	frog	N, I	e.p.p., ΔV	100 µg/ml	↑
Lobeline	Steinberg and Volle (1972)	frog	N	e.p.p.	10—20 µmol/l	↓; may accelerate desensitization
Neomycin	Elmqvist and Josefsson (1962)	rat	N, B	e.p.p., m.e.p.p., ΔV	300 µg/ml	↓ by about 50%
SKF–525 A[f]	Magazanik (1970)	frog	N, I	e.p.p., ΔV	0.2—100 µmol/l	↓; ΔV reduced more than e.p.p.; desensitization enhanced
SKF–525[f] congeners	Terrar (1974)	frog	B(carb)	ΔV	adiphenine 1 µmol/l pipenzolate 10 µmol/l	desensitization enhanced

Table 4 (continued)

Streptomycin	Dretchen et al.(1973)	frog	N, I	m.e.p.p., ΔV	10—500 μg/ml	↓; see also Table 6
Tetraethylammonium	Koketsu (1958)	frog	N, B	e.p.p., ΔV	0.2—3.0 mmol/l	↓; see also Payton and Shand (1966)
Tetraethylammonium	Parsons (1969)	frog	N, I(carb),B(carb)	A.P., e.p.p., ΔV	1—10 mmol/l	→
Tetraethylammonium	Benoit and Mambrini (1970)	frog	N	e.p.p., m.e.p.p.	300 μmol/l	↓; m.e.p.p. reduced by up to 60%
Tetrahydroaminacrine	Karis et al. (1966b)	frog	N	A.P., m.e.p.p.	30, 50, 150 μmol/l	small concentrations ↑, (acetylcholinesterase inhibition), large concentrations ↓

[a] To avoid overlap with Tables 6 and 9, several agents (metal ions, catecholamines, xanthines, adenine nucleosides, some metabolic inhibitors) which have greater pre- than post-junctional actions have not been included. Thus Tables 4, 6 and 9 should be used in conjunction. Also, drugs discussed in detail in the main text have not been listed; for curare alkaloids and congeners, see pages 235, 246, 257, 258, 265, 280—288, 294, 320, Table 3 and Chapter 4B; anticholinesterases, see pages 289, 290, 320, and Chapter 4C; atropine and congeners, see pages 20, 265, 294 also Magazanik (1971a); elapid and other toxins, see pages 258—260, 261, 264, 295, also Datyner and Gage (1973) and Harris et al. (1973); local anaesthetics, see pages 243, 250, 278, 294 also Hirst and Wood (1971a, b).

[b] e.p.p.: end-plate potential; m.e.p.p.: miniature end-plate potential; m.e.p.c.: miniature end-plate current; ΔV: end-plate depolarization in response to externally applied acetylcholine or carbachol; A.P.: action potential.

[c] See also Magazanik (1971b) who has compared the effects of each of these substances on the response to (a) nerve released and (b) ionophoretically-applied acetylcholine in frog muscle. In every instance, the "ionophoretic" depolarization was found to be reduced at concentrations of the drugs which had little if any effect on the end-plate potential. This, it was thought, could reflect an increase in the rate of desensitization (see p. 278). A similar differential sensitivity has been described by Adams et al. (1970) for the actions of thiopentone and amylobarbitone (see also Adams, 1974b, and Seyama and Narahashi, 1975).

[d] 5-(2-cyclohexylideneethyl)-5-ethyl barbituric acid.

[e] 3-(4-amino-2-methyl pyrimidyl-5-methyl) thiazolium bromide hydrobromide.

[f] 2-diethylaminoethyl diphenylpropylacetate.

(FATT and KATZ, 1952; DEL CASTILLO and KATZ, 1956). This is due not to a change in the properties of the chemosensitive membrane but rather to an increase in the duration of the conductance change caused by the transmitter, as might be expected as a consequence of cholinesterase inhibition. However, calculations based on the known dimensions of the synaptic cleft show that the decay of the effect on conductance is often too slow to be accounted for in terms of diffusion of acetylcholine from its site of action to the external solution. Furthermore, application of tubocurarine in the presence of an anticholinesterase is found to increase the rate of decline of the conductance increase, and clearly this would not be expected were simple diffusion alone to determine the time course. One possibility (MAGLEBY and STEVENS, 1972a, b) is that anticholinesterases increase the lifetime of the elementary channels (p. 271) but this has been ruled out by the noise measurements of KATZ and MILEDI (1973b) who have proposed an alternative explanation. They note that only the acetylcholine which is not bound to the receptor is free to diffuse. If the receptors are in sufficient excess, a large proportion (p) of the transmitter will be bound and the effective rate of disappearance by diffusion will be reduced by the factor $1/(1-p)$ as compared with the rate in the absence of binding.

Normally this has no significance because the main route by which the transmitter disappears is local hydrolysis. However, when hydrolysis is inhibited the determining factor becomes diffusion, albeit slowed in the way which has been discussed. This can be considered in another way: under normal circumstances, a single molecule of nerve-released acetylcholine would on average open only one ion channel. However, when hydrolysis is suppressed, the same molecule may open several channels in succession during its passage through the synaptic cleft to the exterior.

The effect of tubocurarine on the time course of the miniature end-plate potentials in the presence of an anticholinesterase can also be explained in these terms. Thus by reducing the number of receptors available to the transmitter, tubocurarine causes p to become smaller, and the factor $1/(1-p)$ to increase. The rate of decay of transmitter action then tends towards that predicted on the basis of simple diffusion (KATZ and MILEDI, 1973b). This presumably accounts for the rather small effect of anticholinesterases on the time course of evoked end-plate potentials in the presence of tubocurarine. By contrast, when the end-plate potentials are evoked in preparations exposed to low-sodium solutions, in the absence of tubocurarine, anticholinesterases have a large effect (FATT and KATZ, 1951; TAKEUCHI and TAKEUCHI, 1959; KORDAŠ, 1968).

2. Local Anaesthetics. Is has been noted on p. 243 that lignocaine and its derivatives increase the duration of the end-plate current. This cannot be attributed to cholinesterase inhibition (STEINBACH, 1968a). One possibility (STEINBACH, 1968a, b) is that these substances might prolong the conductance increase produced by the transmitter, possibly by combining with the acetylcholine-receptor complex to form a longer lasting, though somewhat less active, complex (see KATZ and MILEDI, 1975). Another suggestion (p. 250), based on studies with procaine, is that local anaesthetics produce a time dependent change in the ionic selectivity of the effect of acetylcholine on membrane conductance (MAENO, 1966; MAENO et al., 1971).

3. Atropine and Miscellaneous Substances. Atropine and its congeners cause a striking increase in the rate of decay of the end-plate current as well as a reduction in its amplitude (Beránek and Vyskočil, 1967, 1968; Kordaš, 1968). Again a change in the selectivity of the ion channels may be involved (see p.258). There is, however, evidence that the effect on end-plate current duration is due to a fall in the time for which the elementary channels (p. 271) remain open (Katz and Miledi, 1973d). This is based on a study of the effect of atropine on the power spectrum of acetylcholine "noise". Interestingly, ether (unlike tubocurarine, bungarotoxin and prostigmine) has been reported to have the same effect (unpublished experiments by R. Miledi, quoted in Katz and Miledi, 1973d; see also Katz and Miledi, 1973b, c). It can be expected that application of this new method will throw light on the mechanism of action of other substances listed in Table 4 (see, for example, Ben-Haim et al., 1975; Gage et al., 1975).

C. Pre-Synaptic Events

I. Introduction

The end-plate region of the muscle fibre is characterised not only by the special features of its response to nerve stimulation (see p.234) but also by being the "seat of spontaneous electric discharges which have the character of miniature end-plate potentials" (Fatt and Katz, 1952). Fig.24 illustrates the phenomenon. The miniature discharges can be seen only at the end-plate, their amplitude is increased by anti-cholinesterases and reduced by tubocurarine, and they are not observed after

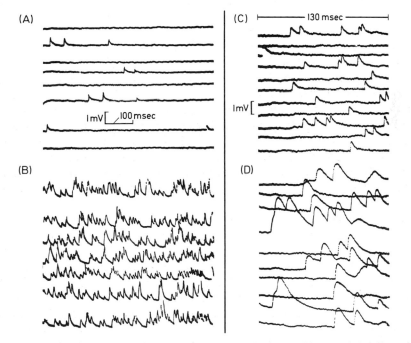

Fig.24 A—D. Discharge of miniature end-plate potentials. Control in A and C. Effect of increase in osmotic pressure in B, same fibre as A: effect of neostigmine in D, same fibre as C. (From Fatt and Katz, 1952)

denervation and degeneration of the nerve terminals (but see p. 299). These results can be explained by supposing that the miniature end-plate potentials are due to the spontaneous release of multimolecular packets or quanta of acetylcholine. A precise estimate of the number of molecules which make up a quantum cannot yet be made. An upper limit of the order of 10^5 is suggested by the fact that ionophoretic application of this amount of acetylcholine would be required to mimic a typical miniature end-plate potential. A lower limit of 10^3 may be derived from estimates of the "elementary" depolarization caused by the molecular action of acetylcholine (see p. 271).

The principal features of the spontaneous discharge as observed at end-plates of frog muscle fibres were described by FATT and KATZ in 1952. The amplitudes were normally distributed, with a mean of between 0.1 to 0.5 mV for different fibres and a coefficient of variation (i.e. standard deviation/mean) of about 0.25. The discharge was random in time, with a mean rate which varied from fibre to fibre from 0.1 to 100 Hz (usually 1 to 10 Hz). The rate could be altered by a number of procedures which had little or no effect on amplitude. These included stretching the preparation and changing the temperature and osmotic pressure. On the other hand the amplitude was affected by tubocurarine and neostigmine without much change in frequency. The distinction is in keeping with the idea that changes in amplitude are related to post-synaptic factors, whereas changes in frequency relate to the nerve terminal and the release process. An extension of this is that the amount of acetylcholine that constitutes a quantum is not readily altered. Another result reported by FATT and KATZ in their paper of 1952 suggested that not only spontaneous release but also nerve stimulus-induced release occurs in the form of quanta. It was already well known that a reduction in the external calcium concentration leads to a reduction in the amount of acetylcholine released by motor nerve stimulation (see Chapter 2) and to a decrease in the amplitude of end-plate potentials recorded extracellularly (FENG, 1937, 1940; KATZ, 1942; DEL CASTILLO and STARK, 1952). When individual end-plates were investigated using intracellular electrodes, a reduction in calcium concentration was found to have little effect on the spontaneous discharge, but to cause a striking change in the response to nerve stimulation. At a sufficiently low concentration of calcium (or high concentration of magnesium — DEL CASTILLO and ENGBAEK, 1954) successive nerve stimuli gave rise to responses that varied greatly, ranging from no larger than a single miniature end-plate potential to some 2 or 3 times that size. This contrasted with the effect of tubocurarine in a concentration which reduced the response to the same mean amplitude; in this case the amplitudes of successive responses were almost constant (Fig. 25). This result foreshadowed the later analysis which showed that normal end-plate potentials could be regarded as being made up of a large number of units each equivalent to a miniature end-plate potential.

The quantal analysis of the evoked response will be discussed in detail in Section C III (see p. 308). It may however, be helpful to summarize the main conclusions at this point. With only a small number of exceptions (see p. 300) quanta are derived from a common pool for both spontaneous and evoked release of transmitter. When the amount of transmitter released by a nerve stimulus is altered by some agent or procedure, the change is almost always in the number of quanta released (usually described as the *quantal content* of the response) and not in the amount of acetylcho-

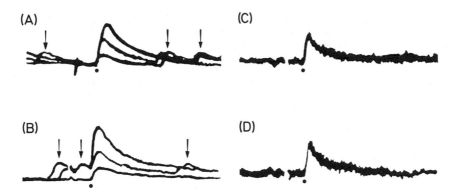

Fig. 25 A—D. Superimposed responses (●) to 3 nerve stimuli recorded from frog muscle fibres in a medium with a low calcium concentration (A and B) or in the presence of tubocurarine (C and D). Arrows indicate spontaneous miniature end-plate potentials. Note their absence in the presence of tubocurarine. The trace length is about 40 msec; the mean response in A and B is about 1 mV and in C and D about 0.5 mV. (From FATT and KATZ, 1952)

line per quantum. The same is true for spontaneous release, experimental treatments generally altering only the rate of discharge of quanta.

So far stress has been placed on the unity of spontaneous and evoked transmitter release. There are also, however, some differences: thus evoked release is easily abolished, for example, by increasing external magnesium levels, whereas spontaneous release persists under almost all conditions. Also, agents which have little effect on evoked release may have a large effect on spontaneous release (e.g. an increase in osmotic pressure). Furthermore, whereas there is strong evidence that evoked release is brought about by the entry of calcium into the nerve terminal, it seems unlikely that this is obligatory for spontaneous release.

The results of electrophysiological recording cannot exclude the possibility that acetylcholine is also released in a non-quantal form. However, what can be stated is that any such release is without detectable effect on the membrane potential of the muscle fibre.

The most attractive hypothesis for the quantal nature of transmitter release is that put forward by DEL CASTILLO and KATZ (1956) who suggested that packets of acetylcholine are contained in the presynaptic vesicles [see also KATZ, 1969 (p. 14); HEUSER and REESE, 1973, and Chapters 1 and 2]. Spontaneous miniature end-plate potentials would then be the result of occasional, random, "successful" collisions occurring between a vesicle and the nerve membrane (perhaps at some strategic position) leading to the discharge of the quantum into the synaptic cleft. From the quantitative point of view, a critical question is whether the acetylcholine content of a vesicle is the same as that of a quantal packet. Although precise estimates are not available for either vesicles or quanta, values of the same order of magnitude (10^4 molecules of acetylcholine) seem reasonable for both.

The relationship between vesicles and quanta will not be discussed further in this chapter. The subject has been reviewed by HUBBARD (1973) and by MARTIN (1975).

Table 5. Miniature end-plate potentials recorded from different muscles

Muscle	Typical rate (per sec)	Reference
Frog sartorius		
Frog ext. dig. longus IV } [a]	1—10	Fatt and Katz (1952)
Lizard and tortoise		
Cat tenuissimus	1—2 (37° C)	Boyd and Martin (1956a)
Rat diaphragm	1—2 (38° C)	Liley (1956a)
Guinea-pig serratus anterior	2—10 (36° C)	Brooks (1956)
Frog iliofibularis slow fibres	[b]	Burke (1957)
Chicken {fast fibres	2—10	
{slow fibres	[b]	Ginsborg (1960)
Human intercostal	0.2 (37° C)	Elmqvist et al. (1960, 1964)
Rat intercostal	15 (37° C)	Hofmann et al. (1962)
Rat diaphragm foetal and newborn	0.01	Diamond and Miledi (1962)
Cat slow extraocular fibres	[b]	Hess and Pilar (1963)
Hagfish {fast fibres	2—10	
{slow fibres	[b]	Alnaes et al. (1964)
Carp "red fibres"	[b]	Hidaka and Toida (1969)
Pigeon iris slow fibres	[b]	Pilar and Vaughan (1969)
Golden hamster	0.5 (20—22° C)	Moravec et al. (1973)

[a] Where no temperature is shown, the experiments were made at room temperature.
[b] Values for rates are not given; they have little significance since the recordings are effectively made from an unknown number of junctions.

II. Miniature End-Plate Potentials

1. Occurrence

Miniature end-plate potentials have been recorded from a wide variety of cells driven by chemical transmission, and their very existence at any particular site is usually regarded as evidence that the transmitter is also released in quanta in response to nerve stimulation. Table 5 illustrates the range of vertebrate skeletal neuromuscular junctions that have been examined. It includes examples from amphibia, reptiles, fish, birds and mammals, not excluding humans.

At all the junctions investigated it has been found that there is no striking regularity in the sequence of the spontaneous discharges (but see following section). However, as was pointed out by Fatt and Katz (1952, p. 123), more powerful methods than the examination of the interval distribution and its comparison with an exponential or Poisson distribution (Gage and Hubbard, 1965) are required to distinguish inherent randomness from a combination of a large number of out of phase regularities. More powerful statistical methods are also required to reveal small interactions such as a marginal increase or decrease in the probability of subsequent spontaneous release caused by particular discharges. Such interaction was first reported by Rotshenker and Rahamimoff (1970) for discharges recorded from muscles bathed in calcium-enriched (15 mmol/l) solutions and it has also been found to occur to a small degree at normal calcium concentrations (Hubbard and Jones, 1973; Cohen et al., 1974a, b, c).

2. Amplitudes of Miniature End-Plate Potentials

As discovered by FATT and KATZ (1952), the amplitudes of miniature end-plate potentials are usually distributed normally. The mean amplitude is determined by the "input impedance" of the muscle fibre which in turn depends in part on fibre diameter. Thus smaller muscle fibres have larger miniature end-plate potentials (see p. 242): this appears to account for the large amplitudes seen in new-born rat diaphragm fibres (DIAMOND and MILEDI, 1962).

An apparent exception to the "normal distribution" is provided by various muscle fibre types which are multiply innervated, each fibre having many junctional regions. Here, miniature end-plate potentials can be recorded wherever the microelectrode is inserted and the amplitudes of those originating from distant junctions tail off into the baseline noise. The distribution therefore, is skewed towards zero. However, there is no reason to suppose that the miniature end-plate potentials from a single junctional region differ in their general properties from those of muscle which is not multiply innervated.

3. Abnormal Miniature End-Plate Potentials

Even in focally innervated fibres occasional transient depolarizations are observed which are several standard deviations removed from the mean. The "giant" miniature end-plate potentials were first reported by LILEY (1956a, 1957) who assumed that they reflected the non-random simultaneous discharge of several quanta (see also MARTIN and PILAR, 1964a). Somewhat at variance with this idea, there appears to be no interaction between quanta in evoked release (LILEY, 1957; MENRATH and BLACKMAN, 1970).

"Subminiature" end-plate potentials, with about one-quarter of the usual amplitudes, were first described in normal muscle (rat diaphragm) by COOKE and QUASTEL (1973a, p. 387). These abnormal miniature end-plate potentials, which presumably reflect the existence of abnormal packets of acetylcholine, would generally go unnoticed: there are however several situations, which will now be considered, in which abnormal spontaneous activity is obvious (see also KRIEBEL and GROSS, 1974).

a) Miniature End-Plate Potentials Recorded from Denervated Muscle Fibres

Section of the motor-nerve to frog muscle is followed by a short period during which miniature end-plate potentials are not seen: subsequently they reappear (see BIRKS et al., 1960), but with very different characteristics. The frequencies were found to range from 1 to 10 per minute as compared with the usual 1 to 10 per second: the amplitude distribution was very skew. Thus while most of the miniature end-plate potentials were less than 1 mV, some, even in the same fibre, might be as large as 10 mV. Furthermore, procedures which cause an increase in frequency of normal miniature end-plate potentials had no effect. From the results of an electron-microscopic study, BIRKS et al. suggested that the Schwann cell could be the origin of the quanta of acetylcholine since this cell was found to replace the degenerated nerve terminal and to occupy a "synaptic" position (see also MILEDI and STEFANI, 1970; HARRIS and MILEDI, 1972).

The situation in rat muscle (the diaphragm, gastrocnemius and plantaris were investigated) is different. MILEDI and SLATER (1968) observed miniature end-plate potentials in only 8 of 1700 fibres examined from 1 day to 2 years after denervation, and in their electron micrographs found that a Schwann cell does not generally replace the nerve terminal in a synaptic position. Even more striking was the finding that in the one of the 8 end-plates at which abnormal miniature potentials did occur a Schwann cell was seen to occupy a synaptic position.

b) Miniature End-Plate Potentials at Regenerating Neuromuscular Junctions

An abnormal discharge of spontaneous depolarizations has also been described (DENNIS and MILEDI, 1971) at regenerating junctions of the cutaneous pectoris muscle of the frog. Nine days after the nerve was crushed, transmission was found to be re-established at some end-plates, and evoked and spontaneous depolarizations could be studied together when a low calcium and high magnesium bathing medium was used (see p. 324). In this way the responses to quanta released by nerve stimuli could be compared with those to spontaneously released quanta. As will be discussed in detail below, in all other situations so far investigated, the evidence is consistent with a common pool of quanta for both spontaneous and evoked release. However, at the regenerating junctions, the miniature end-plate potentials were considerably smaller than the units of the evoked response, with an amplitude distribution which was skewed towards small values. Conceivably they are due to "unripe" quanta whose release is normally suppressed (see also DENNIS and MILEDI, 1974a, b). The possibility that the spontaneous discharge was contaminated by some source of quanta outside the nerve terminals was thought to be unlikely since the frequency of the miniature end-plate potentials was increased by the same agents and in the same way as normal miniature end-plate potentials (see p. 380).

In the mammal the situation seems somewhat different. KOENIG and PÉCOT-DECHAVASSINE (1971) have found that the pattern of spontaneous activity at regenerating junctions in the sternomastoid muscle of the mouse is normal (see also BENNETT et al., 1973). However, at induced end-plates in a previously aneural region, the distribution of amplitudes is considerably broader than usual.

c) Miniature End-Plate Potentials at Junctions Poisoned by Botulinum Toxin

Abnormal miniature end-plate potentials have also been observed at junctions at which transmission was blocked by botulinum toxin. Earlier work had suggested that spontaneous activity was abolished by this toxin (BROOKS, 1956; THESLEFF, 1960) but it was subsequently found by HARRIS and MILEDI (1971) in the frog (using type D toxin), and by SPITZER (1972) in the rat (using type A toxin), that at most end-plates miniature potentials could be observed, although at a low frequency and with an amplitude distribution skewed towards small values. Since their frequency could be increased by tetanic nerve stimulation (see p. 321), it seemed likely that the quanta of transmitter producing the miniature depolarizations were released spontaneously from the nerve terminals (see also BOROFF et al., 1974).

d) The After Effect of Soaking in a High Concentration of Calcium

This provides another example of the persistence of spontaneous release of quanta, though of an abnormal kind, in spite of the abolition of evoked release. On returning frog preparations to normal solution after several hours in isotonic calcium chloride,

HEUSER et al. (1971) found that the response to nerve terminal depolarization had been irreversibly abolished but that spontaneous depolarizations could be observed, varying in amplitude from 0.1 to 35 mV. At the same time electron-microscopic examination showed that prolonged bathing in isotonic calcium chloride caused agglutination of synaptic vesicles. This was only partially reversible. PÉCOT-DECHA-VASSINE (1970) has found similarly abnormal spontaneous activity after restoring to normal solutions preparations which had been bathed in acidic fluid in the presence either of moderate calcium concentrations or of UO_2^{2+} (in which case the presence of calcium was unnecessary).

e) Hemicholinium and Triethylcholine

An interesting exception to the rule that the amplitudes of miniature end-plate potentials reflect only post-synaptic events is provided by the action of hemicholinium and triethylcholine which interfere with the synthesis of the transmitter (see Chapter 2, p. 115). This has been investigated by ELMQVIST and QUASTEL (1965a) on rat diaphragm (cf. JONES and KWANBUNBUMPEN, 1970a, b) and human intercostal neuromuscular junctions. Apart from a small effect due to a post-synaptic reduction in sensitivity to acetylcholine, these substances caused little change in the amplitude of miniature end-plate potentials recorded from resting muscles. However, when the motor nerve was stimulated at a rate above 5/sec, the amplitudes gradually declined until the miniature potentials were submerged in the baseline noise. An analysis of the evoked end-plate potentials showed that the response to nerve stimulation was affected in the same way as the miniature end-plate potentials.

These results therefore suggest that when the total amount of acetylcholine is severely depleted quanta with less than the usual amount of transmitter can be released. JONES and KWANBUNBUMPEN (1970a, b) have also found a small effect of this kind after prolonged repetitive stimulation in the absence of hemicholinium.

4. The Rate of Spontaneous Release

Several studies have been made of the effect of various procedures and agents on the rate of spontaneous release. The most interesting and important effect is the acceleration caused by depolarization of the nerve terminals. This type of release is more usefully regarded as evoked rather than spontaneous, and will be discussed later. However, the effect must be borne in mind since nerve terminal depolarization rather than a direct effect of an agent under investigation may be the cause of an observed increase in miniature end-plate potential frequency.

Another kind of acceleration which will be discussed later is the after effect of nerve stimulation: this too, may be thought of as evoked, though delayed, release. References to other investigations on changes in the rate of spontaneous release are set out in Table 6 and the remainder of this section is provided by way of commentary.

a) Inorganic Ions

FATT and KATZ (1952) and DEL CASTILLO and KATZ (1954a) found that the resting discharge of miniature end-plate potentials in the frog was not affected by a reduction in calcium concentration, or the addition of enough magnesium to decrease

Table 6

Agent	Animal	Reference

A. Agents which increase frequency of miniature end-plate potentials

Inorganic ions

Agent	Animal	Reference
Ca^{2+}	frog	Mambrini and Benoit (1964)
Ca^{2+}, H^+	rat	Hubbard et al. (1968a)
Ba^{2+}, Sr^{2+}	rat	Elmqvist and Feldman (1966)
La^{3+}	frog	Blioch et al. (1968)
		Lambert and Parsons (1970)
		Heuser and Miledi (1971)
		De Bassio et al. (1971)
		Bowen (1972b)
Mn^{2+}	toad	Balnave and Gage (1973)
Pb^{2+}	frog	Manalis and Cooper (1973)
UO_2^{2+}	frog	Benoit and Mambrini (1970)
Co^{2+}	frog	Kita and Van der Kloot (1973), Weakly (1973)
Y^{3+} (yttrium)	frog	Bowen (1972b)
Pr^{3+}	frog	Alnaes and Rahamimoff (1974)

Metabolic inhibitors

Agent	Animal	Reference
2,4-dinitrophenol	frog	Kraatz and Trautwein (1957)
1-fluoro-2,4-dinitrobenzene	frog	Edelson and Nastuk (1973)
Cardiac glycosides	frog	Birks and Cohen (1968a, b)
	rat	Elmqvist and Feldman (1965b)
Uncouplers of oxidative phosphorylation	frog	Glagoleva et al. (1970)

Miscellaneous

Agent	Animal	Reference
Caffeine (0.5 mmol/l)	frog	Mambrini and Benoit (1963)
Theophylline (1.4 mmol/l) Dibutyryl cyclic AMP (4 mmol/l)	rat	Goldberg and Singer (1969)
Noradrenaline (0.01 mmol/l)	frog	Jenkinson et al. (1968)
Adrenaline (0.05 mmol/l)	rat	Kuba (1969)
Catechol (1—100 μmol/l)	cat	Gallagher and Blaber (1973)
Phenol (0.01 mmol/l)	fish	Kuba (1969)
Alcohols (0.5 mol/l)	rat	Gage (1965)
Alcohols, acetone (more than 0.1 mol/l)	frog	Okada (1967, 1970)
Diamide (0.1 mmol/l)	frog	Werman et al. (1971)
CHEB[a] (0.2 mmol/l) Phenobarbitone (0.2 mmol/l)	frog	Thomson and Turkanis (1973)
Methohexital (1 mmol/l)	rat	Westmoreland et al. (1971)
Chlorpromazine (0.02 mmol/l) also, pentobarbitone, ether, chloroform	mouse	Quastel et al. (1971)
Nystatin (0.01 mmol/l)	frog	Crawford and Fettiplace (1971)
Streptomycin (> 1 μmol/l)	frog	Dretchen et al. (1973)
Vinblastine (0.06 mmol/l)	frog	Turkanis (1973b)
Histamine (0.4 mmol/l)	frog	Scuka (1973)
Veratrine (0.01—10 μg/ml)	rat	Hofmann et al. (1962)
Ruthenium red (2.5 μmol/l)	frog	Rahamimoff and Alnaes (1973)
Dimethyl sulphoxide (141 and 282 mmol/l)	frog	Evans and Jaggard (1973)

B. Agents and conditions which reduce the frequency of miniature end-plate potentials

Inorganic ions

Agent	Animal	Reference
Mg^{2+}	rat	Hubbard et al. (1968a)
Be^{2+}	frog	Blioch et al. (1968)

Table 6 (continued)

Agent	Animal	Reference
Toxins		
Tetrodotoxin	rat	LANDAU (1969)
Tetanus	goldfish	MELLANBY and THOMPSON (1972)
	mouse	DUCHEN and TONGE (1973)
Botulinum	frog	HARRIS and MILEDI (1971)
	rat	SPITZER (1972)
Oxyuranus scutellactus venom	mice	KEMENSKAYA and THESLEFF (1974)
Miscellaneous		
Adenosine		GINSBORG and HIRST (1972)
AMP (0.05 mmol/l)	rat	GINSBORG et al. (1973)
ADP, ATP		RIBEIRO and WALKER (1975)
γ-Aminobutyrate	rat	HOFMANN et al. (1962)
Hibernation	hamster	MORAVEC et al. (1973)

C. *Venoms which initially increase and eventually reduce the frequency of miniature end-plate potentials*

Black widow spider	frog	LONGENECKER et al. (1970)
Rattle snake	frog	BRAZIL and EXCELL (1971)
Tiger snake	toad	DATYNER and GAGE (1973); see also LANE and GAGE (1973)
	mouse	HARRIS et al. (1973)
β-bungarotoxin	rat	CHANG et al. (1973c)
	mouse,rat	CHANG and HUANG (1974)

[a] 5-(2-cyclohexylideneëthyl)-5-ethyl barbituric acid.

greatly the evoked release of transmitter. Even in the presence of chelating agents which reduce the calcium concentration in the bathing fluid to less than, say, 10^{-8} mol/l and abolish evoked release, the miniature end-plate potential discharge continues at about half the usual rate (MILEDI and THIES, 1971). In the mammal, the spontaneous rate is somewhat more sensitive to the concentrations of calcium and magnesium (HUBBARD et al., 1968a).

In the virtual absence of calcium spontaneous release is enhanced by the addition of a variety of other cations and BLIOCH et al. (1968) have suggested that this is because such cations enter the nerve terminal where by virtue of their positive charge they promote the vesicle-membrane reaction, which in turn leads to the discharge of quanta. In the presence of calcium they may act as inhibitors because they are in effect competing with calcium which has a higher efficacy (see pp. 267 and 327). This idea cannot be ruled out, but in the light of the rather diverse and complicated effects which have been discovered subsequently it seems likely that some cations at least have specific effects of their own. The most dramatic of these is the acceleration caused by lanthanum, at a concentration of 1 mmol/l or less. A detailed study in the frog relating the changes in the discharge with those in the structure of the terminals has been made by HEUSER and MILEDI (1971). After an enormous increase in rate (to about 1000/sec) there is a slow decline until eventually (probably within 10 hrs at room temperature) the spontaneous discharge ceases. At this stage almost all the synaptic vesicles have disappeared.

Another explanation put forward by Glagoleva et al. (1970) is that certain agents may act by increasing the internal calcium ion concentration as a result of releasing calcium from mitochondria (see p. 305). This might also account for the effect of lithium. The replacement of $3/4$ of the external sodium chloride by sucrose was found by Fatt and Katz (1952) to have no effect on the spontaneous release rate. However, when all the sodium chloride is replaced with lithium chloride there is, in the frog, a delayed increase in the frequency of miniature end-plate potentials (Kelly, 1968) which also persists in the absence of calcium (Carmody and Gage, 1973).

Apart from the delayed abolition observed in lanthanum-containing media, in isotonic calcium chloride (see Heuser et al., 1971) and in the presence of black widow spider venom (Longenecker et al., 1970; see also Clark et al., 1972) associated in each case with late structural changes, spontaneous release is very persistent, continuing for several hours in isotonic calcium chloride and in isotonic potassium sulphate.

The effect of potassium is noteworthy. In addition to the acceleration caused because of the nerve terminal depolarization, this ion has an additional specific action which is apparent as an increase in the slope of the relation between frequency and depolarization. This effect can be abolished by high calcium (Cooke and Quastel, 1973 b).

b) Stretch

Stretch has been found to increase the frequency (up to about three times) of miniature end-plate potentials (Fatt and Katz, 1952; Hutter and Trautwein, 1956) in frog muscle fibres. This is presumably related to the extended nerve terminal branches in this species, since the rat diaphragm, in which the nerve terminals are much more compact, does not respond to stretch in this way (Turkanis, 1973 a). How stretch works is unknown: Turkanis has found that the effect is unaffected by calcium removal.

c) Osmotic Pressure

The experimental treatment producing the most striking increase in the spontaneous release rate was reported by Fatt and Katz (1952) (see Fig. 24) to be an increase in osmotic pressure. Thus in one experiment, a 50% increase changed the rate 45-fold, from 2 to 90 per sec. This effect is not confined to the frog: Boyd and Martin (1956 a) and Liley (1956 a) observed a similar change in the cat tenuissimus and the rat diaphragm. A detailed investigation was made by Furshpan (1956) in the frog. It was found that the effect was not altered by changing the external calcium or magnesium. The direct osmotic effect in the rat diaphragm is similarly insensitive: there is, however, a second phase which *is* affected (Hubbard et al., 1968 c). No satisfactory explanation has been proposed for the osmotic effects.

d) Temperature

In the frog Fatt and Katz (1952) found that an increase from room temperature caused an increased rate of discharge with a Q_{10} of 3. In the rat diaphragm the situation is more complicated, there being a region with a negative temperature coefficient (see Liley, 1956 a; Hubbard et al., 1971).

e) Toxins and Venoms

As might be expected from so diverse a group of substances their effects are by no means uniform. Black widow spider venom (like lanthanum—see p. 303) at first causes a greatly accelerated spontaneous discharge. Only subsequently, and apparently in association with the disappearance of synaptic vesicles, does the discharge cease (CLARK et al., 1970, 1972). The snake venom β-bungarotoxin apparently produces similar effects (see review by LEE, 1972). No initial increase is seen with tetanus toxin and in a chronically poisoned muscle the frequency is less than 1 per 2 min (MELLANBY and THOMPSON, 1972). Tetrodotoxin has only a minor effect on the spontaneous rate, reducing it by about 40% (LANDAU, 1969). Tiger snake venom is of interest because in the mammal it must be applied *in vivo* to be effective, then causing a 5 to 10-fold reduction in the rate of spontaneous release (HARRIS et al., 1973). The inhibitory effect of botulinum toxin on the spontaneous release has already been discussed (p. 300).

f) Metabolic Inhibitors

The substances which for convenience have been grouped together in Table 6 A as metabolic inhibitors may act in diverse ways. Dinitrophenol has been presumed to cause the acceleration of miniature end-plate potentials by depolarization of the nerve terminals (KRAATZ and TRAUTWEIN, 1957). Although such a depolarization does occur, it may, however, not be the cause of the effect. An alternative explanation has been proposed by GLAGOLEVA et al. (1970) who have found that a number of such metabolic poisons increase the rate of spontaneous release even in the virtual absence of calcium. These substances are known to cause the release of calcium from isolated mitochondria, and GLAGOLEVA et al. suggest that they also act in this way on intact nerve terminals. The calcium ions are then supposed to "screen" the surface negative charge and promote vesicle-membrane interaction (see p. 303). It is not impossible that the cardiac glycosides (see BIRKS and COHEN, 1968 a) and a relative of dinitrophenol, the fluoro derivative of di-nitrobenzene (EDELSON and NASTUK, 1973) also increase the rate of spontaneous discharge in this way, although other explanations have been proposed. The problems involved are of considerable interest because their solution may shed light on the whole question of how quantal release is regulated (see BAKER, 1972).

g) Miscellaneous Substances which Increase the Rate of Spontaneous Discharge

Among the more striking of the effects listed in Table 6 A under this heading is that caused by the alcohols, although admittedly the concentrations required are rather high (often greater than 0.1 mol/l). Although it is usually considered that there is no osmotic component, the ascending order of effectiveness is also that of molecular size (methanol, ethanol, propanol). The effect appears to persist in the lowest calcium concentration that can be attained (QUASTEL et al., 1971) but it is nevertheless sensitive to the calcium and magnesium concentrations (OKADA, 1970). In this respect it resembles the delayed osmotic effect (see p. 304).

Another striking increase is that caused by diamide (WERMAN et al., 1971) a substance that oxidises −SH groups. Other information about spontaneous release rates has been obtained as a by-product of investigations of evoked release and will be discussed in a later section (see p. 321).

(A)

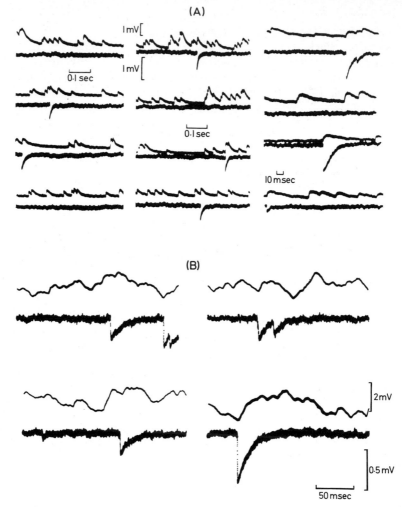

(B)

Fig. 26 A and B. Examples of miniature end-plate potentials recorded simultaneously with intracellular and extracellular electrodes (upper and lower traces respectively). Frog muscle. A: preparations in normal bathing solution, at 20° C. (From DEL CASTILLO and KATZ, 1956.) B: normal bathing solution plus 1 mmol/l lanthanum nitrate. (From HEUSER and MILEDI, 1971)

5. External Recording of Spontaneous Discharge

The miniature depolarizations caused by the spontaneous release of quanta of transmitter are of course associated with end-plate currents in the way described on pp. 245 and 272. As a result an external focal microelectrode placed sufficiently close to a receptor region will signal the action of a quantum by a transient negativity with respect to a distant reference electrode. Such signals, which have been called external miniature end-plate potentials or miniature end-plate currents, were originally recorded by FATT and KATZ (1952) at active spots of frog neuromuscular junctions, and by LILEY (1956a) in the rat diaphragm.

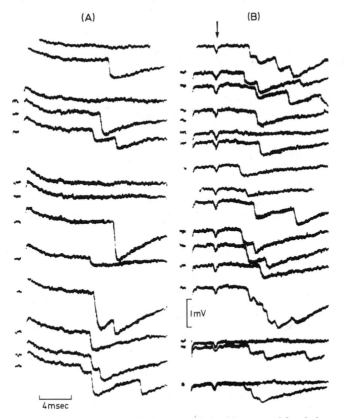

Fig. 27A and B. Responses to nerve stimulation recorded with external focal electrode from two frog muscle fibres at low temperature. Calcium was supplied only to the junctional spot from which the records were made. In B the action potential of the nerve terminal can also be seen (at arrow). (From KATZ and MILEDI, 1965d)

Table 7. Comparison between the observed number of stimuli which release different numbers of quanta and the corresponding number of stimuli predicted on the basis of the Poisson distribution: the predictions are based on a single parameter, namely, the mean number of quanta released per stimulus. (From KATZ and MILEDI, 1965d)

Number of quanta		0	1	2	3	4 or more
Experiment I	Observed number of stimuli	440	195	37	2	0
	Predicted number	448	183	37	5	1
Experiment II	Observed number of stimuli	71	57	13	6	0
	Predicted number	74	51	17	4	1
Experiment III	Observed number of stimuli	64	49	27	8	0
	Predicted number	63	54	23	7	1

A detailed study was made by DEL CASTILLO and KATZ in 1956. An approximate calculation, made on the assumption that the action of the transmitter was analogous to making a small hole in an insulating plate, suggested that the signal would not be detectable further than 20 μm from an active spot. This was in accordance with the observation that a displacement of an electrode by this distance sufficed to attenuate the external miniature end-plate potentials to the recording noise level. Since the neuromuscular junction of the frog extends over a considerable distance (the total length of the unmyelinated nerve fibres is about 600 μm—see Chapter 1), active spots may be widely separated: thus external signals with a focal electrode at a single position represent only a few percent of the total spontaneous activity. This is shown very clearly in the simultaneous external and internal records presented by DEL CASTILLO and KATZ (1956, p. 632) and reproduced in Fig. 26 A.

The method of extracellular focal recording has been much applied to the study of evoked release (see below). It has also been used to establish the nature of the depolarization caused when the frequency of the miniature end-plate potentials becomes so high that intracellular recording does not allow the individual components to be resolved. An example from the work of HEUSER and MILEDI (1971, p. 252) is shown in Fig. 26 B.

It should be mentioned that no electrical signal from the nerve terminal as distinct from the post-synaptic active spot is observed with *spontaneous* transmitter release. This contrasts with the situation during evoked release when the nerve terminal action potential can also be detected (see p. 309).

III. Evidence for the Quantal Nature of Evoked Transmitter Release

1. Intracellular Recording: Counts of "Failures"

As has already been mentioned, when the amount of transmitter released by a nerve impulse is decreased by reduction of external calcium and/or an increase in external magnesium, muscle fibre action potentials are no longer set up and individual responses consist of end-plate potentials which may vary greatly in amplitude. These fluctuations are not associated with any corresponding variation in the nerve terminal action potential (see KATZ and MILEDI, 1965 a, c, d). The analysis which demonstrated the quantal nature of evoked release was reported by DEL CASTILLO and KATZ in 1954 b. The experiments were made on neuromuscular junctions of the extensor muscle of the fourth toe of the frog. A large number of miniature end-plate potentials were recorded (with an intracellular electrode) to allow an accurate determination of their mean amplitude and its standard deviation, and then from the same muscle fibre a large number of "responses" to nerve stimuli were observed. An important point was that the concentration of calcium and magnesium had been adjusted so that a proportion of the stimuli, termed "failures", released no transmitter.

The statistical analysis was based on the hypothesis that there was a fixed population of n units each capable on the arrival of a nerve action potential of releasing a single quantum of the same kind as that released spontaneously. Whether a quantum was released from any particular unit was a matter of chance, but it was supposed that for any one junction the *average* probability (say, $\bar{p}$) of a single unit releasing a quantum remained constant from stimulus to stimulus. Evidently, the expected value for the mean number (say, m) of quanta released per stimulus is equal to $n\bar{p}$. If $\bar{p}$ is less than about 0.1 the expected proportions of stimuli which release 0 (i.e. the proportion of failures), 1, 2, 3 ... quanta are the successive terms of the Poisson distribution, namely $\exp(-m)$, $m \exp(-m)$, $(m^2/2) \exp(-m)$, $(m^3/2.3) \exp(-m)$, ... (see DEL CASTILLO and KATZ, 1954b). Now by hypothesis the value of m is given by the ratio of the mean evoked response (failures being regarded as responses of zero) to the mean amplitude of the miniature end-plate potential. Having been calculated in this way, it may be used to test for a Poisson distribution by comparing the value of $\exp(-m)$ with the proportion of failures actually observed. Excellent agreement was obtained: in ten series of nerve stimuli on six different junctions, 939 failures were predicted and 948 were observed (DEL CASTILLO and KATZ, 1954b). Similar results have been obtained from experiments on transmission at the neuromuscular junctions of the cat tenuissimus (BOYD and MARTIN 1956b) and the rat diaphragm (LILEY, 1956b).

2. Evidence from Extracellular Recording: Counts of Quanta

A further direct test of the quantal hypothesis involving only counts of quanta was reported by KATZ and MILEDI (1965d). The data were obtained by focal external recording from the frog neuromuscular junction (see p. 306). The end of the myelinated part of the motor nerve was located visually (KATZ and MILEDI, 1965a) and by trial and error the electrode was placed close to an active spot. The preparation was bathed in a solution almost devoid of calcium, but the focal electrode contained $CaCl_2$ so that calcium could be released at a convenient rate. This was adjusted so that the local concentration was just sufficient to ensure that only the small fraction of the nerve terminal in the immediate vicinity of the electrode released quanta in response to nerve stimuli. The action of each quantum was signalled in exactly the same way as external miniature end-plate potentials (see p. 308) but the response was preceded by the nerve terminal action potential (or more strictly speaking its 1st or 2nd differential coefficient — see KATZ and MILEDI, 1965a, p.465). The experiments were made at low temperature which caused the release of the quanta to be highly asynchronous and allowed them to be counted individually. Figure 27 reproduces some of KATZ and MILEDI's records, and Table 7 shows the close agreement between the observed and expected distribution.

KATZ and MILEDI point out that although the values for the number of quanta released in their experiments were small, they correspond to relatively large values (of perhaps about 40 or more) when scaled up to the whole of the presynaptic nerve terminal.

3. Amplitude Distribution of Responses

A second successful test of the quantal hypothesis using the data obtained by intracellular recording was made by DEL CASTILLO and KATZ (1954b). This was to compare the observed distribution of amplitudes of the evoked end-plate potentials with that predicted on the basis of the Poisson terms (see above) and the amplitude distribution of the miniature end-plate potentials. This test has also been applied to the neuromuscular junction of the cat tenuissimus (see BOYD and MARTIN, 1956b, where the method is described in detail) and the rat diaphragm (LILEY, 1956b).

4. Variance of the Amplitude Distribution

The third test introduced by DEL CASTILLO and KATZ was based on the equality of the mean and variance of the Poisson distribution. Thus, if the mean amplitude of the miniature end-plate potentials is $\bar{q}$ and the mean quantal content is m, the mean amplitude of the evoked response will be $m\bar{q}$ and its variance should be close to $m\bar{q}^2$, (for further details see p. 318). An estimate for m should therefore be given by dividing the square of the mean response by the variance (alternatively m may be expressed as the reciprocal of the square of the coefficient of variation). This value may then be compared with the ratio of the mean evoked response to the mean miniature end-plate potential. Good agreement was found for values of m less than about 5. For larger values of quantal contents (and hence of responses) it was necessary to take account of non-linear summation of the post-synaptic response (MARTIN, 1955; see p. 240). This test has also been applied satisfactorily to the mammalian junctions investigated (BOYD and MARTIN, 1956b; LILEY, 1956b).

5. Evidence that Fluctuations in Transmitter Release Reflect Variations in the Number of Quanta Released Rather than in the Amount of Transmitter per Quantum during Facilitation and Depression

DEL CASTILLO and KATZ's original results (1954b, c) provided strong evidence that the cause of variation in the evoked output of transmitter was the fluctuation in the number of quanta released per stimulus. Thus, at the single junction in frog muscle, the increased amplitude of the second of pairs of responses was accounted for by an increase in quantal content, as was the 10-fold increase in the amplitude of the end-plate potential during repetitive stimulation at 100 Hz (DEL CASTILLO and KATZ, 1954c). Such facilitation occurs only when the mean quantal content is depressed, for example by low calcium. In normal calcium (and magnesium) repetitive stimulation even at low rates leads to depression in quantal content. Although a quantitative analysis was not made in this situation, DEL CASTILLO and KATZ (1954c) observed that the small mean amplitude of the responses in this condition was associated with large fluctuations, indicative of a small quantal content.

A more detailed analysis of depression was made by THIES (1965) in the guinea-pig, and by ELMQVIST and QUASTEL (1965b) in human muscle preparations. The experiments were made in the presence of tubocurarine, and the results when analysed by the variance method (see p. 318) demonstrated that the decrease in end-plate potential amplitude could be accounted for by the associated decline in quantal content, at least to a first approximation. The possibility that some change might occur in the amount of transmitter per quantum cannot be entirely excluded, but any such change is likely to be small.

As far as spontaneous release is concerned, reference has already been made to the constancy of the mean amount of transmitter in the quanta responsible for the miniature end-plate potentials, in spite of changes in calcium and magnesium. Such changes which do occur in the response may be explained in terms of post-synaptic changes in sensitivity to acetylcholine (see p. 289). Although large changes in the rate of spontaneous release of quanta (see p. 321) take place during and after repetitive nerve stimulation there is no obvious change in the amplitude of the miniature end-plate potentials. A small reduction has been reported (JONES and KWANBUNBUM-

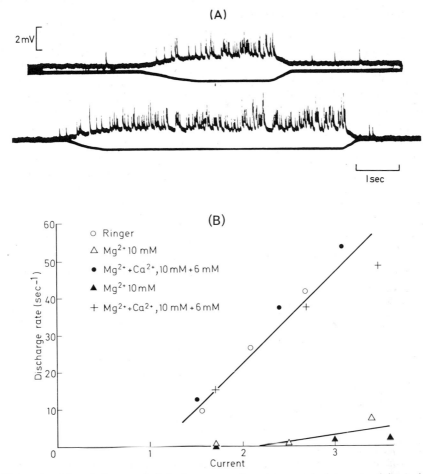

Fig. 28 A and B. Electrical control of the frequency of miniature end-plate potentials. A: in each pair of traces, the upper trace shows the miniature potentials and the lower the current flowing through the terminal part of the motor axon. The cathode was placed near the junction so as to depolarize the nerve endings as in Fig. 29 A. (From KATZ, 1969). B: the effect of calcium and magnesium. Abscissa shows relative current intensity and ordinate shows increment in discharge rate over resting value of 1 to 2 per sec. (From DEL CASTILLO and KATZ, 1954 d)

PEN, 1970 b) but only after very prolonged stimulation (e.g. 30 min at 11.3 Hz) and little is known about acetylcholine sensitivity in this condition. After less drastic stimulation, acetylcholine sensitivity is known not to be obviously depressed (OT-SUKA et al., 1962; see also p. 276).

6. Quantal Nature of Transmitter Release Evoked by Presynaptic Depolarization without Action Potentials

The discovery that there was a graded relationship between the rate of discharge of quanta and the degree of depolarization of the nerve terminals was made by DEL CASTILLO and KATZ (1954 d) in experiments on the toe muscle of the frog. The nerve terminals were depolarized by current passed through the motor nerve and the discharge of quanta was monitored by intracellular recording of miniature end-plate potentials (Fig. 28 A). As the depolarizing current was increased there was an approximately exponential increase in the frequency of miniature end-plate potentials. The effect was greatly diminished by decreasing the external calcium or by increasing magnesium (Fig. 28 B), suggesting a close connection between quantal release evoked by depolarization and by the action potential. The relationship between frequency and depolarization will be discussed further below (see p. 322).

That the essential property of the action potential for causing transmitter release was indeed the associated depolarization was established in later experiments by Katz and Miledi (1967 b). Tetrodotoxin was used to abolish the action potential and thus to allow the effect of relatively large depolarizing pulses to be investigated. Tetrodotoxin does not influence the post-synaptic effect of the transmitter, since the amplitudes of miniature end-plate potentials are unaffected by the drug (Elmqvist and Feldman, 1965a; see also p. 250). The results were completely clear cut: responses indistinguishable from those to nerve stimulation could be obtained (Fig. 29) and the amount of transmitter released was dependent on the calcium concentration.

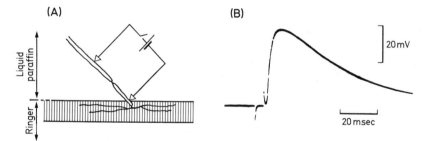

Fig. 29 A and B. Effect of nerve terminal depolarization in the presence of tetrodotoxin. A: method of producing depolarization by electrotonic spread of current; B: "end-plate potential" evoked by a brief but intense current pulse. Temperature, 1.5° C. (From Katz and Miledi, 1967 b)

Other similarities included the demonstration of facilitation, in the form of an increase in amplitude of the response to the second of pairs of pulses. This is of particular interest since in the presence of tetrodotoxin the depolarizing pulse does not give rise to the entry of sodium into the nerve terminal so that this cannot be obligatory for facilitation. The same is true for another form of facilitation, namely post-tetanic potentiation (see Table 11 for references), which has been shown by Weinreich (1971) to occur with responses to depolarizing pulses. Another conclusion which follows from these experiments (see also Martin and Pilar, 1964b), is that facilitation does not in general arise from changes in the amplitude of the presynaptic action potential (although from what follows it will be seen that a change in this would, were other factors to remain constant, give rise to changes in transmitter release). The depression in transmitter release which occurs in response to the second of two appropriately spaced nerve stimuli when the mean quantal content is high (see p. 335) can also be reproduced with depolarizing pulses in the presence of tetrodotoxin (Betz, 1970).

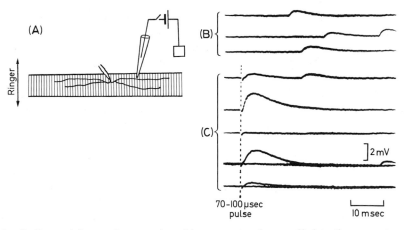

Fig. 30 A—C. Quantal fluctuations produced by current pulses applied to the nerve terminal in the presence of tetrodotoxin. A illustrates the method. B spontaneous miniature end-plate potentials. C responses to stimuli applied at time indicated by dotted line. Room temperature, Neostigmine (2.5 µg/ml) present throughout. (From KATZ and MILEDI, 1967b)

The amplitude of the response is also dependent upon the strength and duration of the pulse. With relatively weak or very short pulses, variations in the amplitudes of successive responses were observed (Fig. 30) and these were shown to be consistent with a Poisson distribution of quantal release. The effects of longer pulses are considered in a later section (p. 317).

IV. Physical and Statistical Models for Quantal Release

There is no simple relationship between the statistical characteristics of release of quanta and the underlying physical processes. DEL CASTILLO and KATZ's original suggestion (1954b) was that each junction contained a population of n units each capable of being released in response to a nerve impulse, with a probability p, which possibly differed for each unit. If $\bar{p}$ is taken as the average probability, the mean quantal content would be given by $m = n\bar{p}$. In general, if the individual values of p differ and $\bar{p}$ is relatively large (greater than 0.1 say), the exact form of the distribution cannot be predicted (but see ZUCKER, 1973, p. 806). If, however, all the p's are small, a Poisson distribution will result. If the p's were larger and equal, a binomial distribution would be followed: it may be noted that for small values of $\bar{p}$ the binomial and Poisson distributions are identical. Thus DEL CASTILLO and KATZ were able to conclude, within the framework of their model, that since a Poisson distribution was followed, the release of acetylcholine could be represented by the effect of a small probability operating on a fixed large population of release sites. These sites might currently be identified with those postulated by electron microscopists (see e.g. COUTEAUX and PÉCOT-DECHAVASSINE, 1970). Other models (see e.g. KATZ and MILEDI, 1965e) may also be envisaged which lead to what could be regarded as inherently Poissonian statistics in which the parameters n and p are indeterminate (in accordance with the fact that the Poisson distribution is completely specified by a single parameter, in this case, the mean quantal content).

Since the discovery of synaptic vesicles, attempts have been made to define n in terms of a certain fraction of the vesicles available for release, and to identify p with the probability of the release of a vesicle. It has however been pointed out that this is not necessarily compatible with the model originally proposed by DEL CASTILLO and KATZ (1954b) (see VERE-JONES, 1966; ZUCKER, 1973). Indeed, if n signifies a population of quanta available for release by the next stimulus (e.g. vesicles close to the membrane), it seems improbable that n is a constant in the relationship $m = np$. It is not unreasonable to suppose that from stimulus to stimulus n would itself be replenished according to Poissonian statistics, and then even for large values of $\bar{p}$ the release would also follow a Poisson distribution (VERE-JONES, 1966). The precise statistical properties of quantal release are therefore of considerable interest. The crux of the matter is that if Poissonian statistics govern transmitter release at all levels of output, there is no unequivocal way of separating m into n and p. Investigators are, however, faced with a number of difficulties. Direct counts of quanta released can be made only in special situations, and furthermore long runs of responses are generally required, during which the underlying parameters may change.

An indirect test of the statistics of release from the rat phrenic nerve has been made by CHRISTENSEN and MARTIN (1970). They made intracellular recordings from the rat diaphragm in the presence of tubocurarine and with two different calcium concentrations. It was assumed that the change in calcium concentration left n unaltered and affected only the value of p, changing it from p_1 say to p_2. The three parameters, n, p_1, and p_2 could then be estimated from the value of the two mean amplitudes and variances (see p.310) after appropriate corrections and on the assumption of binomial statistics (see also BENNETT and FLORIN, 1974; WERNIG, 1975).

In each of nine experiments it was found that the increase in calcium did not increase the variance by as much as would be expected on the basis of Poissonian statistics, the discrepancy being rather too large to be explained by the sources of error described below (on p.318). On the binomial assumption it appeared that the value of n was about 1000 and in 1.5 mmol/l calcium p was about 0.1. One possible interpretation is that the phrenic nerve terminal contains about 1000 release sites. This figure although rather high, is of the same general order as the number of sites suggested on other grounds (see e.g. HUBBARD and JONES, 1973) although it must be stressed that even the idea of a fixed number of sites is at present quite speculative.

Direct tests have been applied to crustacean neuromuscular junctions, where the transmitter is not acetylcholine, but probably glutamate. The most detailed investigations have been made by WERNIG (1972a, b, 1975) and by ZUCKER (1973) who have paid special attention to possible errors (see also BITTNER and HARRISON, 1970; JOHNSON and WERNIG, 1971). The experiments were made by external focal recording from active spots (see DUDEL and KUFFLER, 1961) using much the same method as that described for the frog on p.309. Long series of pairs of responses were recorded, the second having a higher quantal content than the first. The responses consisted of a number of asynchronous signals each corresponding to the release of a quantum which could thus be counted. An extract from ZUCKER's results is shown in Table 8.

The responses to the first stimulus were equally compatible with both the Poisson distribution, derived purely from the mean number of quanta per stimulus, and with the binomial distribution, derived from the mean and variance of the observed counts. The "larger" responses were inconsistent with the Poisson but compatible

Table 8. Observed and predicted distributions of quantal responses: N_0, N_1, ..., N_4 are the number of trials releasing 0, 1, ..., 4 quanta. N is the total number of trials and P is the probability of obtaining the observed responses as a sample from the predicted distribution. The predicted values have been rounded to the nearest integer. (From Table 1 of ZUCKER, 1973)

	N_0	N_1	N_2	N_3	N_4	N	P
Observed 1st stimulus	353	128	18	1	0	500	
Binomial prediction	353	128	18	1	0	500	>0.9
Poisson prediction	358	120	20	2	0	500	>0.3
Observed 2nd stimulus	267	182	47	4	0	500	
Binomial prediction	266	184	45	4	0	499	>0.3
Poisson prediction	281	162	47	9	1	500	<0.005

with the binomial distribution. ZUCKER thus concluded that, in the crayfish at least, the number of release sites is fixed, as in the original model. If this idea is generally true, n in the relationship $m = np$ becomes a constant.

One interpretation of p (see VERE-JONES, 1966) is that it is compounded of two probabilities, p_1, the probability that a release site will be occupied by a quantum between stimuli, and p_2, the probability that a nerve impulse will activate an occupied site. The relationships between the different parameters may be outlined as follows. Suppose n is the number of sites of release and that n' sites are occupied immediately before a stimulus. Immediately after a stimulus, $n' - n'p_2$ sites will be occupied and $n - (n' - n'p_2)$ will be free. At equilibrium when the mean quantal content is stable, the average rate of release must equal the average rate of refilling.

Thus, $p_1(n - n' + n'p_2) = n'p_2$

Whence,
$$n' = \frac{np_1}{p_1 + p_2 - p_1p_2}$$

(this might be regarded as the number of quanta immediately available for release, and it will vary binomially) and

$$m = n'p_2 = n\frac{p_1p_2}{p_1 + p_2 - p_1p_2}.$$

Release will thus vary binomially with parameters n and $p_1p_2/(p_1 + p_2 - p_1p_2)$.

A number of attempts have been made to estimate n and p without explicit reference to a statistical model. The underlying idea, introduced by LILEY and NORTH in 1953, is that there is a pool of readily releasable acetylcholine and the amount released by a stimulus is proportional to the size of the pool. This pool may be significantly depleted by the release caused by a single stimulus and this allows its size, the fraction released per stimulus and the rate of replenishment to be investigated. LILEY and NORTH's hypothesis was extended by ELMQVIST and QUASTEL (1965b) who identified the readily available pool with n and the release factor with p. These ideas have been regarded as almost self-evident by some workers, but it should be emphasized that a particular model is in question (see HUBBARD et al., 1969,

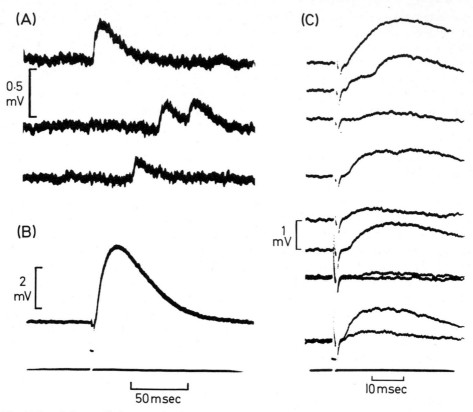

Fig. 31 A—C. Intracellular records of spontaneous and evoked release at the frog neuromuscular junction in isotonic calcium chloride. A: spontaneous activity; B: response to brief focal pulse applied to the nerve terminal; C: quantal fluctuations in the responses to successive applications of such a pulse monitored on the lower traces. (From KATZ and MILEDI, 1969 b)

pp. 143—158), and that it is quite speculative (see e.g. KUNO, 1971; CHRISTENSEN and MARTIN, 1970; BETZ, 1970). Calculation of the pool size and release fraction depends on the way responses evoked during repetitive nerve stimulation vary, and will be discussed later (p. 338).

V. The Calcium Hypothesis

It has already been mentioned that KATZ and MILEDI (1969 b) have shown that spontaneous miniature end-plate potentials, although of reduced amplitude, can be recorded in a solution containing mainly calcium chloride (83 mmol/l, with the usual concentration of potassium chloride, 2 mmol/l). Under these conditions quantal release can also be evoked by focally applied depolarizing pulses (Fig. 31). It seems therefore that the primary requirement for the release of transmitter by nerve terminal depolarization is the presence of calcium.

Other evidence has suggested that the external calcium is necessary because its entry into the nerve terminal plays an important part in the release process. The main experiments on which this idea rests have been made not on neuromuscular junctions but on the giant synapse in the stellate ganglion of the squid (KATZ and MILEDI, 1967e, 1969a, 1971; MILEDI, 1973), where it is possible not only to record intracellularly from the presynaptic terminals but also to alter their internal composition. An important finding which suggests the importance of calcium entry into the terminal (or at least the membrane) is that a large depolarizing pulse causes quantal release to occur with a *longer* latency (measured from the start of the pulse) the *longer* the duration of the pulse. This can be explained by supposing that such pulses displace the membrane potential of the nerve terminal to beyond the equilibrium potential for calcium and, therefore, hinder its entry during the pulse (KATZ and MILEDI, 1967c).

In the same experiments transmitter release was seen to rise in a steep and non-linear manner as the duration of a depolarizing pulse of constant amplitude was increased. This could be explained as the consequence of two different processes (KATZ and MILEDI, 1968a). (1) It is assumed that the calcium permeability, P_{Ca}, increases with depolarization but does not reach its final value instantaneously. At the end of the pulse, P_{Ca} immediately starts to fall. Thus the total calcium entry will be disproportionately small for shorter pulses. (2) It is also supposed that transmitter output is related to the calcium entry raised to some power greater than one. Thus the effect of (1) will be magnified. The second assumption would also help to explain the non-linear relationships between the output of transmitter and (a) the amplitude of pulses of constant duration and (b) the external concentration of calcium. This is discussed further in Section VII.

VI. Estimating Values of the Quantal Content

1. Methods

Experiments of the type that have established the quantal nature of transmitter release have also been made in order to estimate quantal content under different conditions, often with the aim of testing the action of various procedures and agents on evoked quantal release (see p. 324).

a) The Direct Method

The most direct method is to determine the quantal content by dividing the mean amplitude of the evoked response, $\bar{v}$, by that of the miniature end-plate potential, $\bar{q}$. If $\bar{v}$ is more than a small fraction of the resting potential, it is necessary to correct for "non-linear summation" (see p. 240). Each response may be separately corrected or alternatively, the formula:

$$m = \frac{\bar{v}}{\bar{q}} \frac{V_0 + \bar{q}}{V_0 - \bar{v}}$$

where V_0 is the difference between the membrane potential and the transmitter equilibrium potential (see p. 237), may be applied directly to the mean of the observed evoked responses (see HUBBARD et al., 1969, p. 135).

Use of the method also involves the assumption that the quanta produce synchronous post-synaptic effects (see SOUČEK, 1971).

b) Counts of Failures

The method of counting failures is useful where miniature end-plate potentials occur infrequently, where the transmitter equilibrium potential is not known, or where the release may be asynchronous. If m is the average quantal content, the expected proportion of failures is e^{-m}. The method is equivalent to estimating the "concentration" of red cells by counting the proportion of empty haemocytometer squares, or that of live organisms in a fluid by counting the proportion of sterile samples drawn. The precision of such estimates was discussed by R. A. Fisher in the book "Design of Experiments". His calculations show that with an optimal proportion of failures (i.e. between 0.1 and 0.3) the response to about 170 stimuli would have to be observed in order to reduce the standard error of m to about 10 per cent (see also Hubbard et al., 1969, p. 138 et seq.).

c) The Variance Method

The "failure method" is unsuitable for measuring quantal contents above about 3 (the proportion of failures is then less than 5 per cent and subject to large sampling error) and neither it, nor the direct method, can be used in the presence of blocking agents that severely reduce the amplitude of the miniature end-plate potentials. For large quantal contents (since they must in general be estimated in the presence of such a blocking agent because of the need to abolish the action potential and twitch of the muscle) only the "variance method" is available. It should be pointed out that this method is extremely imprecise unless applied to fairly long runs of results. Thus the standard error of m estimated from 50 amplitudes is 20% (see Appendix by Brown to Edwards and Ikeda, 1962, and that by Cormack to Reid, 1972). However, in long runs there is often a systematic change in the amplitude of the response, and this frequently prevents attempts to gain precision (see Reid, 1972).

Apart from this difficulty, there is a particularly vexatious source of systematic error. The calculation of m is made by dividing the square of the mean amplitude by the variance. However, the proper value of the variance is not the observed value but only that component due to the statistical fluctuations in the number of quanta that different stimuli release. Thus from the measured variance must be subtracted not only the variance due to the fluctuations in the responses to single quanta but also that due to recording noise. This latter is usually neglected, but it becomes increasingly important as the mean amplitude is reduced and the signal to noise ratio falls. The result of this is that an agent which has a post-synaptic blocking action may also appear to cause a reduction in transmitter output, and vice versa.

The method of calculation is as follows: if the individual values of the responses are adjusted for non-linear summation (see p. 240) before the mean and variance are computed, the value of m is given by:

$$m = \frac{\bar{v}^2}{\mathrm{var}(v) - \mathrm{var(noise)}} \left(1 + \frac{\sigma^2}{\bar{q}^2}\right).$$

The term in brackets, in which σ^2 is the variance of the miniature endplate potentials, provides the adjustment for fluctuation in response to a single quantum. The original data may also be used, in which case the right hand side of the equation must be multiplied by an extra factor, $(1 - \bar{v}/V_0)^2$, to adjust for non-linear summation (see HUBBARD et al., 1969, p. 135). These expressions are based on the assumption that the release is governed by Poissonian statistics (see pp. 308—309, 313—314).

Where it is possible to record both miniature end-plate potentials and evoked responses, but the direct method cannot be used because the transmitter equilibrium potential is unknown, it is possible to estimate m from the expression:

$$m^3 = \frac{\bar{v}^4(1 + \sigma^2/\bar{q}^2)}{\bar{q}^2 [\mathrm{var}(v) - \mathrm{var}(\mathrm{noise})]}$$

(see MARTIN, 1966; HUBBARD et al., 1969, p. 142).

2. Estimates of Normal Quantal Contents

a) Frog

An approximate value for the number of quanta released by a nerve impulse may be obtained as follows. In sartorius muscle fibres of the frog, with a resting potential of about -90 mV and a transmitter equilibrium potential of about -15 mV, the end-plate potential step corresponds to a depolarization of about 50 mV. Miniature end-plate potentials are about 0.5 mV. Thus applying Martin's correction for non-linear summation (p. 240), the quantal content is about:

$$\frac{-15 - (-90) - 0.5}{-15 - (-90) - 50} \cdot \frac{50}{0.5}, \qquad \simeq 300 .$$

The quantal content of the end-plate potentials in the fourth toe muscle of the frog, in the presence of tubocurarine, was estimated by MARTIN (1955) using the variance method (see p. 318). It will be recalled that the assumption that release follows Poissonian statistics is involved. This will result in an overestimate if release is, in fact, binomial. Experiments on six different fibres gave values of 95, 240, 107, 64, 80, and 106 respectively. Another estimate (TAKEUCHI and TAKEUCHI, 1960) of between 90 and 150 has been made from the ratio of the end-plate current, as measured in voltage clamp experiments, to the miniature end-plate current.

b) Mammal

The variance method has been used on curarized muscles from several mammalian species. BOYD and MARTIN (1956b) obtained values of 220 and 310 quanta for two junctions in the cat tenuissimus. For the rat diaphragm, HUBBARD et al. (1968b) found a mean of 201 (14 experiments); for the guinea-pig serratus anterior, REID (1972) obtained a mean of 156 (13 experiments) and in human muscle, ELMQVIST and QUASTEL (1965b) reported a mean of 100 (26 junctions).

This last result was obtained by a modification of the variance method. The procedure was to evoke a sequence of responses in rapid succession: their amplitudes first decline but eventually reach a relatively steady level. The variance method is then applied to obtain an estimate of the unit response, and the quantal content of the first response of the tetanus is calculated by dividing its amplitude by q. In addition to the sources of error of the standard variance method, there is the further hazard of assuming prematurely that a steady state of quantal release has been reached. The effect of such an error will be to underestimate the quantal content.

3. Errors in Quantal Content Estimates in the Presence of Drugs

a) Possible Effects of Tubocurarine on Quantal Content

The possibility that tubocurarine depresses the quantal content has not yet been excluded but the evidence for such an effect is not at present compelling. Using the "cut" fibre preparation of the rat diaphragm (see below) HUBBARD and WILSON (1973) have reported that 0.5 µmol/l tubocurarine reduces the mean quantal content from a control value of 237 to 165 for the first response of a tetanus whereas BLABER (1973) described an increase from 363 to 617 in comparable experiments on "cut" fibre preparations of the cat tenuissimus with a similar concentration of tubocurarine (0.72 µmol/l). In the frog, MARTIN (1955) and AUERBACH and BETZ (1971) have concluded that tubocurarine in low concentrations does not reduce the quantal content. References to the rather extensive and controversial literature on the possibility that tubocurarine reduces transmitter output will be found in HUBBARD and WILSON's paper. All that can be said here is that in principle there is no reason why such an effect should not occur, but that it is doubtful if any method for measuring large quantal contents is at present sufficiently precise to demonstrate a relatively small presynaptic effect in the face of a concurrent larger post-synaptic effect. The uncertainty is caused by the limited accuracy of the variance method (see p. 318).

b) Possible Effect of Anticholinesterases

When quantal contents are to be determined either by the direct method or by the counting of failures, an anticholinesterase is frequently added to the bath to enhance the amplitudes of both the miniature end-plate potentials and small evoked responses. Attention has recently been paid to the possibility that these substances also affect quantal content. One approach examined by BLABER and CHRIST (1967) was to compare the effect of various cholinesterase inhibitors on miniature end-plate potentials, recorded from cat tenuissimus muscle fibres, with that on evoked end-plate potentials from similar preparations treated with tubocurarine. Several substances increased the evoked responses (although only by small amounts) in concentrations that had little or no effect on the miniature end-plate potentials. This result could be explained by a small increase in quantal content, as BLABER and CHRIST suggest, or perhaps by a post-synaptic interaction between the drugs and tubocurarine. Greater concentrations of the inhibitors caused both the spontaneous and the evoked responses to become larger.

It should be pointed out that there is no necessary link between any effect on quantal content and the action of anticholinesterases in inducing repetitive action potentials in the nerve terminals (MASLAND and WIGTON, 1940) in the absence of tubocurarine. Indeed, some other drugs (e.g. germine acetate) can cause repetitive firing without any change in quantal content or spontaneous release (e.g. DETWILER, 1972).

c) Cut-fibre Preparations

To avoid the need to use a blocking agent in order to abolish the muscle action potential and twitch and reveal the end-plate potentials, the procedure of cutting the muscle (BARSTAD, 1962; BARSTAD and LILLEHEIL, 1968) has been used. The resting potential in such preparations deteriorates continuously and may be as low as – 17 mV (HUBBARD and WILSON, 1973). It is difficult to correct accurately for non-linear summation in this situation: in particular, the "corrected" larger end-plate potentials may be underestimations. Also it is not entirely clear that pre-synaptic function is normal since the usual concentration of potassium for mammalian bathing solutions (5 mmol/l) sometimes induces nerve block in the cut fibre rat diaphragm (RANDIĆ and STRAUGHAN, 1964). A cut fibre preparation of the tenuissimus muscle has also been described, in which higher values for the resting potential have been reported (see e.g. BLABER, 1973).

VII. Studies on Evoked Release of Transmitter

1. Methods of Evoking Release

In general, three different ways of evoking transmitter release have been used, namely (1) nerve stimulation (2) electrical depolarization of the nerve terminals (see also p. 316) and (3) nerve terminal depolarization with high external potassium.

a) Nerve Stimulation

It has already been noted that the essential property of the action potential in causing the release of transmitter is the associated depolarization of the nerve terminal. However, it is interesting that when the action potential in the frog nerve terminals is blocked by locally applied tetrodotoxin, the electrotonic depolarization which remains is not sufficient to cause transmitter release (KATZ and MILEDI, 1968b). Thus, the "safety factor" as far as depolarization is concerned cannot be very great. Similar experiments have not been made in the more compact mammalian junction although there is evidence that in the rat diaphragm the action potential invades the whole of the phrenic nerve terminal (HUBBARD and SCHMIDT, 1963) just as it does in the frog (KATZ and MILEDI, 1965a).

An increased rate of transmitter release also occur not only as the "immediate" result of nerve activity (disregarding the latency), but for a prolonged period afterwards, in the form of an enhanced frequency of miniature end-plate potentials. This is most readily seen after repetitive stimulation at rates greater than 1 per second (DEL CASTILLO and KATZ, 1954c; BROOKS, 1956; LILEY, 1956a; HUBBARD, 1963; MILEDI and THIES, 1971; HARRIS and MILEDI, 1971; HURLBUT et al., 1971; GINS-BORG and HIRST, 1972; BARRETT and STEVENS, 1972b). However, as was first reported by Liley there is also a significant increase in the frequency of miniature end-plate potentials even after a single stimulus (LILEY, 1956a; DODGE et al., 1969; RAHA-MIMOFF and YAARI, 1973). The effect provides a useful "diagnostic" test of treatments (e.g., substitution of magnesium for calcium) which abolish ordinary evoked release.

If repetitive nerve stimulation still increases the rate of miniature end-plate potentials it is evident that the motor nerve terminal has remained excitable (see e.g. HURLBUT et al., 1971).

When using the response to nerve stimulation to assess the effect of an agent on the mechanism of transmitter release, several points must be kept in mind.

1) In general it will be necessary to interfere with neuromuscular transmission to obtain end-plate potentials rather than action potentials and twitches in response to nerve stimulation. If, for example, this is done by bathing the preparation in a medium containing low calcium, so that the quantal content is reduced, it can always be argued that an agent which manifests some effect (or fails to do so) would have a different effect if the control quantal content was normal. On the other hand if a post-synaptic blocking drug such as tubocurarine is used to provide the control end-plate potentials, an agent might appear to have an effect on transmitter release (demonstrated, for example, as an increase in amplitude of the evoked end-plate potential without any effect on miniature end-plate potentials) when its effect could in reality be due to an interaction between the agent and the curare-like substance (see e.g. FERRY and MARSHALL, 1973, and p.285).

2) There appears to be some limitation to the number of quanta that a nerve stimulus can release. This is often attributed to the existence of a limited "store" of immediately available quanta although other explanations (such as a fixed number of release sites) can be envisaged. Whatever the cause, the result is that only if the control quantal content is below this maximal level can increases in release be demonstrated.

3) An agent which makes the motor nerve or its terminal inexcitable, for example tetrodotoxin, will abolish transmitter release although it may not have any fundamental effect on release processes.

Less drastic alterations in the action potential may also change the amount of transmitter released. For this reason effects are often tested on release evoked in ways other than by nerve stimulation.

b) Depolarization by Current

The acceleration of miniature end-plate potentials by current-induced depolarization of the nerve terminals has been repeatedly studied since the discovery of the effect by DEL CASTILLO and KATZ (1954d). Various modifications of the basic method have been described by LILEY (1956c), HUBBARD and WILLIS (1962), KATZ and MILEDI (1967b, c) and LANDAU (1969). In an investigation of the time course of the effect, COOKE and QUASTEL (1973a, b) have found that there is an immediate increase in frequency followed by a more slowly developing and generally less striking rise (see also KATZ and MILEDI, 1967b, p.13). The fast effect is abolished if the calcium concentration is reduced below about 10^{-10} mol/l. At the end of a depolarization, the miniature end-plate potential frequency does not revert to the control value immediately: COOKE and QUASTEL argue that the after-discharge is the counterpart of the slow phase observed at the onset, and that both are reflections of the processes that underlie not only the post nerve-stimulation effect described in the previous section but also facilitation and post-tetanic potentiation (see p.335).

c) High Potassium

This method was introduced by LILEY (1956c) who found that the frequency of miniature end-plate potentials recorded from fibres of the rat diaphragm increased with the fourth power of the potassium concentration over the range 10 to 30 mmol/l (see also KATZ, 1962, p.470): at 30 mmol/l potassium the frequency was greater than 700 per second. On the assumption that potassium acts primarily by depolarizing the nerve terminals, Liley concluded that the frequency rose exponentially with depolarization, to the extent that there was a hundred-fold increase for a 30 mV depolarization.

Liley also pointed out that if the relationship was extrapolated, the depolarization associated with the action potential would be predicted to cause a very large increase in frequency: so much so, in fact, that the "phasic" quantal release caused by an action potential might just represent the instantaneous frequency versus depolarization relationship integrated over the action potential. Further evidence, some of which has already been described (see p.317) has now ruled out this idea. The essential contrary finding is that there is a considerable latency between the release of transmitter and the depolarization (KATZ and MILEDI, 1965b, d, 1967a, b, d).

It may also be mentioned that there is some evidence to suggest that the effect of potassium is not entirely due to the depolarization it causes (p.304).

2. Relationship between the Various Methods of Evoking Release

Other procedures (e.g. increasing the osmotic pressure) which do not involve depolarization of the nerve terminals have also been used to provide a relatively rapid "background" discharge against which various agents can be tested.

This raises the more general question of whether the different methods of evoking quantal release act via a common mechanism. In interpreting their findings that spontaneous quantal release and its acceleration by hyperpolarization of the nerve terminals ("anodic breakdown") were insensitive to changes in calcium and magnesium, in marked contrast to release evoked by depolarization, DEL CASTILLO and KATZ (1954d, p.602) suggested that two separate processes which converged on a final common pathway were involved. A modified version of this idea is that the various procedures that evoke release all reduce the energy required for a quantum to leave the terminal by additive amounts. The contribution made by depolarization is generally held to be a function of calcium concentration, whereas other agents act independently of it (QUASTEL et al., 1971; COOKE et al., 1973). It might be expected on this basis that the various agents should have multiplicative effects when acting simultaneously, but this is not the case. However, the hypothesis can be preserved by supposing that the contribution made by one agent or treatment may be a function of the intensity of other simultaneous treatments. Thus the less than multiplicative effect of an increase in osmotic pressure and nerve stimulation might be accounted for within the hypothesis by the fact that the effect of depolarization is related inversely to the osmotic pressure (COOKE et al., 1973).

The observed interactions can also be explained in terms of the calcium hypothesis (see p.316) by supposing (a) that most if not all procedures which increase quantal release do so by increasing the concentration of calcium (or strontium) at some strategic site within the nerve terminal and (b), that the rate of release is some steep function of this concentration (see also p. 317).

VIII. Factors Affecting Evoked Transmitter Release

1. Calcium and Magnesium

The importance of calcium in evoked transmitter release has already been mentioned (see pp. 296, 316). As noted, most forms of evoked release are abolished in the absence of this ion. Conversely, by raising the external calcium from its normal level, the quantal content can be increased about 3-fold (see e.g. ELMQVIST and QUASTEL, 1965b).

The quantitative relationship between the amplitude of the evoked end-plate potential and the external calcium and magnesium concentrations was investigated by JENKINSON (1957) with extracellular recordings (see p. 230) at the neuromuscular junction of frog muscle (see Fig. 32). More detailed studies based on intracellular recordings have since been made in the frog (DODGE and RAHAMIMOFF, 1967), rat

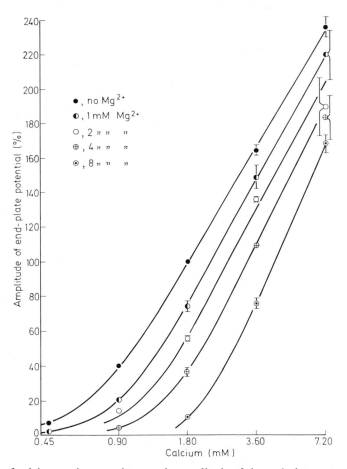

Fig. 32. Effect of calcium and magnesium on the amplitude of the end-plate potential recorded externally from a frog sartorius muscle in tubocurarine. Abscissa: calcium concentration on logarithmic scale. Ordinate: amplitude of end-plate potential as a percentage of that in normal fluid (Ca 1.8 mmol/l, no Mg). (From JENKINSON, 1957)

(HUBBARD et al., 1968 b) and mouse (COOKE, et al., 1973). The general finding is that release rises steeply with increasing calcium (note the logarithmic abscissa in Fig. 32) and varies with the magnesium concentration in a way suggesting simple competition between these two divalent ions. The results were consistent with the suggestion by DEL CASTILLO and KATZ (1954 d) that transmitter release was a function of a concentration of a complex, CaX, between calcium and a membrane component X, and that the complex MgX could also be formed but had no effect on transmitter release. Thus the amplitude of the end-plate potential (v) could be described by:

$$v = f \left(\frac{K_1[Ca]}{1 + K_1[Ca] + K_2[Mg]} \right)$$

where K_1 and K_2 are affinity constants. K_1 is difficult to estimate since the exact form of the function f is unknown, but K_2, the affinity constant for the formation of MgX in the reaction $Mg + X \rightleftharpoons MgX$, could be determined by applying Eq.(24) (p. 281). A value of about $0.25 \, \text{mM}^{-1}$ was derived from the measurements plotted in Fig. 32.

DODGE and RAHAMIMOFF analysed similar results obtained with intracellular electrodes with the aim of determining the particular function of CaX on which release depended. They concluded that a fourth power relationship held between the amplitude of the end-plate potential and the concentration of CaX, and suggested that this implied that 4 calcium ions "co-operated" in some way in the release of a quantum. Thus their results could be fitted by the expression:

$$v = A \left(\frac{K_1[Ca]}{1 + K_1[Ca] + K_2[Mg]} \right)^4$$

where A is a constant. Estimates for the affinity constants of MgX and CaX were about 0.3 and $1 \, \text{mM}^{-1}$ respectively.

Corresponding results obtained with the rat diaphragm (HUBBARD et al., 1968b) have been interpreted more elaborately, in an attempt to find a single relationship which would encompass not only evoked responses but also the effects of calcium and magnesium on spontaneous release in this preparation (HUBBARD et al., 1968a). In order to relate quantal content and frequencies of miniature end-plate potentials it was assumed that a given quantal content, m, was equivalent to a frequency corresponding to the release of m quanta in 1/1600 of a second. In order to fit their results, HUBBARD et al. also assumed the existence of complexes CaX, Ca_2X, Ca_3X, MgX, Mg_2X, and Mg_3X and that together with X itself, all these complexes except MgX and Mg_2X contributed in various degrees to release. While a close fit to the data could be obtained in this way the rather large number of disposable parameters invoked emphasises the need for more direct evidence and suggests that the relationship is at present best regarded as empirical. For high release rates produced either by electrical depolarization, by high potassium (see p. 323 and LANDAU, 1969) or by nerve stimulation, it was assumed that Ca_3X overwhelmingly predominated so that the results could also be interpreted in terms of DODGE and RAHAMIMOFF's concept of co-operativity with the requisite number of calcium ions for evoked quantal release being 3 rather than 4.

The analysis by COOKE et al., (1973) is based on the results obtained from a more detailed study of the effects of graded electrical and "high potassium" depolarizations of the nerve terminals on the frequency of miniature end-plate potentials (COOKE and QUASTEL, 1973a, b, c). After various complications were taken into account, the relationship between the rate of release of quanta and the external concentration of calcium could be fitted by the exponential function of an expression involving three affinity constants and a function of depolarization. As already mentioned on p. 323, this was interpreted on the basis that the probability of release was multiplicatively raised by the presence at particular intracellular sites of each of possibly several molecules of a complex, CaX, and that the intracellular calcium concentration was raised by transport across the membrane of a species Ca_2Y.

A brief description of the underlying theory may be helpful. Suppose that N sites exist and M "molecules" of CaX are distributed between them, the average being $\lambda, = M/N$. Some of the N sites, n_0 say, will be occupied by no molecule at all, and others $n_1, n_2, n_3 \ldots$ will have $1, 2, 3 \ldots$ molecules. If there are no interactions, $n_0, n_1, n_2 \ldots$ will be proportional to the successive terms of the Poisson distribution $\exp(-\lambda), \lambda \exp(-\lambda), \dfrac{\lambda^2}{2} \exp(-\lambda) \ldots$. It is also assumed that the presence of each CaX complex reduces the activation energy required for the release probability by a constant factor $r\{=\exp(\Delta u/RT)\}$. Thus considering all the N sites, if f_0 is the release rate per site in the absence of CaX, then the release rate, F, in its presence is given by:

$$F = n_0 f_0 + n_1 f_0 r + n_2 f_0 r^2 + n_3 f_0 r^3 + \cdots$$

$$= N f_0 \exp(-\lambda) \left\{ 1 + r\lambda + \frac{r^2 \lambda^2}{2} + \frac{r^3 \lambda^3}{2.3} + \cdots \right\}$$

$$= N f_0 \exp\{\lambda(r-1)\}.$$

Since λ is proportional to $[CaX]$,

$$F = N f_0 \exp(a_1 [CaX])$$

This may also be written as:

$$\log F = a_0 + a_1 [CaX] \tag{32}$$

where $a_0 (= \log N f_0)$ and a_1 are constants.

The concentration of CaX is derived as follows.

Let the total concentration of X (assumed to be inside the nerve terminal) be $[X]_T$ and the internal concentration of free calcium be $[Ca]_1$. If the affinity constant of Ca for X is K_3 $\left(\text{i.e. } K_3 = \dfrac{[CaX]}{[Ca][X]} \right)$, the concentration of CaX will be given by

$$[CaX] = \frac{K_3 [Ca]_1 [X]_T}{1 + K_3 [Ca]_1} \tag{33}$$

The internal free calcium concentration is supposed to depend upon the product of the concentration of a compound Ca_2Y and the value v of a function of the membrane potential. Thus

$$[Ca]_1 = v [Ca_2 Y]$$

If the affinity constants for the formation of CaY and Ca_2Y are K_1 and K_2 $\left(\text{i.e. } K_1 = \dfrac{[CaY]}{[Ca][Y]}\right.$
and $K_2 = \dfrac{[Ca_2Y]}{[CaY][Ca]}\left.\right)$ then

$$[Ca_2Y] = \frac{K_1 K_2 [Ca]^2 [Y]_T}{1 + K_1[Ca] + K_1 K_2 [Ca]^2} \tag{34}$$

where $[Ca]$ is the external concentration. Combining Eqs. (33) and (34) gives:

$$[CaX] = \frac{[X]_T [Y]_T}{[Y]_T + 1/K_3 v} \cdot \frac{1}{1 + \dfrac{1}{K}\left\{\dfrac{1}{[Ca]^2} + \dfrac{K_1}{[Ca]}\right\}}$$

where $K = K_1 K_2 (K_3 v [Y]_T + 1)$.
Finally Eq. (32) becomes, in the notation of COOKE et al.

$$\log F = \alpha_0 + \frac{\beta}{1 + \gamma^2 \left\{\dfrac{1}{[Ca]^2} + \dfrac{\varepsilon}{[Ca]}\right\}}$$

where $\alpha_0 = a_0$, $\gamma^2 = 1/K$, $\varepsilon = K_1$, and $\beta = \dfrac{v[X]_T [Y]_T}{v[Y]_T + 1/K_3}$

Magnesium is assumed to compete with calcium for both X and Y.

The main advantage claimed by COOKE et al. for their interpretation over the co-operative model discussed on p. 325 is that the latter does not fit the entire range of data unless it is assumed that the number of CaX complexes required for release varies with the depolarization, being less than 4 for small depolarizations. However, this is not an impossibility, and it seems likely that to distinguish between various models which predict similarly shaped relationships between release rates and external calcium concentration will be extremely difficult.

There is one form of "evoked release" which does not appear to be dependent on calcium. This is the discharge of quanta which occurs during fast repetitive nerve stimulation in virtually calcium-free solution and which is not synchronised to the stimuli. The phenomenon has been found both in the frog (MILEDI and THIES, 1971; BLIOCH et al., 1968; HURLBUT et al., 1971), and in the rat (GINSBORG and HIRST, 1972). MILEDI and THIES, who made the original findings, concluded that the possibility remained that the discharge did depend on calcium accumulation from the external solution, in spite of its low concentration there. The subsequent work of HURLBUT et al. has reduced this likelihood since they found that the effect was not diminished by the addition of a calcium-chelating agent, provided the magnesium concentration was sufficient. Calcium entry would have been seriously reduced by this procedure. The explanation is uncertain, but it is possible that as with spontaneous release (see p. 303), magnesium has the properties of a very weak partial agonist in the release process (cf. BLIOCH et al., 1968).

It has already been pointed out that the actions of calcium and magnesium are mutually antagonistic on the release evoked by depolarizing pulses (p. 312), graded depolarizations (p. 326) and high potassium (p. 326).

At very low concentrations of calcium (less than 0.1 mmol/l), the evoked release of acetylcholine appears to be linearly related to the calcium concentration rather than to its third or fourth power (Crawford, 1974).

Substitutes for Calcium. It was shown by Miledi (1966) that of the ions Cs^+, Ba^{2+}, Ni^{2+}, Co^{2+}, Ce^{3+}, Cu^{2+}, Mn^{2+}, Zn^{2+}, La^{3+}, and Sr^{2+} only Sr^{2+} shared the action of Ca^{2+} in allowing the nerve impulse to release transmitter. The experiments were made by recording focally from frog nerve terminals (Fig. 33) with extracellular electrodes filled with the ions under investigation, the preparation being bathed in a solution virtually free of calcium (see p. 309). Barium occasionally allowed release, but its effect was not consistent and it is possible that it acts indirectly by displacing calcium from the membrane.

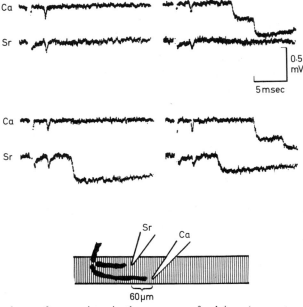

Fig. 33. Quantal release of transmitter in the presence of calcium (upper traces) and strontium (lower traces). Simultaneous extracellular focal recording from two synaptic spots of the same end-plate during a small steady efflux of the divalent ions at 5° C. The diagram shows the position of the two electrodes and their relation to the most distal myelinated segments of the nerve fibre. (From Dodge et al., 1969)

More detailed studies made by Dodge et al. (1969) showed that at low quantal contents, release of acetylcholine in the presence of strontium followed Poissonian statistics in the usual way. In curarized frog muscle (2.5 µmol/l tubocurarine) in solutions with the normal concentration of calcium (1.8 mmol/l) the addition of 2 mmol/l strontium reduced the quantal content of the end-plate potential to about half its control value (Meiri and Rahamimoff, 1972). In general, in the presence of both calcium and strontium, the quantal content, m, could be predicted from the "co-operative model" (see p. 325) on the assumption that both species, SrX and CaX, participate in allowing transmitter release, SrX being less effective. Thus in pharmacological terms strontium has a lower efficacy (see p. 267).

In the presence of calcium, strontium and magnesium the results were fitted by

$$m = A \left(\frac{\beta K_3 [\text{Sr}] + K_1 [\text{Ca}]}{1 + K_3 [\text{Sr}] + K_1 [\text{Ca}] + K_2 [\text{Mg}]} \right)^4 .$$

The relative effectiveness, β, of $\text{Sr}X$ was estimated as about 0.4, and K_3, the affinity constant for $\text{Sr}X$, as about 0.6 mM^{-1}, which is of the same order as that for $\text{Ca}X$.

2. Non-Specific Factors Affecting Evoked Release

a) Stretch

Stretch, which increases the rate of spontaneous release in the frog, but not in the rat (see p. 304), has the same differential effect on evoked release. Furthermore both spontaneous and evoked release in the frog are multiplied by about the same factor, i.e. between 2 and 3, for an increase of about 25% in sarcomere length (HUTTER and TRAUTWEIN, 1956; TURKANIS, 1973a).

b) Osmotic Pressure

Increase in osmotic pressure, which causes such a striking enhancement of spontaneous release (see p. 304) has only a small effect on release evoked by nerve stimulation, both in the frog (FURSHPAN, 1956) and in the rat (HUBBARD et al., 1968c) in which the effect has been studied in the greatest detail. As might be expected, release evoked by applied current or high potassium is also not particularly sensitive to osmotic changes (see also QUASTEL et al., 1971). If the osmotic pressure is raised beyond a critical value (see HUBBARD et al., 1968c, for references), evoked release is diminished and eventually abolished.

c) Temperature

A detailed study of the effect of temperature has been made by HUBBARD et al. (1971). The most striking finding (see also HOFMANN et al., 1966) is that although an increase in temperature between 30 and 37° C leads to an increased rate of spontaneous release, evoked release is reduced.

d) Size of End-Plate

In the frog KUNO, TURKANIS and WEAKLY (1971) have found that in a "standard" bathing solution there is a correlation between the size of the end-plate, the rate of spontaneous release and the evoked quantal content of the end-plate potential. This finding is consistent with the idea that there are particular sites along the terminal branch of the motor nerve from which release occurs (see COUTEAUX and PÉCOT-DECHAVASSINE, 1970). These would naturally be more numerous the longer the terminal branches. The closest correlation is between spontaneous and evoked release: this is also true for neuromuscular junctions of the rat as noted by LILEY (1956c).

e) Depolarization

Nerve terminal depolarization induced by externally applied current (for the effect of potassium see p.323) causes a fall in the amount of transmitter released by nerve stimulation both in the frog (Vladimirova, 1963) and the rat (Hubbard and Willis, 1968). The explanation is uncertain: it is possible that the reduction results from a diminution in the nerve terminal action potential. However, the effect of depolarization can be reduced both by a preceding hyperpolarization and by an increase of magnesium, and neither of these would be likely to affect the change in the nerve terminal action potential caused by the depolarization. This does not rule out a reduction of the action potential amplitude as a contributing factor since preceding hyperpolarization and magnesium might be acting at other stages of the release process. Thus it is conceivable that in high magnesium the amount of transmitter released by a nerve impulse is less sensitive to the amplitude of the nerve terminal action potential.

f) Hyperpolarization

Del Castillo and Katz (1954d) showed that the quantal content of the end-plate potential in the frog was increased both during and after hyperpolarization of the nerve terminal. A detailed study in the curarized rat diaphragm was made by Hubbard and Willis (1962) who reported increases (by a factor as great as 20) as a result of hyperpolarizations lasting about 30 sec. The quantal content of the enhanced end-plate potentials must have been of the order of several thousand. Prolonged hyperpolarization thus seems to be the most potent agent so far discovered affecting evoked transmitter release: its mode of action is completely unknown.

3. Agents which Increase Evoked Transmitter Release

Investigations of agents which increase the evoked release of transmitter are set out in Table 9. The effect of potassium is presumably specific, while that of sodium reduction appears to be due to the fact that sodium competes with calcium in some way (see Colomo and Rahamimoff, 1968). However this competition is neither straight-forward nor specific to sodium. Thus, when sodium is replaced with other monovalent cations the *immediate* effect is a reduction in quantal content (Onodera and Yamakawa, 1966; Kelly, 1968) presumably because removal of sodium reduces the nerve terminal action potential. At calcium concentrations above about 1 mmol/l, replacement of extracellular sodium by sucrose (or glycine) no longer increases the quantal content: the effect of the reduction in the amplitude of the action potential appears thus to have become more important than the reduction of the competitive effect of sodium. The frequency of miniature end-plate potentials accelerated by high potassium, is further increased by sodium reduction (Gage and Quastel, 1966; Birks et al., 1968), by cyclic adenosine monophosphate (cAMP), catecholamines, (Miyamoto and Breckenridge, 1974) and carbachol (Miyamoto and Volle, 1974).

No entirely compelling explanations have been put forward for the way in which most of the agents set out in Table 9 increase the evoked release of transmitter. An exception is tetraethyl-ammonium (TEA), the sole action of which in low concentration is probably to increase the duration of the nerve terminal action potential (as a result of its inhibition of potassium permeability — Armstrong and Binstock, 1965).

Table 9

Agent	Concentration (mmol/l)	Preparation	Potentiation factor[a]	Reference
A. Agents which increase quantal content				
K^+	10	frog[b]	2	TAKEUCHI and TAKEUCHI (1961)
K^+	15	rat[b]	2	PARSONS et al. (1965)
		curarized	2	
Na^+; up to 80% replacement by sucrose or glycine		frog[b]	25	BIRKS and COHEN (1965), KELLY (1965, 1968)
Tetraethyl-ammonium	0.1	frog[b]	3	BENOIT and MAMBRINI (1970)
UO_2^{2+}	0.2		18	
Caffeine	0.5	frog[b]	2	MAMBRINI and BENOIT (1963)
Caffeine	0.2	rat[b]	2	
Theophylline	1.8	rat[b]	5	GOLDBERG and SINGER (1969)
Dibutyryl cyclic AMP	4		2	
Theophylline	1.8	cat (cut fibre)	2	JACOBS and SHINNICK (1973)
Theophylline			2	
Aminophylline	1.0	rat (cut fibre)	2	WILSON (1974)
Dibutyryl cyclic AMP			2	
Noradrenaline	0.01	frog[b]	2	JENKINSON et al. (1968)
Noradrenaline	0.01	rat	2	KUBA (1970) (see also KRNJEVIĆ and MILEDI, 1958a, and KUBA and TOMITA, 1971)
Adrenaline		curarized	2	
Dopamine	0.01	cat (cut fibre)	2	GALLAGHER and KARCZMAR (1973)
Phenol	0.25	frog		
Catechol	0.05	curarized/	2	OTSUKA and NONOMURA (1963)
Hydroquinone	0.5	high Ca		
Catechol	0.01	cat	2	GALLAGHER and BLABER (1973)
Guanidine	5	frog curarized/ high Ca	2	OTSUKA and ENDO (1960)
Guanidine and derivatives	1	rat high Mg	6	BLACKMAN and SKELSEY (1965)
Ethanol	8	rat high Mg	2	GAGE (1965)
Diamide	0.1	frog[b]	6	WERMAN et al. (1971)
Barbiturates	0.2	frog[b]	2	THOMSON and TURKANIS (1973)
2-PAM[c]	1	frog high Mg	2	EDWARDS and IKEDA (1962)
Nystatin	0.01	frog[b]	2	CRAWFORD and FETTIPLACE (1971)
B. Agents which initially enhance but eventually abolish release				
Cs^+	2—10	frog[b]	20	GINSBORG and HAMILTON (1968)
		curarized	3	
Cardiac glycosides	0.01	frog curarized	5	BIRKS and COHEN (1968a)
1-fluoro-2,4-dinitro-benzene	0.4—2	frog[b]	6	EDELSON and NASTUK (1973)
		curarized	2	
Venoms				
Black widow spider		frog		LONGENECKER et al. (1970)
Tiger-snake		toad		DATYNER and GAGE (1973)
β-bungarotoxin		rat		CHANG et al. (1973c, d) CHANG and HUANG (1974)

Table 9 (continued)

Agent	Concen-tration (mmol/l)	Preparation	Poten-tiation factor[a]	Reference

C. Agents which abolish phasic[d] release but not tetanic discharge of min. E.P.P.S.

Botulinum toxin D		frog sartorius in organ culture		Harris and Miledi (1971)
Botulinum toxin A		rat diaphragm		Spitzer (1972)
		frog sartorius		Boroff et al. (1974)
Tetanus toxin		goldfish fin		Mellanby and Thompson (1972)
		mouse limb		Duchen and Tonge (1973)

[a] Where 2 is given, this signifies increase by a factor of 2 or less.
[b] Experiments performed in low Ca^{2+}/high Mg^{2+} solution.
[c] 2-formyl-1-methyl pyridinium chloride oxime.
[d] i.e. release evoked by nerve stimulation after the usual latency.

TEA does not cause an increase in the spontaneous rate of transmitter release or in the potassium induced release. Caesium, whose action was discovered in crustacea (see Gainer et al., 1967), probably also owes its effect to an increase in the duration of the nerve terminal action potential. Unlike TEA, however, caesium eventually blocks evoked transmitter release by abolishing the action potential. This is presumably because replacement of the intracellular potassium by caesium within the nerve terminal leads to depolarization. The eventual abolition of evoked release by the cardiac glycosides and by 1-fluoro-2,4-dinitrobenzene seems also to be consequent on nerve terminal depolarization. With black widow spider venom, there is evidence that evoked release is abolished at the same time as the nerve terminal action potential.

The uranyl ion (UO_2^{2+}) probably owes part of its effect to an increase in the duration of the nerve terminal action potential, but it also increases the frequency of potassium-accelerated miniature end-plate potentials.

At high concentrations TEA has the further effect of allowing the "explosive" release of large amounts of transmitter when depolarizing pulses are applied to the nerve terminal in bathing solutions which do not allow the generation of conventional "sodium" action potentials (see Katz and Miledi, 1969b). In spite of its presynaptic effect, TEA may reduce end-plate responses because of its "curare-like" post-synaptic action (see Table 4). In a similar way, the post-synaptic actions of the barbiturates also greatly outweigh their presynaptic effects, so that they act as neuro-muscular blocking agents, though of low potency.

Some importance has been attached to the enhancement of evoked release by theophylline and caffeine; this has been regarded as evidence that cAMP plays some part in the process of transmitter release. The argument has been based on the view that xanthine derivatives are acting as inhibitors of the phospho-diesterase which can accelerate the hydrolysis of cAMP. At present there is no direct evidence that theophylline, for example, does in fact act in this way on motor nerve terminals, and moreover other substances which are known to enhance cAMP

Table 10. Agents which reduce or abolish evoked release of acetylcholine

Agent	Concentration (mmol/l)	Source of nerve-muscle preparation	Reduction-factor [a]	Reference
Be²⁺	(0.1)	frog	*	BLIOCH and LIBERMAN (1970)
Mn²⁺	(2.5)	frog	*	KAJIMOTO and KIRPEKAR (1972) MEIRI and RAHAMIMOFF (1972) BALNAVE and GAGE (1973)
Pb²⁺	(0.01)	frog	*	MANALIS and COOPER (1973)
Adenosine	0.05	rat	2	GINSBORG and HIRST (1972)
AMP		(low Ca/high Mg)	2	GINSBORG et al. (1973)
ATP		(curarized)	2	
ADP				RIBEIRO and WALKER (1975)
Histamine	0.4	frog (low Ca/high Mg)	2	SCUKA (1973)
Ruthenium red	0.005	frog	4	RAHAMIMOFF and ALNAES (1973)
Tiger snake venom		mouse ext. dig. longus (applied in vivo)	intense	HARRIS et al. (1973)
2,4-dinitrophenol	0.1	frog	▽	KRAATZ and TRAUTWEIN (1957)
La³⁺	<1	frog	▽	HEUSER and MILEDI (1971)
Li⁺	replace Na	frog	initially 0.6, eventually ▽	ONODERA and YAMAKAWA (1966); KELLY (1968)
Pr³⁺	>0.2[b]	frog	▽	ALNAES and RAHAMIMOFF (1974)
Y³⁺	0.3	frog	▽	BOWEN (1972b)

[a] * indicates a Mg-like action; ▽ indicates complete abolition.
[b] 10—30 μmol/l increases release.

in nervous tissue such as adenosine, AMP, ADP, and ATP reduce rather than increase evoked transmitter release (Table 10).

In addition to the investigations listed, that of QUASTEL et al. (1971) should be mentioned. They found that depolarizing current pulses caused an enhanced release from mouse phrenic nerve terminals in the presence of a number of substances including ethanol (0.4 mol/l) and chlorpromazine (20 μmol/l).

4. Substances which Reduce Evoked Transmitter Release

Investigations concerned with substances which reduce transmitter release are set out in Table 10 (see also Table 9, section c). Manganese and beryllium appear to act in much the same way as magnesium. They are however, considerably more potent, causing a significant reduction in transmitter release in concentrations of less than 0.1 mmol/l. Lead is even more effective, reducing output by a factor of about 10 in a concentration of 10 μmol/l (in the presence of low calcium and high magnesium). All three ions have other actions on the neuromuscular junction. Manganese, after a delay, increases spontaneous release, as does lead (but in higher concentration): beryllium reduces spontaneous release. Lead and beryllium also reduce post-synaptic sensitivity to acetylcholine.

The actions of dinitrophenol and lithium are presumably to be explained by depolarization of the nerve terminal resulting in the abolition of the nerve terminal action potential. Lanthanum on the other hand is known *not* to abolish the action potential, and it is clear that this is also true for botulinum and tetanus toxins since repetitive nerve stimulation may result in the restoration of transmission if the block has not been long-established (Brooks, 1956), or to an increase in miniature end-plate potential frequency. It is of interest that high potassium does not enhance miniature end-plate potential frequency in preparations poisoned with either botulinum toxin or tiger snake venom.

Adenosine, AMP, ADP and ATP all appear to act at the same site and with approximately the same potency. Their maximum effect is to reduce the quantal content by a factor of about 2, independent of the concentrations of calcium and magnesium. The same is true of histamine. Evidently none of these substances acts by competing directly with calcium. A difference between adenosine (and its derivatives) and histamine is that adenosine reduces the spontaneous rate of release whereas histamine increases it.

Other substances which interfere with transmitter release include (1) various antibiotics such as neomycin (Elmqvist and Josefsson, 1962) and streptomycin (Dretchen et al., 1973); (2) acetylcholine (Ciani and Edwards, 1963) and succinylcholine (Edwards and Ikeda, 1962), which may act by depolarization of the nerve terminal at the first node of Ranvier and reduction of the action potential (see Hubbard et al., 1965); (3) nickel and zinc, in spite of the fact that they *increase* the duration of the action potential (Benoit and Mambrini, 1970); these ions also reduce the frequency of potassium accelerated miniature end-plate potentials; (4) certain toxins including crotoxin (Brazil and Excell, 1971) and β-bungarotoxin, which initially enhances transmitter release, and which also displays antagonism towards botulinum toxin (Chang et al., 1973d; Chang and Huang, 1974).

5. Relationship between Changes in Evoked and Spontaneous Release of Transmitter

The obvious avenue to explore in seeking to account for changes in evoked transmitter release in terms of the calcium hypothesis is that alterations in the amount of calcium entering the nerve terminal are involved. This would seem to provide a satisfactory explanation for the action of those substances that "compete with calcium" as well as those that alter the motor nerve terminal action potential. There is also evidence that lanthanum prevents the entry of calcium into the squid axon, so that although lanthanum may not compete with calcium at the motor nerve terminal in the same way as magnesium, the end result is similar. It should not be forgotten that there are a number of discrepancies between the effects on evoked and spontaneous release. Thus histamine, 2,4-dinitrophenol, lanthanum and repeated nerve stimulation may all diminish evoked release but augment spontaneous release; hyperpolarization of the nerve terminal may, on the other hand, produce very large increases in evoked release without affecting the spontaneous discharge (see p. 330). Nevertheless, a comparison of Tables 9 and 10 with Table 6 shows that many agents which affect evoked transmitter release alter spontaneous release in the same direction. The finding (Barrett et al., 1974) that after each spontaneous discharge there may be a period of increased probability of evoked release provides a further illustration. It would seem unreasonable to regard the correlation as merely accidental, and it has frequently been suggested that the common factor is an increase in the intracellular calcium concentration within the nerve terminal. This might increase not only spontaneous but also evoked release if the latter depended partly on the intracellular concentration of some calcium fraction as well as on the amount entering as a result of the stimulus (see also CHAPMAN and NIEDERGERKE, 1970). The increase in intracellular calcium might arise indirectly: it has been suggested, for example, that the cardiac glycosides cause the accumulation of internal calcium secondarily to that of sodium (see BAKER, 1972, for review).

Attempts have been made to interpret changes in evoked release in terms of changes in store size, release probability and a number of other factors. It has already been mentioned that in the absence of a well-founded model for the release process the conclusions reached must be regarded with the utmost caution (see p.315).

An elaboration of the calcium hypothesis which appears to be sufficiently flexible to accommodate most phenomena has been put forward by RAHAMIMOFF and YAARI (1973) (see also BAKER, 1972). They suppose that the "significant" internal calcium, Ca*, is derived not only from calcium entry but also from some cellular store. On such a scheme, the amount of transmitter could be envisaged to depend on three parameters, namely 1) the amount of Ca* derived from the nerve stimulus (i.e. from external calcium), 2) the rate of Ca* formation from the internal store, and 3) the rate of inactivation of Ca* (see also MILEDI and THIES, 1971). If, for example, an agent increased 1) and 3), the "phasic" release resulting directly from a stimulus could be enhanced without an increase in the spontaneous release, and the argument can be extended to cater for other situations.

IX. Facilitation and Depression

When several stimuli are applied to a motor nerve in fairly rapid succession, the number of quanta released by the successive stimuli are different; also, a test stimulus given some time after the "conditioning" train releases an abnormal number of quanta (see also pp.310—312). The details of the phenomena are rather complicated, but several generalizations can be made: (1) when the bathing solution contains low calcium and/or high magnesium, so that the quantal content is fairly small, the predominant effect during the train is facilitation; (2) where the quantal content is large, the predominant effect is depression during the train; (3) the after effect of the train is almost always facilitatory; this is now generally referred to as *post-tetanic potentiation*. This term is also used to describe the increase in the mechanical response of the muscle to stimuli applied after a preceding train. The mechanism is quite different, however (see Chapter 4A).

Many investigations of these phenomena have been made. They may be classified in terms of the three groups described above, and for convenience they are listed under those headings in Table 11. It is impossible to give a full account of the diverse results obtained since they depend on particular circumstances. Figure 34 is an attempt at a qualitative summary of the after effects of a single stimulus. It must be remembered that facilitation is statistical, so that for any particular pair of stimuli in reduced calcium (or enhanced magnesium) the second quantal content will sometimes be smaller than the first. For the mammal, curve 2 would apply when the divalent ion concentrations are normal, whereas in the frog, curve 3 would then hold.

Table 11. References to investigations of after effects of nerve stimulation

Short interval facilitation	Short interval depression	Post-tetanic potentiation (presynaptic)
Eccles et al. (1941)	Eccles et al. (1941)	Feng (1941)
Feng (1941)	Liley and North (1953)	Liley and North (1953)
Lundberg and Quillisch (1953a, b)	Lundberg and Quilisch (1953a, b)	Braun et al. (1966)
del Castillo and Katz (1954c)	Takeuchi (1958)	Gage and Hubbard (1966)
Liley (1956b)	Otsuka et al. (1962)	Rosenthal (1969)
Hubbard (1963)	Thies (1965)	Weinreich (1971)
Braun and Schmidt (1966)	Mallart and Martin (1968)	Landau et al. (1973)
Mallart and Martin (1967)	Betz (1970)	Magleby (1973b)
Rahamimoff (1968)	Christensen and Martin (1970)	Magleby and Zengel (1975a, b)
Katz and Miledi (1968a)		
Maeno and Edwards (1969)		
Moran and Rahamimoff (1970)		
Barrett and Stevens (1972a, b)		
Rahamimoff and Yaari (1973)		
Magleby (1973a)		
Younkin (1974)		

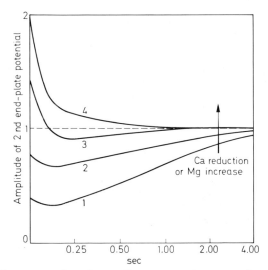

Fig. 34. After-effect of one nerve impulse on the response to a second nerve impulse. Abcissa: interval between stimuli (logarithmic scale). Ordinate: amplitude of second end-plate potential relative to first (linear scale). The change from curve 1 to 4 represents the effect of a reduction in calcium or an increase in magnesium. Schematic.

It may be helpful to give some examples: Lundberg and Quilisch (1953a) found that in normal calcium (and in the presence of tubocurarine) the end-plate potential in frog muscle was larger in response to the second of two stimuli if the delay between the stimuli was not more than 50 msec. The maximum increase was by a factor of about 3. In the rat diaphragm, however, the response to a second stimulus was depressed. The depression reached its peak about 100 msec after the stimulus, the second response being reduced relative to the first by a factor of about 0.75. The normal amplitude was not regained for several seconds. As is shown schematically in Fig. 34, a reduction in calcium concentration made the behaviour of the rat diaphragm resemble that of the frog sartorius, and vice versa (LUNDBERG and QUILISCH, 1953b).

Both the depression that occurs at "normal" quantal contents and the facilitation at low quantal contents are intensified during trains of repetitive stimuli (see e.g. Fig. 35). For example, with stimuli 10 msec apart applied in low calcium or high magnesium, the second response may be about twice the control; however the fiftieth response may be ten times the control (see e.g. DEL CASTILLO and KATZ, 1954c; LILEY, 1956b). Very large increases in miniature end-plate potential frequencies also occur during the period of stimulation. For example, LILEY (1956b) found that after a 17 sec period of stimulation in 12 mmol/l magnesium at 200 Hz, the miniature end-plate potential frequency rose by a factor of 30. The quantal content increased tenfold during the same period.

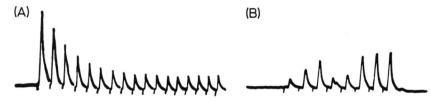

Fig. 35A and B. Depression and facilitation of the responses to nerve stimulation. A End-plate potentials evoked by a train of stimuli at 180 Hz. Extracellular recording from a curarised rat diaphragm preparation; normal calcium and magnesium. B Intracellularly-recorded responses to a train of stimuli at 160 Hz: transmission blocked by magnesium (10 mmol/l). (From LILEY, 1956b)

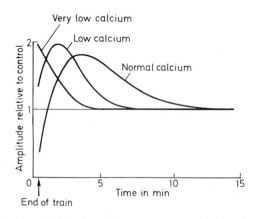

Fig. 36. After-effects of trains of stimuli on the responses to a single stimulus. Abcissa: interval between end of train and test stimulus; ordinate: amplitude of response to test stimulus relative to amplitude of control response. Schematic

The form taken by post-tetanic potentiation is illustrated in Fig. 36. Its special feature is its prolonged time course. In normal calcium, for example, even ten minutes after a 15 sec train of stimuli at 200 Hz a test stimulus will produce a response larger than the control. The phase of potentiation is of course preceded by a phase of depression or facilitation as described above, depending on the control quantal content. The frequency of miniature end-plate potentials is also enhanced during the period of post-tetanic potentiation, in fact by a considerably larger factor than the evoked response.

1. Depression and Depletion of Evoked Transmitter Release

It has frequently been assumed that depression occurs because quanta are released from a small store. Thus if a large number of quanta are released, corresponding to the emptying of a significant part of the store, a subsequent stimulus will not release the same number of quanta unless the store has been refilled. The idea is essentially a variant of one put forward by Liley and North in 1953 before the quantal nature of transmitter release had been established. Suppose that during a train of stimuli, the fraction F which is released of some store S is constant; thus the amount released will be FS. If refilling is slow with respect to the interval between stimuli, the next stimulus will operate on a store containing only S–FS. The amount released on this occasion will therefore be F(S–FS). The ratio of second to first quantal content will therefore be 1–F. Thus F and S can be determined (see also MARTIN, 1966).

The model and its different variants (see HUBBARD et al., 1969, pp. 143—158) should probably be taken as no more than a convenient picture (see also p. 315). The identification of S with n and F with p (n and p being the parameters of the quantal model) is highly speculative and possibly misleading (see also KUNO, 1971).

Direct evidence for depletion would clearly be extremely difficult to obtain, although at one time there seemed to be some experimental support for the idea in that during a train of stimuli the quantal contents of successive responses appeared to decline linearly with the total number of quanta released. However, subsequent investigations (BETZ, 1970; CHRISTENSEN and MARTIN, 1970) showed that within the general framework outlined above, depression is less severe than would be predicted. This could be explained by supposing that as depletion progressed a smaller fraction of the available store was released. If this is so, estimates for the immediately available and total stores, which have been made on the basis of a linear extrapolation, will be too low, and accordingly the number of molecules of acetylcholine calculated to correspond to an average quantum will be too high (see e.g. CHRISTENSEN and MARTIN, 1970).

The possibility that depression is not due to depletion at all but rather to a change in release probability is not excluded. Several alternative explanations have however been eliminated. Thus depression is not post-synaptic (OTSUKA et al., 1962; see also p. 311), nor is it due to changes in the action potential in the motor nerve ending (see e.g. BETZ, 1970).

It is not easy to fit depression into a unitary scheme for evoked and spontaneous release. Apart from a very small diminution of miniature end-plate potential frequency seen at a particular interval after nerve stimulation (RAHAMIMOFF and YAA-

RI, 1973) the predominant effect is an increase in frequency even at times when there is considerable depression of evoked release (see also DEL CASTILLO and KATZ, 1954 c).

2. Short Term Facilitation

When the average quantal content is small successive members of a series of stimuli applied at several per second cause the release of increasing amounts of transmitter, i.e. increasing numbers of quanta. As has already been mentioned (p. 335), the increase is essentially *statistical*. Thus considering pairs of stimuli with the mean quantal content low enough for a proportion of the stimuli to release no transmitter, the facilitation that occurs for the response to the second stimulus is independent of whether or not the first stimulus was "successful" (DEL CASTILLO and KATZ, 1954 c; MORAN and RAHAMIMOFF, 1970; BARRETT and STEVENS, 1972 a).

A detailed investigation has been carried out on frog muscle by MALLART and MARTIN (1967). Two phases of facilitation can be separated. The first phase (which corresponds to a test stimulus giving a response of about twice the control value immediately after a preceding stimulus) decays exponentially with a time constant of 35 msec. The second phase which is much less intense (corresponding to a maximum of less than 1.2) appears about 100 msec after the first stimulus and decays with a time constant of about 250 msec. For a short train of stimuli at 100 per sec, the resultant facilitation could be predicted on the assumptions that each impulse made the same contribution and that the contributions summed linearly. An alternative account by MAGLEBY (1973 a) suggests that both the fast and slow components can be described by exponential processes starting without appreciable delay after a nerve impulse.

As is the case with other aspects of the after effect of nerve stimulation the origin of facilitation is not entirely clear, although it is now apparent that it is not a consequence of an increase in the nerve terminal action potential (HUBBARD and SCHMIDT, 1963; KATZ and MILEDI, 1967 e, 1968 a: see also MARTIN and PILAR, 1964 b). One explanation which has been explored is that facilitation is due to the residuum of the calcium that entered the nerve terminal as a result of the previous stimulus (see p. 335). An important piece of evidence in favour of this idea has been obtained by KATZ and MILEDI (1968 a). They found that in the frog facilitation occurred to the second of two electrical pulses applied to the nerve terminal only if calcium was present (and thus presumably able to enter the nerve terminal) during the first "conditioning" pulse (see also RAHAMIMOFF, 1968; BARRETT and STEVENS, 1972 b; RAHAMIMOFF and YAARI, 1973). An interesting possibility has recently been raised by the finding in *Aplysia* by STINNAKRE and TAUC (1973) that for a certain type of neuronal action potential which depends on the transfer of calcium across the membrane, progressively greater amounts enter in response to successive impulses in a train. As the authors point out, if this also occurs in the presynaptic nerve terminals, it would contribute to facilitation.

It has already been mentioned (p. 321) that a single nerve stimulus is followed by a period in which the frequency of miniature end-plate potentials is increased (though see also RAHAMIMOFF and YAARI, 1973), and that the effect is even more marked after a train of stimuli. It is of interest (see p. 327) that this form of evoked release does not seem critically dependent on external calcium; HURLBUT et al. (1971) have produced evidence that, in the frog at least, magnesium can substitute for calcium (cf. BLIOCH et al., 1968).

3. Post-Tetanic Potentiation (Presynaptic)

There is evidence that post-tetanic potentiation must be related in some way to calcium accumulation. ROSENTHAL (1969) has shown that the magnitude of the effect depends on the number of stimuli in the tetanus, and that calcium must be present during the period of stimulation. WEINREICH (1971) has shown that post-tetanic potentiation occurs when the stimuli are depolarizing pulses applied to the nerve terminal. The effect occurs both when tetrodotoxin (which prevents the entry of sodium but not calcium into the nerve terminals) is present and when all the sodium has been replaced by calcium. Thus external calcium seems both necessary and sufficient for post-tetanic potentiation.

It is tempting to think that there is some relationship between post-tetanic potentiation and facilitation. However it has been found by LANDAU et al. (1973) (see also MAGLEBY, 1973b) that facilitation is essentially unaffected by post-tetanic potentiation; thus in the frog both the control end-plate potential and the facilitated end-plate potential in response to stimuli in low calcium and high magnesium were enhanced to the same extent during post-tetanic potentiation. If calcium accumulation at the same site were responsible for the two processes, it would be expected that facilitation would be reduced during post-tetanic potentiation.

D. Postscript

The main sequence of events during neuromuscular transmission is now well established and can be summarized as follows. The arrival of a motor nerve impulse at the axon endings causes a calcium-dependent release of packets or "quanta" of acetylcholine. Combination of the released acetylcholine with postsynaptic receptors leads to a selective increase in the ionic permeability of the end-plate region of the muscle fibre. The resulting depolarization (the end-plate potential) triggers off a propagated action potential which in turn initiates contraction.

No attempt will be made here to discuss the mechanisms underlying the muscle action potential or contraction. A comprehensive account can be found in the book by ZACHAR (1971); for detailed reviews of the structural, dynamic and biochemical aspects of muscle contraction the reader is referred to articles by HUXLEY (1972), CLOSE (1972) and WEBER and MURRAY (1973) respectively.

References

ADAMIČ, S.: The action of acetylcholine on potassium permeability of denervated rat diaphragm. Biochim. biophys. Acta (Amst.) **102**, 442—448 (1965).

ADAMS, P. R.: Drug concentration—conductance curves at frog end-plates determined by voltage-clamp. J. Physiol. (Lond.) **241**, 7—8 P (1974a).

ADAMS, P. R.: The mechanism by which amylobarbitone and thiopentone block the end-plate response to nictonic agonists. J. Physiol. (Lond.) **241**, 41—42 P (1974b).

ADAMS,P.R., CASH,H.C., QUILLIAM,J.P.: Extrinsic and intrinsic acetylcholine and barbiturate effects on frog skeletal muscle. Brit. J. Pharmacol. **40**, 552—553P (1970).

ADRIAN,R.H.: The effect of internal and external potassium concentration on the membrane potential of frog muscle. J. Physiol. (Lond.) **133**, 631—658 (1956).

ADRIAN,R.H.: Internal chloride concentration and chloride efflux of frog muscle. J. Physiol. (Lond.) **156**, 623—632 (1961).

ADRIAN,R.H., BRYANT,S.H.: On the repetitive discharge in myotonic muscle fibres. J. Physiol. (Lond.) **240**, 505—515 (1974).

ADRIAN,R.H., FREYGANG,W.H.: The potassium and chloride conductance of frog muscle membrane. J. Physiol. (Lond.) **163**, 61—103 (1962).

AGIN,D., HOLTZMAN,D.: Glass microelectrodes: the origin and elimination of tip potentials. Nature (Lond.) **211**, 1194—1195 (1966).

AHMAD,K., LEWIS,J.J.: The influence of drugs which stimulate skeletal muscle and of their antagonists on flux of calcium, potassium and sodium ions. J. Pharmacol. exp. Ther. **136**, 298—304 (1962).

ALBUQUERQUE,E.X., BARNARD,E.A., CHIU,T.H., LAPA,A.J., JOLLY,J.O., JANSSON,S.E., DALY,J., WITKOP,B.: Acetylcholine receptor and ion conductance modulator sites at the murine neuromuscular junction: evidence from specific toxin reactions. Proc. nat. Acad. Sci. (Wash.) **70**, 949—953 (1973).

ALBUQUERQUE,E.X., McISAAC,R.J.: Fast and slow mammalian muscles after denervation. Exp. Neurol. **26**, 183—202 (1970).

ALBUQUERQUE,E.X., SOKOLL,M.D., SONESSON,B., THESLEFF,S.: Studies on the nature of the cholinergic receptor. Europ. J. Pharmacol. **4**, 40—46 (1968).

ALBUQUERQUE,E.X., THESLEFF,S.: Comparative study of membrane properties of innervated and chronically denervated fast and slow skeletal muscles of the rat. Acta physiol. scand. **73**, 471—480 (1968).

ALBUQUERQUE,E.X., WARNICK,J.E., TASSE,J.R., SANSONE,F.M.: Effects of vinblastine and colchicine on neural regulation of the fast and slow skeletal muscles of the rat. Exp. Neurol. **37**, 607—634 (1972).

ALNAES,E., JANSEN,J.K.S., RUDJORD,T.: Spontaneous junctional activity of fast and slow parietal muscle fibres of the hagfish. Acta physiol. scand. **60**, 240—255 (1964).

ALNAES,E., RAHAMIMOFF,R.: Dual action of praseodymium (Pr^{3+}) on transmitter release at the frog neuromuscular synapse. Nature (Lond.) **247**, 478—479 (1974).

ANDERSON,C.R., STEVENS,C.F.: Voltage clamp analysis of acetylcholine produced end-plate current fluctuations at frog neuromuscular junction. J. Physiol. (Lond.) **235**, 655—691 (1973).

ANDERSON,M.J., COHEN,M.W.: Fluorescent staining of acetylcholine receptors in vertebrate skeletal muscle. J. Physiol. (Lond.) **237**, 385—400 (1974).

ARIËNS,E.J., SIMONIS,A.M., VAN ROSSUM,J.M.: Drug-receptor interaction: interaction of one or more drugs with one receptor system. In: ARIËNS,E.J. (Ed.): Molecular Pharmacology, Vol.I. New York: Academic Press 1964.

ARMSTRONG,C.M., BINSTOCK,L.: Anomalous rectification in the squid giant axon injected with tetraethyl ammonium chloride. J. gen. Physiol. **48**, 859—872 (1965).

ARMSTONG,W.McD., KNOEBEL,S.B.: The effect of serum albumin on the efflux of ^{42}K from frog sartorius muscle. J. cell. comp. Physiol. **67**, 211—216 (1966).

ARUNLAKSHANA,O., SCHILD,H.O.: Some quantitative uses of drug antagonists. Brit. J. Pharmacol. **14**, 48—58 (1959).

AUERBACH,A., BETZ,W.: Does curare affect transmitter release? J. Physiol. (Lond.) **213**, 691—705 (1971).

AXELSSON,J., THESLEFF,S.: The "desensitizing" effect of acetylcholine on the mammalian motor end-plate. Acta physiol. scand. **43**, 15—26 (1958).

AXELSSON,J., THESLEFF,S.: A study of supersensitivity in denervated mammalian skeletal muscle. J. Physiol. (Lond.) **147**, 178—193 (1959).

BAKER,P.F.: Transport and metabolism of calcium ions in nerve. Progr. Biophys. molec. Biol. **24**, 177—223 (1972).

BALNAVE,R.J., GAGE,P.W.: The inhibitory effect of manganese on transmitter release at the neuromuscular junction of the toad. Brit. J. Pharmacol. **47**, 339—352 (1973).

BARLOW,R.B.: Introduction to Chemical Pharmacology (2nd Edit). Methuen, London (1964).

BARLOW, R. B., SCOTT, N. C., STEPHENSON, R. P.: The affinity and efficacy of onium salts on the frog rectus abdominis. Brit. J. Pharmacol. **31**, 188—196 (1967).

BARLOW, R. B., THOMPSON, G. M., SCOTT, N. C.: The affinity and activity of compounds related to nicotine on the rectus abdominis muscle of the frog *(Rana pipiens)*. Brit. J. Pharmacol. **37**, 555—584 (1969).

BARNARD, E. A., WIECKOWSKI, J., CHIU, T. H.: Cholinergic receptor molecules and cholinesterase molecules at mouse skeletal muscle junctions. Nature (Lond.) **234**, 207—209 (1971).

BARNARD, E. A., DOLLY, J. O., PORTER, C. W., ALBUQUERQUE, E. X.: The acetylcholine receptor and the ionic conductance modulation system of skeletal muscle. Exp. Neurol. **48**, 1—28 (1975).

BARRETT, E. F., BARRETT, J. N., MARTIN, A. R., RAHAMIMOFF, R.: A note on the interaction of spontaneous and evoked release at the frog neuromuscular junction. J. Physiol. (Lond.) **237**, 453—463 (1974).

BARRETT, E. F., STEVENS, C. F.: Quantal independence and uniformity of presynaptic release kinetics at the frog neuromuscular junction. J. Physiol. (Lond.) **227**, 665—689 (1972a).

BARRETT, E. F., STEVENS, C. F.: The kinetics of transmitter release at the frog neuromuscular junction. J. Physiol. (Lond.) **227**, 691—708 (1972b).

BARSTAD, J. A. B.: Presynaptic effect of the neuromuscular transmitter. Experientia (Basel) **18**, 579—580 (1962).

BARSTAD, J. A. B., LILLEHEIL, G.: Transversally cut diaphragm preparation from rat. Arch. int. Pharmacodyn. **175**, 373—390 (1968).

BELMAR, J., EYZAGUIRRE, C.: Pacemaker site of fibrillation potentials in denervated mammalian muscle. J. Neurophysiol. **29**, 425—441 (1966).

BENDAT, J. S., PIERSOL, A. G.: Random Data: Analysis and Measurement Procedures. New York: Wiley, Interscience 1971.

BEN-HAIM, D., LANDAU, E. M., SILMAN, I.: The role of a reactive disulphide bond in the function of the acetylcholine receptor at the frog neuromuscular junction. J. Physiol. (Lond.) **234**, 305—325 (1973).

BEN-HAIM, D., DREYER, F., PEPER, K.: Acetylcholine receptor: modification of synaptic gating mechanism after treatment with a disulfide bond reducing agent. Pflügers Arch. ges. Physiol. **355**, 19—26 (1975).

BENNETT, M. R., McLACHLAN, E. M., TAYLOR, R. S.: The formation of synapses in reinnervated mammalian striated muscle J. Physiol. (Lond.) **233**, 481—500 (1973).

BENNETT, M. R., FLORIN, T.: A statistical analysis of the release of acetylcholine at newly formed synapses in striated muscle. J. Physiol. (Lond.) **238**, 93—107 (1974).

BENOIT, P. R., MAMBRINI, J.: Modification of transmitter release by ions which prolong the presynaptic action potential. J. Physiol. (Lond.) **210**, 681—695 (1970).

BERÁNEK, R., VYSKOČIL, F.: The action of tubocurarine and atropine on the normal and denervated rat diaphragm. J. Physiol. (Lond.) **188**, 53—66 (1967).

BERÁNEK, R., VYSKOČIL, F.: The effect of atropine on the frog sartorius neuromuscular junction. J. Physiol. (Lond.) **195**, 493—503 (1968).

BERG, D. K., HALL, Z. W.: Increased extrajunctional acetylcholine sensitivity produced by chronic postsynaptic neuromuscular blockade. J. Physiol. (Lond.) **244**, 659—676 (1975).

BERG, D. K., KELLY, R. B., SARGENT, P. B., WILLIAMSON, P., HALL, Z. W.: Binding of α-bungarotoxin to acetylcholine receptors in mammalian muscle. Proc. nat. Acad. Sci. (Wash.) **69**, 147—151 (1972).

BETZ, W. J.: Depression of transmitter release at the neuromuscular junction of the frog. J. Physiol. (Lond.) **206**, 629—644 (1970).

BIRKS, R. I., BURSTYN, P. G. R., FIRTH, D. R.: The form of sodium-calcium competition at the frog myoneural junction. J. gen. Physiol. **52**, 887—907 (1968).

BIRKS, R. I., COHEN, M. W.: Effects of sodium on transmitter release from frog motor nerve terminals. In: PAUL, W. M., DANIEL, E. E., KAY, C. M., MONCKTON, G. (Eds.): Muscle, Oxford: Pergamon Press 1965.

BIRKS, R. I., COHEN, M. W.: The action of sodium pump inhibitors on neuromuscular transmission. Proc. roy. Soc. B **170**, 381—399 (1968a).

BIRKS, R. I., COHEN, M. W.: The influence of internal sodium on the behaviour of motor nerve endings. Proc. roy. Soc. B **170**, 401—421 (1968b).

BIRKS,R.I., KATZ,B., MILEDI,R.: Physiological and structural changes at the amphibian myoneural junction, in the course of nerve degeneration. J. Physiol. (Lond.) **150**, 145—168 (1960).

BITTNER,G.D., HARRISON,J.: A reconsideration of the Poisson hypothesis for transmitter release
at the crayfish neuromuscular junction. J. Physiol. (Lond.) **206**, 1—23 (1970).

BLABER,L.C.: The prejunctional actions of some non-depolarizing blocking drugs. Brit. J. Pharmacol. **47**, 109—116 (1973).

BLABER,L.C., CHRIST,D.D.: The action of facilitatory drugs on the isolated tenuissimus muscle
of the cat. Int. J. Neuropharmacol. **6**, 473—484 (1967).

BLACKMAN,J.G., SKELSEY,M.: Effect of guanidinium, N-methyl and N, N-dimethyl guanidinium
and S-methyl-thiouronium salts on acetylcholine release in the rat isolated diaphragm. Proc.
Univ. Otago med. Sch. **43**, 15—17 (1965).

BLIOCH,Z.L., GLAGOLEVA,I.M., LIBERMAN,E.A., NENASHEV,V.A.: A study of the mechanism of
quantal transmitter release at a chemical synapse. J. Physiol. (Lond.) **199**, 11—35 (1968).

BLIOCH,Z.L., LIBERMAN,E.A.: The influence of beryllium ions on the end-plate potential and
frequency of miniature end-plate potentials at the neuromuscular junction of frogs. Biofizika
15, 468—474 (1970).

BOROFF,D.A., DEL CASTILLO,J., EVOY,W.H., STEINHARDT,R.A.: Observations on the action of
type A botulinum toxin on frog neuromuscular junctions. J. Physiol. (Lond.) **240**, 227—253
(1974).

BOWEN,J.M.: Estimation of the dissociation constant of D-tubocurarine and the receptor for
endogenous acetylcholine. J. Pharmacol. exp. Ther. **183**, 333—340 (1972a).

BOWEN,J.M.: Effects of rare earths and yttrium on striated muscle and the neuromuscular
junction. Canad. J. Physiol. Pharmacol. **50**, 603—611 (1972b).

BOYD,I.A., MARTIN,A.R.: Spontaneous subthreshold activity at mammalian neuromuscular
junctions. J. Physiol. (Lond.) **132**, 61—73 (1956a).

BOYD,I.A., MARTIN,A.R.: The end-plate potential in mammalian muscle. J. Physiol. (Lond.) **132**,
74—91 (1956b).

BOYLE,P.J., CONWAY,E.J.: Potassium accumulation in muscle and associated changes. J. Physiol.
(Lond.) **100**, 1—63 (1941).

BRADLEY,P.B., CANDY,J.M.: Iontophoretic release of acetylcholine, noradrenaline, 5-hydroxy-
tryptamine and D-lysergic acid diethylamide from micropipettes. Brit. J. Pharmacol. **40**,
194—201 (1970).

BRAUN,M., SCHMIDT,R.F.: Potential changes recorded from the frog motor nerve terminal
during its activation. Pflügers Arch. ges. Physiol. **287**, 56—80 (1966).

BRAUN,M., SCHMIDT,R.F., ZIMMERMANN,M.: Facilitation at the frog neuromuscular junction
during and after repetitive stimulation. Pflügers Arch. ges. Physiol. **287**, 41—55 (1966).

BRAZIL,O.V., EXCELL,R.J.: Action of crotoxin and crotactin from the venom of *crotalis durissus
terrificus* (South American rattlesnake) on the frog neuromuscular junction. J. Physiol.
(Lond.) **212**, 34—35P (1971).

BROOKS,V.B.: An intracellular study of the action of repetitive nerve volleys and of botulinum
toxin on miniature end-plate potentials. J. Physiol. (Lond.) **134**, 264—277 (1956).

BROWN,G.L.: The actions of acetylcholine on denervated mammalian and frog's muscle. J.
Physiol. (Lond.) **89**, 438—461 (1937).

BROWN,W.E.L., HILL,A.V.: The oxygen-dissociation curve of blood, and its thermodynamical
basis. Proc. roy. Soc. B **94**, 297—334 (1923).

BRYANT,S.H., CASTILLO,J. DEL, GARCIA,X., GIJON,E., LEE,C.F.: An electrically operated micro-
tap. Electroenceph. clin. Neurophysiol. **23**, 573—576 (1967).

BRYANT,S.H., MORALES-AGUILERA,A.: Chloride conductance in normal and myotonic muscle
fibres and the action of monocarboxylic aromatic acids. J. Physiol. (Lond.) **219**, 367—383
(1971).

BURKE,W.: Spontaneous potentials in slow muscle fibres of the frog. J. Physiol. (Lond.) **135**,
511—521 (1957).

BURKE,W., GINSBORG,B.L.: The electrical properties of the slow muscle fibre membrane. J.
Physiol. (Lond.) **132**, 586—598 (1956a).

BURKE,W., GINSBORG,B.L.: The action of the neuromuscular transmitter on the slow fibre
membrane. J. Physiol. (Lond.) **132**, 599—610 (1956b).

Burns,B.D., Paton,W.D.M.: Depolarization of the motor end-plate by decamethonium and acetylcholine. J. Physiol. (Lond.) 115, 41—73 (1951).

Carmody,J.J., Gage,P.W.: Lithium stimulates secretion of acetylcholine in the absence of extracellular calcium. Brain Res. 50, 476—479 (1973).

Cavanaugh,D.J., Hearon,J.Z.: The kinetics of acetylcholine action on skeletal muscle. Arch. int. Pharmacodyn. 100, 68—78 (1954).

Ceccarelli,B., Hurlbut,W.P., Mauro,A.: Turnover of transmitter and synaptic vesicles at the frog neuromuscular junction. J. Cell Biol. 57, 499—524 (1973).

Chagas,C.: Studies on the mechanism of curarization. Ann. N.Y. Acad. Sci. 81, 345—357 (1959).

Chang,C.C., Chen,T.F., Cheng,H.C.: On the mechanism of neuromuscular blocking action of bretylium and guanethidine. J. Pharmacol. exp. Ther. 158, 89—98 (1967).

Chang,C.C., Chen,T.F., Chuang,S.-T.: N, O−di and N, N, O−tri [^3H] acetyl α-bungarotoxins as specific labelling agents of cholinergic receptors. Brit. J. Pharmacol. 47, 147—160 (1973a).

Chang,C.C., Chen,T.F., Chuang,S.-T.: Influence of chronic neostigmine treatment on the number of acetylcholine receptors and the release of acetylcholine from the rat diaphragm. J. Physiol. (Lond.) 230, 613—618 (1973b).

Chang,C.C., Chen,T.F., Lee,C.Y.: Studies of the presynaptic effect of β-bungarotoxin on neuromuscular transmission. J. Pharmacol. exp. Ther. 184, 339—345 (1973c).

Chang,C.C., Huang,M.C.: Comparison of the presynaptic actions of botulinium toxin and β-bungarotoxin on neuromuscular transmission. Naunyn-Schmiedebergs Arch. exp. Path. Pharmak. 282, 129—142 (1974).

Chang,C.C., Huang,M.C., Lee,C.Y.: Mutual antagonism between botulinum and β-bungarotoxin. Nature (Lond.) 243, 166—167 (1973d).

Chang,C.C., Lee,C.Y.: Isolation of neurotoxins from the venom of Bungarus multicinctus and their modes of neuromuscular blocking action. Arch. int. Pharmacodyn. 144, 241—257 (1963).

Chang,C.C., Su,M.J.: Does α-bungarotoxin inhibit motor end-plate acetylcholinesterase? Nature (Lond.) 247, 480 (1974).

Changeux,J.P., Kasai,M., Lee,C.Y.: Use of a snake venom to characterize the cholinergic receptor protein. Proc. nat. Acad. Sci. (Wash.) 67, 1241—1247 (1970).

Chapman,R.A., Niedergerke,R.: Interaction between heart rate and calcium concentration in the control of contractile strength of the frog heart. J. Physiol. (Lond.) 211, 423—443 (1970).

Chowdhury,T.K.: Techniques of intracellular microinjection. In: Lavallée,M., Schanne,O.F., Hébert,N.C. (Eds.): Glass microelectrodes. New York: Wiley 1969.

Christensen,B.N., Martin,A.R.: Estimates of probability of transmitter release at the mammalian neuromuscular junction. J. Physiol. (Lond.) 210, 933—945 (1970).

Ciani,S., Edwards,C.: The effect of acetylcholine on neuromuscular transmission in the frog. J. Pharmacol. exp. Ther. 142, 21—23 (1963).

Clark,A.J.: The reaction between acetylcholine and muscle cells. J. Physiol. (Lond.) 61, 530—546 (1926a).

Clark,A.J.: The antagonism of acetylcholine by atropine. J. Physiol. (Lond.) 61, 547—556 (1926b).

Clark,A.W., Hurlbut,W.P., Mauro,A.: Changes in the fine structure of the neuromuscular junction of the frog caused by black widow spider venom. J. Cell Biol. 52, 1—14 (1972).

Cark,A.W., Mauro,A., Longenecker,H.E., Hurlbut,W.P.: Effects of black widow spider venom on the frog neuromuscular junction: effects on the fine structure of the frog neuromuscular junction. Nature (Lond.) 225, 703—705 (1970).

Clarke,G., Hill,R.G., Simmonds,M.A.: Microiontophoretic release of drugs from micropipettes: use of ^{24}Na as a model. Brit. J. Pharmacol. 48, 156—161 (1973).

Close,R.I.: Dynamic properties of mammalian skeletal muscles. Physiol. Rev. 52, 129—197 (1972).

Cochrane,D.E., Parsons,R.L.: The interaction between caffeine and calcium in the desensitization of muscle post-junctional membrane receptors. J. gen. Physiol. 59, 437—461 (1972).

Cochrane,D.E., Williams,F.A., Parsons,R.L.: Activation-inactivation of muscle post-junctional membrane receptors in isotonic Mg^{2+} or Ca^{2+} Ringer. Fed. Proc. 31, 305 (1972).

COHEN, I., KITA, H., VAN DER KLOOT, W.: The intervals between miniature end-plate potentials in the frog are unlikely to be independently or exponentially distributed. J. Physiol. (Lond.) 236, 327—339 (1974a).

COHEN, I., KITA, H., VAN DER KLOOT, W.: The stochastic properties of spontaneous quantal release of transmitter at the frog neuromuscular junction. J. Physiol. (Lond.) 236, 341—361 (1974b).

COHEN, I., KITA, H., VAN DER KLOOT, W.: Stochastic properties of spontaneous transmitter release at the crayfish neuromuscular junction. J. Physiol. 236, 363—371 (1974c).

COLOMO, F., RAHAMIMOFF, R.: Interaction between sodium and calcium ions in the process of transmitter release at the neuromuscular junction. J. Physiol. (Lond.) 198, 203—218 (1968).

COLOMO, F., RAHAMIMOFF, R., STEFANI, E.: An action of 5-hydroxytryptamine on the frog motor end-plate. Europ. J. Pharmacol. 3, 272—274 (1968).

COLQUHOUN, D.: The relation between classical and co-operative models for drug actions. In: RANG, H. P. (Ed.): Drug Receptors, pp. 149—182. London: Macmillan 1973.

COLQUHOUN, D.: Mechanisms of drug action at the voluntary muscle end-plate. Ann. Rev. Pharmacol. 15, 307—325 (1975).

COLQUHOUN, D., RANG, H. P., RITCHIE, J. M.: The binding of tetrodotoxin and α-bungarotoxin to normal and denervated mammalian muscle. J. Physiol. (Lond.) 240, 199—226 (1974).

CONWAY, E. J., HINGERTY, D.: The influence of adrenalectomy on muscle constituents. Biochem. J. 40, 561—568 (1946).

COOKE, J. D., OKAMOTO, K., QUASTEL, D. M. J.: The role of calcium in depolarization-secretion coupling at the motor nerve terminal. J. Physiol. (Lond.) 228, 459—497 (1973).

COOKE, J. D., QUASTEL, D. M. J.: Transmitter release by mammalian motor nerve terminals in response to focal polarization. J. Physiol. (Lond.) 228, 377—405 (1973a).

COOKE, J. D., QUASTEL, D. M. J.: Cumulative and persistent effects of nerve terminal depolarization on transmitter release. J. Physiol. (Lond.) 228, 407—434 (1973b).

COOKE, J. D., QUASTEL, D. M. J.: The specific effect of potassium on transmitter release by motor nerve terminals and its inhibition by calcium. J. Physiol. (Lond.) 228, 435—458 (1973c).

COOKSON, J. C., PATON, W. D. M.: Mechanisms of neuromuscular block. Anaesthesia 24, 395—416 (1969).

COUTEAUX, R., PÉCOT-DECHAVASSINE, M.: Vésicules synaptiques et poches au niveau des 'zones actives' de la jonction neuromusculaire. C. R. Acad. Sci. (Paris) 271, 2346—2349 (1970).

COWAN, S. L.: The initiation of all-or-none responses in muscle by acetylcholine. J. Physiol. (Lond.) 88, 3 P (1936).

CRAWFORD, A. C.: The dependence of evoked transmitter release on external calcium ions at very low mean quantal contents. J. Physiol. (Lond.) 240, 255—278 (1974).

CRAWFORD, A. C., FETTIPLACE, R.: A method for altering the intracellular calcium concentration. J. Physiol. (Lond.) 217, 20 P (1971).

CREESE, R.: Sodium fluxes in diaphragm muscle and the effects of insulin and serum proteins. J. Physiol. (Lond.) 197, 255—278 (1968).

CREESE, R., ENGLAND, J. M.: Decamethonium in depolarized muscle and the effects of tubocurarine. J. Physiol. (Lond.) 210, 345—361 (1970).

CREESE, R., MACLAGAN, J.: Entry of decamethonium in rat muscle studied by autoradiography. J. Physiol. (Lond.) 210, 363—386 (1970).

CREESE, R., NORTHOVER, J.: Maintenance of isolated diaphragm with normal sodium content. J. Physiol. (Lond.) 155, 343—357 (1961).

CREESE, R., TAYLOR, D. B., TILTON, B.: The influence of curare on the uptake and release of a neuromuscular blocking agent labelled with radioactive iodine. J. Pharmacol. exp. Ther. 139, 8—17 (1963).

CRONNELLY, R., DRETCHEN, K. L., SOKOLL, M. D., LONG, J. P.: Ketamine: myoneural activity and interaction with neuromuscular blocking agents. Europ. J. Pharmacol. 22, 17—22 (1973).

CUNNINGHAM, J. N. JNR., CARTER, N. W., RECTOR, F. C., SELDIN, D. W.: Resting transmembrane potential difference of skeletal muscle in normal subjects and severely ill patients. J. clin. Invest. 50, 49—59 (1971).

CURTIS, D. R.: Microelectrophoresis. In: NASTUK, W. L. (Ed.): Physical Techniques in Biological Research, Vol. V, Electrophysiological Methods, Part A, pp. 144—190. New York: Academic Press 1964.

Datyner, M. E., Gage, P. W.: Presynaptic and postsynaptic effects of the venom of the Australian tiger snake at the neuromuscular junction. Brit. J. Pharmacol. **49**, 340—354 (1973).

De Bassio, W. A., Schnitzler, R. M., Parsons, R. L.: Influence of lanthanum on transmitter release at the neuromuscular junction. J. Neurobiology **2**, 263—278 (1971).

Deguchi, T., Narahashi, T.: Effects of procaine on ionic conductances of end-plate membranes. J. Pharmacol. exp. Ther. **176**, 423—433 (1971).

del Castillo, J., Engbaek, L.: The nature of the neuromuscular block produced by magnesium. J. Physiol. (Lond.) **124**, 370—384 (1954).

del Castillo, J., Escobar, I., Gijón, E.: Effects of the electrophoretic application of sulfhydryl reagents to the end-plate receptors. International Journal of Neurosciences **1**, 199—209 (1970).

del Castillo, J., Katz, B.: The effect of magnesium on the activity of motor nerve endings. J. Physiol. (Lond.) **124**, 553—559 (1954a).

del Castillo, J., Katz, B.: Quantal components of the end-plate potential. J. Physiol. (Lond.) **124**, 560—573 (1954b).

del Castillo, J., Katz, B.: Statistical factors involved in neuromuscular facilitation and depression. J. Physiol. (Lond.) **124**, 574—585 (1954c).

del Castillo, J., Katz, B.: Changes in end-plate activity produced by pre-synaptic polarization. J. Physiol. (Lond.) **124**, 586—604 (1954d).

del Castillo, J., Katz, B.: The membrane change produced by the neuromuscular transmitter. J. Physiol. (Lond.) **125**, 546—565 (1954e).

del Castillo, J., Katz, B.: On the localization of acetylcholine receptors. J. Physiol. (Lond.) **128**, 157—181 (1955a).

del Castillo, J., Katz, B.: Local activity at a depolarized nerve-muscle junction. J. Physiol. (Lond.) **128**, 396—411 (1955b).

del Castillo, J., Katz, B.: Localization of active spots within the neuromuscular junction of the frog. J. Physiol. (Lond.) **132**, 630—649 (1956).

del Castillo, J., Katz, B.: A study of curare action with an electrical micro-method. Proc. roy. Soc. B **146**, 339—356 (1957a).

del Castillo, J., Katz, B.: The identity of "intrinsic" and "extrinsic" acetylcholine receptors in the motor end-plate. Proc. roy. Soc. B **146**, 357—361 (1957b).

del Castillo, J., Katz, B.: Interaction at end-plate receptors between different choline derivatives. Proc. roy. Soc. B **146**, 369—381 (1957c).

del Castillo, J., Nelson, T. E., Sanchez, V.: Mechanism of the increased acetylcholine sensitivity of skeletal muscle in low pH solutions. J. cell. comp. Physiol. **59**, 35—44 (1962).

del Castillo, J., Stark, L.: The effect of calcium ions on the motor end-plate potentials. J. Physiol. (Lond.) **116**, 507—515 (1952).

Dennis, M., Miledi, R.: Lack of correspondence between the amplitudes of spontaneous potentials and unit potentials evoked by nerve impulses at regenerating neuromuscular junctions. Nature (Lond.) New Biol. **232**, 126—128 (1971).

Dennis, M. J., Miledi, R.: Non-transmitting neuromuscular junctions during an early stage of end-plate reinnervation. J. Physiol. (Lond.) **239**, 553—570 (1974a).

Dennis, M. J., Miledi, R.: Characteristics of transmitter release at regenerating frog neuromuscular junctions. J. Physiol. (Lond.) **239**, 571—594 (1974b).

Detwiler, P. B.: The effects of germine-3-acetate on neuromuscular transmission. J. Pharmacol. exp. Ther. **180**, 244—254 (1972).

Diamond, J., Miledi, R.: A study of foetal and new-born rat muscle fibres. J. Physiol. (Lond.) **162**, 393—408 (1962).

Dockry, M., Kernan, R. P., Tangney, A.: Active transport of sodium and potassium in mammalian skeletal muscle and its modification by nerve and by cholinergic and adenergic agents. J. Physiol. (Lond.) **186**, 187—200 (1966).

Dodge, F. A. Jr., Miledi, R., Rahamimoff, R.: Strontium and quantal release of transmitter at the neuromuscular junction. J. Physiol. (Lond.) **200**, 267—283 (1969).

Dodge, F. A. Jr., Rahamimoff, R.: Co-operative action of Ca ions in the transmitter release at the neuromuscular junction. J. Physiol. (Lond.) **193**, 419—432 (1967).

Drachman, D. B., Witzke, F.: Trophic regulation of acetylcholine sensitivity of muscle: effect of electrical stimulation. Science **176**, 514—516 (1972).

DRETCHEN,K.L., SOKOLL,M.D., GERGIS,S.D., LONG,L.P.: Relative effects of streptomycin on motor nerve terminal and end-plate. Europ. J. Pharmacol. **22**, 10—16 (1973).

DREYER,F., PEPER,K.: The acetylcholine sensitivity in the vicinity of the neuromuscular junction of the frog. Pflügers Arch. ges. Physiol. **348**, 273—286 (1974a).

DREYER,F., PEPER,K.: The spread of acetylcholine sensitivity after denervation of frog skeletal muscle fibres. Pflügers Arch. ges. Physiol. **348**, 287—292 (1974b).

DREYER,F., PEPER,K.: Density and dose-response curve of acetylcholine receptors in frog neuromuscular junction. Nature (Lond.). **253**, 641—643 (1975).

DUCHEN,L.W., STEFANI,E.: Electrophysiological studies of neuromuscular transmission in hereditary "motor end-plate disease" of the mouse. J. Physiol. (Lond.) **212**, 535—548 (1971).

DUCHEN,L.W., TONGE,D.A.: The effect of tetanus toxin on neuromuscular transmission and on the morphology of motor end-plates in slow and fast skeletal muscle of the mouse. J. Physiol. (Lond.) **228**, 157—172 (1973).

DUDEL,J., KUFFLER,S.W.: The quantal nature of transmission and spontaneous miniature potentials at the crayfish neuromuscular junction. J. Physiol. (Lond.) **155**, 514—529 (1961).

DUNIN-BARKOVSKII, V.L., KOVALEV, S.A., MAGAZANIK, L.G., POTAPOVA, T.V., CHAYLAK-HYAN,L.M.: Equilibrium potentials of postsynaptic membrane activated with various cholinomimetics when the extracellular ionic medium is changed. Biofizika **14**, 485—493 (1969). (Also: Neurosciences translations **11**, 41—50; 1970).

ECCLES,J.C.: Specific ionic conductances at synapses. In: AGIN,D.P. (Ed.): Perspectives in Membrane Biophysics. New York: Gordon and Breach 1972.

ECCLES,J.C., KATZ,B., KUFFLER,S.W.: Nature of the "end-plate potential" in curarized muscle. J. Neurophysiol. **4**, 362—387 (1941).

ECCLES,J.C., O'CONNOR,W.J.: Responses which nerve impulses evoke in mammalian striated muscle. J. Physiol. (Lond.) **97**, 44—102 (1939).

EDELSON,A.M., NASTUK,W.L.: Pre- and post-junctional effects of 1-fluoro-2, 4-dinitrobenzene at the frog neuromuscular junction. J. Physiol. (Lond.) **229**, 617—633 (1973).

EDWARDS,C., IKEDA,K.: Effect of 2—PAM and succinylcholine on neuromuscular transmission in the frog. J. Pharmacol. exp. Ther. **138**, 322—328 (1962).

EISENBERG,R.S., HOWELL,J.N., VAUGHAN,P.C.: The maintenance of resting potentials in glycerol treated muscle fibres. J. Physiol. (Lond.) **215**, 95—102 (1971).

ELMQVIST,D., FELDMAN,D.S.: Spontaneous activity at a mammalian neuromuscular junction in tetrodotoxin. Acta physiol. scand. **64**, 475—476 (1965a).

ELMQVIST,D., FELDMAN,D.S.: Effects of sodium pump inhibitors on spontaneous acetylcholine release at the neuromuscular junction. J. Physiol. (Lond.) **181**, 498—505 (1965b).

ELMQVIST,D., FELDMAN,D.S.: Influence of ionic environment on acetylcholine release from the motor nerve terminals. Acta physiol. scand. **67**, 34—42 (1966).

ELMQVIST,D., HOFMANN,W.W., KUGELBERG,J., QUASTEL,D.M.J.: An electrophysiological investigation of neuromuscular transmission in myasthenia gravis. J. Physiol. (Lond.) **174**, 417—434 (1964).

ELMQVIST,D., JOHNS,T.R., THESLEFF,S.: A study of some electrophysiological properties of human intercostal muscle. J. Physiol. (Lond.) **154**, 602—607 (1960).

ELMQVIST,D., JOSEFSSON,J.O.: The nature of the neuromuscular block produced by neomycine. Acta physiol. scand. **54**, 105—110 (1962).

ELMQVIST,D., QUASTEL,D.M.J.: Presynaptic action of hemicholinium at the neuromuscular junction. J. Physiol. (Lond.) **177**, 463—482 (1965a).

ELMQVIST,D., QUASTEL,D.M.J.: A quantitative study of end-plate potentials in isolated human muscle. J. Physiol. (Lond.) **178**, 505—529 (1965b).

ELMQVIST,D., THESLEFF,S.: A study of acetylcholine induced contractures in denervated mammalian muscle. Acta pharmacol. (Kbh.) **17**, 84—93 (1960).

ENGBAEK,L.: Inhibitor ion: magnesium: In: CHEYMOL,J. (Ed.): Neuromuscular blocking and stimulating agents, Chapt. 14, pp. 391—423. Oxford: Pergamon Press 1972.

EVANS,M.H., JAGGARD,P.J.: Some effects of dimethyl sulphoxide (DMSO) on the frog neuromuscular junction. Brit. J. Pharmacol. **49**, 651—657 (1973).

EVANS,R.H.: Accumulation of calcium at motor end-plate. Brit. J. Pharmacol. **43**, 433—434P (1971).

Evans,R.H.: The entry of labelled calcium into the innervated region of the mouse diaphragm muscle. J. Physiol. (Lond.) **240**, 517—533 (1974).

Everett,A.J., Lowe,L.A., Wilkinson,S.: Revision of the structures of (+)-tubocurarine chloride and (+)-chondrocurine. Chem. Commun. **1970**, 1020—1021.

Falk,G., Fatt,P.: Linear electrical properties of striated muscle fibres observed with intracellular electrodes. Proc. roy. Soc. B **160**, 69—123 (1964).

Falk,G., Fatt,P.: Electrical impedance of striated muscle and its relation to contraction. In: Curtis,D.R., McIntyre,A.K. (Eds.): Studies in Physiology, pp.64—70. Berlin-Heidelberg-New York: Springer 1965.

Fambrough,D.M.: Acetylcholine sensitivity of muscle fibre membranes: mechanism of regulation by motoneurons. Science **168**, 372—373 (1970).

Fambrough,D.M., Drachman,D.B., Satyamurti,S.: Neuromuscular junction in myasthenia gravis: decreased acetylcholine receptors. Science **182**, 293—295 (1973).

Fambrough,D.M., Hartzell,H.C.: Acetylcholine receptors: number and distribution at neuromuscular junctions in rat diaphragm. Science **176**, 189—191 (1972).

Fatt,P.: The electromotive action of acetylcholine at the motor end-plate. J. Physiol. (Lond.) **111**, 408—422 (1950).

Fatt,P.: Skeletal neuromuscular transmission. In: Handbook of Physiology, Section 1 (Neurophysiology), Vol. 1, pp.199—213. Washington: Amer. Physiol. Soc. 1959.

Fatt,P.: An analysis of the transverse electrical impedance of striated muscle. Proc. roy. Soc. B **159**, 606—651 (1964).

Fatt,P., Katz,B.: An analysis of the end-plate potential recorded with an intra-cellular electrode. J. Physiol. (Lond.) **115**, 320—370 (1951).

Fatt,P., Katz,B.: Spontaneous subthreshold activity at motor nerve endings. J. Physiol. (Lond.) **117**, 109—128 (1952).

Feltz,A., Jaoul,A.: Direct estimates of chloride activity in muscle fibres depolarized by carbachol. Brit. J. Pharmacol. **51**, 304—306 (1974).

Feltz,A., Mallart,A.: An analysis of acetylcholine responses of junctional and extra-junctional receptors of frog muscle fibres. J. Physiol. (Lond.) **218**, 85—100 (1971a).

Feltz,A., Mallart,A.: Ionic permeability changes induced by some cholinergic agonists on normal and denervated frog muscles. J. Physiol. (Lond.) **218**, 101—116 (1971b).

Feng,T.P.: Studies on the neuromuscular junction. IV. The nature of junctional inhibition. Chin. J. Physiol. **11**, 437—450 (1937).

Feng,T.P.: Studies on neuromuscular transmission. XVIII. The local potentials around N − M junctions induced by single and multiple volleys. Chin. J. Physiol. **15**, 367—404 (1940).

Feng,T.P.: Studies on the neuromuscular junction. XXVI. The changes in the end-plate potential during and after prolonged stimulation. Chin. J. Physiol. **16**, 341—372 (1941).

Ferry,C.B., Marshall,A.R.: An anti-curare effect of hexamethonium at the mammalian neuromuscular junction. Brit. J. Pharmacol. **47**, 353—362 (1973).

Ferry,C.B., Norris,B.: Actions of bretylium tosylate at the neuromuscular junction. Brit. J. Pharmacol. **41**, 607—621 (1971).

Fertuck,H.C., Salpeter,M.M.: Localization of acetylcholine receptor by ^{125}I-labelled α-bungarotoxin binding at mouse motor endplates. Proc. nat. Acad. Sci. (Wash.) **71**, 1376—1378 (1974).

Fisher,R.A.: The design of experiments, 8th Ed. Edinburgh: Oliver and Boyd 1966.

Frank,K., Becker,M.C.: Microelectrodes for Recording and Stimulation. In: Nastuk,W.L. (Ed.): Physical Techniques in Biological Research, Vol.V, Electrophysiological Methods, Part A, pp.23—87. New York: Academic Press 1964.

Furshpan,E.J.: The effects of osmotic pressure changes on the spontaneous activity at motor nerve endings. J. Physiol. (Lond.) **134**, 689—697 (1956).

Furukawa,T., Furukawa,A.: Effects of methyl- and ethyl-derivatives of NH_4^+ on the neuromuscular junction. Jap. J. Physiol. **9**, 130—142 (1959).

Furukawa,T., Sasaoka,T., Hosoya,Y.: Effects of tetrodotoxin on the neuromuscular junction. Jap. J. Physiol. **9**, 143—152 (1959).

Gaddum,J.H.: The quantitative effects of antagonistic drugs. J. Physiol. (Lond.) **89**, 7P (1937).

Gaddum,J.H., Hameed,K.A., Hathway,D.E., Stephens,F.F.: Quantitative studies of antagonists for 5-hydroxytryptamine. Quart. J. exp. Physiol. **40**, 49—74 (1955).

GAGE, P.W.: The effect of methyl, ethyl and n-propyl alcohol on neuromuscular transmission in the rat. J. Pharmacol. exp. Ther. **150**, 236—243 (1965).

GAGE, P.W., EISENBERG, R.S.: Capacitance of the surface and transverse tubular membrane of frog sartorius fibers. J. gen. Physiol. **53**, 265   278 (1969).

GAGE, P.W., HUBBARD, J.I.: Evidence for a Poisson distribution of miniature end-plate potentials and some implications. Nature (Lond.) **208**, 395—396 (1965).

GAGE, P.W., HUBBARD, J.I.: An investigation of the post-tetanic potentiation of end-plate potentials at a mammalian neuromuscular junction. J. Physiol. (Lond.) **184**, 353—375 (1966).

GAGE, P.W., McBURNEY, R.N.: Miniature end-plate currents and potentials generated by quanta of acetylcholine in glycerol-treated toad sartorius fibres. J. Physiol. (Lond.) **226**, 79—94 (1972a).

GAGE, P.W., McBURNEY, R.N.: An analysis of the relationship between the current and potential generated by a quantum of acetylcholine in muscle fibres without transverse tubules. J. Membrane Biol. **12**, 247—272 (1972b).

GAGE, P.W., McBURNEY, R.N., SCHNEIDER, G.T.: Effects of some aliphatic alcohols on the conductance change caused by a quantum of acetylcholine at the toad end plate. J. Physiol. (Lond.) **244**, 409—429 (1975).

GAGE, P.W., QUASTEL, D.M.J.: Competition between sodium and calcium ions in transmitter release at mammalian neuromuscular junctions. J. Physiol. (Lond.) **185**, 95—123 (1966).

GAINER, H., REUBEN, J.P., GRUNDFEST, H.: The augmentation of postsynaptic potentials in crustacean muscle fibres by caesium. A presynaptic mechanism. Comp. Biochem. Physiol. **20**, 877—900 (1967).

GALINDO, A.: Procaine, pentobarbital and halothane: effects on the mammalian myoneural junction. J. Pharmacol. exp. Ther. **117**, 360—368 (1971).

GALLAGHER, J.P., BLABER, L.C.: Catechol, a facilitatory drug that demonstrates only a prejunctional site of action. J. Pharmacol. exp. Ther. **184**, 129—135 (1973).

GALLAGHER, J.P., KARCZMAR, A.G.: A direct facilitatory action for dopamine at the neuromuscular junction. Neuropharmacology **12**, 783—791 (1973).

GEDDES, L.A.: Electrodes and the measurement of bioelectric events. New York: Wiley-Interscience 1972.

GINETZINSKY, A.G., SHAMARINA, N.M.: The tonomotor phenomenon in denervated muscle. Usp. sovrem. Biol. **15**, 283—294 (1942). Available as translation RTS 1710 from the British Library, Boston Spa, England.

GINSBORG, B.L.: Spontaneous activity in muscle fibres of the chick. J. Physiol. (Lond.) **150**, 707—717 (1960).

GINSBORG, B.L.: Ion movements in junctional transmission. Pharmacol. Rev. **19**, 289—316 (1967).

GINSBORG, B.L.: Electrical changes in the membrane in junctional transmission. Biochim. biophys. Acta (Amst.) **300**, 289—317 (1973).

GINSBORG, B.L., HAMILTON, J.T.: The effect of caesium ions on neuromuscular transmission in the frog. Quart. J. exp. Physiol. **53**, 162—169 (1968).

GINSBORG, B.L., HIRST, G.D.S.: The effect of adenosine on the release of the transmitter from the phrenic nerve of the rat. J. Physiol. (Lond.) **224**, 629—645 (1972).

GINSBORG, B.L., HIRST, G.D.S., MAIZELS, J.V., WALKER, J.: Specificity of adenosine on transmitter output at the neuromuscular junction. Brit. J. Pharmacol. **47**, 637P (1973).

GINSBORG, B.L., STEPHENSON, R.P.: On the simultaneous action of two competitive antagonists. Brit. J. Pharmacol. **51**, 287—300 (1974).

GISSEN, A.J., NASTUK, W.L.: The mechanisms underlying neuromuscular block following prolonged exposure to depolarizing agents. Ann. N.Y. Acad. Sci. **135**, 184—194 (1966).

GLAGOLEVA, I.M., LIBERMAN, E.A., KHASHAEV, Z.KH-M.: Effect of uncouplers of oxidative phosphorylation on output of acetylcholine from nerve endings. Biofizika **15**, 76—83 (1970).

GÖPFERT, H., SCHAEFER, H.: Über den direkt und indirekt erregten Aktionsstrom und die Funktion der motorischen Endplatte. Pflügers Arch. ges. Physiol. **239**, 597—619 (1938).

GOLDBERG, A.L., SINGER, J.J.: Evidence for a role of cyclic AMP in neuromuscular transmission. Proc. nat. Acad. Sci. (Wash.) **64**, 134—141 (1969).

GOLDFINE, C.: Dissociation constants of competitive antagonists at the mammalian neuromuscular junction. Thesis, London University (1973).

GOLDMAN,D.E.: Potential, impedance and rectification in membranes. J. gen. Physiol. **27**, 37—60 (1943).

GRAMPP,W., HARRIS,J.B., THESLEFF,S.: Inhibition of denervation changes in skeletal muscle by blockers of protein synthesis. J. Physiol. (Lond.) **221**, 743—754 (1972).

GUTH,L.: "Trophic" influences of nerve on muscle. Physiol. Rev. **48**, 645—687 (1968).

HALL,Z.W.: Multiple forms of acetylcholinesterase and their distribution in end-plate and non-end-plate regions of rat diaphragm muscle. J. Neurobiol. **4**, 343—361 (1973).

HARRINGTON,L.: A linear dose-response curve at the motor end-plate. J. gen. Physiol. **62**, 58—76 (1973).

HARRIS,A.J., MILEDI,R.: The effect of type D botulinum toxin on frog neuromuscular junctions. J. Physiol. (Lond.) **217**, 497—515 (1971).

HARRIS,A.J., MILEDI,R.: A study of frog muscle maintained in organ culture. J. Physiol. (Lond.) **221**, 207—226 (1972).

HARRIS,E.J.: Anion interaction in frog muscle. J. Physiol. (Lond.) **141**, 351—365 (1958).

HARRIS,E.J., NICHOLLS,J.G.: The effect of denervation on the rate of entry of potassium into frog muscle. J. Physiol. (Lond.) **131**, 473—476 (1956).

HARRIS,E.J., OCHS,S.: Effects of sodium extrusion and local anaesthetics on muscle membrane resistance and potential. J. Physiol. (Lond.) **187**, 5—21 (1966).

HARRIS,J.B., KARLSSON,E., THESLEFF,S.: Effects of an isolated toxin from Australian Tiger Snake (*Notechis scutatus scutatus*) venom at the mammalian neuromuscular junction. Brit. J. Pharmacol. **47**, 141—146 (1973).

HARTZELL,H.C., FAMBROUGH,D.M.: Acetylcholine receptors: distribution and extrajunctional density in rat diaphragm after denervation correlated with acetylcholine sensitivity. J. gen. Physiol. **60**, 248—262 (1972).

HARTZELL,H.C., KUFFLER,S.W., YOSHIKAMI,D.: Postsynaptic potentiation: interaction between quanta of acetylcholine at the skeletal neuromuscular synapse. J. Physiol. (Lond.). **251**, 427—463 (1975).

HEAD,S.D.: Depolarising neuromuscular blocking drugs: an electrophysiological investigation in mammalian skeletal muscle. Thesis. University of London, 1975.

HEILBRONN,E., MATTSON,CH.: The nicotinic cholinergic receptor protein: improved purification method, preliminary amino acid composition and observed auto-immune response. J. Neurochem. **22**, 315—317 (1974).

HENDERSON,E.G., HANCOCK,J.C.: Nicotine-induced depolarization and stimulation of potassium efflux in striated muscle. J. Pharmacol. exp. Ther. **177**, 377—388 (1971).

HESS,A., PILAR,G.: Slow fibres in the extraocular muscles of the cat. J. Physiol. (Lond.) **169**, 780—798 (1963).

HEUSER,J., KATZ,B., MILEDI,R.: Structural and functional changes of frog neuromuscular junctions in high calcium solutions. Proc. roy. Soc. B **178**, 407—415 (1971).

HEUSER,J., MILEDI,R.: Effect of lanthanum ions on function and structure of frog neuromuscular junctions. Proc. roy. Soc. B **179**, 247—260 (1971).

HEUSER,J.E., REESE,T.S.: Evidence for recycling of synaptic vesicle membrane during transmitter release at the frog neuromuscular junction. J. Cell Biol. **57**, 315—344 (1973).

HIDAKA,T., TOIDA,N.: Neuromuscular transmission and excitation-contraction coupling in fish red muscle. Jap. J. Physiol. **19**, 130—142 (1969).

HILL,A.V.: The mode of action of nicotine and curari, determined by the form of the contraction curve and the method of temperature coefficients. J. Physiol. (Lond.) **39**, 361—373 (1909).

HIRST,G.D.S., WOOD,D.R.: On the neuromuscular paralysis produced by procaine. Brit. J. Pharmacol. **41**, 94—104 (1971a).

HIRST,G.D.S., WOOD,D.R.: Changes in the time course of transmitter action produced by procaine. Brit. J. Pharmacol. **41**, 105—112 (1971b).

HODGKIN,A.L.: Ionic movements and electrical activity in giant nerve fibres. Proc. roy. Soc. B **148**, 1—37 (1958).

HODGKIN,A.L., HOROWICZ,P.: Movements of sodium and potassium in single muscle fibres. J. Physiol. (Lond.) **145**, 405—432 (1959a).

HODGKIN,A.L., HOROWICZ,P.: The influence of potassium and chloride ions on the membrane potential of single muscle fibres. J. Physiol. (Lond.) **148**, 127—160 (1959b).

HODGKIN, A. L., KATZ, B.: The effect of sodium ions on the electrical activity of the giant axon of the squid. J. Physiol. (Lond.) **108**, 37—77 (1949).

HODGKIN, A. L., NAKAJIMA, S.: The effect of diameter on the electrical constants of frog skeletal muscle fibres. J. Physiol. (Lond.) **221**, 105—120 (1972a).

HODGKIN, A. L., NAKAJIMA, S.: Analysis of the membrane capacity in frog muscle. J. Physiol. (Lond.) **221**, 121—136 (1972b).

HOFMANN, W. W., FEIGEN, G. A., GENTHER, G. H.: Effects of veratrine, nitrate ion and γ-aminobutyric acid on mammalian miniature end-plate potentials. Nature (Lond.) **193**, 175—176 (1962).

HOFMANN, W. W., PARSONS, R. L., FEIGEN, G. A.: Effects of temperature and drugs on mammalian motor nerve terminals. Amer. J. Physiol. **211**, 135—140 (1966).

HOFMANN, W. W., THESLEFF, S.: Studies on the trophic influence of nerve on skeletal muscle. Europ. J. Pharmacol. **20**, 256—260 (1972).

HOH, J. F. Y., SALAFSKY, B.: Effects of nerve cross-union on rat intracellular potassium in fast-twitch and slow-twitch rat muscles. J. Physiol. (Lond.) **216**, 171—179 (1971).

HOWELL, J. N., JENDEN, D. J.: T-tubules of skeletal muscle: morphological alterations which interrupt excitation-contraction coupling. Fed. Proc. **26**, 553 (1967).

HUBBARD, J. I.: Repetitive stimulation at the mammalian neuromuscular junction and the mobilization of transmitter. J. Physiol. (Lond.) **169**, 641—662 (1963).

HUBBARD, J. I.: Microphysiology of vertebrate neuromuscular transmission. Physiol. Rev. **53**, 674—723 (1973).

HUBBARD, J. I., JONES, S. F.: Spontaneous quantal transmitter release: a statistical analysis and some implications. J. Physiol. (Lond.) **232**, 1—21 (1973).

HUBBARD, J. I., JONES, S. F., LANDAU, E. M.: On the mechanism by which calcium and magnesium affect the spontaneous release of transmitter from mammalian motor nerve terminals. J. Physiol. (Lond.) **194**, 355—380 (1968a).

HUBBARD, J. I., JONES, S. F., LANDAU, E. M.: On the mechanism by which calcium and magnesium affect the release of transmitter by nerve impulses. J. Physiol. (Lond.) **196**, 75—86 (1968b).

HUBBARD, J. I., JONES, S. F., LANDAU, E. M.: An examination of the effects of osmotic pressure changes upon transmitter release from mammalian motor nerve terminals. J. Physiol. (Lond.) **197**, 639—657 (1968c).

HUBBARD, J. I., JONES, S. F., LANDAU, E. M.: The effect of temperature change upon transmitter release, facilitation and post-tetanic potentiation. J. Physiol. (Lond.) **216**, 591—609 (1971).

HUBBARD, J. I., LLINÁS, R., QUASTEL, D. M. J.: Electrophysiological analysis of synaptic transmission. London: Edward Arnold 1969.

HUBBARD, J. I., SCHMIDT, R. F.: An electrophysiological investigation of mammalian motor nerve terminals. J. Physiol. (Lond.) **166**, 145—167 (1963).

HUBBARD, J. I., SCHMIDT, R. F., YOKOTA, T.: The effect of acetylcholine upon mammalian motor nerve terminals. J. Physiol. (Lond.) **181**, 810—829 (1965).

HUBBARD, J. I., WILLIS, W. D.: Hyperpolarization of mammalian motor nerve terminals. J. Physiol. (Lond.) **163**, 115—137 (1962).

HUBBARD, J. I., WILLIS, W. D.: The effects of depolarization of motor nerve terminals upon the release of transmitter by nerve impulses. J. Physiol. (Lond.) **194**, 381—405 (1968).

HUBBARD, J. I., WILSON, D. F.: Neuromuscular transmission in a mammalian preparation in the absence of blocking drugs and the effect of D-tubocurarine. J. Physiol. (Lond.) **228**, 307—325 (1973).

HUBBARD, S. J.: The electrical constants and the component conductances of frog skeletal muscle after denervation. J. Physiol. (Lond.) **165**, 443—456 (1963).

HURLBUT, W. P., LONGENECKER, H. B., MAURO, A.: Effects of calcium and magnesium on the frequency of miniature end-plate potentials during prolonged tetanization. J. Physiol. (Lond.) **219**, 17—38 (1971).

HUTTER, O. F., PADSHA, S. M.: Effect of nitrate and other ions on the membrane resistance of frog skeletal muscle. J. Physiol. (Lond.) **146**, 117—132 (1959).

HUTTER, O. F., TRAUTWEIN, W.: Neuromuscular facilitation by stretch of motor nerve endings. J. Physiol. (Lond.) **133**, 610—625 (1956).

HUTTER, O. F., WARNER, A. E.: The pH sensitivity of the chloride conductance of frog skeletal muscle. J. Physiol. (Lond.) **189**, 403—425 (1967a).

Hutter,O. F., Warner,A. E.: The effect of pH on the ^{36}Cl efflux from frog skeletal muscle. J. Physiol. (Lond.)**189**, 427—443 (1967b).

Hutter,O. F., Warner,A. E.: Action of some foreign cations and anions on the chloride permeability of frog muscle. J. Physiol. (Lond.) **189**, 445—460 (1967c).

Huxley,H. E.: Molecular basis of contraction in cross-striated muscles. In: Bourne,G. H. (Ed.): The structure and function of muscle, Vol. I, 2nd Ed. New York: Academic Press 1972.

Ing,H. R., Wright,W. M.: The curariform action of quaternary ammonium salts. Proc. roy. Soc. B **109**, 337—353 (1932).

Jacobs,R. S., Shinnick,P. L.: Facilitatory sites of action of theophylline in isolated cat tenuissimus muscle. Int. J. Neuropharmacol. **12**, 885—895 (1973).

Jenkinson,D. H.: The nature of the antagonism between calcium and magnesium ions at the neuromuscular junction. J. Physiol. (Lond.) **138**, 434—444 (1957).

Jenkinson,D. H.: The antagonism between tubocurarine and substances which depolarize the motor end-plate. J. Physiol. (Lond.) **152**, 309—324 (1960).

Jenkinson,D. H., Nicholls,J. G.: Contractures and permeability changes produced by acetylcholine in depolarized denervated muscle. J. Physiol. (Lond.) **159**, 111—127 (1961).

Jenkinson,D. H., Stamenović,B. A., Whitaker,B. D. L.: The effect of noradrenaline on the endplate potential in twitch fibres of the frog. J. Physiol. (Lond.) **195**, 743—754 (1968).

Jenkinson,D. H., Terrar,D. A.: Influence of chloride ions on changes in membrane potential during prolonged application of carbachol to frog skeletal muscle. Brit. J. Pharmacol. **47**, 363—376 (1973).

Johnson,E. W., Parsons,R. L.: Characteristics of postjunctional carbamycholine receptor activation and inhibition. Amer. J. Physiol. **222**, 793—799 (1972).

Johnson,E. W., Wernig,A.: The binomial nature of transmitter release at the crayfish neuromuscular junction. J. Physiol. (Lond.) **218**, 757—767 (1971).

Jones,R., Vrbová,G.: Effect of muscle activity on denervation hypersensitivity. J. Physiol. (Lond.) **210**, 144—145 P (1970).

Jones,R., Vrbová,G.: Two factors responsible for the development of denervation hypersensitivity. J. Physiol. (Lond.) **236**, 517—538 (1974).

Jones,S. F., Kwanbunbumpen,S.: The effects of nerve stimulation and hemicholinium on synaptic vesicles at the mammalian neuromuscular junction. J. Physiol. (Lond.) **207**, 31—50 (1970a).

Jones,S. F., Kwanbunbumpen,S.: Some effects of nerve stimulation and hemicholinium on quantal transmitter release at the mammalian neuromuscular junction. J. Physiol. (Lond.) **207**, 51—61 (1970b).

Josefsson,J. O., Thesleff,S.: Electromyographic findings in experimental botulinum intoxication. Acta physiol. scand. **51**, 163—168 (1961).

Kahn,R., LeYaouanc,A.: Appendix to: Feltz,A. and A.Mallart: An analysis of acetylcholine responses of junctional and extrajunctional receptors of frog muscle fibres. J. Physiol. (Lond.)**218**, 85—100 (1971).

Kajimoto,N., Kirpekar,S. M.: Effect of manganese and lanthanum on spontaneous release of acetylcholine at frog motor nerve terminals. Nature (Lond.) New Biol. **235**, 29—30 (1972).

Karis,J. H., Gissen,A. J., Nastuk,W. L.: Mode of action of diethyl ether in blocking neuromuscular transmission. Anesthesiology **27**, 42—51 (1966a).

Karis,J. H., Gissen,A. J., Nastuk,W. L.: The effect of volatile anaesthetic agents on neuromuscular transmission. Anesthesiology **28**, 128—134 (1967).

Karis,J. H., Nastuk,W. L., Katz,R. L.: The action of tacrine on neuromuscular transmission: a comparison with hexafluorenium. Brit. J. Anaesth. **38**, 762—774 (1966b).

Karlin,A.: On the application of "a Plausible Model" of allosteric proteins to the receptor for acetylcholine. J. theor. Biol. **16**, 306—320 (1967).

Kasai,M., Changeux,J. P.: In vitro excitation of purified membrane fragments by cholinergic agonists. 11. The permeability change caused by cholinergic agonists. J. Membrane Biol. **6**, 24—57 (1971).

Katz,B.: Impedance changes in frog's muscle associated with electronic and "end-plate" potentials. J. Neurophysiol. **5**, 169—184 (1942).

Katz,B.: The transmission of impulses from nerve to muscle, and the subcellular unit of synaptic action. Proc. roy. Soc. B **155**, 455—477 (1962).

KATZ,B.: Nerve, muscle and synapse. New York: McGraw-Hill 1966.

KATZ,B.: The release of neural transmitter substances. Liverpool: University Press 1969.

KATZ,B., MILEDI,R.: The localized action of "end-plate drugs" in the twitch fibres of the frog. J. Physiol. (Lond.) **155**, 399—415 (1961).

KATZ,B., MILEDI,R.: Further observations on the distribution of acetylcholine-reactive sites in skeletal muscle. J. Physiol. (Lond.) **170**, 379—388 (1964a).

KATZ,B., MILEDI,R.: The development of acetylcholine sensitivity in nerve-free segments of skeletal muscle. J. Physiol. (Lond.) **170**, 389—396 (1964b).

KATZ,B., MILEDI,R.: Propagation of electric activity in motor nerve terminals. Proc. roy. Soc. B **161**, 453—482 (1965a).

KATZ,B., MILEDI,R.: The measurement of synaptic delay, and the time course of acetylcholine release at the neuromuscular junction. Proc. roy. Soc. B **161**, 483—495 (1965b).

KATZ,B., MILEDI,R.: The effect of calcium on acetylcholine release from the motor nerve terminals. Proc. roy. Soc. B **161**, 496—503 (1965c).

KATZ,B., MILEDI,R.: The effect of temperature on the synaptic delay at the neuromuscular junction. J. Physiol. (Lond.) **181**, 656—670 (1965d).

KATZ,B., MILEDI,R.: The quantal release of transmitter substances. In: CURTIS,D.R., MCINTYRE,A.K. (Eds.): Studies in Physiology, pp.118—124. Berlin-Heidelberg-New York: Springer 1965e.

KATZ,B., MILEDI,R.: Modification of transmitter release by electrical interference with motor nerve endings. Proc. roy. Soc. B **167**, 1—7 (1967a).

KATZ,B., MILEDI,R.: Tetrodotoxin and neuromuscular transmission. Proc. roy. Soc. B **167**, 8—22 (1967b).

KATZ,B., MILEDI,R.: The release of acetylcholine from nerve endings by graded electric pulses. Proc. roy. Soc. B **167**, 23—38 (1967c).

KATZ,B., MILEDI,R.: The timing of calcium action during neuromuscular transmission. J. Physiol. (Lond.) **189**, 535—544 (1967d).

KATZ,B., MILEDI,R.: A study of synaptic transmission in the absence of nerve impulses. J. Physiol. (Lond.) **192**, 407—436 (1967e).

KATZ,B., MILEDI,R.: The role of calcium in neuromuscular facilitation. J. Physiol. (Lond.) **195**, 481—492 (1968a).

KATZ,B., MILEDI,R.: The effect of local blockage of motor nerve terminals. J. Physiol. (Lond.) **199**, 729—741 (1968b).

KATZ,B., MILEDI,R.: Tetrodotoxin-resistant electrical activity in presynaptic terminals. J. Physiol. (Lond.) **203**, 459—487 (1969a).

KATZ,B., MILEDI,R.: Spontaneous and evoked activity of motor nerve endings in calcium ringer. J. Physiol. (Lond.) **203**, 689—706 (1969b).

KATZ,B., MILEDI,R.: Further study of the role of calcium in synaptic transmission. J. Physiol. (Lond.) **207**, 789—801 (1970).

KATZ,B., MILEDI,R.: The effect of prolonged depolarization on synaptic transfer in the stellate ganglion of the squid. J. Physiol. (Lond.) **216**, 503—512 (1971).

KATZ,B., MILEDI,R.: The statistical nature of the acetylcholine potential and its molecular components. J. Physiol. (Lond.) **224**, 665—699 (1972).

KATZ,B., MILEDI,R.: The characteristics of "end-plate noise" produced by different depolarizing drugs. J. Physiol. (Lond.) **230**, 707—717 (1973a).

KATZ,B., MILEDI,R.: The binding of acetylcholine to receptors and its removal from the synaptic cleft. J. Physiol. (Lond.) **231**, 549—574 (1973b).

KATZ,B., MILEDI,R.: The effect of α-bungarotoxin on acetylcholine receptors. Brit. J. Pharmacol. **49**, 138—139 (1973c).

KATZ,B., MILEDI,R.: The effect of atropine on acetylcholine action at the neuromuscular junction. Proc. roy. Soc. B **184**, 221—226 (1973d).

KATZ,B., MILEDI,R.: The effect of procaine on the action of acetylcholine at the neuromuscular junction. J. Physiol. (Lond.) **249**, 269—284 (1975).

KATZ,B., THESLEFF,S.: On the factors which determine the amplitude of the "miniature end-plate potential". J. Physiol. (Lond.) **137**, 267—278 (1957a).

KATZ,B., THESLEFF,S.: A study of the "desensitization" produced by acetylcholine at the motor end-plate. J. Physiol. (Lond.) **138**, 63—80 (1957b).

KELLY, J.S.: Antagonism between Na$^+$ and Ca^{2+} at the neuromuscular junction. Nature (Lond.) **205**, 296—297 (1965).

KELLY, J.S.: The antagonism of Ca^{2+} by Na$^+$ and other monovalent ions at the frog neuromuscular junction. Quart. J. exp. Physiol. **53**, 239—249 (1968).

KEMENSKAYA, M.A., THESLEFF, S.: The neuromuscular blocking action of an isolated toxin from the elapid *(Oxyuranus scutellactus)*. Acta physiol. scand. **90**, 716—724 (1974).

KERNAN, R.P.: Membrane potential changes during sodium transport in frog sartorius muscle. Nature (Lond.) **193**, 986—987 (1962).

KERNAN, R.P.: Resting potential of isolated rat muscles measured in plasma. Nature (Lond.) **200**, 474—475 (1963).

KERNAN, R.P.: Membrane potential and chemical transmitter in active transport of ions by rat skeletal muscle. J. gen. Physiol. **51**, 204—210 (1968).

KERNAN, R.P.: Active transport and ionic concentration gradients in muscle. In: HARRIS, E.J. (Ed.): Transport and accumulation in biological systems, 3rd Ed. London: Butterworth 1972.

KHROMOV-BORISOV, N.V., MICHELSON, M.J.: The mutual disposition of cholinoreceptors of locomotor muscles and the changes in their disposition in the course of evolution. Pharmacol. Rev. **18**, 1051—1090 (1966).

KIM, K.C., KARCZMAR, A.G.: Adaptation of the neuromuscular junction to constant concentrations of acetylcholine. Int. J. Neuropharmacol. **6**, 51—61 (1967).

KIRSCHNER, L.B., STONE, W.E.: Action of inhibitors at the myoneural junction. J. gen. Physiol. **34**, 821—834 (1951).

KITA, H., VAN DER KLOOT, W.: Action of Co and Ni at the frog neuromuscular junction. Nature (Lond.) New Biology **245**, 52—53 (1973).

KLAUS, W., LÜLLMANN, H., MUSCHOLL, E.: Der Kalium-Flux des normalen und denervierten Rattenzwerchfells. Pflügers Arch. ges. Physiol. **271**, 761—775 (1960a).

KLAUS, W., LÜLLMANN, H., MUSCHOLL, E.: Der Einfluß von Acetylcholin auf die ^{42}Kalium-Abgabe postnataler denervierter und reinnervierter Skeletmuskulatur. Experientia (Basel) **16**, 498 (1960b).

KLAUS, W., LÜLLMANN, H., MUSCHOLL, E.: Die Wirkung von Acetylcholin auf den K- und Na-Flux und ihre pharmakologische Beeinflussung am denervierten Rattenzwerchfell. Arch. exp. Path. Pharmak. **241**, 281—292 (1961).

KOENIG, J., PÉCOT-DECHAVASSINE, M.: Relations entre l'apparition des potentials miniaturs spontanés et l'ultrastructure des plaques motrices en voie de reinnervation et de néoformation chez le rat. Brain Res. **27**, 43—57 (1971).

KOESTER, J., NASTUK, W.L.: Reversal potentials of cholinergic partial agonists. Fed. Proc. **29**, 716 (1970).

KOKETSU, K.: Action of tetraethylammonium chloride on neuromuscular transmission in frogs. Amer. J. Physiol. **193**, 213—218 (1958).

KOKETSU, K., NISHI, S.: Restoration of neuromuscular transmission in sodium-free hydrazinium solution. J. Physiol. (Lond.) **147**, 239—252 (1959).

KORDAŠ, M.: The effect of atropine and curarine on the time course of the end-plate potential in frog sartorius muscle. Int. J. Neuropharmacol. **7**, 523—530 (1968).

KORDAŠ, M.: The effect of membrane polarization on the time course of the end-plate current in frog sartorius muscle. J. Physiol. (Lond.) **204**, 493—502 (1969).

KORDAŠ, M.: The effect of procaine on neuromuscular transmission. J. Physiol. (Lond.) **209**, 689—699 (1970).

KORDAŠ, M.: An attempt at an analysis of the factors determining the time course of the end-plate current. I. The effect of prostigmine and of the ratio of Mg^{2+} to Ca^{2+}. J. Physiol. (Lond.) **224**, 317—332 (1972a).

KORDAŠ, M.: An attempt at an analysis of the factors determining the time course of the end-plate current. II. Temperature. J. Physiol. (Lond.) **224**, 333—348 (1972b).

KRAATZ, H.G., TRAUTWEIN, W.: Die Wirkung von 2,4-Dinitrophenol (DNP) auf die neuromuskuläre Erregungsübertragung. Arch. exp. Path. Pharmak. **231**, 419—439 (1957).

KRIEBEL, M.E., GROSS, C.E.: Multimodal distribution of frog miniature endplate potentials in adult, denervated and tadpole leg muscle. J. gen. Physiol. **64**, 85—103 (1974).

KRNJEVIĆ, K., MILEDI, R.: Some effects produced by adrenaline upon neuromuscular propagation in rats. J. Physiol. (Lond.) **141**, 291—304 (1958a).

KRNJEVIĆ,K., MILEDI,R.: Acetylcholine in mammalian neuromuscular transmission. Nature (Lond.) **182**, 805—806 (1958 b).

KRNJEVIĆ,K., MITCHELL,J.F., SZERB,J.C.: Determination of iontophoretic release of acetylcholine from micropipettes. J. Physiol. (Lond.) **165**, 421—436 (1963).

KRUCKENBERG,P., BAUER,H.: Die Dissoziation-konstante zwischen Curare und dem Acetylcholin-Receptor. Pflügers Arch. ges. Physiol. **326**, 184—192 (1971).

KUBA,K.: The action of phenol on neuromuscular transmission in the red muscle of fish. Jap. J. Physiol. **19**, 762—774 (1969).

KUBA,K.: Effects of catecholamines on the neuromuscular junction in the rat diaphragm. J. Physiol. (Lond.) **211**, 551—570 (1970).

KUBA,K., TOMITA,T.: Noradrenaline action on nerve terminal in the rat diaphragm. J. Physiol. (Lond.) **217**, 19—31 (1971).

KUFFLER,S.W., YOSHIKAMI,D.: The distribution of acetylcholine sensitivity at the post-synaptic membrane of vertebrate skeletal twitch muscles: iontophoretic mapping in the micron range. J. Physiol. (Lond.) **244**, 703—730 (1975).

KUNO,M.: Quantum aspects of central and ganglionic synaptic transmission in vertebrates. Physiol. Rev. **51**, 647—678 (1971).

KUNO,M., TURKANIS,S.A., WEAKLY,J.N.: Correlation between nerve terminal size and transmitter release at the neuromuscular junction of the frog. J. Physiol. (Lond.) **213**, 545—556 (1971).

LAMBERT,D.H., PARSONS,R.L.: Influence of polyvalent cations on the activation of muscle end-plate receptors. J. gen. Physiol. **56**, 309—321 (1970).

LANDAU,E.M.: The interaction of presynaptic polarization with calcium and magnesium in modifying spontaneous transmitter release from mammalian motor nerve terminals. J. Physiol. (Lond.) **203**, 281—299 (1969).

LANDAU,E.M., SMOLINSKY,A., LASS,Y.: Post-tetanic potentiation and facilitation do not share a common calcium-dependent mechanism. Nature (Lond.) New Biol. **244**, 155—157 (1973).

LANDOWNE,D., POTTER,L.T., TERRAR,D.A.: Structure-function relationship in excitable membranes. Ann. Rev. Physiol. **37**, 485—508 (1975).

LANE,N.J., GAGE,P.W.: Effects of Tiger snake venom on the ultrastructure of motor nerve terminals. Nature (Lond.) New Biology **244**, 94—96 (1973).

LANGLEY,J.N.: On the reaction of cells and of nerve endings to certain poisons, chiefly as regards the reaction of striated muscle to nicotine and to curari. J. Physiol. (Lond.) **33**, 374—413 (1905).

LANGLEY,J.N.: On the contraction of muscle, chiefly in relation to the presence of "receptive" substances. J. Physiol. (Lond.) **36**, 347—384 (1907).

LANGLEY,J.N.: The antagonism of curari and nicotine in skeletal muscles. J. Physiol. (Lond.) **48**, 73—108 (1914).

LAVALLÉE,M., SCHANNE,O.F., HÉBERT,N.C.: Glass microelectrodes. New York: Wiley 1969.

LEE,C.Y.: Chemistry and pharmacology of polypeptide toxins in snake venoms. Ann. Rev. Pharmacol. **12**, 265—286 (1972).

LEE,C.Y., CHANG,C.C., CHEN,Y.M.: Reversibility of neuromuscular blockade by neurotoxins from elapid and sea snake venoms. J. Formosan Med. Ass. **71**, 344—349 (1972).

LEE,C.Y., TSENG,L.F., CHIU,J.H.: Influence of denervation on localization of neurotoxins from elapid venoms in rat diaphragm. Nature (Lond.) **215**, 1177—1178 (1967).

LESTER,H.A.: Blockade of acetylcholine receptors by cobra toxin: electrophysiological studies. Molec. Pharmacol. **8**, 623—631 (1972a).

LESTER,H.A.: Vulnerability of desensitized or curare-treated acetylcholine receptors to irreversible blockade by cobra toxin. Molec. Pharmacol. **8**, 633—644 (1972b).

LI,C.L., SHY,G.M., WELLS,J.: Some properties of mammalian skeletal muscle fibres with particular reference to fibrillation potentials. J. Physiol. (Lond.) **135**, 522—535 (1957).

LIÈVREMONT,M., CZAJKA,M., TAZIEFF-DEPIERRE,F.: Étude in situ d'une fixation de calcium et de sa libération á la jonction neuromusculaire. C.R. Acad. Sci. (Paris) **267**D, 1988—1991 (1968).

LILEY,A.W.: An investigation of spontaneous activity at the neuromuscular junction of the rat. J. Physiol. (Lond.) **132**, 650—666 (1956a).

LILEY,A.W.: The quantal components of the mammalian end-plate potential. J. Physiol. (Lond.) **133**, 571—587 (1956b).

Liley,A.W.: The effects of presynaptic polarization on the spontaneous activity at the mammalian neuromuscular junction. J. Physiol. (Lond.) **134**, 427—443 (1956c).

Liley,A.W.: Spontaneous release of transmitter substance in multiquantal units. J. Physiol. (Lond.) **136**, 595—605 (1957).

Liley,A.W., North,K.A.K.: An electrical investigation of effects of repetitive stimulation on mammalian neuromuscular junction. J. Neurophysiol. **16**, 509—527 (1953).

Ling,G., Gerard,R.W.: The normal membrane potential of frog sartorius fibers. J. cell. comp. Physiol. **34**, 383—396 (1949).

Lipicky,R.J., Bryant,S.H., Salmon,J.H.: Cable parameters, sodium, potassium, chloride and water content, and potassium efflux in isolated external intercostal muscle of normal volunteers and patients with myotonia congenita. J. clin. Invest. **50**, 2091—2103 (1971).

Lømo,T., Rosenthal,J.: Control of acetylcholine sensitivity by muscle activity in the rat. J. Physiol. (Lond.) **221**, 493—513 (1972).

Longenecker,H.E., Hurlbut,W.P., Mauro,A., Clark,A.W.: Effects of black widow spider venom on the frog neuromuscular junction. Nature (Lond.) **225**, 701—703 (1970).

Lu,T.-C.: Affinity of curare-like compounds and their potency in blocking neuromuscular transmission. J. Pharmacol. exp. Ther. **174**, 560—566 (1970).

Lubińska,L., Zeleńa,J.: Acetylcholinesterase at muscle-tendon junctions during postnatal development in rats. J. Anat. (Lond.) **101**, 295—308 (1967).

Lundberg,A., Quilisch,H.: Presynaptic potentiation and depression of neuromuscular transmission in frog and rat. Acta physiol. scand. **30**, Suppl. III, 111—120 (1953a).

Lundberg,A., Quilisch,H.: On the effect of calcium on presynaptic potentiation and depression at the neuromuscular junction. Acta physiol. scand. **30**, Suppl. III, 121—129 (1953b).

Lunt,G.G., Stefani,E., De Robertis,E.: Increased incorporation of [G−^{3}H] Leucine into a possible "receptor" proteolipid in denervated muscle *in vivo*. J. Neurochem. **18**, 1545—1553 (1971).

Mackay,D.: A new method for the analysis of drug-receptor interactions. Advanc. Drug Res. **3**, 1—19 (1966).

Maclagan,J.: A comparison of the responses of the tenuissimus muscle to neuromuscular blocking drugs *in vivo* and *in vitro*. Brit. J. Pharmacol. **18**, 204—216 (1962).

Maclagan,J., Vrbová,G.: A study of the increased sensitivity of denervated and reinnervated muscle to depolarizing drugs. J. Physiol. (Lond.) **182**, 131—143 (1966).

Maeno,T.: Analysis of sodium and potassium conductances in the procaine end-plate potential. J. Physiol. (Lond.) **183**, 592—606 (1966).

Maeno,T., Edwards,C.: Neuromuscular facilitation with low frequency stimulation and effects of some drugs. J. Neurophysiol. **32**, 785—792 (1969).

Maeno,T., Edwards,C., Hashimura,S.: Differences in effects on end-plate potentials between procaine and lidocaine as revealed by voltage-clamp experiments. J. Neurophysiol. **34**, 32—46 (1971).

Magazanik,L.G.: Mechanism of desensitization of the post-synaptic membrane of the muscle fibre. Biofizika **13**, 199—203 (1968).

Magazanik,L.G.: Effect of sympathomimetic amines on the desensitization of the frog motor end-plate to acetylcholine. Sechenov physiol. J. U.S.S.R. **55**, 1147—1155 (1969).

Magazanik,L.G.: On the mechanism of influence of the diethylaminoethyl ether of diphenyl-propylacetic acid (SKF-525A) on neuromuscular synapses. (In Russian). Bull. Biol. Méd. Exp. URSS **69**, (3) 10—13 (1970).

Magazanik,L.G.: On the mechanism of antiacetylcholine effects of some mononitrogen anticholinergics in the neuromuscular synapse. Farmakol. i Toksikol. **3**, 292—296 (1971a).

Magazanik,L.G.: Influence of certain membrane stabilizers on the function of a neuromuscular synapse. Sechenov physiol. J. U.S.S.R. **57**, 1313—1321 (1971b).

Magazanik,L.G., Potapova,T.V.: Effect of changes in extracellular ionic medium on equilibrium potentials of the extrasynaptic membrane of denervated muscle. Biofizika **14**, 658—661 (1969) (English version in Neurosciences Translations **12**, 1—4, 1970).

Magazanik,L.G., Shekhirev,N.N.: Desensitization to acetylcholine in various frog muscles. Sechenov physiol. J. U.S.S.R. **56**, 582—588 (1970).

Magazanik,L.G., Vyskočil,F.: Different action of atropine and some analogues on the end-plate potentials and induced acetylcholine potentials. Experientia (Basel) **25**, 618—619 (1969).

MAGAZANIK,L.G., VYSKOČIL,F.: Dependence of acetylcholine desensitization on the membrane potential of frog muscle fibre and on the ionic changes in the medium. J. Physiol. (Lond.) **210**, 507—518 (1970).

MAGAZANIK,L.G., VYSKOČIL,F.: The loci of α-bungarotoxin action on the muscle postjunctional membrane. Brain Res. **48**, 420—423 (1972).

MAGAZANIK,L.G., VYSKOČIL,F.: Desensitization at the motor end-plate. In: RANG,H.P. (Ed.): Drug receptors, pp. 105—119. London: Macmillan 1973.

MAGAZANIK,L.G., VYSKOČIL,F.: The effect of temperature on desensitization kinetics at the post-synaptic membrane of the frog muscle fibre. J. Physiol. (Lond.) **249**, 285—300 (1975).

MAGLEBY,K.L.: The effect of repetitive stimulation on facilitation of transmitter release at the frog neuromuscular junction. J. Physiol. (Lond.) **234**, 327—352 (1973a).

MAGLEBY,K.L.: The effect of tetanic and post-tetanic potentiation on facilitation of transmitter release at the frog neuromuscular junction. J. Physiol. (Lond.) **234**, 353—371 (1973b).

MAGLEBY,K.L., STEVENS,C.F.: The effect of voltage on the time course of end-plate currents. J. Physiol. (Lond.) **223**, 151—171 (1972a).

MAGLEBY,K.L., STEVENS,C.F.: A quantitative description of end-plate currents. J. Physiol. (Lond.) **223**, 173—197 (1972b).

MAGLEBY,K.L., ZENGEL,J.E.: A dual effect of repetitive stimulation on post-tetanic potentiation of transmitter release at the frog neuromuscular junction. J. Physiol. (Lond.) **245**, 163—182 (1975a).

MAGLEBY,K.L., ZENGEL,J.E.: A quantitative description of tetanic and post-tetanic potentiation of transmitter release at the frog neuromuscular junction. J. Physiol. (Lond.) **245**, 183—208 (1975b).

MAHLER,H.R., CORDES,E.H.: Biological Chemistry. 2nd ed. New York: Harper and Row 1971.

MALLART,A., MARTIN,A.R.: An analysis of facilitation of transmitter release at the neuromuscular junction of the frog. J. Physiol. (Lond.) **193**, 679—694 (1967).

MALLART,A., MARTIN,A.R.: The relation between quantum content and facilitation at the neuromuscular junction of the frog. J. Physiol. (Lond.) **196**, 593—604 (1968).

MALLART,A., TRAUTMANN,A.: Ionic properties of the neuromuscular junction of the frog: effects of denervation and pH. J. Physiol. (Lond.) **234**, 553—567 (1973).

MAMBRINI,J., BENOIT,P.R.: Action de la caféine sur les jonctions neuro-musculaires de la grenouille. C.R. Soc. Biol. (Paris) **157**, 1373—1377 (1963).

MAMBRINI,J., BENOIT,P.R.: Action du calcium sur la jonction neuro-musculaire chez la grenouille. C.R. Soc. Biol. (Paris) **158**, 1454—1458 (1964).

MANALIS,R.S., COOPER,G.P.: Presynaptic and postsynaptic effects of lead at the frog neuromuscular junction. Nature (Lond.) **243**, 354—355 (1973).

MANTHEY,A.A.: The effect of calcium on the desensitization of membrane receptors at the neuromuscular junction. J. gen. Physiol. **49**, 963—976 (1966).

MANTHEY,A.A.: Further studies of the effect of calcium on the time course of the action of carbamylcholine at the neuromuscular junction. J. gen. Physiol. **56**, 407—419 (1970).

MANTHEY,A.A.: The antagonistic effects of calcium and potassium on the time course of action of carbamylcholine at the neuromuscular junction. J. Membrane Biol. **9**, 319—340 (1972).

MARTIN,A.R.: A further study of the statistical composition of the end-plate potential. J. Physiol. (Lond.) **130**, 114—122 (1955).

MARTIN,A.R.: Quantal nature of synaptic transmission. Physiol. Rev. **46**, 51—66 (1966).

MARTIN,A.R.: Synaptic Transmission. In: HUNT,C.C. (Ed.): MTP International Review of Science. Physiology Series I: Neurophysiology, Vol. 3, pp. 53—80. London: Butterworths 1975.

MARTIN,A.R., PILAR,G.: Quantal components of the synaptic potential in the ciliary ganglion of the chick. J. Physiol. (Lond.) **175**, 1—16 (1964a).

MARTIN,A.R., PILAR,G.: Presynaptic and postsynaptic events during post-tetanic potentiation and facilitation in the avian ciliary ganglion. J. Physiol. (Lond.) **175**, 17—30 (1964b).

MASLAND,R.L., WIGTON,R.S.: Nerve activity accompanying fasciculation produced by prostigmine. J. Neurophysiol. **3**, 269—275 (1940).

MEIRI,U., RAHAMIMOFF,R.: Neuromuscular transmission: inhibition by manganese ions. Science **176**, 308—309 (1972).

MELDRUM, B.S.: The actions of snake venoms on nerve and muscle. The pharmacology of phospholipase A and of polypeptide toxins. Pharmacol. Rev. **17**, 393—445 (1965).

MELLANBY, J., THOMPSON, P.A.: The effect of tetanus toxin at the neuromuscular junction of the goldfish. J. Physiol. (Lond.) **224**, 407—419 (1972).

MENRATH, R.L.E., BLACKMAN, J.G.: Observations on the large spontaneous potentials which occur at end-plates of the rat diaphragm. Proc. Univ. Otago med. Sch. **48**, 72—73 (1970).

MICHELSON, M.J., ZEIMAL, E.V.: Acetylcholine: an approach to the molecular mechanism of action. Oxford: Pergamon Press 1973.

MILEDI, R.: The acetylcholine sensitivity of frog muscle fibres after complete or partial denervation. J. Physiol. (Lond.) **151**, 1—23 (1960a).

MILEDI, R.: Junctional and extra-junctional acetylcholine receptors in skeletal muscle fibres. J. Physiol. (Lond.) **151**, 24—30 (1960b).

MILEDI, R.: Induction of receptors. In: MONGAR, J.L., DE REUCK, A.V.S. (Eds.): Enzymes and drug action, pp. 220—235. London: Churchill 1962.

MILEDI, R.: Strontium as a substitute for calcium in the process of transmitter release at the neuromuscular junction. Nature (Lond.) **212**, 1233—1234 (1966).

MILEDI, R.: Transmitter release induced by injection of calcium ions into nerve terminals. Proc. roy. Soc. B **183**, 421—425 (1973).

MILEDI, R., MOLINOFF, P., POTTER, L.T.: Isolation of the cholinergic receptor protein of *Torpedo* electric tissue. Nature (Lond.) **229**, 554—557 (1971a).

MILEDI, R., POTTER, L.T.: Acetylcholine receptors in muscle fibres. Nature (Lond.) **233**, 599—603 (1971).

MILEDI, R., SLATER, C.R.: Electrophysiology and electronmicroscopy of rat neuromuscular junction after nerve degeneration. Proc. roy. Soc. B **169**, 289—306 (1968).

MILEDI, R., STEFANI, E.: Miniature potentials in denervated slow muscle fibres of the frog. J. Physiol. (Lond.) **209**, 179—186 (1970).

MILEDI, R., STEFANI, E., STEINBACH, A.B.: Induction of the action potential mechanism in slow muscle fibres of the frog. J. Physiol. (Lond.) **217**, 737—754 (1971b).

MILEDI, R., STEFANI, E., ZELENÁ, J.: Neural control of acetylcholine-sensitivity in rat muscle fibres. Nature (Lond.) **220**, 497—498 (1968).

MILEDI, R., THIES, R.: Tetanic and post-tetanic rise in frequency of miniature end-plate potentials in low-calcium solutions. J. Physiol. (Lond.) **212**, 245—257 (1971).

MILEDI, R., TROWELL, O.A.: Acetylcholine sensitivity of rat diaphragm maintained in organ culture. Nature (Lond.) **194**, 981—982 (1962).

MILEDI, R., ZELENÁ, J.: Sensitivity to acetylcholine in rat slow muscle. Nature (Lond.) **210**, 855—856 (1966).

MIYAMOTO, M.D., BRECKENRIDGE, B.McL.: A cyclic adenosine monophosphate link in the catecholamine enhancement of transmitter release at the neuromuscular junction. J. gen. Physiol. **63**, 609—624 (1974).

MIYAMOTO, M.D., VOLLE, R.L.: Enhancement by carbachol of transmitter release from motor nerve terminals. Proc. nat. Acad. Sci. (Wash.) **71**, 1489—1492 (1974).

MONOD, J., WYMAN, J., CHANGEUX, J.-P.: On the nature of allosteric transitions: a plausible model. J. molec. Biol. **12**, 88—118 (1965).

MOORE, R.D.: Effect of insulin upon the sodium pump in frog skeletal muscle. J. Physiol. (Lond.) **232**, 23—45 (1973).

MORAN, N., RAHAMIMOFF, R.: Some statistical properties of neuromuscular facilitation. Israel J. med. Sci. **6**, 201—208 (1970).

MORAVEC, J., MELICHAR, I., JANSKÝ, L., VYSKOČIL, F.: Effect of hibernation and noradrenaline on the resting state of neuromuscular junction of Golden Hamster *(Mesocricetus auratus)*. Pflügers Arch. ges. Physiol. **345**, 93—106 (1973).

MUCHNIK, S., YARYURA, A.: The action of chlorpromazine on the neuromuscular junction. Acta physiol. lat.-amer. **19**, 94—100 (1969).

NASLEDOV, G.A., THESLEFF, S.: Denervation changes in frog skeletal muscle. Acta physiol. scand. **90**, 370—380 (1974).

NASTUK, W.L.: Membrane potential changes at a single muscle end-plate produced by transitory application of acetylcholine with an electrically controlled microjet. Fed. Proc. **12**, 102 (1953).

NASTUK,W.L.: Some ionic factors that influence the action of acetylcholine at the muscle end-plate membrane. Ann. N.Y. Acad. Sci. **81**, 317—327 (1959).

NASTUK,W.L.: Mechanisms of neuromuscular blockade. Ann. N.Y. Acad. Sci. **183**, 171—182 (1971).

NASTUK,W.L., HODGKIN,A.L.: The electrical activity of single muscle fibers. J. cell. comp. Physiol. **35**, 39—73 (1950).

NASTUK,W.L., KARIS,J.H.: The blocking action of hexafluorenium on neuromuscular transmission and its interaction with succinylcholine. J. Pharmacol. exp. Ther. **144**, 236—252 (1964).

NASTUK,W.L., LIU,J.H.: Muscle postjunctional membrane: changes in chemosensitivity produced by calcium. Science **154**, 266—267 (1966).

NASTUK,W.L., PARSONS,R.L.: Factors in the inactivation of postjunctional membrane receptors of frog skeletal muscle. J. gen. Physiol. **56**, 218—249 (1970).

NASTUK,W.L., POPPERS,P.J.: The effect of a thiamine analog on neuromuscular transmission. J. Pharmacol. exp. Ther. **154**, 441—448 (1966).

NICHOLLS,J.G.: The electrical properties of denervated skeletal muscle. J. Physiol. (Lond.) **131**, 1—12 (1956).

NIEDERGERKE,R.: The potassium chloride contracture of the heart and its modification by calcium. J. Physiol. (Lond.) **134**, 584—599 (1956).

NIEDERGERKE,R., ORKAND,R.K.: The dependence of the action potential of the frog's heart on the external and intracellular sodium concentration. J. Physiol. (Lond.) **184**, 312—334 (1966).

O'BRIEN,R.D., ELDEFRAWI,M.E., ELDEFRAWI,A.T.: Isolation of acetylcholine receptors. Ann. Rev. Pharmacol. **12**, 19—34 (1972).

OCHS,S.: Action of choline on frog sartorius muscle. J. Physiol. (Lond.) **182**, 244—254 (1966).

OCHS,S., MUKHERJEE,A.K.: Action of acetylcholine, choline and D-tubocurarine on the membrane of frog sartorius muscle. Amer. J. Physiol. **196**, 1191—1196 (1959).

OKADA,K.: Effects of alcohols and acetone on the neuromuscular junction of frog. Jap. J. Physiol. **17**, 245—261 (1967).

OKADA,K.: Effects of divalent cations on the spontaneous transmitter release at the amphibian neuromuscular junction in the presence of ethanol. Jap. J. Physiol. **20**, 97—111 (1970).

ONODERA,K., YAMAKAWA,K.: The effects of lithium on the neuromuscular junction of the frog. Jap. J. Physiol. **16**, 541—550 (1966).

OTSUKA,M., ENDO,M.: The effect of guanidine on neuromuscular transmission. J. Pharmacol. exp. Ther. **128**, 273—282 (1960).

OTSUKA,M., ENDO,M., NONOMURA,Y.: Presynaptic nature of neuromuscular depression. Jap. J. Physiol. **12**, 573—584 (1962).

OTSUKA,M., NONOMURA,Y.: The action of phenolic substances on motor nerve endings. J. Pharmacol. exp. Ther. **140**, 41—45 (1963).

PARKER,R.B., GOLDFINE,C.: Stoichiometry of the drug nicotinic receptor interaction. J. Pharmacol. exp. Ther. **185**, 649—652 (1973).

PARSONS,R.L.: Mechanism of neuromuscular blockade by tetraethylammonium. Amer. J. Physiol. **216**, 925—931 (1969).

PARSONS,R.L., HOFMANN,W.W., FEIGEN,G.A.: Presynaptic effects of potassium ion on the mammalian neuromuscular junction. Nature (Lond.) **208**, 590—591 (1965).

PARSONS,R.L., JOHNSON,E.W., LAMBERT,D.H.: Effects of lanthanum and calcium on chronically denervated muscle fibres. Amer. J. Physiol. **220**, 401—405 (1971).

PARSONS,R.L., NASTUK,W.L.: Activation of contractile system in depolarized skeletal muscle fibres. Amer. J. Physiol. **217**, 364—369 (1969).

PATON,W.D.M., WAUD,D.R.: The margin of safety of neuromuscular transmission. J. Physiol. (Lond.) **191**, 59—90 (1967).

PATRICK,J., LINDSTROM,J.: Autoimmune response to acetylcholine receptor. Science **180**, 871—872 (1973).

PATRICK,J., LINDSTROM,J., CULP,B., McMILLAN,J.: Studies on purified eel acetylcholine receptor and anti-acetylcholine receptor antibody. Proc. nat. Acad. Sci. (Wash.) **70**, 3334—3338 (1973).

PAYTON,B.W.: Use of the frog neuromuscular junction for assessing the action of drugs affecting synaptic transmission. Brit. J. Pharmacol. **28**, 35—43 (1966).

PAYTON, B. W., SHAND, D. G.: Actions of gallamine and tetraethylammonium at the frog neuro-muscular junction. Brit. J. Pharmacol. **28**, 23—24 (1966).

PÉCOT-DECHAVASSINE, M.: Effets conjugués du pH et des cations divalents sur la libération spontanée d'acétylcholine au niveau de la plaque motrice de la grenouille. C. R. Acad. Sci. (Paris) **271**, 674—677 (1970).

PEPER, K., MCMAHAN, U. J.: Distribution of acetylcholine receptors in the vicinity of nerve terminals on skeletal muscle of the frog. Proc. roy. Soc. B **181**, 431—440 (1972).

PILAR, G., VAUGHAN, P. C.: Electrophysiological investigations of the pigeon iris neuromuscular junctions. Comp. Biochem. Physiol. **29**, 51—72 (1969).

PORTELA, A., PEREZ, R. J., VACCARI, J., PEREZ, J. C., STEWART, P.: Muscle membrane depolarization by acetylcholine, choline and carbamylcholine, near and remote from motor end-plates. J. Pharmacol. exp. Ther. **175**, 476—482 (1970).

PORTER, C. W., BARNARD, E. A.: The density of cholinergic receptors at the endplate post-synaptic membrane: ultrastructural studies in two mammalian species. J. membrane Biol. **20**, 31—49 (1975).

PORTER, C. W., BARNARD, E. A., CHIU, T. H.: The ultrastructural localization and quantitation of cholinergic receptors at the mouse motor end-plate. J. Membrane Biol. **14**, 383—402 (1973a).

PORTER, C. W., CHIU, T. H., WIECKOWSKI, J., BARNARD, E. A.: Types and locations of cholinergic receptor-like molecules in muscle fibres. Nature (Lond.) New Biology **241**, 3—7 (1973b).

PORTER, R., O'CONNOR, M.: The molecular properties of drug receptors. London: Churchill 1970.

POTTER, L. T.: Synthesis, storage and release of [^{14}C] acetylcholine in isolated rat diaphragm muscles. J. Physiol. (Lond.) **206**, 145—166 (1970).

PURVES, D., SAKMANN, B.: The effect of contractile activity on fibrillation and extrajunctional acetylcholine-sensitivity in rat muscle maintained in organ culture. J. Physiol. (Lond.) **237**, 157—182 (1974).

QUASTEL, D. M. J., HACKETT, J. T., COOKE, J. D.: Calcium: is it required for transmitter secretion? Science **172**, 1034—1036 (1971).

RAHAMIMOFF, R.: A dual effect of calcium ions on neuromuscular facilitation. J. Physiol. (Lond.) **195**, 471—480 (1968).

RAHAMIMOFF, R., ALNAES, E.: Inhibitory action of ruthenium red on neuromuscular transmission. Proc. nat. Acad. Sci. (Wash.) **70**, 3613—3616 (1973).

RAHAMIMOFF, R., YAARI, Y.: Delayed release of transmitter at the frog neuromuscular junction. J. Physiol. (Lond.) **228**, 241—257 (1973).

RANDIĆ, M., STRAUGHAN, D. W.: Antidromic activity in the rat phrenic nerve-diaphragm preparation. J. Physiol. (Lond.) **173**, 130—148 (1964).

RANG, H. P.: The kinetics of action of acetylcholine antagonists in smooth muscle. Proc. Roy. Soc. B **164**, 488—510 (1966).

RANG, H. P.: Drug receptors and their function. Nature (Lond.) **231**, 91—96 (1971).

RANG, H. P.: Drug receptors. London: Macmillan 1973a.

RANG, H. P.: Receptor mechanisms (Fourth Gaddum Memorial Lecture). Brit. J. Pharmacol. **48**, 475—495 (1973b).

RANG, H. P.: In: Receptor Biochemistry and Biophysics. Neurosci. Res. Program Bull. **11**, 220—224 (1973c).

RANG, H. P.: Acetylcholine receptors. Quart. Rev. Biophys. **7**, 283—399 (1975).

RANG, H. P., RITTER, J. M.: A new kind of drug antagonism: evidence that agonists cause a molecular change in acetylcholine receptors. Molec. Pharmacol. **5**, 394—411 (1969).

RANG, H. P., RITTER, J. M.: On the mechanism of desensitization at cholinergic receptors. Molec. Pharmacol. **6**, 357—382 (1970a).

RANG, H. P., RITTER, J. M.: The relationship between desensitization and the metaphilic effect of cholinergic receptors. Molec. Pharmacol. **6**, 383—390 (1970b).

RANG, H. P., RITTER, J. M.: The effect of disulfide bond reduction on the properties of cholinergic receptors in chick muscle. Molec. Pharmacol. **7**, 620—631 (1971).

RAS, R., DEN HERTOG, A., LAMMERS, W.: The effect of suxamethonium on the striated muscle fibre outside the end-plate region. Pflügers Arch. ges. Physiol. **333**, 187—196 (1972).

RAS, R., MOOIJ, J. J. A.: The depolarizing effect of suxamethonium on the membrane potential of striated muscle fibres at endplate-free regions. Europ. J. Pharmacol. **23**, 217—222 (1973).

REDFERN, P., THESLEFF, S.: Action potential generation in denervated rat skeletal muscle. Acta physiol. scand. **82**, 70—78 (1971).

REID, J.: Quantum content in guinea-pig serratus anterior. Quart. J. exp. Physiol. **57**, 120—130 (1972).

RIBEIRO, J. A., WALKER, J.: The effects of ATP and ADP on transmission at the rat and frog neuromuscular junctions. Brit. J. Pharmacol. **54**, 213—218 (1975).

ROBERT, E. D., OESTER, Y. T.: Absence of supersensitivity to acetylcholine in innervated muscle subjected to a prolonged pharmacoligic nerve block. J. Pharmacol. exp. Ther. **174**, 133—140 (1970).

ROSENBLUETH, A., LUCO, J. V.: A study of denervated skeletal muscle. Amer. J. Physiol. **120**, 781—797 (1937).

ROSENTHAL, J.: Post-tetanic potentiation at the neuromuscular junction of the frog. J. Physiol. (Lond.) **203**, 121—133 (1969).

ROTSHENKER, S., RAHAMIMOFF, R.: Neuromuscular synapse: stochastic properties of spontaneous release of transmitter. Science **170**, 648—649 (1970).

RÜDEL, R., SENGES, J.: Mammalian skeletal muscle: reduced chloride conductance in drug-induced myotonia and induction of myotonia by low-chloride solution. Arch. exp. Path. Pharmak. **274**, 337—347 (1972).

SALAFSKY, B., BELL, J., PREWITT, M. A.: Development of fibrillation potentials in denervated fast and slow skeletal muscle. Amer. J. Physiol. **215**, 637—643 (1968).

SALPETER, M. M., ELDEFRAWI, M. E.: Sizes of end-plate compartments, densities of acetylcholine receptor and other quantitative aspects of neuromuscular transmission. J. Histochem. Cytochem. **21**, 769—778 (1973).

SCHILD, H. O.: pAx and competitive drug antagonism. Brit. J. Pharmacol. **4**, 277—280 (1949).

SCHMIDT, H., TONG, E. Y.: Inhibition by actinomycin D of the denervation-induced action potential in frog slow muscle fibres. Proc. roy. Soc. B **184**, 91—95 (1973).

SCHNEIDER, M. F.: Linear electrical properties of the transverse tubules and surface membrane of skeletal muscle fibres. J. gen. Physiol. **56**, 640—671 (1970).

SCHWAN, H. P.: Electrical properties of tissue and cell suspensions. Advanc. biol. med. Phys. **5**, 147—209 (1957).

SCUKA, M.: Analysis of the effects of histamine on the end-plate potential. Neuropharmacology **12**, 441—450 (1973).

SEVCIK, C., NARAHASHI, T.: Electrical properties and excitation contraction coupling in skeletal muscle treated with ethylene glycol. J. gen. Physiol. **60**, 221—236 (1972).

SEYAMA, I., NARAHASHI, T.: Mechanism of blockade of neuromuscular transmission by pentobarbital. J. Pharmacol. exp. Ther. **192**, 95—104 (1975).

SIMPSON, L. L.: The use of neuropoisons in the study of cholinergic transmission. Ann. Rev. Pharmacol. **14**, 305—317 (1974).

SOUČEK, B.: Complete model for the statistical composition of the end-plate potential. J. theor. Biol. **30**, 631—645 (1971).

SPITZER, N.: Miniature end-plate potentials at mammalian neuromuscular junctions poisoned by botulinum toxin. Nature (Lond.) New Biol. **237**, 26—27 (1972).

SRÉTER, F. A., WOO, G.: Cell water, sodium and potassium in red and white mammalian muscles. Amer. J. Physiol. **205**, 1290—1294 (1963).

STALČ, A., ŽUPANČIČ, A. O.: Effect of α-bungarotoxin on acetylcholinesterase bound to mouse diaphragm endplates. Nature (Lond.) New Biology **239**, 91—92 (1972).

STAMENOVIĆ, B. A.: The influence of adrenaline on the maintenance of the acetylcholine effect on the subsynaptic membrane of the isolated frog skeletal muscle. Jugoslav. Physiol. Pharmacol. Acta **1**, Suppl. 1, 101—106 (1968).

STANFIELD, P. R.: The differential effects of tetraethylammonium and zinc ions on the resting conductance of frog skeletal muscle. J. Physiol. (Lond.) **209**, 231—256 (1970).

STEFANI, E., STEINBACH, A. B.: Resting potential and electrical properties of frog slow muscle fibres. Effect of different external solutions. J. Physiol. (Lond.) **203**, 383—401 (1969).

STEINBACH, A. B.: Unusual endplate potentials which reflect the complexity of muscle structure. Nature (Lond.) **216**, 1331—1333 (1967).

STEINBACH, A. B.: Alteration by xylocaine (lidocaine) and its derivatives of the time course of the end-plate potential. J. gen. Physiol. **52**, 144—161 (1968 a).

STEINBACH, A. B.: A kinetic model for the action of xylocaine on the receptors for acetylcholine. J. gen. Physiol. **52**, 162—180 (1968 b).

STEINBERG, M. I., VOLLE, R. L.: A comparison of lobeline and nicotine at the frog neuromuscular junction. Arch. Pharmacol. **272**, 16—31 (1972).

STEPHENSON, R. P.: A modification of receptor theory. Brit. J. Pharmacol. **11**, 379—393 (1956).

STEPHENSON, R. P., GINSBORG, B. L.: Potentiation by an agonist. Nature (Lond.) **222**, 790—791 (1969).

STEVENS, C. F.: Inferences about membrane properties from electrical noise measurements. Biophys. J. **12**, 1028—1047 (1972).

STINNAKRE, J., TAUC, L.: Calcium influx in active *Aplysia* neurones detected by injected aequorin. Nature (Lond.) New Biology **242**, 113—115 (1973).

SUAREZ-KURTZ, G., PAULO, L. G., FONTELES, M. C.: Further studies on the neuromuscular effects of β-diethylaminoethyl-diphenyl propylacetate hydrochloride (SKF-525-A). Arch. int. Pharmacodyn. **177**, 185—195 (1969).

SUGIYAMA, H., BENDA, P., MEUNIER, J.-C., CHANGEUX, J.-P.: Immunological characterisation of the cholinergic receptor protein from *Electrophorus electricus*. FEBS Letters **35**, 124—128 (1973).

TAKEUCHI, A.: The long-lasting depression in neuromuscular transmission of the frog. Jap. J. Physiol. **8**, 102—113 (1958).

TAKEUCHI, A., TAKEUCHI, N.: Active-phase of frog's end-plate potential. J. Neurophysiol. **22**, 395—411 (1959).

TAKEUCHI, A., TAKEUCHI, N.: On the permeability of end-plate membrane during the action of transmitter. J. Physiol. (Lond.) **154**, 52—67 (1960).

TAKEUCHI, A., TAKEUCHI, N.: Changes in potassium concentration around motor nerve terminals, produced by current flow, and their effects on neuromuscular transmission. J. Physiol. (Lond.) **155**, 46—58 (1961).

TAKEUCHI, N.: Some properties of conductance changes at the end-plate membrane during the action of acetylcholine. J. Physiol. (Lond.) **167**, 128—140 (1963 a).

TAKEUCHI, N.: Effects of calcium on the conductance change of the end-plate membrane during the action of transmitter. J. Physiol. (Lond.) **167**, 141—155 (1963 b).

TAYLOR, D. B.: The role of inorganic ions in ion exchange processes at the cholinergic receptor of voluntary muscle. J. Pharmacol. exp. Ther. **186**, 537—551 (1973).

TAYLOR, D. B., CREESE, R., NEDERGAARD, O. A., CASE, R.: Labelled depolarizing drugs in normal and denervated muscle. Nature (Lond.) **208**, 901—902 (1965).

TAYLOR, D. B., DIXON, W. J., CREESE, R., CASE, R.: Diffusion of decamethonium in the rat. Nature (Lond.) **215**, 989 (1967).

TAYLOR, D. B., NEDERGAARD, O. A.: Relation between structure and action of quaternary ammonium neuromuscular blocking agents. Physiol. Rev. **45**, 523—554 (1965).

TAYLOR, D. B., STEINBORN, J., LU, T.-C.: Ion exchange processes at the neuromuscular junction of voluntary muscle. J. Pharmacol. exp. Ther. **175**, 213—227 (1970).

TERRAR, D. A.: Influence of SKF-525 A congeners, strophanthidin and tissue-culture media on desensitization in frog skeletal muscle. Brit. J. Pharmacol. **51**, 259—268 (1974).

THESLEFF, S.: The mode of neuromuscular block caused by acetylcholine, nicotine, decamethonium and succinylcholine. Acta physiol. scand. **34**, 218—231 (1955 a).

THESLEFF, S.: The effects of acetylcholine, decamethonium and succinylcholine on neuromuscular transmission in the rat. Acta physiol. scand. **34**, 386—392 (1955 b).

THESLEFF, S.: Supersensitivity of skeletal muscle produced by botulinum toxin. J. Physiol. (Lond.) **151**, 598—607 (1960).

THESLEFF, S.: Functional properties of receptors in striated muscle. In: RANG, H. P. (Ed.): Drug Receptors, pp. 121—133. London: Macmillan 1973.

THIES, R. E.: Neuromuscular depression and apparent depletion of transmitter in mammalian muscle. J. Neurophysiol. **28**, 427—442 (1965).

THOMAS, R. C.: Electrogenic sodium pump in nerve and muscle cells. Physiol. Rev. **52**, 563—594 (1972).

THOMSON, T. D., TURKANIS, S. A.: Barbiturate-induced transmitter release at a frog neuromuscular junction. Brit. J. Pharmacol. **48**, 48—58 (1973).

THRON, C. D.: On the analysis of pharmacological experiments in terms of an allosteric receptor model. Molec. Pharmacol. **9**, 1—9 (1973).

TRUOG, P., WASER, P. G.: Einflüsse der Denervation von Muskelendplatten auf die Lokalisation der Acetylcholinesterase und die Bindung von Decamethonium. Arch. exp. Path. Pharmak. **266**, 101—112 (1970).

TURKANIS, S. A.: Effects of muscle stretch on transmitter release at end-plates of rat diaphragm and frog sartorius muscle. J. Physiol. (Lond.) **230**, 391—403 (1973 a).

TURKANIS, S. A.: Some effects of vinblastine and colchicine on neuromuscular transmission. Brain Res. **54**, 324—329 (1973 b).

VAN MAANEN, E. F.: The antagonism between acetylcholine and the curare alkaloids D-tubocurarine, c-curarine-I, c-toxiferine-II and β-erythroidine in the rectus abdominis of the frog. J. Pharmacol. exp. Ther. **99**, 255—264 (1950).

VERE-JONES, D.: Simple stochastic models for the release of quanta of transmitter from a nerve terminal. Aust. J. Stat. **8**, 53—63 (1966).

VERVEEN, A. A., DE FELICE, L. J.: Membrane noise. In: BUTLER, J. A. V., NOBLE, D. (Eds.): Progr. Biophys. Mol. Biol., Vol. 28. Oxford: Pergamon 1974.

VINCENT, A.: Turnover of motor end-plate. Nature (Lond.) **254**, 182—184 (1975).

VLADIMIROVA, A. T.: Effect of electric polarization of motor nerve terminals on the transmission of single impulses. Bull. Biol. Méd. Exp. URSS **11**, 11—14 (1963).

VOGEL, Z., SYTKOWSKI, A. J., NIRENBERG, M. W.: Acetylcholine receptors of muscle grown in vitro. Proc. nat. Acad. Sci. (Wash.) **69**, 3180—3184 (1972).

VRBOVÁ, G.: Induction of an extrajunctional chemosensitive area in intact innervated muscle fibres. J. Physiol. (Lond.) **191**, 20—21 P (1967).

VYSKOČIL, F., MAGAZANIK, L. G.: The desensitization of post-junctional muscle membrane after intracellular application of membrane stabilizers and snake venom polypeptides. Brain Res. **48**, 417—419 (1972).

WASER, P. G.: On receptors in the post-synaptic membrane of the motor end-plate. In: PORTER, R., O'CONNOR, M. (Eds.): Molecular Properties of Drug Receptors. London: Churchill 1970.

WASER, P. G.: Localization of ^{14}C-pancuronium by histo- and wholebody-autoradiography in normal and pregnant mice. Arch. Pharmacol. **279**, 399—412 (1973).

WASER, P. G., LÜTHI, U.: Autoradiographische Lokalisation von ^{14}C-Calebassen—curarin I und ^{14}C—Decamethonium in der Motorischen Endplatte. Arch. int. Pharmacodyn. **112**, 272—296 (1957).

WAUD, B. E., WAUD, D. R.: The relation between the response to "train of four" stimulation and receptor occlusion during competitive neuromuscular block. Anesthesiology **37**, 413—416 (1972).

WAUD, B. E., CHENG, M. C., WAUD, D. R.: Comparison of drug-receptor dissociation constants at the mammalian neuromuscular junction in the presence and absence of halothane. J. Pharmacol. exp. Ther. **187**, 40—46 (1973).

WAUD, D. R.: The rate of action of competitive neuromuscular blocking agents. J. Pharmacol. exp. Ther. **158**, 99—114 (1967).

WAUD, D. R.: On the measurement of the affinity of partial agonists for receptors. J. Pharmacol. exp. Ther. **170**, 117—122 (1969).

WAUD, D. R.: A review of pharmacological approaches to the acetylcholine receptors at the neuromuscular junction. Ann. N.Y. Acad. Sci. **183**, 147—157 (1971).

WAUD, D. R.: Adsorption isotherm vs. ion exchange models for the drug-receptor relation. J. Pharmacol. exp. Ther. **188**, 520—528 (1974).

WAUD, D. R., WAUD, B. E.: The relationship between tetanic fade and receptor occlusion in the presence of competitive neuromuscular block. Anesthesiology **35**, 456—464 (1971).

WEAKLY, J. N.: The action of cobalt ions on neuromuscular transmission in the frog. J. Physiol. (Lond.) **234**, 597—612 (1973).

WEBER, A., MURRAY, J. M.: Molecular control mechanisms in muscle contraction. Physiol. Rev. **53**, 612—673 (1973).

WEINREICH, D.: Ionic mechanism of post-tetanic potentiation at the neuromuscular junction of the frog. J. Physiol. (Lond.) **212**, 431—446 (1971).

WERMAN, R.: An electrophysiological approach to drug-receptor mechanisms. Comp. Biochem. Physiol. **30**, 997—1017 (1969).

WERMAN, R., CARLEN, P. L., KUSHNIR, M., KOSOWER, E. M.: Effect of thiol-oxidizing agent, diamide, on acetylcholine release at the frog end-plate. Nature (Lond.) **233**, 120—121 (1971).

WERMAN, R., MANALIS, R. S.: Reversal potential measurements for strong and weak agonists of acetylcholine at the frog neuromuscular junction. Israel J. med. Sci. **6**, 320—321 (1970).

WERMAN, R., WISLICKI, L.: Propranolol, a curariform and cholinomimetic agent at the frog neuromuscular junction. Comp. Gen. Pharmacol. **2**, 69—81 (1971).

WERNIG, A.: Changes in statistical parameters during facilitation at the crayfish neuromuscular junction. J. Physiol. (Lond.) **226**, 751—759 (1972 a).

WERNIG, A.: The effects of calcium and magnesium on statistical release parameters at the crayfish neuromuscular junction. J. Physiol. (Lond.) **226**, 761—768 (1972 b).

WERNIG, A.: Estimates of statistical release parameters from crayfish and frog neuromuscular junctions. J. Physiol. (Lond.) **244**, 207—221 (1975).

WESTMORELAND, B. F., WARD, D., JOHNS, T. R.: The effect of methohexital at the neuromuscular junction. Brain Res. **26**, 465—468 (1971).

WILSON, D. F.: The effects of dibutryl cyclic adenosine 3', 5'-monophosphate, theophylline and aminophylline on neuromuscular transmission in the rat. J. Pharmacol. exp. Ther. **188**, 447—452 (1974).

WOODBURY, J. W., MILES, P. R.: Anion conductance of frog muscle membranes: one channel, two kinds of pH dependence. J. gen. Physiol. **62**, 324—353 (1973).

YOUNKIN, S. G.: An analysis of the role of calcium in facilitation at the frog neuromuscular junction. J. Physiol. (Lond.) **237**, 1—14 (1974).

ZACHAR, J.: Electrogenesis and contractility in skeletal muscle cells. Baltimore: University Park Press 1971.

ZAIMIS, E.: Transmission and block at the motor end-plate and in autonomic ganglia. The interruption of neuromuscular transmission and some of its problems. Pharmacol. Rev. **6**, 53—57 (1954).

ZAIMIS, E.: Experimental hazards and artefacts in the study of neuromuscular blocking drugs. In: DE REUCK, A. V. S. (Ed.): Curare and Curare-like Agents, pp. 75—82. London: Churchill 1962.

ZIERLER, K. L., ROGUS, E., HAZELWOOD, C. F.: Effect of insulin on potassium flux and water and electrolyte content of muscles from normal and from hypophysectomised rats. J. gen. Physiol. **49**, 433—456 (1966).

ZUCKER, R. S.: Changes in the statistics of transmitter release during facilitation. J. Physiol. (Lond.) **229**, 787—810 (1973).

CHAPTER 4 A

Depolarising Neuromuscular Blocking Drugs

ELEANOR ZAIMIS and S. HEAD

Since the publication of the review by PATON and ZAIMIS on the "Methonium Compounds" (1952), the pharmacology of depolarising neuromuscular blocking drugs has been covered from various vantage points by a number of other authors, including BOVET (1972), BOWMAN (1964), BOWMAN and MARSHALL (1972), BOWMAN and WEBB (1972), CHAGAS et al. (1972), CHEYMOL and BOURILLET (1972), FOLDES (1960), FOLDES and DUNCALF (1972), KARCZMAR (1967), MICHELSON and ZEIMAL (1973), PATON (1956), COOKSON and PATON (1969), THESLEFF and QUASTEL (1965), VOURC'H (1972). Because of this, the present chapter will not aim at the orthodox overall coverage, but will concentrate instead on areas of especial relevance to the actions of these drugs and particularly on certain recent developments.

A. General Introduction

In 1850 PELOUZE and BERNARD made an observation which marks the first step towards our understanding of neuromuscular transmission. They noticed that while stimulation of motor nerves in animals killed by toxic doses of a variety of substances still produced muscle contractions, this was not the case with animals poisoned with curare. Their own description was:« sur l'animal encore chaud et mort depuis une minute les nerfs sont inertes comme sur un animal qui serait froid et mort depuis longtemps». However, it was not until comparatively recently that sufficient information became available to allow coherent theories on the mechanism of transmission to be developed. The most important discovery during this period has been the demonstration by DALE and his co-workers (DALE and FELDBERG, 1934; DALE et al., 1936; BROWN et al., 1936), that transmission at the neuromuscular junction is brought about by the action of acetylcholine. "Our observations", they said, "seem to us to be compatible with a form of chemical transmission, in which the direct stimulant of the muscle fibre at its end-plate, acetylcholine, is liberated by arrival of the nerve impulses at the nerve ending, and destroyed during the refractory period by a local concentration of cholinesterase". Curare has been an invaluable tool in such studies, which have also shed light on how curare itself exerts its action. Many disciplines have contributed, but it is to pharmacological analyses, histochemistry, biochemistry, electron microscopy and the development of valuable electrophysiological techniques that progress is primarily due.

For many years the only well-known neuromuscular blocking drug was curare which has the property of being sufficiently like acetylcholine to have an affinity for the specific receptors normally reacting to acetylcholine at the neuromuscular junction, but is so unlike acetylcholine that it cannot activate the receptors. In 1937, however, it was demonstrated for the first time that competition with acetylcholine is not the only mechanism by which a substance can produce a neuromuscular block. Bacq and Brown reported in that year that acetylcholine itself can produce an interruption of neuromuscular transmission if made to accumulate under the influence of an anticholinesterase drug. Almost ten years later synthetic substances were discovered whose action can be regarded as similar to that of acetylcholine, except that their action is spread out over a much longer period.

As a consequence of the observation made by W.D.M.Paton that octamethylene-bistrimethylammonium chloride (prepared by Harold King) was remarkably effective in causing neuromuscular block, a number of bisquaternary ammonium salts were synthetized by Zaimis (1950). They are all polymethylene bistrimethylammonium di-iodides of the general type I $[(CH_3)_3 N(CH_2)n-N(CH_3)_3]$ I where n is from 2 to 13 and 18. At the same time, Barlow and Ing (1948a and b) independently prepared the dibromides, with the exception of the hexamethylene member. The name "methonium compounds" was approved by the British Pharmacopoeia Commission for the members of the polymethylene bistrimethylammonium series, and it is under this name, preceded by the appropriate numerical prefix, that they have since been known.

One of the most remarkable properties of the members of this series, and especially of decamethonium, was the very great variation in their activity depending on the species of animal on which they were tested. Variation of this sort has been described for many other onium salts, but in the case of decamethonium its magnitude was unprecedented, and sufficient for great activity to be found in the cat but only slight activity in the rat. This observation led Paton and Zaimis (1949b) to conclude that in future any investigations of new "curarizing" agents must necessarily be made with more than one species.

B. An Introduction to the Pharmacological Actions of Decamethonium at the Neuromuscular Junction

The early pharmacological experiments described by Paton and Zaimis (1948a and b, 1949a and b, 1950, 1951a and b) demonstrated that although decamethonium possessed some of what were classically regarded as "curarizing" properties (i.e. paralysed neuromuscular transmission leaving nervous conduction unaltered; permitted the muscle to respond to direct stimulation; prevented the effect of a close-arterial injection of acetylcholine; did not interfere with the release of acetylcholine), there were also important differences. For example: 1) a phase of potentiation of the muscle twitch with fasciculations of the muscle and repetitive responses to single nerve volleys preceded the block; 2) tetanization of the motor nerve or injection of acetylcholine or potassium neither diminished nor deepened the block; 3) during a partial block tetanization of the muscle gave rise to a well-sustained contraction; 4) sensitivity to decamethonium varied greatly according to species; in order of decreasing sensitivity, the order is cat-man-rabbit-monkey-mouse-rat. Using the same tests, the variation in sensitivity with tubocurarine was much smaller, the order being rat-mouse-rabbit-cat; 5) the action of decamethonium was not antagonized by anticholinesterase drugs; 6) previous administration of tubocurarine reduced the effectiveness of decamethonium; 7) penta- and hexamethonium provided effective antagonists and the antagonism appeared to be by competitive inhibition; 8) decamethonium elicited a contraction of the frog's rectus abdominis muscle, and did not antagonize the contraction elicited by acetylcholine; 9) decamethonium could also elicit a twitch of the cat's tibialis muscle if a small dose was given by close-arterial injection.

It was concluded, therefore, that decamethonium produced neuromuscular block by initiating some active response in the end-plate or muscle fibre and that the differences between tubocurarine and decamethonium were so striking as to indicate the possibility of a fundamental divergence in their mode of action.

An analysis of these stimulant effects by ZAIMIS (1951) established that they cannot be attributed to the weak anticholinesterase activity of decamethonium, and emphasized the similarities between decamethonium and acetylcholine. The evidence against an action through anticholinesterase activity was (1) that the stimulant action was still demonstrable in the presence of a known anticholinesterase in concentrations sufficient to inactivate all the enzymes; (2) that the stimulant action did not parallel the anticholinesterase actions when these were compared in a series of compounds, including tetramethylammonium; (3) that the stimulant effects were transient and different from those elicited by anticholinesterases in many respects.

The strongest evidence that the potentiation of the twitch and the spontaneous fasciculations were not due to the weak anticholinesterase activity but to the active acetylcholine-like action of decamethonium was obtained from denervated cat muscle. The close-arterial injection of decamethonium into the tibialis anterior muscle, denervated by the section of its nerve supply 15 to 20 days previously, produced a double mechanical response consisting of a quick initial contraction followed by a prolonged contracture. The quick response was accompanied by an outburst of action potentials, greatly in excess of any previous spontaneous activity; this outburst of action potentials was cut short with the onset of slow contracture during which no more rapid action potentials could be detected. Acetylcholine, in doses similar to those of decamethonium (2 to 10 µg) produced the same effect.

The conclusion was therefore drawn that decamethonium possesses many of the properties of acetylcholine at the neuromuscular junction, but differs from it in being a stable substance unaffected by the local enzyme.

C. End-Plate Depolarisation
by Decamethonium and Suxamethonium in vivo

BURNS and PATON (1951), using the gracilis muscle of the cat and recording with external electrodes, demonstrated that this likeness of decamethonium to acetylcholine rests in the ability of decamethonium to cause a persistent depolarisation of the end-plate region. They showed, moreover, that all the principal features of block by decamethonium can be reproduced with acetylcholine in the presence of an anticholinesterase drug. The depolarisation produced by decamethonium, although limited to the end-plate region, always extended slightly beyond the area in which end-plate potentials could be recorded. The extent of this spatial distribution increased with time. After an initial transient increase of excitability which was associated with random spontaneous fasciculations, the end-plate region depolarised by decamethonium became inexcitable to direct stimulation, although the muscle remote from the end-plate region remained normally excitable. With intravenous administration of doses of the order of 30 µg/kg the development of local depolarisation was comparatively slow; the peak value was reached only 3 to 5 min after injection, and was followed by a steady repolarisation to the normal value, taking 30 to 40 min for its completion. Intra-arterial injection, on the other hand, caused an immediate depolarisation of the end-plate region, and recovery was continuous from a few moments after injection. Moreover, the greatest depolarisations that BURNS and PATON had produced by intravenous administration of decamethonium had never exceeded about 40% of the maximal depolarisation following arterial injection.

BURNS and PATON concluded that the inexcitability of the muscle membrane around the point at which the end-plate potential is set up was a principal cause of the neuromuscular block produced by decamethonium. Successive doses of decamethonium produced progressively smaller depolarisations, even if time was allowed for full recovery from each dose. It was suggested, therefore, that a new mechanism of block was present, namely a decrease in the electrical excitability of the membrane of the end-plate region as a result of the persisting depolarisation.

All the principal features of block by decamethonium could be reproduced with acetylcholine, or by tetanization of the motor nerve in the presence of an anticholinesterase. Removal of the end-plate depolarisation, by passing an anodal current at the end-plate region, restored neuromuscular transmission in a muscle blocked by decamethonium. Cathodal currents, on the other hand, intensified the decamethonium block. BURNS and PATON concluded that the characteristic features of block by decamethonium and acetylcholine at the neuromuscular junction are simply those of any persistent cathode.

Similar results were obtained with suxamethonium, another depolarising drug introduced by BOVET and BOVET-NITTI in 1955. Using the same method of recording, PATON and WAUD (1962) demonstrated that when suxamethonium was given to a cat to produce between 90 and 100% block for a period up to one hour, the end-plates do indeed remain depolarised throughout, but that the peak depolarisation falls to a steady level of about half the maximum.

D. Effect of Decamethonium, Suxamethonium and Acetylcholine on the Electrical Properties of Single Mammalian Muscle Cells

More recently the electrical properties of single mammalian muscle cells were studied in the presence of concentrations of decamethonium or suxamethonium similar to those required to produce neuromuscular block. The cat tenuissimus muscle was chosen for these experiments because cat and human skeletal muscles are very similar in their responses to neuromuscular blocking drugs. Moreover, the tenuissimus muscle is very similar in its physiological characteristics and its responses to neuromuscular blocking drugs to the well studied tibialis anterior muscle (PATON and ZAIMIS, 1952; ZAIMIS, 1953; MACLAGAN, 1962). On a practical level, the muscle is thin and covered by a layer of connective tissue which is easily removed; the muscle is thus readily accessible and can be dissected easily, so that it can be isolated together with its nerve for *in vitro* experiments.

Experiments were first performed *in vivo* using slow intravenous infusions of tritiated decamethonium. To a solution of unlabelled decamethonium iodide, tritiated decamethonium (methyl-H^3) chloride was added to give a final concentration equivalent to 10 µg/ml decamethonium iodide and possessing radioactivity of 4.44×10^6 d.p.m./ml. The plasma concentration of decamethonium was measured by liquid scintillation counting from blood samples which were taken at regular intervals, while the degree of neuromuscular block was assessed by recording the contractions of the indirectly stimulated tenuissimus muscle. The upper part of Fig. 1 shows the plasma concentration that was achieved in three individual experiments during prolonged infusions of tritiated decamethonium at the rate of 5 to 7 µg/kg per min. Muscle fasciculations and an increase in twitch tension ($> 70\%$) became obvious at a concentration of decamethonium of 0.53 µmol/l. When the plasma concentration of decamethonium reached 0.88 µmol/l, reduction in twitch tension could be observed. The infusion rate was then adjusted and maintained for a further period of 58 to 70 min at a constant rate. The results showed that a plasma concentration of 1 to 1.4 µmol/l decamethonium was sufficient to produce an 80 to 90% block. This is similar to the concentration of radioactive decamethonium found necessary by CREESE and MACLAGAN (1972) to maintain a neuromuscular block in the tibialis anterior muscle of the cat.

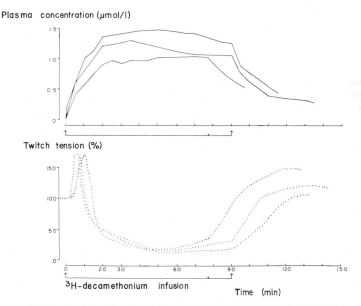

Fig. 1. Cat; anaesthetised with chloralose. Lower trace: neuromuscular blockade produced in three animals by tritiated decamethonium (slow intravenous infusion, 5 to 7 µg/kg per min). The graphs show the twitch tension of indirectly elicited maximal contractions of the tenuissimus muscle expressed as a percentage of the control value. Upper trace; plasma concentrations of tritiated decamethonium during the infusion, measured by liquid scintillation counting

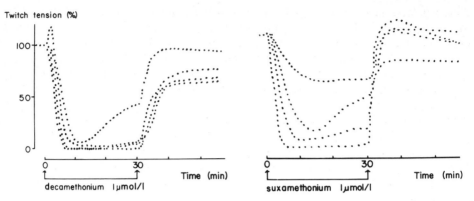

Fig. 2. Cat; isolated tenuissimus muscle. Neuromuscular block produced by decamethonium and suxamethonium (1 µmol/l) applied for 30 min in different preparations. The graphs show the twitch tension of the indirectly elicited contractions expressed as a percentage of the control value

Suxamethonium chloride was infused intravenously at a constant rate of 14 to 17 µg/kg per min for 30 min. Although plasma suxamethonium concentrations have not been measured in the intact animal, the range of blood levels in man during a suxamethonium infusion was found to be between 0.25 and 10 µmol/l (KVISSEL-GAARD and MOYA, 1961). Two minutes after the infusion started an increase in twitch tension and generalised muscle fasciculations could be seen which lasted for about 2 min. This period of potentiation gave way to neuromuscular block. When the infusion was stopped after 30 min the twitch started to recover within one min. Recovery was complete within 4 to 8 min, and was followed by a period during which potentiation of the twitch occurred ($28 \pm 9\%$). Figure 4A illustrates these results.

This increase in twitch tension above the control levels following recovery from a neuromuscular block produced by decamethonium or suxamethonium is a well recognised phenomenon. The size of this increase is always greater following the first dose in each experiment. MACLAGAN and VRBOVÁ (1966) demonstrated that this potentiation is not the result of repetitive firing of the muscle fibres and suggested that the phenomenon could be the consequence of the hyperpolarisation of the muscle membrane which they recorded with external electrodes during this phase. Decisive proof, however, is not yet available. A similar increase was found by NASTUK and GISSEN (1965) in isolated frog muscle which had been blocked by acetylcholine or carbachol. However, the increase in muscle contraction did not follow the block when the muscle was bathed in solutions containing low calcium concentrations. NASTUK and GISSEN suggested that exposure to depolarising drugs increases calcium uptake and that this extra calcium potentiates the tension developed by the muscle fibres as soon as neuromuscular transmission is restored.

For the *in vitro* work (recording the muscle contractions or measurement of the electrical properties of single muscle cells) great care was taken to ensure that the muscle was rapidly dissected and that adequate oxygenation and a steady temperature where maintained. After dissection the muscle was placed within 5 sec into a beaker containing about 100 ml of oxygenated Krebs solution at 37° C. Within

30 sec the muscle was transferred to a recording chamber (volume 2 to 3 ml) situated in a Faraday cage. Oxygenated Krebs solution at 37.5° C ± 0.5° C flowed through the chamber at a rate of 12 to 15 ml/min for the whole duration of the experiment.

With the tenuissimus muscle *in vitro* it was found that at a concentration of 1 µmol/l, both decamethonium and suxamethonium produced an 80 to 98% neuromuscular block. Thus it was established that similar concentrations give rise to the same degree of neuromuscular block in both the *in vivo* and *in vitro* preparations. Application of both decamethonium and suxamethonium was maintained for 30 min. In all preparations the neuromuscular block became maximal in about 10 min. In three out of four experiments the neuromuscular block was well maintained during the exposure of the muscle to either decamethonium or suxamethonium. In only one experiment with either drug was there a partial recovery of the twitch tension (Fig. 2).

In order to test the extent to which the depolarisation was sustained during continued application of decamethonium or suxamethonium, changes in membrane potential and input resistance at the end-plate region of single surface muscle cells of the tenuissimus muscle were recorded using intracellular microelectrodes.

1. Membrane Potential

Prolonged application of 1 µmol/l suxamethonium or decamethonium produced a depolarisation at the end-plate region. The drugs were always applied in a continuously flowing solution. From a value of about −85 mV the membrane potential decreased to about −42 mV in the presence of either drug. Contraction of the muscle did not occur when the membrane potential reached the threshold value for action potential generation of −55 mV (BOYD and MARTIN, 1956). It appears that the rate of depolarisation at this concentration is too slow to initiate an action potential. When a higher concentration of decamethonium was used (6 µmol/l), causing a faster initial depolarisation, action potentials were generated and contraction of the muscle occurred.

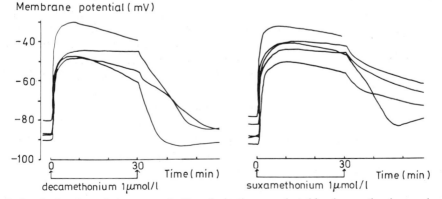

Fig. 3. Cat; isolated tenuissimus muscle. Depolarisations produced by decamethonium and suxamethonium (1 µmol/l) and recorded from the end-plate region of surface muscle cells in different preparations. Continuous recording for up to 60 min. During this period the drugs were applied for 30 min

Figure 3 shows continuous recordings of membrane potential over periods of up to 60 min in preparations considered technically satisfactory. The replacement of the normal Krebs solution with a solution containing 1 µmol/l decamethonium or suxamethonium caused an almost immediate depolarisation at an initial rate of 100 to 200 mV/min, over a period of 15 to 20 sec. This rapid phase of depolarisation was followed by a slower one, maximal depolarisation being reached in about 5 to 8 min.

In four experiments with decamethonium and five with suxamethonium the depolarising drug was applied continuously for 30 min. During this period a depolarisation of about 43 mV was well maintained in 4 out of 9 fibres. In the other five fibres while depolarisation tended to diminish with time, it was still substantial after 30 min. In the preparation which showed the largest repolarisation the membrane was still depolarised by 28 mV after 30 min of continuous application of decamethonium. Maintained depolarisation was recorded for periods of up to 50 min under continuous application of decamethonium.

In seven experiments higher concentrations of decamethonium (2 and 4 µmol/l) were used for periods of 15 and 30 min; depolarisation was once more well maintained. In order to exclude distortions that could be ascribed to mechanical movements the microelectrode was removed and re-implanted in the same fibre several times in some experiments, before and during the decamethonium application. The time-course of the depolarisation was the same as with the continuous recording. In

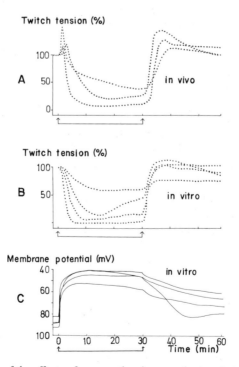

Fig. 4A—C. Comparison of the effects of suxamethonium on the tenuissimus muscle: (A) recording of muscle contractions *in vivo;* (B) recording of muscle contractions *in vitro;* (C) recording of membrane potential from single muscle fibres *in vitro.* (See text for details). In (A) and (B), twitch tension is expressed as a percentage of the control value

conclusion, there was a good correlation between (a) neuromuscular block measured *in vivo* and *in vitro* by means of indirectly elicited contraction of the tenuissimus muscle and (b) the changes in membrane potential at the end-plate region. Figure 4 illustrates this correlation for suxamethonium.

2. Input Resistance

In experiments in which membrane potential and input resistance were recorded simultaneously, a second microelectrode, carrying pulses of current of constant duration and magnitude, was inserted into the fibre within 70 μm of the recording electrode. Thus not only membrane potential but also electrotonic potentials were measured through the recording electrode. Figure 5A illustrates such an experiment. Changes in membrane potential (in mV) are shown by the continuous line, while the interrupted vertical lines represent electrotonic potentials. It is known that the size of the electrotonic potentials (also expressed in mV) is proportional to the input resistance of the cell, which may be derived from the formula $R = V/I$, and is expressed in ohms. Figure 5B is a graphical representation of the input resistance of the muscle fibre of Fig. 5A plotted against the membrane potential during the initial phase of depolarisation (until depolarisation reached its maximum). It is clear that the depolarisation is linearly related to the decrease in input resistance, i.e. the increase in input conductance.

From the results of the present experiments it was possible to obtain a potential value corresponding to the reversal potential. Extrapolation of the line formed by the plot of the input resistance versus membrane potential to the potential axis gives reversal potential. For the plot illustrated in Fig. 5B, the extrapolated line bisects the potential axis at a value of -16.5 mV. In the experiments with decamethonium ($n = 19$), this value was found to be -21 ± 3.5 mV (mean $\pm$ S.E. of mean). The theory underlying this method of determining reversal potential is that in order to get a depolarisation to the reversal point, the conductance produced by the decamethonium would have to be infinite, thus the input resistance would then be zero.

Measurements of input resistance were made for both short and prolonged applications of decamethonium and suxamethonium. Input resistance decreased on applying either drug, and this decrease lasted as long as the drug was present in the bathing solution. Only after the removal of the drug did input resistance begin to return towards its previous level.

After the removal of the depolarising drug from the bathing solution, recovery of the input resistance proceeded at a faster rate than did recovery of the membrane potential. This is illustrated in Fig. 6. The difference in recovery times is independent of the time the muscle was exposed to the drug. A lack of linearity between the two processes has been noted previously during the application of carbachol to frog sartorius muscle (NASTUK and PARSONS, 1970) and it was suggested that this might be the result of chloride ion redistribution.

3. Effect of Acetylcholine on Membrane Potential

Concentrations of acetylcholine similar to those of decamethonium and suxamethonium had no effect on the resting potential of the tenuissimus muscle. In the presence of an anticholinesterase drug, however, the same concentration of acetyl-

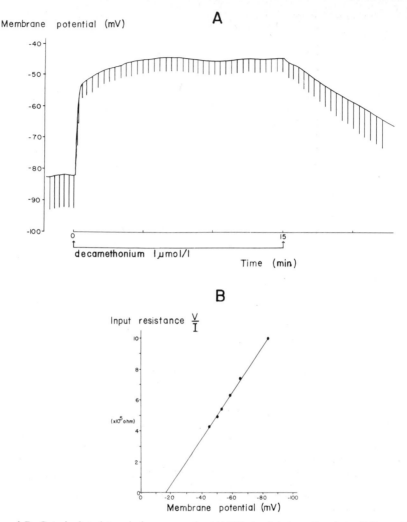

Fig. 5A and B. Cat; isolated tenuissimus muscle. (A) Effect of decamethonium (1.0 μmol/l), applied for 15 min, on the membrane potential and electrotonic potentials of a single surface muscle cell recorded at the end-plate region. Electrotonic potentials were produced by pulses of hyperpolarising current passed through a second microelectrode 70 μm away from the recording electrode. Current intensity: 100 nA; pulse duration: 500 msec. (B) Graph of input resistance (ordinate) plotted against membrane potential (abscissa). The input resistance was calculated from the values shown in (A). On application of decamethonium there was a linearly related decrease in input resistance and the depolarisation of the end-plate region. The line joining the points, when extrapolated, crosses the membrane potential axis at a value of − 16.5 mV

choline induced a depolarisation of the end-plate region. When the membrane potential reached about − 60 mV, muscle contractions occurred and the microelectrode was expelled. The addition of tetrodotoxin to the bathing fluid prevented the muscle from contracting. The following procedure was thus adopted: an end-plate region was first located in normal Krebs solution; this solution was then replaced by

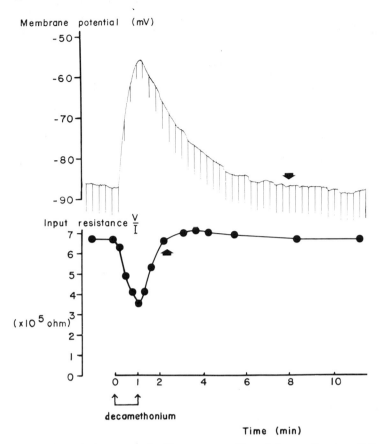

Fig.6. Cat; isolated tenuissimus muscle. Upper trace: effect of decamethonium $(1.0\,\mu mol/l)$ applied for one min on membrane potential and electrotonic potentials of a single surface cell,
recorded at the end-plate region. (Intensity of hyperpolarising current: 10 nA; duration of current pulses: 500 msec; stimulating electrode 70 µm away from the recording electrode). Lower
trace: graphical representation of the input resistance, derived by dividing the amplitude of the
electrotonic potential by the intensity of the applied current. The arrows indicate the point of
recovery of input resistance and membrane potential

one containing 250 nmol/l tetrodotoxin. Five min later this second solution was
replaced by one containing the same concentration of tetrodotoxin and in addition
eserine at a concentration of 3 µmol/l; after another five min acetylcholine was added
at a concentration of 1.1 µmol/l. This final solution was allowed to flow over the
muscle preparation for up to 30 min. Figure 7 shows that in six experiments acetylcholine produced substantial depolarisation from a resting potential of
-85.7 ± 2.0 mV (mean $\pm$ S.E. of mean) to a depolarisation in the presence of acetylcholine of -51.7 ± 3.0 mV. In three of these experiments the drug was applied for
30 min. While depolarisation tended to diminish with time, it was still substantial by
the end of the drug application. Complete recovery of the membrane potential
occurred only on removal of acetylcholine from the bathing solution.

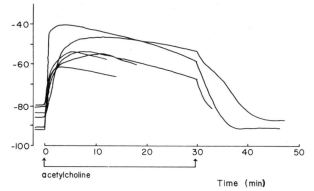

Fig. 7. Cat; isolated tenuissimus muscle. Depolarisations produced by acetylcholine (1.1 µmol/l in the presence of eserine, 3 µmol/l; and tetrodotoxin, 250 nmol/l) and recorded from the end-plate region of surface muscle cells in different preparations

4. The Effect of Decamethonium in Chloride-Free Solution

JENKINSON and TERRAR (1973) suggested that chloride ions influence the change in membrane potential during the prolonged application of a depolarising drug, pointing out that the marked increase in membrane permeability to potassium and sodium at the end-plate causes the membrane potential to fall below the chloride equilibrium potential. Thus the inward sodium current is opposed not only by the outward potassium current but also by an outward chloride current caused by the net inward movement of chloride ions.

In order to determine the influence of chloride ions on the time-course of the depolarisation induced by decamethonium on the tenuissimus muscle, the chloride ions in the Krebs solution were replaced by a less permeant anion. Commercial preparations of methylsulphate have been found to vary in quality (HUTTER and WARNER, 1967) and it was decided to try the slightly larger ethylsulphate anion, which is commercially available in a fairly pure form. Preliminary experiments showed that mammalian skeletal muscle is not readily permeable to ethylsulphate, and this anion was therefore used to replace chloride ions. Tetrodotoxin at a concentration of 250 nmol/l was also present to prevent the generation of action potentials, easily initiated in the absence of chloride ions. Decamethonium was applied for five min in two preparations, for three min in one and for one min in five. The rate of decamethonium-induced depolarisation was much faster in a chloride-free solution than in a chloride-containing one, reaching its maximum in about 15 to 30 sec; repolarisation after removal of the drug was also faster. Figure 8 A and B shows the time-course of the depolarisation induced by a 1 µmol/l concentration of decamethonium in two fibres, one in normal Krebs solution, the other in chloride-free solution. In three experiments when decamethonium was applied for more than one min, the depolarisation was well maintained with no more than 3 mV recovery of potential occurring during the presence of the depolarising drug. Fig. 8 C shows the result of a five min application of decamethonium in chloride-free solution.

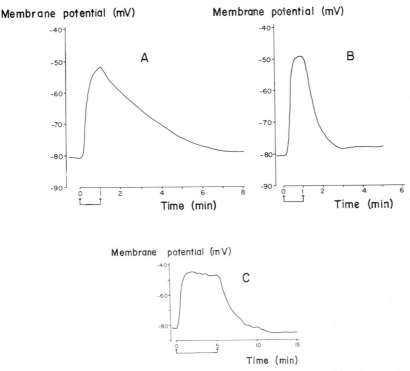

Fig. 8 A—C. Cat; isolated tenuissimus muscle. Depolarisations produced by decamethonium (A and B) 1 µmol/l for one min and (C) 1 µmol/l for five min, in the presence of tetrodotoxin 250 nmol/l, and recorded from the end-plate region of three separate muscle fibres bathed in: (A) normal Krebs solution; (B and C) chloride-free solution

JENKINSON and TERRAR (1973) suggested that changes in fibre chloride content might complicate the assessment of desensitisation, particularly when the muscle is exposed to a depolarising drug over a long period. In particular they state that the absence of desensitisation probably "cannot be inferred from the occurrence of a stable plateau of depolarisation in response to a steady concentration of agonist since this may merely indicate that the opposing influence of desensitisation and chloride redistribution are in balance". Indeed, their results in the frog showed that in the absence of chloride movement, carbachol-induced depolarisation was not well maintained. In our experiments on the tenuissimus muscle, however, the depolarisation was well maintained in a chloride-free solution. Thus a difference appears between frog and cat muscle.

5. The Effect of Ouabain

Another difference between frog and mammalian muscle was found when the effect of ouabain was studied. It is generally accepted that almost all cells, including erythrocytes, nerve and muscle, possess a Na^+-K^+ATP-ase, which is located at the cell surface. The prime action of this Na^+-K^+ATP-ase is to expel sodium ions from the cell as fast as they are able to enter through the cell membrane. The enzyme is

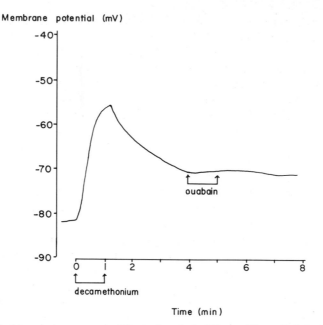

Fig. 9. Cat; isolated tenuissimus muscle. Effect of ouabain (50 μmol/l) applied during the repolarisation of the membrane following the removal of decamethonium from the bathing solution. Depolarisation induced by 1.0 μmol/l decamethonium and recorded at the end-plate region

activated by external potassium and internal sodium (Glynn, 1962). Furthermore, it is inhibited by low concentrations of cardiac glycosides, which are known to be potent inhibitors of the active "uphill" transport of sodium and potassium in erythrocytes (Glynn, 1957; Post et al., 1960), nerve (Caldwell and Keynes, 1959) and muscle (Matchett and Johnson, 1954; Conway et al., 1961).

Depolarising drugs such as decamethonium or carbachol when applied for prolonged periods are likely to increase the internal sodium concentration at the end-plate region, thus stimulating the active extrusion of sodium. It was therefore of interest to find out how a mammalian muscle under the influence of decamethonium is affected by the cardiac glycoside ouabain. It was found in the isolated tenuissimus of the cat that if the glycoside was applied during the repolarisation phase after the removal of decamethonium it slowed or halted the recovery of the membrane potential. This is illustrated in Fig. 9. These results suggest that in the cat tenuissimus muscle at 37° C, there is a mechanism of sodium extrusion which is sensitive to ouabain. In contrast, Terrar (1974) found that in frog muscle at 20° C strophanthidin did not greatly influence carbachol-induced changes in membrane potential. This difference in results suggests that the contribution of active sodium extrusion to repolarisation is much less in frog muscle than it is in cat muscle.

E. Depolarisation Versus Desensitisation

The results just described appear to be in disagreement with those asserting that the neuromuscular block produced by decamethonium and suxamethonium is mainly

due to receptor desensitisation. In 1955(a) THESLEFF reported that prolonged neuromuscular block by acetylcholine in the sartorius muscle of the frog was not due to a
persistent depolarisation of the end-plate region but to a decrease in its sensitivity to
acetylcholine. Subsequently, THESLEFF (1955b) compared the effects of decamethonium and suxamethonium with that of acetylcholine on frog muscle. In the presence of
neostigmine bromide 3.3 to 6.6 μmol/l, acetylcholine iodide in a concentration of 55
to 110 μmol/l depolarised the end-plate region, but this depolarisation subsided
spontaneously without the removal of acetylcholine. However, the neuromuscular
block which had developed in the presence of acetylcholine persisted despite repolarisation of the membrane to the normal level. The subsequent addition of acetylcholine did not significantly change the membrane potential. The same pattern was
observed with both decamethonium (78 to 156 μmol/l) and suxamethonium (25 to
50 μmol/l). Complete neuromuscular block did not develop until the membrane
potential of the end-plate region was restored to approximately its normal value.
THESLEFF concluded that in his experiments in the frog it was not possible to show
any relationship between the membrane depolarisation and the neuromuscular
block. This work was later repeated on isolated mammalian muscle by THESLEFF and
his colleagues. In 1958, AXELSSON and THESLEFF studied the effect of acetylcholine at
the end-plate of isolated muscles removed from several mammalian species (including the tenuissimus muscle of the cat) and THESLEFF (1959) compared the effect of
acetylcholine with that of decamethonium and suxamethonium, confining this investigation to the tenuissimus muscle. The experiments were made with ionophoretic
application of the drugs to single end-plates, recording the resulting potential
changes by an intracellular electrode. By using a twin drug pipette, in which each
barrel was filled with a different solution, it was possible to compare drug effects on
the same receptors or to study their local interaction.

In the first group of experiments twin micro-pipettes were used containing a
concentrated solution of acetylcholine chloride. The sensitivity of the end-plate
membrane was tested by releasing acetylcholine by means of a series of positive
voltage pulses of constant intensity and 10 msec duration applied to one barrel of the
twin pipette. The other barrel of the pipette was used to apply a "conditioning" dose,
i.e. generally a prolonged and steady release of acetylcholine. In the second group of
experiments one of the barrels was filled with a concentrated solution of acetylcholine while the other contained one of the two depolarising drugs. The effect of the
depolarising drug on the sensitvity of the membrane was found by recording the
amplitude of brief acetylcholine pulses administered at regular intervals during the
steady efflux of either decamethonium or suxamethonium. In all the various mammalian muscles a steady application of acetylcholine produced a loss of sensitivity of
the motor end-plate membrane. This was demonstrated by the observation that
during the steady release of acetylcholine the effect of successive test pulses diminished (Fig. 10A). The degree of this desensitisation and its speed of onset was graded
and increased with the applied concentration of acetylcholine while the rate of
recovery was relatively constant. Marked species variations in the intensity and time-
course of desensitisation were observed. Whereas in the guinea-pig and the rabbit a
steady efflux of acetylcholine for several seconds was needed to produce desensitisation, the same effect was obtained in the rat and particularly in the tenuissimus
muscle of the cat within a few tenths of a second using smaller conditioning doses.

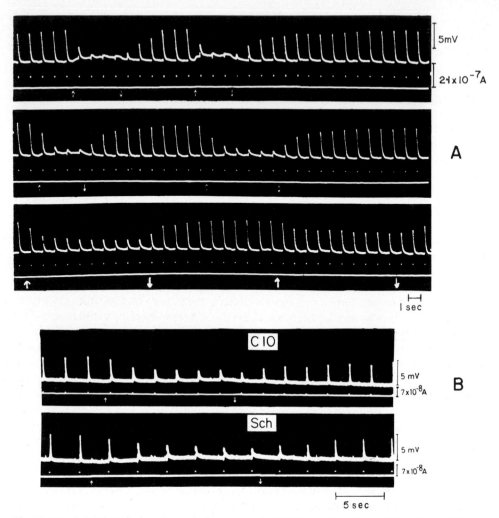

Fig. 10 A and B. Cat; isolated tenuissimus muscle. (A) Desensitisation produced by different conditioning doses of acetylcholine at a single end-plate spot. The onset and with-drawal of the conditioning dose is marked with arrows and its strength increases successively from down upwards. Current pulses through pipette are registered in lower trace. (B) Desensitisation produced at the end-plate by decamethonium and suxamethonium. Note that also with these agents receptor desensitisation develops without a concomitant membrane depolarisation. (From: (A) Axelsson and Thesleff, 1958; (B) Thesleff, 1959)

Similar results were obtained with the two depolarising drugs. The release of decamethonium or suxamethonium produced a depolarisation of the end-plate region. This depolarisation was marked during brief applications of either drug to the end-plate. During continuous application the depolarisation, however, was slowly abolished; instead desensitisation developed as evidenced by the reduced amplitude of the acetylcholine potential (Fig. 10 B). The degree and speed of onset was once more graded and increased with the dose. Furthermore, Thesleff (1959) showed that during this period of desensitisation, the well-known phenomenon of antagonism between competitive and depolarising drugs did not occur.

In 1962, ELMQVIST and THESLEFF defined desensitisation as "a condition in which application of a depolarising drug has made the chemoreceptors of the end-plate refractory to chemical stimulation". On the grounds of these results THESLEFF questioned whether a block could be due solely to depolarisation and put forward the view that a major part of the block produced by decamethonium and suxamethonium was due to desensitisation, even in the intact animal.

The phenomenon of desensitisation has been the subject of much discussion in recent years. A great number of factors have been suggested as likely to influence the rate of its development. The concentration of the drug, however, appears to be one of the most important factors. FATT (1950) was the first to describe a decrease in sensitivity of the motor end-plate after the application of acetylcholine and to state that the rate of its development is concentration-dependent. In 1955, DEL CASTILLO and KATZ pointed out that "with the ionophoretic applications complications occur because nearby and more distant receptors within a single end-plate are not equally affected by the discharge of acetylcholine from a point source. With a given dose, receptors at very close range may be saturated, or even damaged, by the momentary attainment of an excessive concentration, while more distant receptors are acted upon more slowly and at a lower concentration". They added, "this situation differs from the normal process of transmission and also from the more conventional methods of drug application in which the whole receptor area is subject to a uniform dose". AXELSSON and THESLEFF themselves (1958) concluded that the degree of desensitisation and the speed of its onset were graded and increased with the applied concentration of acetylcholine. Moreover, THESLEFF (1959) pointed out that the duration of the initial depolarisation is inversely related to drug concentration.

Differences in drug concentration might therefore explain the very substantial differences between the results of our own experiments and those of THESLEFF and his group. Using the same species (cat) and the same isolated muscle (tenuissimus) we were able to demonstrate a well-maintained depolarisation to acetylcholine, decamethonium and suxamethonium, while in the experiments of THESLEFF and his colleagues depolarisation was short-lived and desensitisation was put forward as the mechanism behind the neuromuscular block. In our experiments the concentration of the depolarising drug was very similar to that necessary to produce an almost complete block in the intact animal. In this way unnecessarily large concentrations were avoided. In contrast, in the studies of THESLEFF and his colleagues the depolarising drugs were applied either ionophoretically or in concentrations much larger than those necessary to produce an interruption of neuromuscular transmission.

F. Species Differences and Depolarising Neuromuscular Blocking Drugs

I. Man and Cat

The use of decamethonium and suxamethonium in man made it quite clear that both drugs interrupt neuromuscular transmission by long-lasting depolarisation. Stimulant effects associated with random spontaneous fasciculations often precede the block. Action potential records show that these effects are the result of repetitive firing of the muscle fibres. Tetanic stimulation applied during a partial block, produces a contraction that, though reduced in tension, is fairly well sustained throughout the period of stimulation. After the tetanus, transmission is not restored. Anticholinesterase substances are ineffective against the neuromuscular block produced by either decamethonium or suxamethonium and the previous administration of tubocurarine reduces the action of both drugs. All these characteristics correspond to an interruption of neuromuscular transmission produced by prolonged depolarisation of the end-plate region. The activity of decamethonium or suxamethonium corresponds closely to that in the cat.

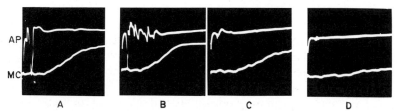

Fig. 11 A—D. Anaesthetised man. Action potentials (AP) and muscle contractions (MC) recorded during a chest operation from the diaphragm with concentric needle electrodes in response to stimulation of the phrenic nerve. (A) record taken during control period; (B) 30 sec, and (C) 3 min, after the intravenous administration of 20 mg suxamethonium; (D) 2 min after the intravenous administration of 5 mg edrophonium. (From: C. B. B. DOWNMAN and E. ZAIMIS, unpublished record)

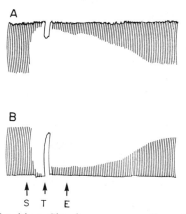

Fig. 12A and B. Anaesthetised subject. Simultaneous recording of maximal twitches from the tibialis anterior muscle (B) and the adductor pollicis muscle (A) in response to indirect stimulation delivered one per 10 sec. At (S) suxamethonium, 10 mg I.V.; at (T) tetanus 60 Hz; at (E) edrophonium 5 mg I.V.

Figure 11 shows action potentials and muscle contractions recorded during a chest operation from the diaphragm of a patient with concentric needle electrodes in response to stimulation of the phrenic nerve. The intravenous administration of 20 mg of suxamethonium was followed by an outburst of repetitive muscle action potentials lasting for a few seconds. Edrophonium (5 mg) administered intravenously two min later had no effect whatsoever on the suxamethonium block. The same failure of edrophonium to antagonise a suxamethonium block is shown in Fig. 12. In this patient maximal twitches of the tibialis anterior and of the adductor pollicis muscle, elicited by indirect stimulation, were recorded simultaneously. A tetanus at 60 Hz, delivered during the suxamethonium block was well maintained and did not antagonise the block; edrophonium (5 mg I.V.) administered a little later intensified the block.

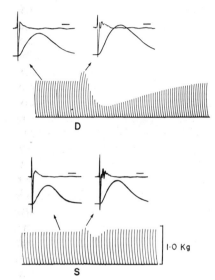

Fig. 13. Cat; 4.8 kg. The upper trace of each section shows simultaneously recorded muscle action potentials (by means of concentric needle electrodes) and muscle contractions from the tibialis anterior elicited by indirect stimulation of the sciatic nerve every 10 sec, and photographed from an oscilloscope. Horizontal bars: 10 msec. In the lower trace, the same muscle contractions were recorded on a slow moving paper. D decamethonium, 200 μg I.V., S suxamethonium, 150 μg I.V

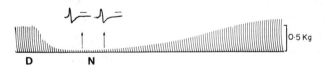

Fig. 14. Cat; 4.6 kg. Maximal twitches of the tibialis anterior muscle elicited by indirect stimulation of the sciatic nerve every 10 sec. D decamethonium 125 μg I.V., N neostigmine 100 μg I.V. Insert: muscle action potential recorded at the points indicated by the arrows. Horizontal bars: 10 msec

Similar results are obtained in the cat. In the experiment illustrated in Fig. 13 the intravenous administration of either decamethonium (150 μg I.V.) or suxamethonium (200 μg I.V.) was followed by a short-lasting potentiation of the maximal twitch which preceded the onset of the block. The simultaneous recording of muscle action potentials shows that this potentiation was the result of repetitive firing of the muscle fibres. The administration of neostigmine (100 μg I.V.) during a decamethonium block was ineffective (Fig. 14).

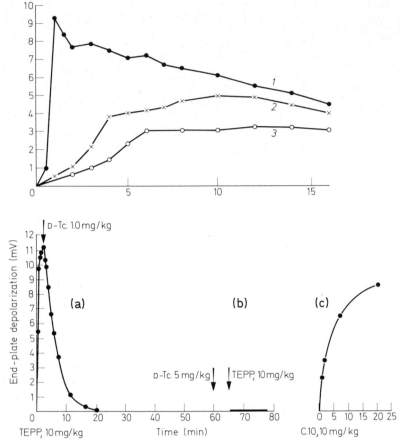

Fig. 15a—c. Cat; gracilis muscle. Upper trace: End-plate depolarisations with successive doses of TEPP (10 mg/kg repeated at 1 to 1 ¼ hrs intervals). The nerve to the muscle had been tied shortly before recording. Lower trace: Graph of end-plate depolarisation produced (a) by TEPP 10 mg/kg, followed by D-tubocurarine 1.0 mg/kg; (b) by TEPP 10 mg/kg, after 5 mg/kg D-tubocurarine, 50 min later; (c) by decamethonium (C. 10) 10 mg/kg, 30 min later. (From: DOUGLAS and PATON, 1954)

Studies in the intact animal show that desensitisation is not a normal phenomenon. In the experiments of BURNS and PATON (1951) after the intravenous administration of 30 µg/kg of decamethonium the peak value of the local depolarisation was reached 3 to 5 min after the injection and was followed by a steady repolarisation to the normal value, taking 30 to 40 min for its completion. "Since recovery never took less than half an hour" BURNS and PATON pointed out, "it was not possible to carry out more than a few tests during the course of a day's work". PATON and WAUD (1962), using electrodes which traversed the length of the fibres, showed that if suxamethonium is given to a cat to produce between 90 and 100% block for up to 1 hr, the end-plates do indeed remain depolarised throughout, but the peak depolarisation falls to a steady level of about half the maximum. In 1954, DOUGLAS and PATON studied the mechanism of motor end-plate depolarisation due to tetraethyl-

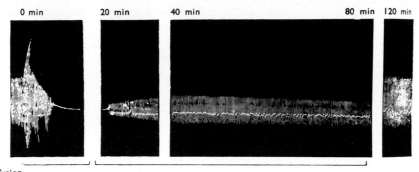

Fig. 16. Cat; tenuissimus muscle. Record of maximal twitches *in vivo*. Suxamethonium infusion started at rate of 2.8 µg/kg/min and later reduced to 0.7 µg/kg/min. The infusion rate was then maintained constant throughout the experiment. Artificial respiration given during the infusion. (From: MACLAGAN, 1962)

pyrophosphate (TEPP)—an anticholinesterase drug. It was concluded that TEPP lacks a direct action and that its effects at the motor end-plate are all attributable to acetylcholine accumulating there from local or distant sources. "With doses of 2 to 20 mg/kg", they reported, "a rapid, large unfluctuating depolarisation always occurred". The upper trace of Fig. 15 illustrates end-plate depolarisations with successive doses of TEPP (recorded with external electrodes). The lower trace of Fig. 15 illustrates that even after tubocurarine, decamethonium given in sufficiently large doses produced a typical depolarisation of the end-plate region lasting for more than 15 min. Figure 16 is a record of maximal twitches of the tenuissimus muscle *in vivo*. Suxamethonium infusion was given at a rate of 2.8 µg/kg/min was later reduced to 0.7 µg/kg/min. The infusion rate was then maintained constant for more than 80 min, during which time the degree of paralysis remained constant.

There are other findings which underline the mechanism of action of decamethonium and suxamethonium. Temperature, as we have already seen, increases the magnitude and especially the duration of a block produced by a depolarising drug. In contrast, cooling reduces the magnitude of a block produced by tubocurarine. Figures 28 and 29 show this effect of muscle temperature on a block produced by suxamethonium and decamethonium in man, and illustrate once more the ineffectiveness of edrophonium in antagonising a suxamethonium block.

One of the consequences of the long-lasting depolarisation produced by decamethonium and suxamethonium is an efflux of potassium from the depolarised area of the muscle cell. As described later (p. 396, Fig. 25), PERRY and ZAIMIS using ^{42}K, found a 30% increase in the rate of loss of potassium from perfused muscle following a dose of decamethonium which completely blocked neuromuscular transmission. Moreover, in man (MAZZE et al., 1969), in cats (PATON, 1956) and in dogs (KLUPP and KRAUPP, 1954; STEVENSON, 1960) it was found that the amount of potassium released during a suxamethonium blockade is sufficient to raise the plasma potassium level. In 60 patients free of neuromuscular, cardiovascular, acid-base and electrolyte disorder, FAHMY et al. (1975) found significant increases in serum potassium after the intravenous administration of either decamethonium (0.1 mg/kg) or suxamethonium

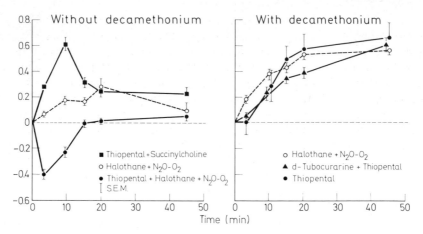

Fig. 17. Anaesthetised man. Serum potassium changes (mEq/1) without, and in the presence of, decamethonium (0.1 mg/kg I.V.). (From: FAHMY et al., 1975)

(1 mg/kg). The increase in serum potassium after decamethonium ranged from 0.1 to 0.9 mEq/l and that induced by suxamethonium between 0.2 and 0.6 mEq/l. The mean increase in the 30 patients who received decamethonium was +8%. Figure 17 is a graphic representation of these results.

In denervated muscles and in any situation where the muscle is undergoing atrophy the chemosensitive area is known to extend beyond the end-plate region. In such cases, during the action of a depolarising drug, both the rate of loss of potassium (PERRY and ZAIMIS, p. 396) and the plasma potassium concentration (STONE et al., 1970) are greatly increased in comparison with normal muscle. These results in animals correlate well with some clinical observations (ELLIS, 1974; see also Chapter 5B). From 1958 onward many papers have appeared reporting cardiac arrest in convalescing burned patients immediately after induction of anaesthesia and injection of suxamethonium. The pattern of the response found in burned patients has also been observed in patients with extensive injuries of soft tissues, or in patients whose muscles have been paralysed either by lesions of the upper motor neurone or by spinal cord injury. A common mechanism, the result of an increase in the chemosensitivity of the muscle membrane present in these clinical conditions, has been considered the cause of this almost lethal efflux of potassium after the administration of a depolarising drug. In a recent review (1975) GRONERT and THEYE discuss these clinical cases in detail and analyse the hyperkalaemic responses against a background of the physiology of normal muscle. The reader will find the review a good source of references also.

II. Other Mammalian Species

The study of the effects produced by neuromuscular blocking drugs in various mammalian species has led to the discovery that whereas the response of all mammalian skeletal muscles to competitive neuromuscular blocking drugs is uniform, the response to depolarising drugs is not. In reviewing past work with decamethonium one comes across accounts of experiments on many varieties of species which cannot be explained in terms of a single mode of action. BOVET et al. (1951) found that in the rabbit the block produced by decamethonium can be antagonised by eserine, and they concluded that an absolute distinction between a depolarisation block and a competitive block cannot be drawn. JARCHO et al. (1951), experimenting in rats, noted that "in normally innervated rat muscle, decamethonium appeared to act in some ways like acetylcholine, in others, like curare". PHILIPPOT and DALLEMAGNE (1952) reached the same conclusion for work done on dogs, finding that neostigmine and adrenaline antagonise a decamethonium block. In many mammals, including the monkey, dog, rabbit, hare (ZAIMIS, 1953) and guinea-pig (HALL and PARKES, 1953) it was found that decamethonium and suxamethonium initially exhibit a depolarising action but during the blocking process their action changes into that of a substance competing with acetylcholine. When first observed, this mode of action was described as a "dual" one (ZAIMIS, 1953). More recently, BOWMAN (1962) found that the "dual" mode of action of decamethonium is particularly well marked in the ferret.

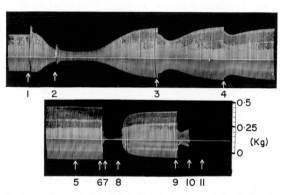

Fig. 18. Rabbit, 3 kg. Contractions of tibialis excited by supramaximal shocks to the sciatic nerve, every 10 sec. At (1), (3), and (4) intravenous injection of 0.6 mg of decamethonium iodide. At (2) and (7), tetanic stimulus to motor nerve, 50 Hz. At (5) 2 mg atropine sulphate i.v. At (6) 1.8 mg decamethonium iodide i.v. At (8) and (11) intravenous injection of 0.5 mg neostigmine methylsulphate. At (9) 1 mg decamethonium iodide and at (10) 0.5 mg tubocurarine chloride i.v. (From: ZAIMIS, 1953)

An analysis of the characteristics of the dual block shows that it has two components, one due to the intial "acetylcholine-like" action, the other to a "curare-like" action (ZAIMIS, 1953). The block is preceded by potentiation of the maximal twitch, a feature peculiar to a substance capable of depolarising the motor end-plates. However, a tetanus produced during the block is not well sustained and antagonises it. Finally, the block is deepened by tubocurarine and is readily antagonised by neostigmine. In other words, one is confronted with a type of block which has some of the characteristics of a depolarisation block and some of the characteristics of a competitive one. Figure 18 shows the characteristics of the "dual" mode of action of decamethonium in the rabbit and Fig. 19 illustrates the "dual" effect of suxamethonium and decamethonium in two experiments in the dog. In the first one (A) neuromuscular block was measured by recording action potentials from the diaphragm elicited by

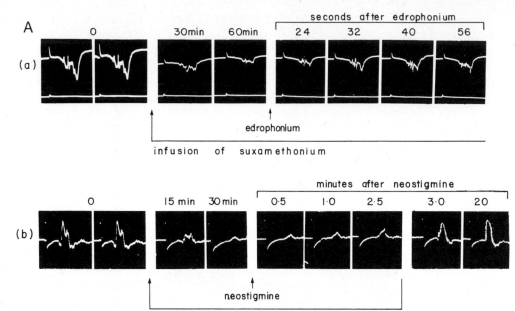

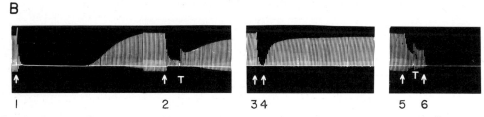

Fig. 19. (A) Dog; diaphragm. Action potentials recorded with concentric needle electrodes in response to stimulation of the phrenic nerve once every 10 sec. Experiment (a) Records taken before and during a slow continuous infusion of suxamethonium diiodide. At arrow, 2 mg edrophonium given intravenously. Experiment (b) Effect of 500 µg neostigmine methylsulphate administered during a continuous infusion of suxamethonium diiodide. (B) Dog; tibialis. At 1, 2, 3, and 5, 1 mg decamethonium diiodide. At 4, 0.5 mg of neostigmine methylsulphate. At 6, 300 µg of tubocurarine chloride. T tetanus, 50 Hz. (From: ZAIMIS, 1959)

stimulation of the phrenic nerve. In the second one (B) neuromuscular block was measured by recording the contraction of the tibialis muscle elicited by stimulation of the sciatic nerve. In both experiments anticholinesterase drugs readily antagonised the action of either decamethonium or suxamethonium.

   The muscles which are blocked by the "dual" mechanism of action are relatively insensitive to decamethonium and suxamethonium. Moreover, not only are they relatively insensitive to the first dose, but they exhibit a rapidly decreasing sensitivity to repeated doses. This striking decrease in the sensitivity of the muscles to subsequent doses is a totally new feature, being absent in either of the two basic mechanisms when they appear in their pure form (for details see ZAIMIS, 1953; JEWELL and ZAIMIS, 1954a).

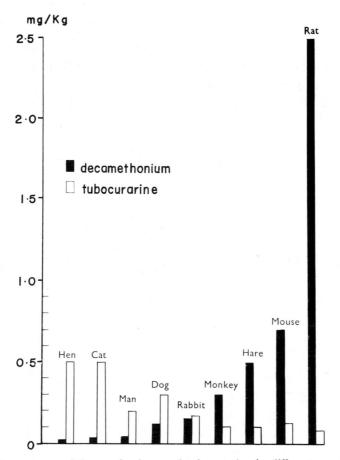

Fig.20. Relative potency of decamethonium and tubocurarine in different species. The dose indicated in mg/kg is that required to produce a 90 to 100% neuromuscular block in all species but mouse where it represents the ED_{50} using the righting reflex test. (From: Zaimis, 1953)

The "dual" mode of action provides an explanation for the varying sensitivity of different species to decamethonium and suxamethonium (Fig.20). Sensitivity is at its highest where the compounds interrupt neuromuscular transmission by depolarisation. Immediately the "dual" mode of action appears, the muscles become more resistant to the same drugs, most probably because the two modes of action are antagonistic. The phases of depolarisation and competition in muscles in which suxamethonium and decamethonium exhibit a "dual" mode of action are not always the same. In some muscles the depolarisation phase predominates, in others the competitive one. Nor is the "dual" mode of action which decamethonium and suxamethonium exhibit the same. The balance between the depolarising and competitive propensities of suxamethonium appears weighted in favour of the former action, whereas with decamethonium it is the competitive tendency which appears dominant. In other words, of the two, it is suxamethonium which mimics acetylcholine more faithfully.

This idea of a "dual" mechanism of action arose from a study of the effects produced by tridecamethonium, a higher member of the polymethylene bistrimethyl-ammonium series, on chicks (ZAIMIS, 1953). As discussed later (p. 395), in birds tubocurarine produces the usual flaccid paralysis, while decamethonium and suxa-methonium, like acetylcholine, produce a contracture characterised by extension of the limbs and retraction of the head. If the dose of decamethonium is small, recovery is abrupt; if large, the animal dies in contracture and never exhibits paralysis. How-ever, when an injection of tridecamethonium is given, a completely different picture is produced. First contracture appears, albeit slowly, then while the legs are still extended the head drops forward in paralysis and finally the paralysis extends to the leg muscles so that the whole animal becomes flaccid. From this result it is obvious that tridecamethonium acts initially as a depolarising substance but changes during the blocking process to a competitive inhibitor. On observing these results in the chicks it was decided that it might be useful to test tridecamethonium in the cat (ZAIMIS, 1953). The effect produced by tridecamethonium on the tibialis muscle of the cat was similar to that obtained with decamethonium and suxamethonium on the tibialis muscle of the monkey, dog and hare. Thus it appears that the muscles of different species may have widely different properties, and that the mode of action of a quaternary molecule is determined not only by its own structure but also by the properties of the muscle concerned.

Rat skeletal muscle, as Fig. 20 shows, is particularly insensitive to depolarising neuromuscular blocking drugs and the characteristics of the blockade by both deca-

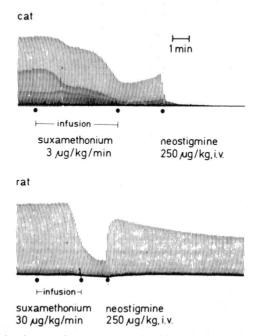

Fig. 21. Effect of neostigmine on the neuromuscular block induced by suxamethonium in the tibialis anterior muscle of the cat and the rat. Vertical bars indicate infusion of suxamethonium, while neostigmine was administered as a single dose. (From: DERKX et al., 1971)

methonium and suxamethonium *in vivo* (DERKX et al., 1971; IRESON et al., 1969) and *in vitro* indicate that a maintained end-plate depolarisation is not the cause of the interruption of neuromuscular transmission. DERKX and his colleagues showed that while neostigmine potentiates the action of suxamethonium in the cat, it antagonises the blockade in the rat (Fig. 21). The competitive tendency in the rat is so powerful that IRESON et al. (1969) concluded that suxamethonium blocks neuromuscular transmission in this animal species, only by competition with acetylcholine and that it has none of the normal characteristics of depolarisation blockade. Similar results were obtained with decamethonium. HUMPHREY (1973), using the isolated rat diaphragm, studied the time-course of the neuromuscular block produced over a range of concentrations of decamethonium and also measured membrane potential changes at the end-plate region by means of external electrodes. His very interesting results showed that both the time-course and the concentration of decamethonium required for depolarisation were very different from those required for neuromuscular block and concluded that the interruption of neuromuscular transmission produced by decamethonium in rat muscle is not the result of a prolonged depolarisation. Indeed, by recording membrane potential and input resistance from surface fibres of the isolated extensor digitorum longus muscle of the rat HEAD (1975) showed that

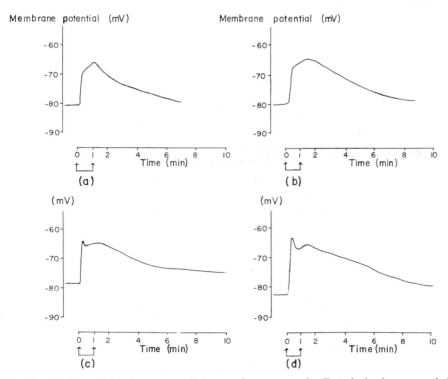

Fig. 22a—d. Rat; isolated extensor digitorum longus muscle. Depolarisations recorded with intracellular microelectrodes at the end-plate region of surface cells during one min applications of decamethonium at the following concentrations: (a) 20 µmol/l; (b) 50 µmol/l; (c) 100 µmol/l; (d) 390 µmol/l

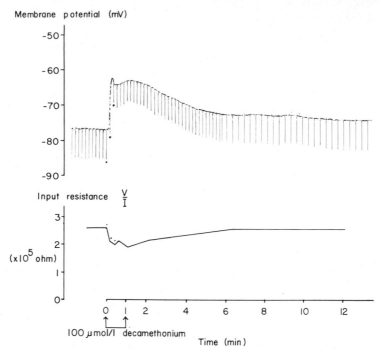

Fig. 23. Rat; isolated extensor digitorum longus muscle. Upper trace: effect of decamethonium
100 μmol/l, applied for one min, on membrane potential and electrotonic potentials of a single
surface cell, recorded at the end-plate region. (Intensity of applied current: 30 nA; duration of
pulses: 500 msec; stimulating electrode about 50 μm away from the recording microelectrode).
Lower trace: graphical representation of the input resistance to hyperpolarising current, derived
by dividing the amplitude of the electrotonic potentials by the intensity of the applied current

the responses to decamethonium in the rat differed fundamentally from those in the
cat. Membrane potential and input resistance changes were recorded from the end-
plate region of surface cells of the muscle over a wide range of decamethonium
concentrations. The results showed a) that on increasing the concentration of decamethonium from 2.5 to 390 μmol/l maximal depolarisation remained the same; and
b) that at no concentration of decamethonium did depolarisation exceed 25 mV—in
other words the membrane potential never reached a value more positive than
− 60 mV. This is illustrated in Fig. 22 which shows the effect of increasing concentrations of decamethonium on four different preparations. In all preparations the removal of the depolarising drug was followed within 8 min by recovery of the membrane potential to a value almost equal to its previous level. Input resistance measurements were made in six experiments. A stimulating electrode inserted into the
fibre at a distance of 50 μm or less from the recording electrode carried a pulse of
current of constant duration and amplitude. Thus changes in both electrotonic
potentials and membrane potential were recorded simultaneously. Figure 23 shows
membrane potential and input resistance changes which occurred on the exposure of
the muscle to 100 μmol/l decamethonium. Comparable results were obtained in five
other experiments from which it can be concluded that input resistance changes were

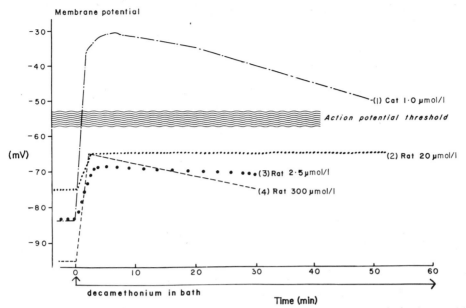

Fig. 24. Graphical representation of measurements by several authors on depolarisations produced by decamethonium in isolated muscles of cat and rat and recorded from single fibres with intracellular microelectrodes. References: (1) HEAD, 1975; (2) GALINDO, 1971; (3) HEAD, 1975; (4) THESLEFF, 1955c

related to membrane potential changes. The reversal potential, derived as previously described (p. 373) for decamethonium on the digitorum longus muscle of the rat was found to be -41.7 ± 1.3 mV (mean $\pm$ S.E. of mean $n = 6$).

In rat skeletal muscle, as in other mammalian muscles, the threshold for muscle action potential generation is about -55 mV (THESLEFF, 1955c). Therefore, it would appear that no concentration of decamethonium produces a depolarisation of the end-plate region large enough to trigger action potentials. Figure 24 summarises the published results of several authors who studied decamethonium in rat muscle. The figure also includes the contrasting results obtained in the tenuissimus muscle of the cat by HEAD (1975) who demonstrated that decamethonium produces dose-dependent depolarisations and that the concentration necessary to produce a neuromuscular block also causes a depolarisation exceeding the threshold value for action potential generation. It appears, therefore, that there is a correlation between a drug's ability to cause a neuromuscular block by depolarisation and its capacity to produce a depolarisation exceeding the threshold value for action potential generation. This explains the results of HUMPHREY (1973) who found that while a small depolarisation can occur in the rat at relatively low concentrations of decamethonium (average concentration 4.7 µmol/l), neuromuscular block required much larger concentrations (in excess of 100 µmol/l). THESLEFF (1955c) also found that the concentration of decamethonium necessary to produce a block of neuromuscular transmission of the rat diaphragm muscle was in the order of 300 to 400 µmol/l. Thus the twin facts that in rat muscle no concentration of decamethonium can cause depolarisation exceeding 25 mV and that only large concentrations can produce a neuromuscular block, suggest that a mechanism different from that by which decamethon-ium interrupts neuromuscular transmission in the cat is involved.

In 1953, and on the basis of pharmacological analysis Zaimis discussed the "dual" block as follows: "The impression obtained is that when a block with such character-istics is produced the neuromuscular-blocking substance starts its action as a depo-larizing agent but subsequently changes into a competitive inhibitor. The molecules when first injected apparently adhere in the specific way necessary to produce a depolarization at the motor end-plate. As a result they produce some stimulant actions. However, their grip changes so that they now become molecules competing with acetylcholine and in doing so they raise the threshold to any depolarizing substance. The non-uniform response of the cat, monkey, dog, rabbit and hare muscles to the same neuromuscular blocking substance suggests that there must be distinct physical differences between the muscle membranes of these mammalian species in spite of the apparent similarity of their reaction to acetylcholine." It appears, therefore, that there is a good correlation between the pharmacological results of Zaimis and the electrophysiological analysis of Humphrey and Head.

Two examples can be quoted which provide direct electrical evidence to support the idea that depolarisation block may give way to competitive block by the same drug. Paton and Perry (1953) have shown that a transition from the picture of depolarisation block to that of competitive block can be seen with nicotine in the superior cervical ganglion. With nicotine the depolarisation is always transient, ending much before the actual block. During the period of block, in the absence of depolarisation, a further similar dose of nicotine produces only a small fraction of the original depolarisation. Paton and Perry therefore concluded that nicotine has a dual mode of action, being initially a depolarising and later a competitive blocking drug. In the cat's gracilis muscle Paton (personal communication) observed a simi-lar situation with the higher members of the alkyltrimethyl ammonium series, stu-died for the first time by Philippot and Dallemagne (1951). An injection first produced a typical end-plate depolarisation, which then waned, although block persisted. More recently, however, Paton and Savini (1968) studied the action of nicotine at the neuromuscular junction in the cat and found that its blocking action can for the most part be simply characterised as that of an end-plate depolarising drug with a prolonged action. The authors concluded that the difference in the mechanisms of action of nicotine at the motor end-plate and at the ganglionic synapse "provides another example of the manner in which the type of action as well as the potency of a drug may change when it is tested in different cholinergic synapses".

Further work has shown that a single substance may produce different types of neuromuscular block in the various skeletal muscles of an individual animal. In the cat, as far as the muscles of the hind-limbs are concerned, the red muscles (exempli-fied by soleus) are slow and the white muscles (examplified by tibialis) are fast-contracting. Jewell and Zaimis (1954a) demonstrated a further difference between the two types of muscle by pharmacological means. In tibialis, decamethonium produced a typical depolarisation block while the block in soleus had all the charac-teristics of a "dual" block.

Hitherto it has generally been assumed that results obtained from experiments upon one mammal could safely be regarded as typical for mammals in general. It is now clear that results obtained from the muscle of any one mammalian species are valid only for this species, and perhaps for the particular muscle upon which the experiment was made.

In experiments in which the tibialis and soleus muscle had been tenotomized in order to cause a disuse atrophy, decamethonium blocked the atrophied soleus by depolarisation alone, the competitive phase of its action having disappeared (JEW-ELL and ZAIMIS, 1954b). This change in mode of action was accompanied by a marked increase in the sensitivity of the atrophied muscle to the drug. The atrophied tibialis showed no change in response to decamethonium except for a small increase in sensitivity.

The results obtained by JEWELL and ZAIMIS also offered evidence that the changes in the atrophied muscle were in the muscle fibre membrane, since the time-course of the twitch, and the development of tetanus, which are presumably properties of the contractile elements, appeared to remain unaltered. The atrophied tibialis retained the contraction characteristics of fast white muscle and the atrophied soleus those of slow red muscle. The changes in response to neuromuscular blocking agents which occurred with disuse would appear, then, to be primarily referable to changes in the muscle membrane, and the experiments revealed an interesting relationship between the two types of fibre. The fact that the red muscle when atrophied loses its dual mode of response to depolarising agents and comes to resemble white muscle suggests that the white fibre membrane possesses the less differentiated structure; the red fibre reverts to this state with disuse.

Myasthenic Muscle. These normally occurring differences between certain species and between different muscles may appear as pathological changes in the muscles of any one species. Myasthenia gravis is a disease characterised by a gradually developing weakness of the muscles of the body (see Chapter 5B). CHURCHILL-DAVIDSON and RICHARDSON (1952a, 1953) have obtained convincing evidence that unlike the normal human muscle the neuromuscular block produced by decamethonium in myasthenics has all the characteristics of the dual block. The block is rapidly and completely reversed by anticholinesterase substances and tetanic rates of stimulation are not well sustained. This means that in the myasthenic, as in the monkey and dog, we are confronted with a transition from the picture of a depolarising block to that of a competitive block. Consequently, a change has occurred in the muscle membrane of the myasthenic patient. This explained their previous finding (CHURCHILL-DAVIDSON and RICHARDSON, 1952b) that the myasthenic muscle exhibits a diminished sensitivity to decamethonium and that while the mildly myasthenic patient is extremely resistant to the drug, the severely affected one is only slightly more resistant than the normal muscle.

III. Avian Muscle

A particular type of avian muscle responds in a characteristic way to substances possessing an acetylcholine-like action at the neuromuscular junction. For example, while tubocurarine produces the usual flaccid paralysis in adult fowls and chicks, an intravenous injection of decamethonium or suxamethonium causes a rigid extension of the limbs and retraction of the head, as does acetylcholine. This is a peripheral effect, the muscles reacting to the depolarising drugs with a true "contracture". If the dose of the depolarising drug is small recovery is abrupt; if large the animal dies in contracture and never exhibits flaccid paralysis.

In the first publication by BUTTLE and ZAIMIS which described this action of decamethonium in birds in 1949, the suggestion was made that avian muscle might be used as a test in differentiating substances with a "curare-like" action from those interrupting neuromuscular transmission by prolonged depolarisation. The advantage of using this test is the ease with which the difference in the action of these two groups of drugs can be strikingly illustrated, and indeed, the "chick test" has been widely used for both research and teaching purposes from that day to this.

In 1938, BROWN and HARVEY demonstrated that the close-arterial injection of acetylcholine into the gastrocnemius muscle of the hen evokes a double mechanical response consisting of a quick initial response followed by a "contracture", which becomes more evident as the concentration of the drug is increased. The quick response was associated with an outburst of action potentials which was cut short by the onset of the slow contracture, during which no rapid action potentials could be detected. Such a contracture is also produced by both decamethonium and suxamethonium (ZAIMIS, 1959). After denervation both decamethonium and suxamethonium continue to produce a typical contracture. However, while denervation markedly increases the sensitivity of mammalian muscle to decamethonium (ZAIMIS, 1951), the sensitivity of denervated avian muscle to both depolarising drugs is only modestly increased.

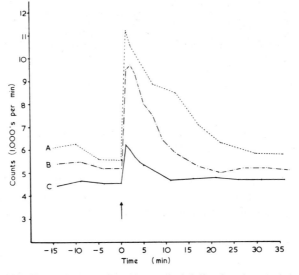

Fig.25A—C. ^{42}KCl in effluent from perfused lower limb following the administration of decamethonium. (A) Normal hen, 100 µg decamethonium (contracture); (B) Denervated cat, 100 µg decamethonium (contracture); (C) Normal cat, 500 µg decamethonium (complete block). (for details, see text p.379). (From an unpublished experiment by W.L.M.PERRY and E.ZAIMIS, 1953)

One of the consequences of the long-lasting depolarisation produced by decamethonium or suxamethonium is an efflux of potassium ions from the depolarised area of the muscle cell. In the early 1950s, W.L.M.PERRY and ZAIMIS (reported by ZAIMIS

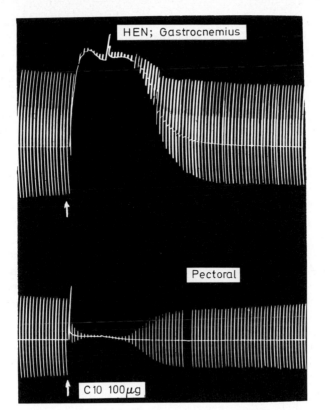

Fig. 26. Hen; pentobarbitone anaesthesia. Maximal contractions of the gastrocnemius and pectoral muscles elicited indirectly every 10 sec and recorded simultaneously. At arrow, 100 μg decamethonium injected intravenously

in 1954) measured the potassium output of normal and denervated mammalian muscle and normal avian muscle under the influence of a depolarising substance, the animals having first been loaded with radioactive potassium. The following results were obtained: a) In the normal cat a dose of decamethonium in excess of that necessary to block neuromuscular transmission completely, produced a 30% increase in the rate of loss of potassium. It was considered that such a dose of decamethonium was quite sufficient to depolarise all the end-plates and part of the surrounding membrane and that the observed rise in output could be attributed to an increased exit of potassium across this zone. b) In denervated mammalian muscle and some innervated avian muscles, all of which respond to acetylcholine and other depolarising drugs with a "contracture", the rate of loss of potassium was greatly increased after decamethonium. For example, when decamethonium was injected in a dose sufficient to induce a contracture in the denervated mammalian muscle or in the innervated gastrocnemius of the hen, an increase of 70 to 80% in the potassium loss was observed (see Fig. 25). From the results obtained in normally innervated mammalian muscle it was concluded that any loss of potassium in excess of 30% must represent an increased flux across membrane other than that of the end-plate

region. The results with denervated mammalian muscle and normally innervated
avian muscles therefore strongly suggested that the chemosensitive area in these
muscles extended beyond the end-plate region. GINSBORG (1960b) and GINSBORG
and MACKAY (1961) subsequently showed that avian muscles contain different proportions of focally and multiply innervated fibres. For example, the anterior latissimus dorsi of the domestic fowl and the latissimus dorsi of the pigeon are composed
almost entirely of multiply innervated fibres, whereas both focally and multiply
innervated fibres are present in the biventer cervicis, semispinalis cervicis, gastrocnemius and sartorius muscles. In contrast, the posterior latissimus dorsi and the pectoral muscles of the fowl are composed mainly of focally innervated fibres. This morphological variation, as will be discussed below, explains why a particular type of
avian muscle responds with a "contracture" to injected acetylcholine or other depolarising drugs. It also explains why the intravenous administration of decamethonium to an adult hen produces a "contracture" of the gastronemius muscle but a
flaccid paralysis of the pectoral muscle (Fig. 26 and ZAIMIS, 1954).

All fibres of the anterior latissimus dorsi of the adult hen possess multiple "en
grappe" innervation points at intervals of about 1 mm along them (GINSBORG and
MACKAY, 1961; HESS, 1961, 1967; MAYR, 1967). In contrast, most fibres of the
posterior latissimus dorsi muscle possess a single innervation point with an "en
plaque" type of junction (HESS, 1961, 1967). GINSBORG (1960a) pointed out, however,
that the available evidence does not exclude the possibility that more than one end-
plate may exist on focally innervated fibres. What is certain, however, is that if more
than one neuromuscular junction does exist on such fibres, the interval between
them is much greater, by a factor of ten at least, than the intervals between the
neuromuscular junctions on multiply innervated fibres. The fibres with multiple
neuromuscular junctions are innervated by several motor axons and respond to
direct and to maximal indirect stimulation with propagated action potentials (GINS-
BORG, 1960b). On repetitive stimulation of the nerve, at frequencies varying from 15
to 35 Hz, multiply innervated muscles respond with maximal sustained tension
throughout the period of stimulation. Moreover, the amplitude of the maximal
contraction produced by decamethonium, suxamethonium and carbachol was found
to be almost identical with that produced by the tetanic stimulation of the nerve.
According to GINSBORG these results suggest that all the fibres in this muscle were
taking part in the response.

GINSBORG (1960a) studied the spontaneous activity in the muscle fibres of the
chick and found that miniature end-plate potentials (m.e.p.p.s) could be recorded at
almost every location along fibres of the anterior latissimus dorsi. The same results
were obtained by FEDDE (1969). In contrast, m.e.p.p.s could not be found at all, even
after hours of searching, in many fibres of the posterior latissimus dorsi. FEDDE also
found that peaks of acetylcholine sensitivity occurred at intervals of about 740 μm
along the multiply innervated anterior latissimus dorsi muscle of 3 to 6 months old
chickens, with areas of low sensitivity between the peaks. In contrast, only one peak
of acetylcholine sensitivity was detected in the focally innervated posterior latissimus
dorsi muscle. Sensitivity to acetylcholine was studied by recording transmembrane
potentials with an intracellular micropipette while applying acetylcholine ionophoretically to the membrane surface with another micropipette filled with approximately 2 mol/l acetylcholine chloride solution. In addition, FEDDE found that the

membranes of these two muscle fibre types differ widely in some of their electrical properties. It appears, therefore, that these two avian muscles provide a unique opportunity for studying the possible relationships between the type of motor innervation and the membrane characteristics of skeletal muscles.

In mammals, suxamethonium is rapidly hydrolysed by plasma butyrocholinesterase (WHITTAKER and WIJESUNDERA, 1952) while decamethonium is mainly excreted unchanged (ZAIMIS, 1951). Because of this, the duration of the suxamethonium block in both man and cat is very short and a larger dose is necessary to produce a particular degree of neuromuscular block than would be needed if decamethonium were used. In birds, however, the two substances have the same duration of action and they are equipotent. The findings of BOWMAN and his colleagues throw light on these differences. In 1962 BLABER and BOWMAN reported that the plasma cholinesterase in the fowl appeared unable to hydrolyse the bisquaternary substrate suxamethonium. Moreover, the enzyme present in hen skeletal muscle was only slightly inhibited by ambenonium, another bisquaternary compound usually considered to be a specific inhibitor of mammalian acetylcholinesterase. Later, BLABER and CUTHBERT (1962) found that the plasma of the domestic fowl does not possess a typical butyrylcholinesterase, but a cholinesterase with intermediate properties somewhere between fowl acetylcholinesterase and mammalian butyrocholinesterase. Fowl skeletal muscle on the other hand was found to contain acetylcholinesterase and a small amount of a second enzyme with properties similar to those of the plasma enzyme. BLABER and CUTHBERT pointed out the possible fallacies that might arise if results obtained with inhibitors in one species were used to interpret results in another.

When muscle containing multiply innervated fibres is isolated from a chick which is a few days old it responds to a depolarising drug with a sustained contracture. Having observed this, CHILD and ZAIMIS (1960) investigated several muscles of the chick *in vitro* in the hope of obtaining a sensitive and specific method for the quantitative determination of depolarising drugs. This work led to the introduction of a new biological method for the assay of depolarising substances using the isolated semispinalis of a 3 to 10 days old chick. This preparation has three main advantages over the rectus abdominis of the frog: (a) quick relaxation without any artificial stretching of the muscle; (b) greater sensitivity to depolarising drugs, and (c) no falling off in sensitivity for at least two hours.

At the same time a rapid and accurate assay of acetylcholine was developed by TYLER (1960). The semispinalis cervicis muscle of two to three week old chicks was used and the preparation was sensitised to acetylcholine by adding edrophonium chloride to the bath to give a concentration of 4 to 8 µg per ml before acetylcholine was added. This method has definite advantages over the frog rectus abdominis preparation. First, the sensitivity of the chick muscles stays constant for several hours, whereas in the frog muscle preparation there is often a slow steady decrease in sensitivity. Secondly, biological fluids such as blood plasma or urine have little effect on the tone of the chick muscle, and acetylcholine contained in such fluids need not be extracted before the assay. Thirdly, the speed with which an assay can be carried out is much greater than is the case with the frog muscle preparation. This is because the chick muscle relaxes rapidly; artificial stretching is never required.

GINSBORG and WARRINER (1960) were able to obtain an isolated nerve-muscle preparation by using the innervated lower belly of the biventer cervicis muscle of the chick. This preparation can be used to test both competitive neuromuscular blocking drugs (producing a reduction of the contractions induced by nerve stimulation) and depolarising drugs (producing "contractures").

G. Factors which May Modify the Action of Depolarising Neuromuscular Blocking Drugs and Variations Due to Experimental Conditions

I. The Effect of Lowered Muscle Temperature

The study of the effects of muscle temperature on the action of neuromuscular blocking drugs has brought to light a new factor which once more underlines the differences between the modes of action of competitive and depolarising neuromuscular blocking drugs. It was found that, in both cats and man, lowered muscle temperature increases the magnitude of the effect of depolarising drugs and markedly prolongs their duration of action (Bigland et al., 1958; Cannard and Zaimis, 1959; Alderson and Maclagan, 1964). In contrast, cooling reduces the magnitude of a block produced by substances interrupting neuromuscular transmission by competition with acetylcholine. On rewarming, these effects are reversed. Figure 27 illustrates the results of an experiment in which suxamethonium was administered by a slow intravenous infusion to a cat after the body temperature had been lowered to 29° C. The rate of infusion was adjusted to produce complete neuromuscular block, and kept constant while the animal was rewarmed. It can be clearly seen that the magnitude of the neuromuscular block followed the temperature variations faithfully. Figure 28 illustrates the same effect in an anaesthetised man. After premedication with atropine sulphate, quinalbarbitone and pethidine hydrochloride, anaesthesia was induced with thiopentone sodium and maintained with a mixture of oxygen and nitrous oxide. For the recording of muscle contractions in man a method was used which provided experimental conditions under which uniform isometric contractions could be elicited and recorded for long periods of time (for details see

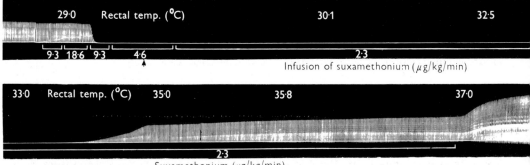

Fig. 27. Records of maximal twitches of the tibialis anterior muscle of a 2.3 kg cat in response to indirect stimulation at a frequency of 0.1 Hz. Effect of raising body temperature during intravenous infusion of suxamethonium diiodide. Before infusion the body temperature had been lowered to 29° C. (From: Bigland et al., 1958)

CANNARD and ZAIMIS, 1959). The temperature of one limb was lowered by the use of ice packs and thin plastic bags containing crushed ice. Muscle temperature was measured by means of a thermistor needle inserted into either the tibialis anterior or the gastrocnemius muscle of each leg. Muscle temperature was almost always 1 to 2° C lower than rectal temperature and this difference usually increased after immobilization of the limbs. Because of this, the temperature of the control leg had to be maintained at normal levels by means of hot-water bottles. In anaesthetised cats the temperature of the limb muscles is also lower than that of the general body temperature (BIGLAND and ZAIMIS, 1958). Figure 28 shows a section of a record taken in an anaesthetised subject while the muscle temperature of the two legs differed by 6.5° C. The intravenous injection of 2 mg of decamethonium produced a neuromuscular block in both legs but in the colder leg the magnitude of the effect was increased and the duration of action prolonged.

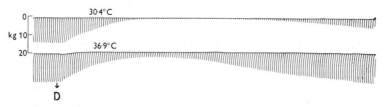

Fig. 28. Anaesthetised man. Simultaneous recordings of maximal twitches from the right (upper trace) and left (lower trace) tibialis anterior muscles in response to indirect stimulation delivered once per 10 sec. At the arrow 2 mg decamethonium diiodide intravenously. (From: CANNARD and ZAIMIS, 1959)

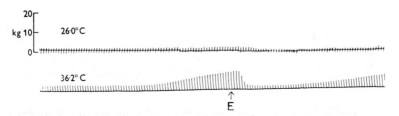

Fig. 29. Anaesthetised man. Simultaneous recordings of maximal twitches from the right (upper trace) and left (lower trace) tibialis anterior muscles in response to indirect stimulation delivered once per 10 sec during a slow continuous infusion of suxamethonium diiodide. The figure starts at a point when the block was 85% in warm muscle and 95% in the cold one. At the arrow 5 mg of edrophonium chloride intravenously. (From: CANNARD and ZAIMIS, 1959)

Although cooling prolongs the action of depolarising drugs the nature of the blockade does not appear to be affected, however long the paralysis lasts. For example, anticholinesterase drugs are ineffective or prolong the block and tubocurarine antagonizes it. Figure 29 illustrates that 5 mg of edrophonium injected intravenously into an anaesthetised subject potentiated the action of suxamethonium in both the warm and the cold leg. Furthermore, in several experiments the depolarising drug was administered after one or several injections of tubocurarine. The previous administration of tubocurarine did not alter the effect of cooling on the depolarising drug.

Decamethonium is a substance which is not destroyed in the body and is almost entirely excreted in the urine in unchanged form (Zaimis, 1951). On the other hand, suxamethonium is rapidly hydrolysed, mainly by plasma pseudo-cholinesterase. The fact that a block produced by decamethonium is more, or at least as much, affected by decreased temperature as one produced by suxamethonium suggests that the effect cannot be due only to inactivation of the enzyme at the lower temperature, for if this were so the block produced by suxamethonium should be the most affected. It was concluded, therefore, by Bigland et al. (1958) that the recovery processes following depolarisation, which are dependent on a supply of metabolic energy, are slowed at lower temperatures. Such a suggestion is supported by the findings of Csapo and Wilkie (1956) who, studying the effect of potassium on frog's skeletal muscles, found that at low temperatures the recovery from the depolarisation produced by potassium is very slow and that a brief period of rewarming leads to a sudden and dramatic recovery.

Maclagan (1960), using the domestic fowl, studied the time-course of the "contracture" of the gastrocnemius muscle produced by successive doses of suxamethonium at various body temperatures. As the temperature was lowered, the size of the contracture was slightly increased but the duration of action of the drug was considerably prolonged. The conclusion was reached that cooling has the same effect on the action of depolarising drugs in both avian and mammalian muscle.

Cooling reduced the action of tubocurarine in both cat and man (Bigland et al., 1958; Cannard and Zaimis, 1959). A lowering of muscle temperature would logically be expected to have the same influence on the action of acetylcholine as on that of suxamethonium and decamethonium. Thus, an increase in the effectiveness of acetylcholine might be expected to reduce the action of drugs competing with it. This is also suggested by the observation that cooling reduced only the magnitude of the tubocurarine block, leaving the duration almost unaltered, since the magnitude depends on the ease with which the drug can compete with acetylcholine, while the duration, however, is governed by factors such as its rate of redistribution, excretion and destruction. Holmes et al. (1951) studied the action of tubocurarine in the isolated rat diaphragm muscle at various temperatures. They also found that a reduction of temperature from 40° C to 26° C reduced the neuromuscular blocking action of tubocurarine.

A lowering of body temperature is usually accompanied by bradycardia and a fall in blood pressure. Such effects will tend to slow the blood flow through skeletal muscles. However, the experimental results suggest that the changes in the action of neuromuscular blocking drugs occurring at lower muscle temperatures are independent of changes in blood flow. Such a conclusion was reached by Bigland et al. (1958) because (a) a lowering of muscle temperature affects the action of depolarising and competitive neuromuscular blocking drugs in opposite directions; (b) in isolated preparations, where there is no blood supply, the effect of lowered muscle temperature is just the same—increased activity of depolarising drugs and reduced activing of tubocurarine; (c) the results obtained have always been dependent on local muscle temperature—for example, the same results have been obtained in animals whose muscle temperature changes have been produced by altering body temperature, and in those where the temperature of one limb only was altered; (d) the increased or decreased activity of neuromuscular blocking drugs at lowered muscle temperature

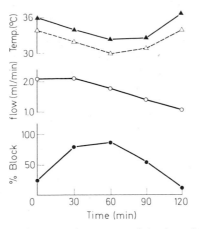

Fig. 30. Cat 3.5 kg. In this experiment an intravenous injection of 50 μg of decamethonium was administered every 30 min. The graph shows the percentage paralysis of the left tibialis anterior muscle produced by each dose and the venous outflow from the same leg recorded simultaneously as the body temperature was lowered and restored to normal again. (From: MACLAGAN, 1960)

is independent of the effect of cooling on the blood pressure and heart rate. MACLAGAN (1960) studied in cats the effect of cooling on the blood flow through a limb while at the same time observing the effect on the action of several neuromuscular blocking drugs. No correlation could be found between the magnitude and duration of a blockade produced by decamethonium or suxamethonium and changes in blood flow. For example, in the experiment illustrated in Fig. 30, blood flow was recorded from the tibialis muscle in the anaesthetised cat while body temperature was lowered and then restored to normal. The magnitude and duration of the block followed the changes in muscle temperature faithfully but in contrast, the blood flow continued to decrease even when the animal was rewarmed. The only effect which can be attributed to changes in blood flow is the more gradual onset of the blockade in the cold muscle, an effect seen with both depolarising and competitive neuromuscular blocking drugs.

The demonstration of the effect of muscle temperature on the action of neuromuscular blocking drugs not only underlines the differences between competitive and depolarising substances but also explains some of the clinical results. Neuromuscular blocking drugs are extensively used during surgery under a variety of conditions (general hypothermia, cold operating theatres, etc.) when the body temperature of the anaesthetised patient consistently falls. Decreases in muscle temperature may therefore provide an explanation for some cases of prolonged apnoea following the use of depolarising drugs and for cases of "recurarisation" where the patient had received tubocurarine as a muscle relaxant and was taken, at the end of the operation, from a cold operating theatre to a warm recovery room.

WOLLMAN and CANNARD (1960) measured the skeletal muscle, oesophageal and rectal temperatures of 23 adult patients undergoing general anaesthesia. Temperatures decreased in all cases, particularly during intra-thoracic operations. In these operations the mean temperature of the exposed intercostal muscles decreased to

32.0° C and that of the diaphragm to 33.7° C. In other words, the temperature of the respiratory muscles reached levels at which the action of suxamethonium and deca-methonium should be increased and prolonged. They concluded that heat loss in patients under anaesthesia is perhaps more common than has been recognised and suggested rewarming of the patient as a reasonable procedure if apnoea persists. The same conclusions were reached by SMITH (1962) who found that rectal and oesopha-geal temperatures were unreliable indicators of the course of muscle temperatures. Thus the effect of temperature on neuromuscular block has considerable practi-cal importance, and should certainly be kept in mind by anaesthetists.

II. Tachyphylaxis

Decreased sensitivity which develops rapidly after the administration of only a few doses of a drug is known as tachyphylaxis. Such a phenomenon has been described for both decamethonium and suxamethonium.

In 1954(a), JEWELL and ZAIMIS found that when small doses of decamethonium (producing less than complete block) are given, the muscle shows increased sensitiv-ity to the second and usually to the third dose; subsequent doses, however, have a progressively smaller effect (Fig. 31). When on the other hand, the initial dose of decamethonium is so large as to produce a prolonged and complete block of tibialis, a progressive diminution in the response may begin with the second dose. This has been found to be so even if the time interval between doses is lengthened to 75 min. In the results illustrated in Fig. 31, the depth and duration of block have been combined to give a more adequate single measurement of the block produced, but these factors may be to some extent independent. The first manifestation of a reduced sensitivity of tibialis to repeated doses of decamethonium is a shortening of the duration of the block, the degree of depression being the same. With subsequent doses both the degree of depression and the duration of the block are reduced. No evidence could be obtained which would suggest that the mode of action of decame-thonium on tibialis had changed during an experiment, and the interruption of neuromuscular transmission produced by the later doses of decamethonium always retained the characteristics of a depolarisation block. The action on tibialis of succes-sive doses of suxamethonium was also studied by JEWELL and ZAIMIS. It was found that the characteristics of a depolarisation block were retained throughout all the experiments but that at the dose level they used the sensitivity of the muscle did not decrease (Fig. 31).

Similar results were reported by THESLEFF (1952) in cats and VON DARDEL and THESLEFF in man (1952). Tachyphylaxis to suxamethonium, however, has been re-ported. For example, PAYNE (1959) found that suxamethonium has a progressive diminishing effect in most patients when given repeatedly at short intervals. The intervals in this study were really short—only 10 min. It appears, therefore, that under certain conditions tachyphylaxis to successive administrations of suxametho-nium can develop.

Further evidence that the mode of action of decamethonium does not change during tachyphylaxis was obtained by ALDERSON and MACLAGAN (1964). Five successive injections of 40 µg/kg of decamethonium were administered to anaesthe-tised cats at 60 min intervals. The block in the tibialis muscle diminished with each

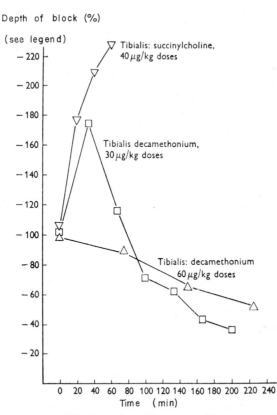

Fig. 31. Changes in the depth of block produced by repeated intravenous injections of succinyl-choline and decamethonium given at regular intervals. Tibialis ▽ — ▽ succinylcholine 40 μg/kg every 20 min; tibialis □—□ decamethonium 30 μg/kg every 33 min; tibialis △— △ decamethonium 60 μg/kg every 75 min. Ordinates: area of the depression caused in the tracings during neuromuscular block (planimeter measurements). The measurements are expressed as a percentage of the block produced by the first dose of each series. Abscissae: time after injection of the first dose in min. (From: JEWELL and ZAIMIS, 1954a)

successive dose (Fig. 32). In addition, ALDERSON and MACLAGAN found that tachyphylaxis also occurred to a comparable extent in the diaphragm muscle and that the time to half recovery from neuromuscular block was very similar in both muscles when the temperatures were the same (doses 1, 2, 4, and 5). Between the second and third injections, when tachyphylaxis was well developed, the tibialis muscle was allowed to cool to the level which is normally found in an anaesthetised cat, and when the third dose was given, the neuromuscular block in the tibialis muscle was much greater than that in the diaphragm. As cooling increases only a block by depolarisation and not that produced by competition with acetylcholine, we can conclude once more that during tachyphylaxis the characteristics of a depolarisation blockade are maintained.

An understanding of the changes occurring in the muscle fibre during a prolonged depolarisation would appear to be vital to an interpretation of the effects of

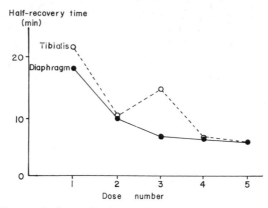

Fig. 32. Cat, 2.5 kg. The graph shows the time to half recovery of successive blockades produced by I.V. injections of 40 μg/kg of decamethonium di-iodide administered at 60 min intervals. Diaphragm temperature was 38.5 to 39° C throughout the experiment. Tibialis temperature was also maintained at 38.5 to 39° C for doses 1, 2, 4, and 5 but was 3° C colder during dose 3. (From: ALDERSON and MACLAGAN, 1964)

decamethonium. After a dose of decamethonium the muscle twitch returns to its previous height, demonstrating that the excitability of the motor end-plate to acetylcholine has returned. But, as BURNS and PATON (1951) have shown, the return of excitability at the end-plate regions does not necessarily run parallel with the return of excitability of the adjacent membrane, the latter lagging behind the former. The degree of block produced by decamethonium is a result of both depolarisation of the motor end-plate and of spread of inexcitability in the surrounding membrane. During the period of depolarisation blockade the muscle may lose significant amounts of potassium and gain significant amounts of sodium, calcium and chloride. The fact that these ionic movements are so big means that during and after a block by a drug depolarising the end-plate, the ionic concentrations on either side of the muscle membrane may be significantly altered. The implications of these changes on the state of block are not simple, but it is clear that the reaction of the end-plate and of the muscle membrane adjacent to the end-plate will be radically conditioned by them. There would be, then, a possible explanation of the phenomenon of decreasing sensitivity; the magnitude of response of a further injection of decamethonium is less because the drug finds a normal end-plate but adjacent regions of reduced excitability.

Another suggestion made by BURNS and PATON (1951) was that the progressively smaller depolarisations produced by successive doses of decamethonium could be explained if the entry of decamethonium into the interior of the fibre was an essential part of the depolarisation process, for depolarisation would then depend upon the concentration difference of the drug across the membrane. Repolarisation of the membrane would occur as soon as there was the same amount inside as outside, but the drug remaining within the muscle would reduce the rate of entry of (and hence the depolarisation) produced by a subsequent dose of decamethonium. Recently, TAYLOR and CRESSE, 1966; TAYLOR et al., 1967a; CREESE and MACLAGAN, 1967, using labelled decamethonium, confirmed that the drug enters the muscle fibres. This penetration of decamethonium is prevented by tubocurarine. However, this theory relies on an increase in the intracellular concentration of "free" decamethonium and it has recently been shown (TAYLOR et al., 1967b) that the drug becomes firmly bound within the cell. Consequently, there is at present no conclusive experimental support for this suggestion and in fact PATON has publicly disowned it (PATON, 1962).

III. "Potentiation" of a Maximal Twitch

A single supramaximal stimulus applied to a nerve is followed by the depolarisation of each individual motor end-plate in response to the released acetylcholine. When this depolarisation of the end-plate region reaches the excitation threshold of the adjacent membrane a muscle action potential is generated and the whole muscle responds with a twitch.

Post-Tetanic Potentiation. When a series of single stimuli is delivered to a motor nerve at intervals of 5 to 10 sec and a period of tetanic stimulation is then applied, the subsequent muscular twitches undergo typical changes. In fast mammalian muscles they become larger than the control twitches; finally they subside slowly to the initial level. This effect is known as "post-tetanic" potentiation and is not accompanied by repetitive firing of the muscle fibres (BROWN and VON EULER, 1938). BOTELHO and CANDER (1953) made a quantitative study of the post-tetanic potentiation in man and found that the phenomenon is not accompanied by changes in the associated muscle action potential. The only change was a decrease in the latent period of the contraction and a slowing followed by a speeding up in the rate of contraction.

In slow muscles, such as the soleus muscle of the cat, repetitive responses can be recorded after a tetanus (FENG et al., 1939; BOWMAN et al., 1969) only when prolonged tetani of high frequency are applied. After brief tetani within the physiological range of frequencies the soleus response is the opposite of that obtained in a fast-contracting muscle, twitch tension being slightly decreased for a short time (BROWN and VON EULER, 1938; BOWMAN et al., 1962).

The phenomenon of post-tetanic potentiation is not simple and probably is made up of several events. Calcium distribution within the sarcoplasmic reticulum must play an important, if not the only, role in the increase of the isometric twitch after a tetanus. WINEGRAD (1970) found that during the period immediately after a tetanus the calcium distribution within the sarcoplasmic reticulum differs from that before the tetanus. The influence of calcium distribution was also demonstrated by CONNOLLY et al. (1971). The post-tetanic repetitive firing in the soleus muscle of the cat was studied by BOWMAN et al. (1969). They concluded that an increase in trasmitter output, coupled with a weaker cholinesterase activity in this muscle, probably accounts for the repetitive responses seen after prolonged tetani of high frequency.

Recruitment of Muscle Fibres. An increase in the muscle tension in response to single nerve shocks following a tetanus also occurs during partial competitive neuromuscular block. This increase, however, is the result of a greater number of muscle fibres responding to the nerve impulse and therefore the increase in muscle contraction is accompanied by an increase in the size of the action potential. The difference between post-tetanic potentiation and the effect of a tetanus during a neuromuscular block by tubocurarine is shown in Fig. 33 A and B. This "recruitment" of muscle fibres is seen under conditions in which neuromuscular block can be overcome by the presence of increased amounts of acetylcholine as occurs during a tetanus, or after the administration of an anticholinesterase drug (Fig. 33 D). The term post-tetanic potentiation is being used by many anaesthetists to refer to both (a) the physiological increase in muscle contraction seen after a tetanus when the size of the compound action potential does not alter, and (b) the "decurarisation" induced by a tetanus that is accompanied by a simultaneous increase in muscle contraction and action potential. Other workers prefer the term "post-tetanic facilitation" for both phenomena. This is confusing because the mechnisms underlying the increase in muscle contraction in these two situations are fundamentally different. It is therefore essential to use terms which distinguish clearly between them. Since a tetanus anta-gonizes a block induced by drugs competing with acetylcholine, the terms "decurar-isation" or (even simpler) "the tetanus antagonizes the block" are preferable to "post-tetanic potentiation" or "post-tetanic facilitation" and are unlikely to be misinter-preted (see also Chapter 3 B).

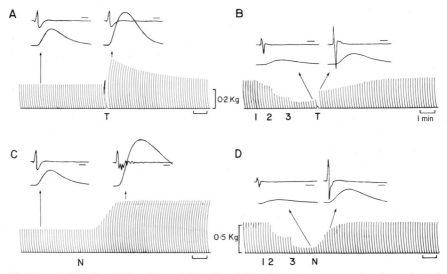

Fig. 33. (A) and (C): Cat 2.3 kg. (B) and (D): Cat 4.6 kg. The upper trace of each section shows simultaneously recorded muscle action potentials (by means of concentric needle electrodes) and muscle contractions from the tibialis anterior elicited by indirect stimulation of the sciatic nerve every 10 sec, and photographed from an oscilloscope. Horizontal bars: 10 msec. In the lower trace the same muscle contractions were recorded on a slow moving paper. (A) Effect of a tetanus. (During the tetanus amplifier sensitivity was reduced 2.5 times.) (B) Effect of a tetanus on a block induced by tubocurarine. (C) Effect of neostigmine on a normal muscle. (D) Effect of neostigmine on a block induced by tubocurarine. T tetanus, 30 Hz for 5 sec; N neostigmine, 100 µg I.V.; 1, 2, 3 three successive intravenous injections of tubocurarine, 750 µg each

Repetitive Firing of Muscle Fibres. Following the administration of an anticho-linesterase drug a single indirect stimulus produces a short burst of muscle action potentials and consequently the muscle responds as if stimulated at a high frequency.

This explains the increase in twitch tension illustrated in Fig. 33C following the administration of neostigmine. Thus, a repetitive firing of the muscle fibres without increase in the peak voltage of the individual action potentials represents yet another mechanism for potentiation of the maximal twitch.

IV. Frequency of Stimulation

It is well known that during voluntary contractions there is a progressive increase in the number of active motor units, and, over a certain range of tensions, an increase in the frequency of discharge of each unit (ADRIAN and BRONK, 1929; SMITH, 1934; SEYFFARTH, 1940; DENNY-BROWN, 1949). Evidence was also obtained that units in normal muscle do not fire at frequencies much above 20 to 50 Hz, even for comparatively short periods. In a maintained tetanic contraction, the frequency of firing is quite low. The longest steady sequence observed by SMITH (1934) in voluntary contractions of human muscle lasted 13 min: its frequency was only 9 Hz. "The efficiency of muscle", as BRONK said in 1930, "reaches its maximum level when the frequency of stimulation of its fibres is just sufficient to produce maximum tetanic tension; at frequencies above and below this, the muscle fibre is less efficient."

In 1954, BIGLAND and LIPPOLD studied motor unit activity in voluntary contractions of human muscle (a) by stimulating a muscle artificially and determining the relation between frequency response and tension produced—a method previously used in anaesthetised animals (ADRIAN and BRONK, 1929; BROWN and BURNS, 1949); and (b) by recording the frequency response of a single unit during a voluntary contraction. In all experiments the tension exerted by the muscle increased with the frequency of stimulation and the tension was directly proportional to frequency until this reached a value between 35 and 45 Hz. At this frequency the tension increased no further and the plotted curve reached a plateau (Fig. 34). On increasing the frequency of stimulation still further, the usual result was a slight decrease in tension, although in a few cases the plateau remained flat or fell steeply. In the second group of experiments frequencies above 50 Hz were never observed and frequencies between 40 and 50 Hz occurred only when the tension was above 75% of the maximum voluntary contraction. Over a greater range of tensions (25 to 75% of the maximum voluntary contraction) most of the fastest units responded at frequencies between 25 and 35 Hz (Fig. 34).

MERTON (1954) also compared maximal voluntary strength with a single maximal twitch and with tetani ranging from 10 to 50 Hz. At frequencies above 30 Hz the tension rate curve had clearly flattened out. At these frequencies the contraction was completely fused. Only in paretic human muscle was a wider range of frequencies found, with a maximum up to 70 to 80 Hz (SEYFFARTH, 1940). This may indicate a functional adaptation to the greater load on the surviving motor units.

The tetanic tension developed by a muscle excited through the motor nerve with repeated maximal stimuli declines as stimulation continues or if the frequency of stimulation is high. This is a poorly understood phenomenon. Although deficient muscle contraction may result from failure at several points in a long chain of events, it seems likely, in the light of more recent work, that presynaptic events play an important role. There is evidence that under certain conditions a nerve impulse will not be propagated down the distributing line to all the muscle fibres. KRNJEVIĆ and

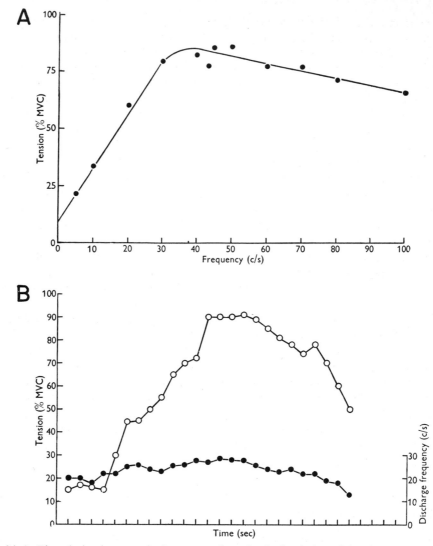

Fig. 34. A: The relation between the frequency of maximal stimulation of the ulnar nerve and the tension produced in the human adductor pollicis muscle. B: The frequency response of a single unit measured a 1 sec intervals during a voluntary contraction of abductor digiti minimi brevis. Open circles ○ show changes in tension between 15 and 92% MVC, while filled circles ● are the corresponding discharge frequencies, varying between 10 and 30/sec. MVC: maximal voluntary contraction. (From: BIGLAND and LIPPOLD, 1954)

MILEDI (1958 and 1959) demonstrated that repetitive indirect stimulation of rat muscle *in vitro* or *in vivo* leads to a presynaptic block of nerve conduction which may be intermittent or complete, but which is reversed when the stimulation is stopped or continued at a lower rate. With an intracellular microelectrode in the region of the end-plate, they were able to recognise presynaptic failures easily, since unlike the other types of block no local end-plate potentials could be recorded. According to

KRNJEVIĆ and MILEDI, the most likely sites for the presynaptic block seemed to be branching points of the fibre where the safety factor of transmission is sharply reduced. In both *in vitro* and *in vivo* preparations, stimulation of the nerve at 50 Hz usually caused intermittent failure of many fibres within 2 to 5 min. As a rule, however, the frequency needed for the appearance of failure was lower *in vitro* (very often 10 to 30 Hz) than *in vivo*. Furthermore, presynaptic block, especially *in vitro*, was precipitated by anoxia and was found to be very sensitive to changes in temperature. The influence of such variables must therefore be carefully considered as they can easily alter the results obtained from experiments in which the magnitude of the muscle action potentials to repetitive stimulation is measured.

During a maintained contraction the blood flow through a muscle may well be inadequate, and hypoxia is likely to develop. In discussing this possibility KRNJEVIĆ and MILEDI (1959) pointed out that although nerve fibres are protected from changes in their environment by the low permeability of their sheaths, the sheaths cannot protect them from anoxia.

A prejunctional block which occurs at prolonged or high frequencies of stimulation is not likely to be of any advantage during investigations of drug action at the neuromuscular junction. In far too many studies, however, frequencies of up to 300 Hz have been used in both animal and man. But frequency above 50 Hz is clearly outside the physiological range and carries with it a great number of experimental dangers which make interpretation of the results difficult indeed. We find the use of high frequencies of stimulation in man puzzling. Most of these studies are performed in anaesthetised patients with the object (a) of analysing the mechanism of action of various neuromuscular blocking drugs, and (b) of assessing the magnitude of the neuromuscular block during or at the end of an operation. However, under anaesthesia, or with the arm completely at rest (SMITH, 1934), motor neurone activity is almost absent. If we really want to find out what a drug does at the neuromuscular junction in an anaesthetised patient, frequencies of stimulation inside the physiological range would be more than adequate.

H. Concluding Remarks

Neuromuscular block by prolonged depolarisation of the end-plate presents a complex picture, for a sequence of excitation followed by depression of transmission is always detectable. The depolarisation, although limited to the end-plate region, spreads slightly beyond the area in which end-plate potentials can normally be recorded, the extent of this spread of depolarisation increasing with time. The manifestations of this sequence vary with different species and with different muscles in the same species so that the same process may give rise, as we have already seen, to a situation in which either repetitive firing, or contracture or block of transmission predominates.

Uncertainties of interpretation arise because different effects have been observed under different experimental conditions. For example, KATZ and MILEDI (1973) compared end-plate depolarisation and associated "membrane noise" due to decamethonium, acetylthiocholine and suberyldicholine with the effects of acetylcholine and carbachol. Their experiments were made on the isolated sartorius muscle of the

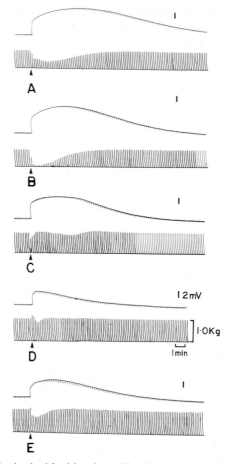

Fig. 35 A—E. Cat; anaesthetised with chloralose. Simultaneous recordings of the depolarisation of the end-plate region of the tibialis anterior muscle measured with an external electrode, and of neuromuscular block measured by recording muscle contractions, elicited by indirect stimulation of the sciatic nerve (0.1 Hz). At (A), 50 μg decamethonium; (B), 75 μg suxamethonium; (C); 250 μg suberyldicholine; (D), 200 μg acetylthiocholine; (E), 100 μg carbachol. All drugs administered close-arterially

frog and the drugs were applied ionophoretically. The results showed that decamethonium exhibited little depolarising power and that the development of depolarisation was a very slow process. They concluded therefore that decamethonium can be described as a "partial agonist" forming with the receptor a compound which has a much higher probability of being in the inactive (i.e. competitively blocking) rather than the depolarising conformation. Carbachol, but not acetylthiocholine, proved more effective than decamethonium. Finally suberyldicholine proved as effective, if not more so, than acetylcholine.

We compared the four substances, and in addition suxamethonium, using the tibialis anterior muscle of the cat *in vivo*. All drugs were administered close-arterially into the circulation of the muscle. Simultaneous recordings of the depolarisation of the end-plate region recorded with external electrodes and neuromuscular block measured by recording muscle contractions elicited by indirect stimulation of the sciatic nerve confirmed our previous results with decamethonium and suxamethonium in the cat—a fast and effective depolarisation of the end-plate region—and these two drugs were not less effective than carbachol and suberyldicholine. Figure 35 illustrates the results obtained.

Therefore, decamethonium may well be a "partial agonist" in the frog as it is in the rat or the dog but it is an "agonist" in the cat, having a potency very similar to that of acetylcholine.

During a prolonged depolarisation of the end-plate region the muscle may lose significant amounts of potassium and gain significant amounts of sodium, calcium and chloride. The ionic concentrations, therefore, on either side of the muscle must be significantly altered. These rather "unphysiological" changes produced by a prolonged depolarisation reduce the functional reserve at the neuromuscular junction and therefore the motor end-plate region becomes vulnerable. At the same time these "unphysiological" changes may be easily magnified by a variety of experimental conditions.

A two-phase action of decamethonium was described in muscle preparations isolated from several species such as the rabbit lumbrical muscle, the guinea-pig diaphragm and human intercostal muscle (JENDEN et al., 1954; JENDEN, 1955; DILLON and SABAWALA, 1959; TAYLOR, 1962). The first phase consists of neuromuscular block of rapid onset which reaches a maximum in 4 to 6 min and then recovers spontaneously in spite of the continued presence of decamethonium in the same concentration. Maximum recovery occurs in 15 to 30 min, after which the second phase begins. This consists of a slow progressive neuromuscular block which reaches a steady state after 3 to 6 hrs; this "remains constant for hours if undisturbed" (JENDEN, 1955). Suxamethonium and carbachol produce effects qualitatively similar to those of decamethonium. After 25 µg of neostigmine, acetylcholine also produces a similar action. Therefore the effects of depolarising drugs on isolated muscle preparations may differ according to the conditions of the experiment and the method of applying the drug. And, without any doubt, these effects differ from those obtained in the intact animal. In the rabbit and guinea-pig in vivo, decamethonium has a dual mode of action (see p. 387) possibly acting as a partial agonist, whereas in the cat and man the neuromuscular block has all the features of a block due to long-lasting depolarisation.

It appears, therefore, that once the same muscles are studied in vitro the differences disappear; and the time-course of the two-phase blockade is almost identical in all of them.

Reviewing the clinical reports on the use of depolarising drugs during anaesthesia, it becomes very clear that certain general anaesthetics can alter the mechanism of action of these drugs. For example, when nitrous oxide, oxygen and thiopentone are used, the neuromuscular block produced by either decamethonium or suxamethonium exhibits all the characteristics of a block by depolarisation. However, when ether is used, and especially fluorinated anaesthetics, the mechanism of action of depolarising drugs is changed. For example, a tetanus is no longer well maintained and anticholinesterase drugs readily antagonise the block. We must infer that, in the presence of a particular type of anaesthetic drug, a change takes place in the muscle membrane—a change which is brought to light by the changing pattern of the neuromuscular block produced by depolarising drugs. See introductory chapter for details.

Considering the two processes of neuromuscular block (a) competition with acetylcholine, (b) depolarisation, it may be said that a block produced by long-lasting depolarisation has provided a great deal of information not accessible through the study of a block produced by competition with acetylcholine. However, while the interpretation of the results obtained with a competitive substance is relatively straightforward, since the response of skeletal muscles to such a substance is apparently uniform, the handling of a depolarising substance, or of a substance having a depolarising element, is much more difficult and the interpretation of the results obtained from different species and from different muscles needs great care.

References

Adrian, E. D., Bronk, D. W.: The discharge of impulses in motor nerve fibres. Part 2. The frequency of discharge in reflex and voluntary contractions. J. Physiol. (Lond.) **67**, 119—151 (1929).

Alderson, A. M., MacLagan, J.: The action of decamethonium and tubocurarine on the respiratory and limb muscle of the cat. J. Physiol. (Lond.) **173**, 38—56 (1964).

Axelsson, J., Thesleff, S.: The desensitizing effect of acetylcholine on mammalian motor endplate. Acta physiol. scand. **43**, 15—26 (1958).

Bacq, Z. M., Brown, G. L.: Pharmacological experiments on mammalian voluntary muscle, in relation to the theory of chemical transmission. J. Physiol. (Lond.) **89**, 45—60 (1937).

Barlow, R. B., Ing, H. R.: Curare-like action of polymethylene bis-quaternary ammonium salts. Nature (Lond.) **161**, 718 (1948a).

Barlow, R. B., Ing, H. R.: Curare-like action of polymethylene bis-quaternary ammoniam salts. Brit. J. Pharmacol. **3**, 298—304 (1948b).

Bigland, B., Goetzee, B., MacLagan, J., Zaimis, E.: The effect of lowered muscle temperature on the action of neuromuscular blocking drugs. J. Physiol. (Lond.) **141**, 425—434 (1958).

Bigland, B., Lippold, O. C. J.: Motor unit activity in the voluntary contraction of human muscle. J. Physiol. (Lond.) **125**, 322—335 (1954).

Bigland, B., Zaimis, E.: Factors influencing limb temperature during experiments on skeletal muscle. J. Physiol. (Lond.) **141**, 420—424 (1958).

Blaber, L. C., Bowman, W. C.: A comparison between the responses of avian and mammalian muscles to substances which facilitate neuromuscular transmission. Arch. int. Pharmacodyn. **138**, 185—208 (1962).

Blaber, L. C., Cuthbert, A. W.: Cholinesterases in the domestic fowl and the specificity of some reversible inhibitors. Biochem. Pharmacol. **11**, 113—124 (1962).

Botelho, S. Y., Cander, L.: Post-tetanic potentiation before and during ischemia in intact human skeletal muscle. J. appl. Physiol. **6**, 221—228 (1953).

Bovet, D.: Synthetic inhibitors of neuromuscular transmission. In: Cheymol, J. (Ed.): Neuromuscular Blocking and Stimulating Agents. International Encyclopedia of Pharmacology and Therapeutics, Section 14, Vol. I, pp. 243—294. Oxford: Pergamon Press 1972.

Bovet, D., Bovet-Nitti, F.: Succinylcholine chloride, curarising agent of short duration of action. Pharmaco-dynamic activity and clinical application. Sci. med. ital. **3**, 484 (1955).

Bovet, D., Bovet-Nitti, F., Guarino, S., Longo, V. G., Fusco, R.:Recherches sur les poisons curarisants de synthèse. Arch. int. Pharmacodyn. **88**, 1—50 (1951).

Bowman, W. C.: Mechanisms of neuromuscular blockade. In: West, G. B., Ellis, G. P. (Eds.): Progress in Medicinal Chemistry, Vol. 2, pp. 88—131. London: Butterworth 1962.

Bowman, W. C.: Neuromuscular blocking agents. In: Laurence, D. R., Bacharach, A. L. (Eds.): Evaluation of Drug Activities: Pharmacometrics, Vol. 1, pp. 325—351. London: Academic Press 1964.

BOWMAN, W. C., GOLDBERG, A. A. J., RAPER, C.: A comparison between the effects of a tetanus and the effects of sympathomimetic amines on fast- and slow-contracting mammalian muscles. Brit. J. Pharmacol. **19**, 464—484 (1962).

BOWMAN, W. C., GOLDBERG, A. A. J., RAPER, C.: Post-tetanic and drug-induced repetitive firing in the soleus muscle of the cat. Brit. J. Pharmacol. **35**, 62—78 (1969).

BOWMAN, W. C., MARSHALL, I. G.: Inhibitors of acetylcholine synthesis. In: CHEYMOL, J. (Ed.): Neuromuscular Blocking and Stimulating Agents. International Encyclopedia of Pharmacology and Therapeutics, Section 14, Vol. I, pp. 357—390. Oxford: Pergamon Press 1972.

BOWMAN, W. C., WEBB, S. N.: Acetylcholine and anticholinesterase drugs. In: CHEYMOL, J. (Ed.): Neuromuscular Blocking and Stimulating Agents. International Encyclopedia of Pharmacology and Therapeutics, Section 14, Vol. II, pp. 427—502. Oxford: Pergamon Press 1972.

BOYD, I. A., MARTIN, A. R.: The end-plate potential in mammalian muscle. J. Physiol. (Lond.) **132**, 74—91 (1956).

BRONK, D. W.: The energy expended in maintaining a muscular contraction. J. Physiol. (Lond.) **69**, 306—315 (1930).

BROWN, G. L., BURNS, B. D.: Fatigue and neuromuscular block in mammalian skeletal muscle. Proc. roy. Soc. B **136**, 182—195 (1949).

BROWN, G. L., DALE, H. H., FELDBERG, W.: Reactions of the normal mammalian muscle to acetylcholine and to eserine. J. Physiol. (Lond.) **87**, 394—424 (1936).

BROWN, G. L., HARVEY, A. M.: Reaction of avian muscle to acetylcholine and eserine. J. Physiol. (Lond.) **94**, 101—117 (1938).

BROWN, G. L., VON EULER, U. S.: The after effects of a tetanus on mammalian muscle. J. Physiol. (Lond.) **93**, 39—60 (1938).

BURNS, B. D., PATON, W. D. M.: Depolarisation of the motor end-plate by decamethonium and acetylcholine. J. Physiol. (Lond.) **115**, 41—73 (1951).

BUTTLE, G. A. H., ZAIMIS, E.: The action of decamethonium iodide in birds. J. Pharm. Pharmacol. **1**, 991—992 (1949).

CALDWELL, P. C., KEYNES, R. D.: The effect of ouabain on the efflux of sodium from a squid giant axon. J. Physiol. (Lond.) **148**, 8 P (1959).

CANNARD, T. H., ZAIMIS, E.: The effect of lowered muscle temperature on the action of neuromuscular blocking drugs in man. J. Physiol. (Lond.) **149**, 112—119 (1959).

CHAGAS, G., SOLLERO, L., SUAREZ-KURTZ, G.: Synthetic neuromuscular blocking agents: Absorption—distribution—metabolism—excretion. In: CHEYMOL, J. (Ed.): Neuromuscular Blocking and Stimulating Agents. International Encyclopedia of Pharmacology and Therapeutics, Section 14, Vol. I, pp. 409—423. Oxford: Pergamon Press 1972.

CHEYMOL, J., BOURILLET, F.: Inhibitors of post-synpatic receptors. In: CHEYMOL, J. (Ed.): Neuromuscular Blocking and Stimulating Agents. International Encyclopedia of Pharmacology and Therapeutics, Section 14, Vol. I, pp. 297—356. Oxford: Pergamon Press 1972.

CHILD, K. G., ZAIMIS, E.: A new biological method for the assay of depolarizing substances using the isolated semispinalis muscle of the chick. Brit. J. Pharmacol. **15**, 412—416 (1960).

CHURCHILL-DAVIDSON, H. C., RICHARDSON, A. T.: Motor end-plate differences as a determining factor in the mode of action of neuromuscular blocking substances. Nature (Lond.) **170**, 617—618 (1952a).

CHURCHILL-DAVIDSON, H. C., RICHARDSON, A. T.: Decamethonium iodide (ClO): Some observation on its action using electromyography. Proc. roy. Soc. Med. **45**, 179—185 (1952b).

CHURCHILL-DAVIDSON, H. C., RICHARDSON, A. T.: Neuromuscular transmission in myasthenia gravis. J. Physiol. (Lond.) **122**, 252—263 (1953).

CONNOLLY, R., GOUGH, W., WINEGRAD, S.: Characteristics of the isometric twitch of skeletal muscle immediately after a tetanus: A study of the influence of the distribution of calcium within the sarcoplasmic reticulum on the twitch. J. gen. Physiol. **57**, 697—704 (1971).

CONWAY, E. J., KERNAN, R. P., ZADUNAISKY, J. A.: The sodium pump in skeletal muscle in relation to energy barriers. J. Physiol. (Lond.) **155**, 263—279 (1961).

COOKSON, J. C., PATON, W. D. M.: Mechanisms of neuromuscular block. Anaesthesia **24**, 395—416 (1969).

CREESE, R., MACLAGAN, J.: Autoradiography of decamethonium in rat muscle. Nature (Lond.) **215**, 988—989 (1967).

CREESE, R., MACLAGAN, J.: Uptake of ^{3}H-decamethonium in cat muscle fibres. V. International Congress on Pharmacology 864. San Francisco 1972.

CSAPO, A., WILKIE, D. R.: Dynamics of the effect of potassium on frog's muscle. J. Physiol. (Lond.) **134**, 479—514 (1956).

DALE, H. H., FELDBERG, W.: Chemical transmission at motor nerve endings in voluntary muscle. J. Physiol. (Lond.) **81**, 39—40 P (1934).

DALE, H. H., FELDBERG, W., VOGT, M.: Release of acetylcholine at voluntary motor nerve endings. J. Physiol. (Lond.) **86**, 353—380 (1936).

DEL CASTILLO, J., KATZ, B.: On the localization of acetylcholine receptors. J. Physiol. (Lond.) **128**, 157—181 (1955).

DENNY-BROWN, D.: Interpretation of the electromyogram. Arch. Neurol. Psychiat. (Chic.) **61**, 99—128 (1949).

DERKX, F. H. M., BONTA, I. L., LAGENDIJK, A.: Species-dependent effect of neuromuscular blocking agents. Europ. J. Pharmacol. **16**, 105—108 (1971).

DILLON, J. B., SABAWALA, P. B.: The mode of action of depolarizing drugs. Acta anaesth. scand. **3**, 83—101 (1959).

DOUGLAS, W. W., PATON, W. D. M.: The mechanisms of motor end-plate depolarization due to a cholinesterase-inhibiting drug. J. Physiol. (Lond.) **124**, 325—344 (1954).

ELLIS, F. R.: Neuromuscular disease and anaesthesia. Brit. J. Anaesth. **46**, 603—612 (1974).

ELMQUIST, D., THESLEFF, S.: Ideas regarding receptor desensitization at the motor end-plate. Rev. canad. Biol. **21**, 229—234 (1962).

FAHMY, N. R., GISSEN, A. J., SAVARESE, J. J., KITZ, R. J.: Decamethonium and serum potassium in man. Anesthesiology **42**, 692—697 (1975).

FATT, P.: Electromotive action of acetylcholine at the motor end-plate. J. Physiol. (Lond.) **111**, 408—422 (1950).

FEDDE, M. R.: Electrical properties and acetylcholine sensitivity of singly and multiply innervated avian muscle fibers. J. gen. Physiol. **53**, 624—637 (1969).

FENG, T. P., LI, T. H., TING, Y. C.: Studies on the neuromuscular junction. XII. Repetitive discharges and inhibitory after-effect in post-tetanically facilitated responses of cat muscle to single nerve volleys. Chin. J. Physiol. **14**, 55—79 (1939).

FOLDES, F.: The pharmacology of neuromuscular blocking agents in man. Clin. Pharmacol. Ther. **1**, 345—395 (1960).

FOLDES, F. F., DUNCALF, D.: Clinical applications of peripheral inhibitors and stimulants of neuromuscular transmission. In: CHEYMOL, J. (Ed.): Neuromuscular Blocking and Stimulating Agents. International Encyclopedia of Pharmacology and Therapeutics. Section 14, Vol. II, pp. 545—559. Oxford: Pergamon Press 1972.

GALINDO, A.: Depolarizing neuromuscular block. J. Pharmacol. exp. Ther. **178**, 339—349 (1971).

GINSBORG, B. L.: Spontaneous activity in muscle fibres of the chick. J. Physiol. (Lond.) **150**, 707—717 (1960a).

GINSBORG, B. L.: Some properties of avian skeletal muscle fibres with multiple neuromuscular junctions. J. Physiol. (Lond.) **154**, 581—598 (1960b).

GINSBORG, B. L., MACKAY, B.: A histochemical demonstration of two types of motor innervation in avian skeletal muscle. Bibl. anat. (Basel) **2**, 174—181 (1961).

GINSBORG, B. L., WARRINER, J.: The isolated chick biventer cervicis nerve-muscle preparation. Brit. J. Pharmacol. **15**, 410—411 (1960).

GLYNN, I. M.: The action of cardiac glycosides on sodium and potassium movements in human red cells. J. Physiol. (Lond.) **136**, 148—173 (1957).

GLYNN, I. M.: Activation of adenosine-triphosphates activity in a cell membrane by external potassium and internal sodium. J. Physiol. (Lond.) **160**, 18—19 P (1962).

GRONERT, G. A., THEYE, R. A.: Pathophysiology of hyperkalemia induced by succinylcholine. Anesthesiology **43**, 89—99 (1975).

HALL, R. A., PARKES, M. W.: The effect of drugs upon neuromuscular transmission in the guinea-pig. J. Physiol. (Lond.) **122**, 274—281 (1953).

HEAD, S. D.: Depolarising neuromuscular blocking drugs; an electrophysiological investigation in mammalian skeletal muscle. Ph. D. Thesis, University of London, 1975.

HESS, A.: Structural differences of fast and slow extrafusal muscle fibres and their nerve endings in chickens. J. Physiol. (Lond.) **157**, 221—231 (1961).

HESS, A.: The structure of vertebrate slow and twitch muscle fibers. Invest. Opthal. **6**, 217—228 (1967).

HOLMES, P. E. B., JENDEN, D. J., TAYLOR, D. B.: The analysis of the mode of action of curare on neuromuscular transmission: the effect of temperature changes. J. Pharmacol. exp. Ther. **103**, 382—402 (1951).

HUMPHREY, P. P. A.: Depolarisation and neuromuscular block in the rat. Brit. J. Pharmacol. **48**, 636—637 P (1973).

HUTTER, O. F., WARNER, A. E.: The pH sensitivity of the chloride conductance of frog skeletal muscle. J. Physiol. (Lond.) **189**, 403—425 (1967).

IRESON, T. D., FORD, R., LOVEDAY, C.: The neuromuscular blocking action of suxamethonium in the anaesthetised rat. Arch. int. Pharmacodyn. **181**, 283—286 (1969).

JARCHO, L. W., BERMAN, B., EYZAGUIRRE, C., LILIENTHAL, J. L., JR.: Curarization of denervated muscle. Ann. N.Y. Acad. Sci. **54**, 337—346 (1951).

JENDEN, D. J.: Effect of drugs upon neuromuscular transmission in the isolated guinea-pig diaphragm. J. Pharmacol. exp. Ther. **114**, 398—408 (1955).

JENDEN, D. J., KAMIJO, K., TAYLOR, D. B.: The action of decamethonium on isolated rabbit lumbrical muscle. J. Pharmacol. exp. Ther. **111**, 229—240 (1954).

JENKINSON, D. H., TERRAR, D. A.: Influence of chloride ions on changes in membrane potential during prolonged application of carbachol to frog skeletal muscle. Brit. J. Pharmacol. **47**, 363—376 (1973).

JEWELL, P. A., KEEN, P., TONG, E. H.: The use of the muscle relaxant suxethonium to immobilize captive animals with the projectile-syringe rifle. J. Zool. **146**, 263—271 (1965).

JEWELL, P. A., ZAIMIS, E.: A differentiation between red and white muscle in the cat based on responses to neuromuscular blocking agents. J. Physiol. (Lond.) **124**, 417—428 (1954a).

JEWELL, P. A., ZAIMIS, E.: Changes at the neuromuscular junction of red and white muscle fibres in the cat induced by disuse atrophy and by hypertrophy. J. Physiol. (Lond.) **124**, 429—442 (1954b).

KARCZMAR, A. G.: Neuromuscular pharmacology. Ann. Rev. Pharmacol. **7**, 241—276 (1967).

KATZ, B., MILEDI, R.: The characteristics of end-plate noise produced by different depolarizing drugs. J. Physiol. (Lond.) **230**, 707—713 (1973).

KLUPP, H., KRAUPP, O.: Über die Freisetzung von Kalium aus der Muskulatur unter der Einwirkung einiger Muskelrelaxantien. Arch. int. Pharmacodyn. **98**, 340—354 (1954).

KRNJEVIĆ, K., MILEDI, R.: Failure of neuromuscular propagation in rats. J. Physiol. (Lond.) **140**, 440—461 (1958).

KRNJEVIĆ, K., MILEDI, R.: Presynaptic failure of neuromuscular propagation in rats. J. Physiol. (Lond.) **149**, 1—22 (1959).

KVISSELGAARD, L., MOYA, F.: Estimation of succinylcholine blood levels. Acta anaesth. scand. **5**, 1—11 (1961).

MAGLAGAN, J.: Factors influencing the action of neuromuscular blocking drugs. Ph. D. Thesis, University of London, 1960.

MACLAGAN, J.: A comparison of the responses of the tenuissimus muscle to neuromuscular blocking drugs *in vivo* and *in vitro*. Brit. J. Pharmacol. **18**, 204—216 (1962).

MACLAGAN, J., VRBOVÁ, G.: A study of the increased sensitivity of denervated and re-innervated muscle to depolarising drugs. J. Physiol. (Lond.) **182**, 131—143 (1966).

MATCHETT, P. A., JOHNSON, J. A.: Inhibition of sodium and potassium transport in frog santorii in the presence of ouabain. Fed. Proc. **13**, 384 (1954).

MAYR, R.: Zur elektronenmikroskopischen Unterscheidbarkeit eines einfach und eines multipel innervierten Hühnermuskels. Naturwissenschaften **54**, 22 (1967).

MAZZE, R. E., ESCUE, H. M., HOUSTON, J. B.: Hyperkalaemia and cardiovascular collapse following administration of succinylcholine to the traumatised patient. Anesthesiology **31**, 540—547 (1969).

MERTON, P. A.: Voluntary strength and fatigue. J. Physiol. (Lond.) **123**, 553—564 (1954).

MICHELSON, M. J., ZEIMAL, E. V.: Acetylcholine: an approach to the molecular mechanism of action. Oxford: Pergamon Press 1973.

NASTUK, W. L., GISSEN, A. J.: Actions of acetylcholine and other quaternary ammonium compounds at the muscle post junctional membrane. In: PAUL, W. M., DANIEL, E. E., KAY, C. M., MONCKTON, G. (Eds.): Muscle, pp. 389—402. Oxford: Pergamon Press 1965.

NASTUK, W. L., PARSONS, R. L.: Factors in the inactivation of postjunctional membrane receptors of frog skeletal muscle. J. gen. Physiol. **56**, 218—249 (1970).

PATON, W. D. M.: Mode of action of neuromuscular blocking agents. Brit. J. Anaesth. **28**, 470—480 (1956).

PATON, W. D. M.: In: DE REUCK, A. V. S. (Ed.): Curare and Curare-like Agents. Ciba Foundation Study Group No. 12, p. 33. London: Churchill 1962.

PATON, W. D. M., PERRY, W. L. M.: The relationship between depolarization and block in the cat's superior cervical ganglion. J. Physiol. (Lond.) **119**, 43—57 (1953).

PATON, W. D. M., SAVINI, E. C.: The action of nicotine on the motor end-plate in the cat. Brit. J. Pharmacol. **32**, 360—380 (1968).

PATON, W. D. M., WAUD, D. R.: Drug-receptor interactions at the neuromuscular junction. In: DE REUCK, A. V. S. (Ed.): Curare and curare-like Agents. Ciba Foundation Study Group No. 12, pp. 34—54. London: Churchill 1962.

PATON, W. D. M., ZAIMIS, E.: Curare-like action of polymethylene bis-quaternary ammonium salts. Nature (Lond.) **161**, 718—719 (1948a).

PATON, W. D. M., ZAIMIS, E.: Clinical potentialities of certain bisquaternary salts causing neuromuscular and ganglionic block. Nature (Lond.) **162**, 810 (1948b).

PATON, W. D. M., ZAIMIS, E.: The properties of polymethylene bistrimethylammonium salts. J. Physiol. (Lond.) **108**, 55—57 P (1949a).

PATON, W. D. M., ZAIMIS, E.: The pharmacological actions of polymethylene bistrimethylammonium salts. Brit. J. Pharmacol. **4**, 381—400 (1949b).

PATON, W. D. M., ZAIMIS, E.: Actions and clinical assessment of drugs which produce neuromuscular block. Lancet 1950 **2**, 568—570.

PATON, W. D. M., ZAIMIS, E.: The action of d-tubocurarine and of decamethonium on respiratory and other muscles in the cat. J. Physiol. (Lond.) **112**, 311—331 (1951a).

PATON, W. D. M., ZAIMIS, E.: Paralysis of autonomic ganglia by methonium salts. Brit. J. Pharmacol. **6**, 155—168 (1951b).

PATON, W. D. M., ZAIMIS, E.: The methonium compounds. Pharmacol. Rev. **4**, 219—253 (1952).

PAYNE, J. P., SON HOLMDAHL, M. H.: The effect of repeated doses of suxamethonium in man. Brit. J. Anaesth. **31**, 341—347 (1959).

PELOUZE, T. J. P., BERNARD, C.: Recherches sur le curare. C.R. Acad. Sci. **31**, 533 (1850).

PHILIPPOT, E., DALLEMAGNE, M. J.: Synergies et antagonismes à la junction neuromusculaire. Action de sels d'alkyltrimethyl-ammonium. Arch. int. Physiol. **59**, 357—373 (1951).

PHILIPPOT, E., DALLEMAGNE, M. J.: Les inhibiteurs de la transmission neuro-musculaire étudiés chez le chien. Experientia (Basel) **8**, 273—274 (1952).

POST, R. L., MERRITT, C. R., KINSOLVING, C. R., ALBRIGHT, C. D.: Membrane adenosine-tri-phosphatase as a participant in the active transport of sodium and potassiom in the human erythrocyte. J. biol. Chem. **235**, 1796—1802 (1960).

POULSEN, H., HOUGS, W.: The effect of some curarizing drugs in unanesthetized man II. Succinylcholine iodide and its bis-monoethylsubstituted derivative in continuous intravenous infusion. Acta anaesth. scand. **2**, 107—115 (1958).

SEARS, T. A.: Efferent discharges in alpha and fusimotor fibres of intercostal nerves of the cat. J. Physiol. (Lond.) **174**, 295—315 (1964).

SEYFFARTH, H.: The behaviour of motor-units in voluntary contraction. Skr. norske Vidensk A Kad. (1. Mat. Naturw. Kl. 4), pp. 1—63, 1940.

SMITH, N: TY.: Subcutaneous, muscle, and body temperatures in anesthetized man. J. appl. Physiol. **17**, 306—310 (1962).

SMITH, O. C.: Action potentials from single motor units in voluntary contraction. Amer. J. Physiol. **108**, 629—638 (1934).

STEVENSON, D. E.: Changes in the blood electrolytes of anaesthetized dogs caused by suxamethonium. Brit. J. Anaesth. **32,** 364—371 (1960).

STONE, W. A., BEACH, T. P., HAMELBERG, W.: Succinylcholine-induced hyperkalemia in dogs with transected sciatic nerves or spinal cords. Anesthesiology **32**, 515—520 (1970).

TAYLOR, D. B.: Influence of curare on uptake and release of a neuromuscular blocking agent labelled with iodine-131. In: DE REUCK, A. V. S. (Ed.): Curare and Curare-like Agents. Ciba Foundation Study Group No. 12, p. 21. London: Churchill 1962.

TAYLOR, D. B., CREESE, R.: Uptake of labelled transmitter analogues and their blockade by antagonists. Lecture to New York Academy of Sciences. Conference on cholinergic Mechanisms May 1966. Ann. N.Y. Acad. Sci. (1966).

TAYLOR, D. B., CREESE, R., LU, T. C., CASE, R.: Uptake of labelled transmitter analogues and their blockade by antagonists. Ann. N.Y. Acad. Sci. 144, 768—771 (1967a).

TAYLOR, D. B., DIXON, W. J., CREESE, R., CASE, R.: Diffusion of decamethonium in the rat. Nature (Lond.) 215, 989 (1967b).

TERRAR, D. A.: Influence of SKF 525A congeners, strophanthidin and tissue-culture media on desensitization in frog skeletal muscle. Brit. J. Pharmacol. 51, 259—268 (1974).

THESLEFF, S.: Succinylcholine iodide: Studies on its pharmacological properties and clinical use. Acta physiol. scand. 27, Suppl. 99, 1—36 (1952).

THESLEFF, S.: Neuromuscular block caused by acetylcholine. Nature (Lond.) 175, 594—595 (1955a).

THESLEFF, S.: The mode of neuromuscular block caused by acetylcholine, nicotine, decamethonium and succinylcholine. Acta physiol. scand. 34, 218—231 (1955b).

THESLEFF, S.: The effects of acetylcholine, decamethonium and succinylcholine on neuromuscular transmission in the rat. Acta physiol. scand. 34, 386—392 (1955c).

THESLEFF, S.: Interactions between neuromuscular blocking agents and acetylcholine at the mammalian motor end-plate. Atti Congresso Societa Italiana di Anestesiologa 1959, 37—42.

THESLEFF, S., QUASTEL, D. M. J.: Neuromuscular pharmacology. Ann. Rev. Pharmacol. 5, 263—284 (1965).

TYLER, C.: The assay of acetylcholine with the isolated semispinalis cervicis muscle of the chick. Analyst 85, 8—11 (1960).

VON DARDEL, O., THESLEFF, S.: Succinylcholine iodide as a muscular reflexant. A report of 500 surgical cases. Acta chir. scand. 103, 322—336 (1952).

VOURC'H, G.: Depressants and stimulants of neuromuscular transmission. A clinical and therapeutic study in anesthesia. In: CHEYMOL, J. (Ed.): Neuromuscular Blocking and Stimulating Agents. International Encyclopedia of Pharmacology and Therapeutics, Section 14, Vol. II, pp. 517—543. Oxford: Pergamon Press 1972.

WHITTAKER, V. P., WIJESUNDERA, S.: The hydrolysis of succinyldicholine by cholinesterase. Biochem. J. 51, 348—351 (1952).

WINEGRAD, S.: The intracellular site of calcium activation of contraction in frog skeletal muscle. J. gen. Physiol. 55, 77—88 (1970).

WOLLMAN, H., CANNARD, T. H.: Skeletal muscle, esophageal and rectal temperatures in man during general anesthesia and operation. Anesthesiology 21, 476—481 (1960).

ZAIMIS, E.: The synthesis of methonium compounds, their isolation from urine and their photometric determination. Brit. J. Pharmacol. 5, 424—430 (1950).

ZAIMIS, E.: The action of decamethonium on normal and denervated mammalian muscle. J. Physiol. (Lond.) 112, 176—190 (1951).

ZAIMIS, E.: Motor end-plate differences as a determining factor in the mode of action of neuromuscular blocking substances. J. Physiol. (Lond.) 122, 238—251 (1953).

ZAIMIS, E.: The interruption of neuromuscular transmission and some of its problems. Pharmacol. Rev. 6, 53—57 (1954).

ZAIMIS, E.: Factors influencing the action of neuromuscular blocking substances. In: Lectures on scientific basis of medicine. Vol. 6. London: Athlone Press 1956.

ZAIMIS, E.: Mechanisms of neuromuscular blockade. In: BOVET, D., BOVET-NITTI, F., MARINI-BETTOLO, G. B. (Eds.): Curare and Curare-Like Agents, pp. 191—203. Amsterdam: Elsevier 1959.

ZAIMIS, E.: Experimental hazards and artefacts in the study of neuromuscular blocking drugs. In: DE REUCK, A. V. S. (Ed.): Curare and Curare-like Agents, Ciba Foundation Study Group No. 12, pp. 75—82. London: Churchill 1962.

Competitive Neuromuscular Blocking Drugs

JENNIFER MACLAGAN

A. Introduction and Terminology

The first neuromuscular blocking drug to be introduced into general anaesthetic use was tubocurarine (GRIFFITH and JOHNSON, 1942). In man, a single intravenous injection of a dose which caused adequate relaxation of the abdominal muscles, produced paralysis lasting for 30 to 40 min. This proved to be unduly long for convenient use during anaesthesia and the search began for neuromuscular blocking drugs with a shorter duration of action.

Both gallamine (BOVET et al., 1947) and decamethonium (PATON and ZAIMIS, 1949) had a slightly shorter duration of action than tubocurarine but suxamethonium (HUNT and TAVEAU, 1906; BOVET et al., 1955) was the first drug found to cause a paralysis which lasted for five minutes or less. In fact the drug's duration of action was at first thought to be too short for practical use in anaesthesia. The modes of action of these drugs were found to differ. Decamethonium and suxamethonium were shown to act by causing depolarisation of the muscle end-plate region (BURNS and PATON, 1951) in complete contrast to the competitive action of tubocurarine (JENKINSON, 1960) and gallamine (MUSHIN et al., 1949). During the ten years following 1949, most of the neuromuscular blocking drugs which were introduced for clinical use belonged to the depolarising group. However, the action of the depolarising neuromuscular blocking drugs was found to be influenced by a wide variety of factors. Thus these drugs were more unpredictable in clinical use than were the competitive neuromuscular blocking drugs. By 1960 the frequent complications encountered with depolarising drugs were well documented in the literature. It had become clear that the ideal neuromuscular blocking drug would belong to the competitive group while also having a short duration of action. An active search for such a compound began in the 1960's and is still continuing today.

In this chapter a general account will be given of the pharmacological actions and pharmacokinetics of a number of competitive neuromuscular blocking drugs. Preferences vary from country to country so a total of 10 of the most interesting drugs are considered; they are shown in Table 1. Four of them are chemically related to tubocurarine, while six are based on the steroid nucleus. Their chemical formulae are shown in the third column and the proprietary names as well as names of the manufacturers are given in the fourth column. In addition, their chemical structures are shown in Fig. 1. A few general points can be made at this stage about the terms used to describe their action, their formulae and chemical properties.

Table 1. Competitive neuromuscular blocking drugs

Name	Molecular weight of salt	Chemical name	Proprietary names, code names and manufacturers	Number of quaternary nitrogen groups
Tubocurarine chloride (BP, USP, EurP)[a]	771.6[c]	Tubocuraranium, 7′, 12′-dihydroxy-6, 6′-dimethoxy-2, 2′, 2′-trimethyl chloride	Tubarine (Burroughs Wellcome) Tubadil (ENDO) Intocostrin-T. (Squibb)	one
Dimethyl-tubocurarine iodide (BAN, INN)[a]	906.7	Tubocuraranium, 6,6′, 7′, 12′ tetramethoxy 2, 2, 2′, 2′-tetramethyl-, iodide[b]	Metubine iodide (LILLY) Mecostrin chloride (Squibb) Diamethine bromide (Burroughs Wellcome)	two
Gallamine Triethiodide (BP, USP, EurP)[a]	891.5	1, 2, 3-Tri (triethyl-ammoniummethoxy) benzene triiodide	Flaxedil (May & Baker) Relaxan (Gea) Sincurarina (Farmitalia) Syntubin (Heilmittelwerke)	three
Alcuronium chloride (BAN, INN, USAN)[a]	827.9	N, N′-Diallyl bisnortoxiferine dichloride pentahydrate	Ro-4-3816 Alloferin (Roche) Toxiferene (Roche)	two
Dipyrandium chloride	499	$3\beta, 17\beta$-di-pyrrolidin-1′-γ1-5α androstane dichloride	M & B 9105A Dipyrandium (May & Baker)	two
Pancuronium bromide (BAN, INN, USAN)[a]	750	$2\beta, 16\beta$-dipiperidino-5a-androstane-3α, 17β-dioldiacetate dimethobromide monohydrate	NA 97 (Organon) Pavulon (Organon) Myoblock (Sankyo)	two
Dacuronium bromide (BAN, INN)[a]	698	$2\beta, 16\beta$-dipiperidino-5α-androstane, 17β-diol 3α acetate dimethobromide	NB 68 (Organon) Dacuronium (Organon)	two
N, N′-dimethyl-conessine diiodide	639	(19-methylcona-4, 6-dienin-3-β-γ1) trimethylammonium iodide	N, N′-dimethyl-conessine di-iodide (Glaxo)	two
Stercuronium iodide (INN)[a]	510	(cona-4, 6-dienin-3β-γ1) dimethylethyl ammonium iodide	MYC 1080 (Gist-Brocades) Stercuronium (Gist-Brocades)	one
AH 8165 dibromide	604.38	1, 1′-azobis [3-methyl-2-phenyl-1H-imidazo (1, 2α) pyridinium] dibromide	AH 8165 D (Allen & Hanburys) (base denoted by AH 8165)	two

[a] Approved name listed in one of following sources: BP = British Pharmacopoeia, USP = United States Pharmacopoeia, EurP = European Pharmacopoeia, BAN = British Approved Names, INN = International Non-proprietary names (WHO), USAN = United States Adopted Names.
[b] Due to altered formula of tubocurarine this is more correctly described as trimethyl-tubocurarine, not dimethyltubocurarine (see p. 425).
[c] Corrected for new structure (EVERETT et al., 1970).

The drugs listed in Table 1 have been referred to by various authors as "non-depolarising", "curare-like" and "competitive" neuromuscular blocking drugs. There is some controversy about which of these terms is preferable.

"Non-depolarising" is a clumsy term, relying upon the *absence* of a pharmacological action to describe a substance. It is also insufficiently precise as it must include those substances which act by preventing the release of transmitter from the nerve. "Curare-like", on the other hand, is a vague term which has been applied in the past to a wide spectrum of effects, ranging from the action of depolarising drugs on isolated muscles (JENDEN et al., 1954) to the entirely non-specific depressant actions of ether (AUER and MELTZER, 1914) and the pre-synaptic blocking action of streptomycin (FELDMAN, 1973). The term "competitive neuromuscular blocking drug" seems more satisfactory.

The concept of "competitive antagonism" involves the idea that a substance reduces the proportion of receptors occupied by another agent by becoming attached to the same site, so that the binding of the two agents is mutually hindered. In this case, the log dose-response curves for an agonist determined in the presence and absence of antagonist should be parallel. This is indeed the case *in vitro* for tubocurarine (JENKINSON, 1960), gallamine (LU, 1970), pancuronium (WAUD et al., 1973; GOLDFINE, 1972) and alcuronium (GOLDFINE, 1972) (for further discussion see p. 280 of Chapter 3). At present, however, similar direct experimental evidence is not available for the remaining drugs in Table 1.

In the intact animal the inhibitory effect of these compounds can be abolished over a wide range of concentrations by increasing the local concentration of neurotransmitter, either by close-arterial injections of acetylcholine or by applying anticholinesterase drugs. This in itself provides evidence for a "competitive" neuromuscular blocking action although *in vitro* experiments probably provide more conclusive proof. Dimethyltubocurarine seems to be in a rather anomalous position; *in vivo* it behaves like tubocurarine, yet *in vitro* experiments on frog muscles show that the block is not strictly competitive (PAYTON, 1966).

Despite these difficulties it seems justifiable to use the term "competitive" when referring to the entire group of drugs, provided that one realises that definitive proof of competitive antagonism at the receptor level is not yet available for all the substances listed.

Because of the continuing search for a short-lasting neuromuscular blocking drug particular emphasis will be placed on the factors which influence the duration of action of this type of compound.

The last section includes a brief description of the action of a wide variety of miscellaneous drugs which cause neuromuscular blockade and which are either general anaesthetics themselves or are used as adjuncts to anaesthesia. Although they are not competitive antagonists of acetylcholine using the strict definition of that term, they have been included because their action bears a superficial similarity to the action of the competitive neuromuscular blocking drugs whose actions they modify.

B. Chemical Structure

Figure 1 shows that all of the competitive neuromuscular blocking drugs are quaternary ammonium compounds. The majority of them have two quaternary nitrogen

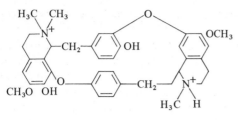

Tubocurarine

Gallamine

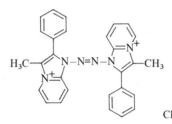

AH 8165

Alcuronium

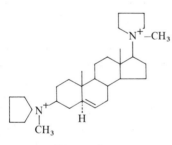

Dipyrandium

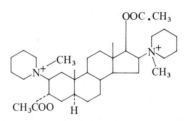

Pancuronium

NN′ Dimethylconessine

Stercuronium

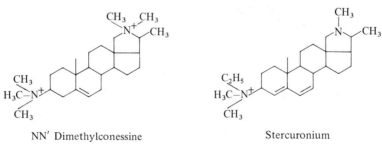

Fig. 1. Chemical structure of eight of the competitive blocking drugs listed in Table 1. The structure of dimethyltubocurarine is not included; it is similar to that of tubocurarine except that both hydroxyl groups and the tertiary nitrogen group are methylated. Dacuronium differs from pancuronium by the replacement of both acetoxy groups by hydroxyl groups. Note similarity of NN′-dimethylconessine and stercuronium

groups, the exceptions being tubocurarine and stercuronium which are monoquaternary, and gallamine which is triquaternary.

Until recently, tubocurarine was thought to contain two quaternary nitrogen groups (KING, 1935). However, EVERETT et al. (1970) have shown that the formula of tubocurarine was incorrect, and it is now thought to have one quaternary and one tertiary nitrogen group. This has been confirmed by CODDING and JAMES (1973) in a thorough crystallographic analysis. The molecular weight has accordingly been reduced to allow for this change in the formula (Table 1). KING prepared dimethyltubocurarine by methylation of tubocurarine with methyl iodide and it is not immediately obvious whether the formula of dimethyltubocurarine should also be modified. However, recent work by SOBELL et al. (1972) on the steriochemistry of the dimethylderivative has shown that during methylation the tertiary nitrogen centre becomes methylated at the same time as methylation of the two hydroxyl groups occurs. Thus King's formula for dimethyltubocurarine was correct and it is a diquaternary compound. SOBELL et al. (1972) point out, however, that dimethyltubocurarine should more correctly be described as trimethyltubocurarine. However, in this chapter we have thought it preferable to retain the name dimethyltubocurarine until such time as the approved name of the compound is altered.

Many neuromuscular blocking drugs were known to possess two quaternary nitrogen groups, and for many years the distance between the quaternary centres was thought to be a critical factor in determining the affinity of the drug for the acetylcholine receptors. It was generally accepted that optimal competitive neuromuscular blocking activity occurred when the two quaternary groups were 1.25 nm apart (BARLOW, 1960; KOELLE, 1970).

This belief has been progressively weakened in three ways. First, it was found that tubocurarine was a monoquaternary compound and secondly other powerful neuromuscular blocking drugs with only one (stercuronium) or with three quaternary groups (gallamine) were discovered. Thirdly, diquaternary neuromuscular blocking drugs were synthesised with their quaternary groups less than 1.25 nm apart. For example, in the case of pancuronium the inter-quaternary distance is 1.108 nm (SAVAGE et al., 1971), while for AH 8165 it is 0.75 nm and for alcuronium 0.97 nm (POINTER and WILFORD, 1972).

The position today is that while a distance of 1.25 nm between quaternary nitrogen atoms may confer optimal *depolarising* activity it is not considered a critical factor in competitive blockade (KOELLE, 1970).

C. Methods Used to Measure Neuromuscular Blockade

I. Muscle Contractions Evoked by Stimulation of the Motor Nerve

Neuromuscular block can be measured by recording muscle contractions evoked by stimulation of the motor nerves. This is a reliable method provided that certain precautions are taken.

A maximal stimulus should be applied to the nerve to ensure that all nerve fibres are activated; this in turn ensures contraction of all the muscle fibres. In animal experiments the motor nerve should be shielded to prevent stimulation of underlying muscles, but in man, where such a procedure is obviously impossible, a large nerve trunk is stimulated per-cutaneously using surface electrodes and a much higher current intensity.

The electrodes should be made of a metal which is biochemically inert and non-polarisable; silver and platinum are most commonly used.

When the intact nerve is stimulated impulses pass in the orthodromic direction towards the muscle in motor nerve fibres. At the same time, low-threshold afferent nerve fibres are also stimulated and this elicits reflex activation of motor-neurones which causes delayed activation of muscle motor units. This phenomenon has been called the H reflex (MAGLADERY and McDOUGALL, 1950). The F-wave, which can also be recorded from the muscle (MAGLADERY and McDOUGALL, 1950), is due to a reflex elicited by antidromic impulses travelling in the motor fibres (DAWSON and MERTON, 1956; McLEOD and WRAY, 1966). Theoretically this reflex activation of the muscle should result in distortion of the recorded twitch.

In animal experiments this complication is always prevented by cutting the nerve proximal to the electrode. In human experiments the H reflex can be abolished by using *maximal* motor nerve stimulation (MAGLADERY et al., 1951). There remains the F-wave which is always small and inconsistent. MARSDEN and MEADOWS (1970) compared the contractions of human calf muscles before and after applying a pressure block to the intact sciatic nerve central to the electrodes. This method, which abolished the H and F reflexes, did not significantly affect the size and shape of the twitch, so neither reflex appears to affect the recorded muscle contraction to any appreciable extent in this type of experiment. However, the influence of these reflexes should always be assessed in any experiment involving the stimulation of intact nerves.

A square wave stimulating pulse of short duration (less than 0.5 msec) must be used. If the pulse duration is greater than the refractory period of the muscle membrane a second action potential will be triggered by the falling phase of the stimulating pulse.

When a muscle is activated by a single maximal shock applied to its nerve, the resulting twitch may differ markedly from that produced by slightly asynchronous activation of the same muscle fibres. This was first observed by MERTON (1950, 1954) who showed that in conscious humans a "synchronous" twitch is larger and lasts longer than a "desynchronised" twitch. Later BROWN and MATTHEWS (1960) extended these observations in a careful study in the cat and suggested that the difference between the synchronous and asynchronous twitches might be that the synchronous activation produced a brief tetanic contraction of some muscle fibres. This was because the large action potential of the muscle fibres excited the motor nerve fibres within the muscle and this ephaptically induced "back-response" of the nerve fibres re-excited the muscle fibres.

These authors recorded isometric contractions of the soleus and gastrocnemius muscles in the cat developed in response to stimulation of their respective intact motor nerves using stimuli of short duration. The antidromic compound action potential in the motor nerve fibres was recorded from the peripheral end of an appropriate ventral root and displayed on an oscilloscope together with a record of muscle contraction. At the same time action potentials were recorded from the muscle. The method used is shown in the upper section of Fig. 2. A stimulus applied to the motor nerve travels simultaneously to the muscle and in the antidromic direction, to the ventral root. The lower section of Fig. 2 shows the resulting muscle contraction (top trace) and the antidromic action potential from the ventral root (lower trace). Following the large nerve action potential which resulted from the synchronous stimulation of all the fibres in the nerve, there is a second wave of nerve activity. This "back-response" was set up by ephaptic stimulation of the α-motor fibres by the summed action potential of the muscle fibres. The back response was shown to be conducted in the α-motor fibres, for it could be abolished by rendering these fibres refractory by exciting them with an appropriately timed second shock applied at an interval which was less than the absolute refractory period of the muscle fibres. This second shock has no effect on the muscle fibres but renders the

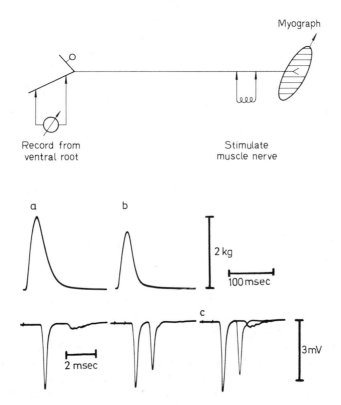

Fig. 2. Top section. The experimental arrangement used for simultaneously recording the contraction of the soleus or gastrocnemius muscles of the cat and the back-response of their motor nerves. The nerve to each muscle was dissected free from other nerve branches for several cm central to the muscle and all other nerves were cut. On stimulation of the motor nerve the compound action potential which travelled in the antidromic direction was recorded from the peripheral end of the appropriate ventral root.

The lower section shows the reduction of the back-response produced by re-exciting the nerve during the refractory period of the muscle. Above, contraction of the medial head of gastrocnemius; below, the action potential of its nerve fibres. (a) single maximal shock; (b) two maximal shocks separated by 0.7 msec; (c) superimposed records of the action potentials set up by single and double stimulation. The nerve action potential initiated by the second stimulus was too early to re-excite the muscle, but by reducing the back-response, it made the muscle contraction smaller. From Brown and Matthews (1960).

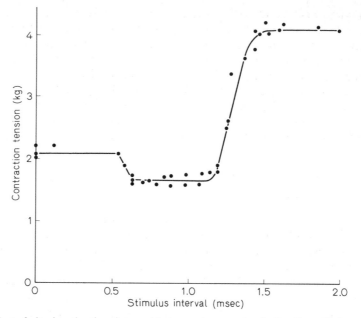

Fig. 3. The effect of altering the time interval between two maximal stimuli applied to the nerve. When the second stimulus excited a second nerve action potential, but the muscle was still refractory, the contraction was reduced, because the back response was then reduced (Same experiment as Fig. 2, both stimuli were about twice the strength required to excite all the large motor fibres when they were not refractory). From Brown and Matthews (1960)

intramuscular nerve fibres refractory to any ephaptic stimulation by the muscle action potential. The effects of such a second volley are illustrated in Fig. 2 (b), and it may be seen that the twitch is smaller and has a shorter time to peak and to half-relaxation. The graph of the muscle tension against the interval between the two stimuli (Fig. 3) shows that with stimulus intervals of less than 0.5 msec the motor nerve is refractory to the second excitation wave which therefore has no effect on the size of the twitch. With intervals of more than 0.5 msec and less than 1.5 msec the nerve conducts the second volley but the muscle fibres are refractory. The second nerve volley therefore leads to a reduction in the twitch response in the manner described above. With intervals in excess of 1.5 msec the muscle fibres are no longer refractory to the second nerve volley and summation of mechanical responses occurs. These results have been confirmed by Buller and Lewis (1963).

It is perhaps not generally realised that this "back response" is not a rare phenomenon. Brown and Matthews (1960) found it in all their recordings from the cat gastrocnemius muscle and in 50% of the experiments on the cat soleus muscle. Epstein and Jackson (1970) applied the double-shock test of Brown and Matthews to the adductor pollicis muscle in man and obtained similar results. They reported repetitive firing in response to single shock stimulation in 16 patients out of a group of 50 patients. An exactly similar effect was noticed with human calf muscle and in the adductor pollicis muscle by Marsden and Meadows (1970).

BROWN and MATTHEWS found that the back response was abolished by increasing the depth of pentobarbitone anaesthesia and this has led to be idea that this phenomenon may not play an important role in experiments on anaesthetised animals or man. However, the recent work of EPSTEIN and JACKSON does not support this assumption, since in their series the effect occurred in one-third of the deeply anaesthetised patients. Thus it appears that in animals and man the "back-response" is a hazard which has to be taken into account when attempting to record synchronous muscle twitches evoked by nerve stimulation. As the effect is due to restimulation of terminals of motor nerve fibres it may occur with both intact and cut nerve trunks.

II. Recording of Muscle Contraction

1. Selection of Strain Gauge

The recording of muscle tension requires either a strain gauge or a myograph whose characteristics are appropriately chosen to match the force of contraction and the rate of development of tension of the muscle twitch. Table 2 shows the time to peak (in msec) of single twitches for a large range of muscles from various species. Obviously a strain gauge with a frequency response of 50 Hz would be suitable for the slowly contracting soleus muscle in the cat but it would severely attenuate a twitch recorded in the same animal from one of the rapidly contracting external eye muscles. The force developed by a single contraction is also shown in Table 2. In order to select a suitable recording device one also needs to know the maximal tetanic tension and this can be calculated from the column showing the tetanus-twitch ratio.

2. Optimal Muscle Length

In all striated muscles, the rate of development of tension and the force developed during both twitch and tetanic contractions is related to the initial resting length of the muscle. For this reason it is important to adopt some standard for the resting length. The influence of resting length has been studied in detail for cat hind-limb muscles by BULLER et al. (1960) and for the rat extensor longus digitorum and soleus muscles by CLOSE (1964). Figure 4 shows the results obtained by CLOSE. The standard adopted by these authors, which is now universally used, is to make all recordings with the muscle length adjusted so that the peak twitch tension evoked by nerve stimulation, in excess of initial resting tension, is maximal. This length is called the optimal resting length.

3. Influence of Temperature

The rate of development of tension by a muscle has a fairly high temperature coefficient; the Q_{10} is 1.53 according to GORDON and PHILLIPS (1953). The tension developed in a twitch is also affected by temperature, although there is considerable disagreement between authors about the direction and magnitude of this effect.

In many mammalian muscles, a fall in muscle temperature produces a reduction in twitch tension, but has little or no effect on maximal tetanic tension. This effect was recorded in the tibialis (MACLAGAN and ZAIMIS, 1957) and intercostal muscles (BISCOE, 1962) of the cat, and in the tibialis anterior and calf muscle in man (CAN-

Table 2

Species	Muscle	Temperature (°C)	Contraction[a] time (msec)	Half-relaxation time (msec)	Force of single contraction (g)	Tetanus: twitch ratio[b]	References
Cat	tibialis anterior	36—37	11—18	15—20	500—1000	—	(m)(d)
	soleus	37—38	60—80	70—90	300—800	9	(m)(d)
	lateral gastrocnemius	37—38	30	20—30	—	5	(d)
	flexor longus digitorum	37—38	30	20—30	1000	4	(d)
	gracilis	37—38	30	15—30	—	—	(d)
	tenuissimus	35	30	35	5	—	(l)
	external intercostal	37—38	33	34	200	3	(b)
	inferior oblique	37.5	fast fibres 5—7 / slow fibres 20—27	7—8 / 38—44	2—3	9—10	(a)
	internal rectus	34—37	7.5—10.0	—	9	10	(g)
	obicularis oculi	34—39	8.5	—	6	7	(k)
	obicularis oris	34—39	33	—	55	4.5	(k)
	thyroarytenoid	36—38	9—13	—	—	10	(o)
	cricothyroid	36—38	30—35	—	—	5	(o)
Rat	soleus	35—36	30—35	30—40	40	4	(f)
	extensor longus digitorum	35—36	10	10	40	5.4	(f)
Rabbit	thyroarytenoid	37—38	6.5	—	—	—	(j)
	cricothyroid	37—38	24—30	—	—	—	(j)
	tibialis	37—38	24—28	—	—	—	(j)
Fowl (chick)	ant. latissimus dorsi	37	100	100	5	5	(i)
	post. latissimus dorsi	37	15	15	12	5	(i)
Man	gastrocnemius	not stated	110	60	—	—	(c)
	soleus	not stated	120	60	—	—	(e)
	tibialis anterior	not stated	120—150	112	1500—2000	—	(e)
	"calf" (soleus plus gastrocnemius)	not stated	64—136	162—225	7000—8000	—	(n)
	adductor pollicis	not stated	46—69	90—127	750—1000	—	(n)
	external oblique	36—37	140	290	—	—	(h)
	internal oblique	36—37	60—88	110—140	—	—	(h)
	rectus abdominis	36—37	58—140	68—285	—	—	(h)

a "Contraction time" is the time from the end of the latent period to the peak of the isometric twitch response evoked by supramaximal nerve stimulation.

b Tetanus: twitch ratio is obtained by dividing the maximal tetanic tension by the twitch tension.

References: (a) BACH-Y-RITA and ITO, 1966; (b) BISCOE, 1962; (c) BULLER et al. 1959; (d) BULLER et al. 1960; (e) CANNARD and ZAIMIS, 1959; (f) CLOSE, 1964; (g) COOPER and ECCLES, 1930; (h) EBERSTEIN and GOODGOLD, 1968; (i) GINSBORG, 1960b; (j) HALL-CRAGGS, 1968; (k) LINDQVIST, 1973; (l) MACLAGAN, 1962; (m) MACLAGAN and VRBOVÁ, 1966a and b; (n) MARSDEN and MEADOWS, 1970; (o) MARTENSSON and SKOGLUND, 1964.

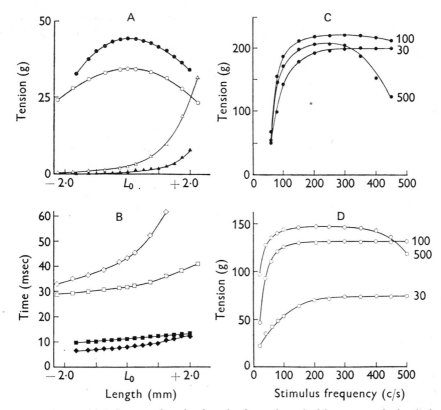

Fig. 4. Rat; 72-day old. Influence of resting length of muscle and of frequency of stimulation on isometric contractions in slow and fast muscles; soleus (open symbols) and extensor longus digitorum muscle (closed symbols). A. Initial tension ($\triangle$, $\blacktriangle$) and the maximum twitch tension ($\bigcirc$, $\bullet$) developed in excess of the initial tension at various muscle lengths. B. Times for contraction ($\square$, $\blacksquare$) and half-relaxation times ($\diamondsuit$, $\blacklozenge$) for twitches at various muscle lengths. The graphs in C and D are for the isometric tension (ordinate) developed at various times after the onset of contraction in response to different frequencies of repetitive stimulation (abscissae). The numbers at the right of each curve refer to the times in msec after the onset of the contractions. From CLOSE (1964)

NARD and ZAIMIS, 1959). BULLER et al. (1968) obtained different results according to which cat muscle they used. A fall in temperature produced a reduction in the twitch tension of the soleus but an increase in twitch tension of the flexor longus digitorum muscle. Twitch tension also increased as the temperature was reduced in two isolated preparations, rat diaphragm (HOLMES et al., 1951) and frog sartorius muscle (HILL, 1951).

The size and shape of the isometric myogram is determined by the contractile and the "series-elastic" components of the muscle. Both these factors would be expected to vary with temperature in a complicated manner, and it is perhaps not surprising that the effect of temperature appears to vary from muscle to muscle and to be influenced by the experimental technique used. The importance of the recording method was shown by JEWELL and WILKIE (1958). Using frog sartorius muscle, they found that in a preparation where the twitch tension increased as the temperature was raised, the addition of an extra compliance, between the tendon and the recording apparatus, reversed the effect. In other words, the extensibility of the apparatus greatly influenced the contribution of the "series-elastic" component to the size of the recorded twitch.

4. Correlation between Twitch Size and Receptor Occlusion

PATON and WAUD (1967) have shown that in cats and dogs, about 75% of the receptors have to be occupied by tubocurarine before there is any reduction in the size of muscle twitch elicited by infrequent nerve stimulation. If the dose of tubocurarine is increased beyond this level, the size of the twitch is then directly related to receptor occupancy. The existence of such a "safety margin" must be borne in mind in interpreting the results obtained with this method. This is particularly important under conditions where the safety margin may have been eroded by rapid frequency stimulation, by general anaesthetics, or by other drugs.

III. Recording of Action Potentials

Electrical recordings of muscle action potentials can be obtained either by using small concentric needle electrodes inserted into the muscle, or with surface electrodes secured to the skin overlying the muscle. With both these methods, the electrical recording obtained represents only a small group of muscle fibres. The difficulties encountered in human experiments when e.m.g. records obtained from a few fibres are compared with tension records obtained from the entire muscle have been discussed in Chapter 5B by SMITH. Exactly similar problems occur in animal experiments, but in this case it is possible to increase the number of fibres from which the electrical recording is being made by using belly-tendon electrodes (BROWN and VON EULER, 1938). The only disadvantage of this method is that large movement artifacts may occur due to the resultant contraction of the muscle under study.

Lack of correlation between electrical and mechanical recordings is the probable explanation for the long drawn out controversy which centered on the basic issue of whether the amplitude of the muscle action potential increases or decreases during post-tetanic potentiation, (i.e. BROWN and VON EULER, 1938; HUGHES and MORELL, 1957). One can only conclude that in a whole muscle, the relationship between e.m.g. and tension recordings is always difficult to establish, particularly when drugs which act at the neuromuscular junction are present.

IV. Measurements of Membrane Potential

1. Extracellular Recording

These methods are suitable for recording from many muscle fibres simultaneously but have the disadvantage that absolute values for membrane potential cannot be obtained. *Changes* in potential can, however, usefully be recorded by these techniques.

a) In vivo

BURNS and PATON (1951) developed a method for recording from the surface of the gracilis muscle in anaesthetised cats using non-polarisable electrodes. The muscle was exposed and immersed in paraffin contained in a pool formed from skin flaps. One electrode was placed over the end-plate region of the muscle while the reference electrode was positioned on an inactive tendon or bone. The method was used to record the changes in membrane potential produced by various depolarising neuromuscular blocking drugs and to record the injury potential. Later PATON and WAUD (1967) modified the method so that the spatial distribution of the potential could be mapped by moving the recording electrode along the fibre. The potential at each point is recorded against the distance from the tendon.

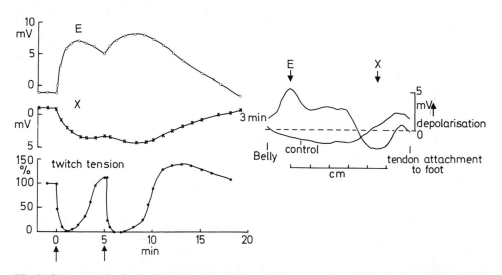

Fig. 5. Cat; anaesthetised with chloralose. Extracellular recording of depolarisation in tibialis anterior muscle. A non-polarisable electrode was moved along the surface of the muscle which was covered with paraffin at 37° C. The potential difference between the moving electrode and a reference electrode placed on the patellar tendon, was recorded using a DC amplifier and displayed on an X-Y plotter. The distribution of potential along the muscle from belly to tendon is shown in the right hand section of the diagram, before (control) and 3 min after injection of 30 μg/kg of decamethonium diiodide. After the drug, a depolarisation is recorded at the end-plate region (E), but the potential change at X, close to the musculo-tendinous junction, is in the opposite direction. The left-hand section shows the change of potential with time at E and X, measured from the records on the X-Y plotter. At all stages, the change in potential at X is in the opposite direction to that recorded at the end-plate region. The lower graph shows the size of the indirectly elicited twitches

One hazard encountered with this method is that when the end-plate becomes depolarised, an apparent "hyperpolarisation" can be recorded very close to the musculo-tendinous junction (see Fig. 5). The reasons for this are unclear; it could be due to the fact that this position is very close to a secondary chemosensitive area near the end of the fibres where the conductance might be increased. Alternatively, it may be related to the geometrical arrangement of the fibres in the tibialis anterior muscle. Whatever the explanation of these results, the inference is that the reference electrode should not be placed near the muscle-tendinous junction otherwise an overestimate of the depolarisation at the end-plate region will be obtained.

b) In vitro

An extracellular recording method was described by FATT (1950) for use with isolated frog muscle immersed in physiological saline. The liquid-air interface was used as the recording electrode and the level of fluid surrounding the muscle was raised and lowered to scan the distribution of potential along the muscle fibres. This method was also used in the frog by JENKINSON (1960) and with guinea-pig diaphragm by LU (1970).

One disadvantage of the method, particularly critical when mammalian muscle is studied at 37° C, is that the muscle is deprived of oxygenating medium and warmth for an appreciable length of time during each scan.

2. Intracellular Microelectrode Recording

This technique is used to measure membrane potential in individual fibres. It has the great advantage of providing quantitative measurement of membrane potential but has the disadvantage that only one fibre at a time can be impaled by the electrode. In addition, it is necessary to avoid or prevent muscle contraction as this breaks the electrode. This means that the effect of a drug on membrane potential cannot be recorded simultaneously with its effects on muscle contractions evoked by nerve stimulation; studies in parallel are necessary.

For full details of microelectrode recording the reader is referred to the chapter by GINSBORG and JENKINSON.

D. Distribution of Competitive Neuromuscular Blocking Drugs

I. General Properties

The neuromuscular blocking drugs like all the quaternary ammonium compounds are strong bases which are fully ionised at physiological pH. For this reason they have low lipid solubilities and can only penetrate cell membranes with difficulty. Consequently they are poorly absorbed from the digestive tract, do not cross the placental or blood brain barriers and are excreted in the urine without undergoing reabsorption in the renal tubules.

II. Transport of Neuromuscular Blocking Drugs across Cell Membranes

1. Entry into Liver Cell and Biotransformation

In the case of the liver, the general rule of cell membrane impermeability to cations does not apply. The endothelium of the blood sinusoids of the liver, like that of blood capillaries in general, behaves as an extremely porous membrane permitting the ready equilibration between plasma and the extracellular fluid of virtually all molecules and ions whose size is less than that of protein molecules. The membrane of the hepatic parenchymal cell acts as a lipoid membrane containing fairly large aqueous pores; the pores, although smaller than those of the sinusoidal endothelium, are large enough to admit a number of lipid-insoluble substances that do not penetrate many other cells (SCHANKER, 1962b).

Two of the competitive neuromuscular blocking drugs, AH 8165 and pancuronium, are able to enter the hepatic parenchymal cells where they are metabolished by the microsomal enzymes. By this mechanisms AH 8165 (TYERS, personal communication) and pancuronium (AGOSTON et al., 1973a and b) undergo hydroxylation in several species including man. (See Fig.6 for metabolite of AH 8165). In addition, the hydroxyl group of AH 8165 then undergoes conjugation with glucuronide (TYERS, 1975).

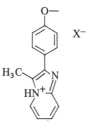

Fig. 6. Formula of the neutral metabolite of AH 8165. Note that this is not a quaternary ammonium compound. It was obtained from canine urine by the addition of acid and β-glucuronidase. The product was extracted into pentan-1-ol. The results indicate that the metabolite is probably excreted as a glucuronide or another conjugate

There is some disagreement in the literature on the biotransformation of tubocurarine and dimethyltubocurarine. MARSH (1952) found that only a fraction of an injected dose of tubocurarine could be recovered from the urine and suggested that it was metabolised to a considerable extent in the rat and to a lesser extent in guinea-pigs, rabbits and dogs. He postulated that N-demethylation or oxidation of the aromatic ring to give quinone-like structures might occur. MARSH performed similar experiments with dimethyltubocurarine and the results suggested that metabolism occurred in rats but not in the other three species studied. Later work using chromatography to identify the drugs and their metabolites has not confirmed these results. MEIJER and WEITERING (1970) could not detect any metabolites of tubocurarine in the isolated perfused rat liver using thin layer chromatography although significant quantities of the drug appeared in the bile in an unchanged form. Similarly, COHEN et al. (1967) were unable to detect any metabolites of tubocurarine in anaesthetised dogs. In the case of dimethyltubocurarine MEIJER and WEITERING (1970) were again unable to confirm Marsh's claim for metabolism in the rat.

Various workers have looked for evidence of metabolism of stercuronium (HESPE and WIERIKS, 1971) alcuronium (MEIJER and WEITERING, 1970) and gallamine (MEIJER and WEITERING, 1970; FELDMAN et al., 1969), and they have shown that these substances do not undergo metabolic transformation in animals.

In the case of alcuronium, gallamine and dimethyltubocurarine it is not clear from the present experimental data whether these drugs lack the ability to penetrate the hepatic parenchymal cell or whether they do penetrate, but have no suitable reactive groups for degradation by the microsomes. Stercuronium and tubocurarine certainly gain access to the liver cells, as they are excreted into the bile in an unchanged form (HESPE and WIERIKS, 1971), so we must assume a lack of suitable reactive groups. In the case of dipyrandium and dacuronium no evidence is available.

At the present time, therefore, it appears that AH 8165 and pancuronium are the only competitive neuromuscular blocking drugs for which conclusive evidence of metabolism by the liver microsomal enzymes exists. See Table 3 for a summary of the published results.

2. Excretion into Bile

The membrane of the liver cell appears to possess special transport mechanisms for certain organic cations which are actively transported into bile despite their apparent lipid insolubility (SCHANKER, 1962a). In the case of the neuromuscular blocking drugs, it is mainly those belonging to the competitive group which are transported into the bile canaliculus. The depolarising drugs do not appear to be able to cross this membrane (SCHANKER, 1962a; BROEN-CHRISTENSEN, 1965).

AH 8165 and pancuronium are metabolised in the liver, and it is not surprising that their metabolites appear in the bile. This was demonstrated for pancuronium in both cat and man (HESPE and WIERIKS, 1971). Similarly, when tritiated AH 8165 was injected into cats, dogs and rabbits, radioactivity was detected in the faeces and the authors assumed that this indicated biliary excretion of a conjugated metabolite (BOLGER et al., 1972). However, tubocurarine (COHEN et al., 1967; MEIJER and WEITERING, 1970) and stercuronium (HESPE and WIERIKS, 1971), which are not metabolised in the liver, are transported from the liver parenchymal cell into the bile canaliculus and are excreted unchanged in the bile. For tubocurarine the ratio of the concentration of the drug in the bile to that in the plasma is 40:1 in dogs (COHEN et al., 1967) and 100:1 in rats (MEIJER and WEITERING, 1970). This suggests that an active transport process is involved. With normally functioning kidneys approximately 5.9% of an injected dose of tubocurarine can be recovered from the bile within three hours, while in animals with ligated renal pedicles biliary excretion increases to 15.6% over the same period (COHEN et al., 1967) (see Fig. 12).

When attempting to predict whether biliary excretion is feasible for a particular quaternary neuromuscular blocking drug the rules suggested by SCHANKER (1962b; 1972) are particularly useful. He pointed out that all the quaternary amines that are known to be actively transported into bile seem to have certain structural characteristics in common; a single quaternary ammonium group at one end of the molecule and one or more nonpolar ring structures at the opposite end. The evidence quoted in the preceeding paragraph shows that tubocurarine and stercuronium are excreted into the bile unchanged, while pancuronium and AH 8165 appear in a metabolised form. The monoquaternary structure of the first two of these drug fits in with Schanker's hypothesis. The neutral metabolite of AH 8165, whose formula is shown in Fig. 6, is not a quaternary compound so that Schanker's rule is not relevant. Similarly, the metabolite of pancuronium appears to be suitable for biliary excretion. The remaining competitive neuromuscular blocking drugs all have more than one quaternary ammonium group and thus their chemical structure does not appear to meet the requirements for biliary transport. Indeed, biliary excretion has been sought but not detected for gallamine (FELDMAN et al., 1969) alcuronium (MEI-

Table 3

Drugs	Lipid solubility	Plasma protein binding	Metabolism	Biliary excretion
Tubocurarine	octanol/Krebs 15:85 (a) olive oil or heptane insoluble (m)	bovine, 72h dialysis 50% (c) human, 6h dialysis 45% (h) human, 5h dialysis 40—50%(d) human 30% (e)	rat nil (a); dog nil (e); rat demethylation and oxidation (l); guinea-pig, rabbit, dog nil (l)	rat considerable (a); dog 5% in 3h (e); dog 10—20% in 24h (m)
Dimethyl-tubocurarine	octanol/Krebs 1:99(a) organic solvents insoluble(m)	human, 48h ultrafiltration 70%(f)	rat nil (a); guinea-pig, rabbit, dog nil(l); rat demethylation (l)	rat nil(a)
Gallamine	octanol/Krebs 3:97 (a) olive oil 10% soluble (m) organic solvents insoluble(m)		rat nil(a); dog nil(b)	rat nil(a); dog nil(k)
Alcuronium	octanol/Krebs 1:99 (a)		rat nil (a)	rat nil(a); cat 10% in 2h (n)
Pancuronium	octanol/Krebs 1:99(a)		cat, rat, man hydroxylation (i)	rat nil(a); cat, man metabolite in bile (i)
Stercuronium		rat nil(b)	rat nil(b)	rat considerable (b)
AH 8165		human 17% (g); rat, 24h dialysis <10%(g)	cat, rat, rabbit and dog hydroxylation and glucuronide(g) conjugation	cat, dog, rat and rabbit metabolite in bile (j)

(a) MEIJER and WETTERING (1970); (b) HESPE and WIERIKS (1971); (c) ALADJEMOFF et al. (1958); (d) COHEN et al. (1965); (e) COHEN et al. (1967); (f) DAL SANTO (1964); (g) TYERS (personal communication); (h) GHONEIM et al. (1973); (i) AGOSTON et al. (1973a and b); (j) BOLGER et al. (1972); (k) FELDMAN et al. (1969); (l) MARSH (1952); (m) COHEN (1974); (n) LÜTHI (1966).

JER and WEITERING, 1970) and dimethyltubocurarine (MARSH, 1952). No information is available on dipyrandium and dacuronium. These results are summarised in Table 3.

3. Entry into Muscle Cells

The experimental situation in muscle is much more complicated than in the liver cell because many of the quaternary ammonium compounds cause an increase in the permeability of the muscle to sodium and other ions, and such a permeability change could facilitate the entry of the drug. In addition, once inside the muscle cell the drugs may become bound.

a) Competitive Neuromuscular Blocking Drugs

As these drugs do not depolarise the cell membrane they are easier to study in this respect, and it has in fact been shown that they do not penetrate muscle cells. This was first demonstrated for tubocurarine by WASER (1966) using an autoradiographic method. Scintillation counting methods with isotopically labelled polymethylene bistrimethylammonium(methonium) compounds has shown that the C 2, C 4, and C 6 derivatives, which also have no depolarising action at the neuromuscular junction, are accumulated by the isolated rat diaphragm to the same extent as inulin. This clearly suggests that these compounds do not penetrate the muscle cells (MACKAY and TAYLOR, 1970).

b) Depolarising Drugs

Many of these substances can be shown to enter the muscle cells. Slow entry along the entire length of the fibre has been shown for the neurotransmitter ACh (POTTER, 1970; ADÀMIC, 1970), for choline (RENKIN, 1961) and for carbachol (TAYLOR et al., 1965). In the last-named case uptake was not affected by a prior dose of tubocurarine, sufficient to prevent the pharmacological effects of carbachol.

In contrast, the higher members of the methonium series, octamethonium, decamethonium and its di-ethyl derivative known as decaethonium (MACKAY and TAYLOR, 1970), and the related drug iodocholinium (CREESE et al., 1963), enter specifically at the end-plate region of skeletal muscle, where they become concentrated.

The first suggestion that decamethonium could accumulate at the end-plate region of muscle stemmed from the results of WASER and LÜTHI (1957). Using a method of contact autoradiography, they found that after decamethonium the darkening of the autoradiograph in the end-plate region was about 100 times greater than after tubocurarine and had a more diffuse distribution. Their method, however, could not distinguish between extracellular adsorbtion of the drug and intracellular penetration. Later work with iodocholinium (TAYLOR et al., 1964a) showed that each gram of muscle removed the drug from 4 to 5 ml of bathing solution in 12 hrs. This uptake was markedly inhibited by tubocurarine in pharmacological concentrations. The curare-sensitive portion of iodocholinium uptake at the end-plate was reduced by a fall in temperature with an activation energy of 21,000 cal/mole. Similar results were obtained with decamethonium in both rat (TAYLOR et al., 1965) and guinea-pig muscle (CREESE et al., 1971). Although the evidence was inconclusive the authors suggested that these depolarising drugs were entering the cells. CREESE and MACLA-

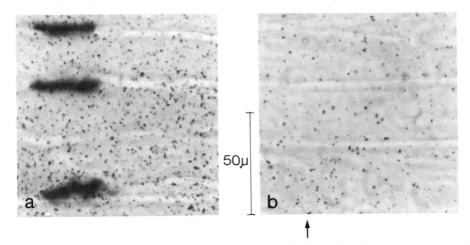

Fig. 7a and b. Autoradiograms prepared from a longitudinal section of rat peroneus muscle removed and frozen 2 hrs after intravenous injection of tritiated decamethonium dichloride (0.82 mg/kg). On the left hand side (a) the position of the end-plates is shown by the dark azo-dye stain of the esterase. There is a high grain density. Right hand side (b) shows the same fibres at a distance of 600 μm from the end-plates, as indicated by the arrow. The grain density is much reduced. Calibration 50 μm. From CREESE and MACLAGAN (1970)

GAN (1970) were able to demonstrate the presence of decamethonium inside the cells at the end-plate region in rat and cat muscle (MACLAGAN and CREESE, 1972) either following application of the drug *in vitro* or after close-arterial injection *in vivo*. Autoradiograms of frozen sections of muscle were used to prevent movement of the water soluble drug during processing. The resolution of the method was good enough to distinguish whether the drug was in the intracellular or extracellular compartment. Decamethonium was found to enter the cells at the end-plate region and for several hundred microns on either side (Fig. 7). The end-plate uptake could be prevented by prior administration of tubocurarine, whereas uptake along the rest of the fibre was unaffected and therefore assumed to be non-specific (see Fig. 8). Entry of decamethonium could be demonstrated as early as 30 sec after close-arterial injection. This pattern of distribution of decamethonium corresponded with the chemosensitive area as determined by iontophoretic application of ACh (MILEDI, 1962) but was more widespread than the distribution of receptors shown by bungarotoxin labelling (BARNARD et al., 1971).

The results could be interpreted as showing entry of the drug over the entire chemosensitive area. Alternatively entry might be restricted to the end-plate area and followed by rapid lateral diffusion of the drug within the following 30 sec. Unfortunately the experimental method used cannot distinguish between these two possibilities.

No change in the distribution of decamethonium was detected in a period of two hours following its injection. This suggested intracellular binding of the drug but the resolution of the method was not sufficient to permit localisation of the binding structures within the cell. Binding is also indicated by the fact that decamethonium is only slowly released from the cell and can still be demonstrated intracellularly up to three weeks after its administration (TAYLOR et al., 1965; CREESE and MACLAGAN, 1970). Intracellular binding seems to be the most likely explanation of these results as it is known that the drug is not metabolised in muscle (WASER et al., 1954; LÜTHI and WASER, 1965).

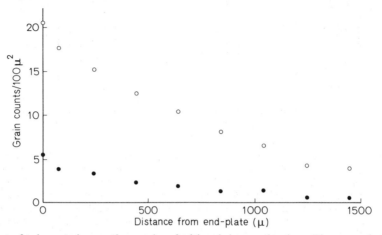

Fig. 8. Effect of tubocurarine on the uptake of tritiated decamethonium. The open circles show the distribution of radioactivity in four fibres of peroneus longus from a rat which had received an intravenous injection of labelled decamethonium dichloride (1.64 mg/kg). The closed circles show six fibres from the peroneus muscle of another rat which had received tubocurarine dichloride (0.8 mg/kg) prior to injection of labelled decamethonium. Ordinate: grain count/100 μm^2, minus background. Abscissa: distance from the centre of the end-plate in μm. From CREESE and MACLAGAN (1970)

In this connection it is interesting to note that the monovalent quaternary compounds carbachol and acetylcholine, which are potent depolarising substances, have not been shown to accumulate at the end-plate region of muscle. The methods used, however, do not rule out the possibility that these compounds enter the cell at the end-plate but are rapidly lost because they do not become bound.

Denervation considerably increases the uptake of decamethonium so that the radioactivity in the extra-junctional regions approaches that of the end-plate. This has been shown in the isolated muscles of the rat (Fig. 9) and guinea-pig (CREESE et al., 1971) and in cat muscle *in vivo* (CREESE and MACLAGAN, 1972). As in the innervated muscle, tubocurarine prevented the uptake.

TAYLOR and his colleagues have emphasised the correlation between the entry of decamethonium and its pharmacological effect and considered that the kinetics of uptake suggested a carrier-like system. The main evidence for a carrier is the demonstration that there is a saturable component of the influx and also that unlabelled decamethonium or high concentrations of acetylcholine can inhibit the uptake of labelled decamethonium. Saturation has been shown in depolarised rat muscle, where half-saturation occurred at a concentration of 400 mmol/l (CREESE and ENGLAND, 1970). When the uptake was expressed as a clearance, half saturation occurred at a concentration of 2.5 µmol/l (sufficient to elicit the pharmacological effects of decamethonium) and again at a much higher concentration of 2 mmol/l (HUMPHREY, 1970).

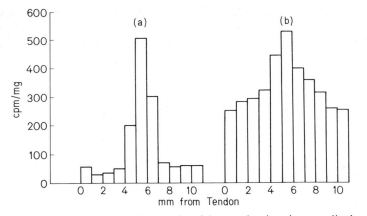

Fig. 9a and b. Effect of denervation on the uptake of decamethonium into rat diaphragm muscle. Tritiated decamethonium (1.64 mg/kg) was injected intravenously and 2 hrs later the diaphragm was rapidly removed, frozen and divided into 1 mm strips which were weighed and dissolved. The concentration of decamethonium in each strip was measured by scintillation counting methods. The arrows indicate the slice of tissue containing the band of end-plates. (a) left hemidiaphragm with normal innervation, (b) right hemidiaphragm which had been denervated eight days before the injection of decamethonium. (a) and (b) from same rat. The distribution of radioactivity is more widespread in the denervated muscle. From CREESE et al. (1971)

As there is evidence that decamethonium becomes bound inside the cell, the interpretation of the experiments showing saturation and competitive inhibition is more difficult. Since the characteristics of binding within the cell (saturation of binding sites, competition between cations for binding sites and apparent concentration gradients between tissue and medium) are similar to those expected for carrier-mediated transport, such experiments cannot distinguish the latter process from one combining passive diffusion and intracellular binding. It is unfortunate that the evidence for a carrier in the muscle cell is not as clear-cut as it is in the liver (COHEN et al., 1967), renal tubule cells (McISAAC, 1965; 1969) or choroid plexus (TOCHINO and SCHANKER, 1964; 1965).

There have been two other explanations for the entry of decamethonium at the end-plate region. PATON and RANG (1965) suggested that the entry was a secondary consequence of the depolarisation which is produced by the drug. This hypothesis, however, cannot account for the fact that a curare-sensitive uptake at the end-plate can be demonstrated in muscles already completely depolarised by potassium. The second explanation is that the accumulation of decamethonium inside the cells is simply due to the non-specific increase in permeability which is produced by the drug (PATON and RANG, 1965; COOKSON and PATON, 1969). In this context it would be interesting to know whether a cation such as hexamethonium, which has no depolarising action and which does not normally enter the cells, could be made to enter when the cell permeability is increased using decamethonium. Such an experiment was attempted by MACKAY and TAYLOR (1970) but the design of the experiment makes interpretation of the results difficult. They did not select the muscle end-plate region for their scintillation counting method but made their measurements from the entire muscle. Considering the small size of the end-plate area relative to the rest of the fibre, any uptake of hexamethonium at the end-plate would have been swamped by the non-specific uptake in the rest of the fibre and would probably not have been detected.

In the absence of such evidence it is difficult to decide on the exact mechanism underlying the entry of depolarising neuromuscular blocking drugs into the muscle cell.

III. Plasma Protein Binding

There is evidence that some of the competitive neuromuscular blocking drugs bind to plasma proteins. DUNDEE and GRAY (1953) were the first to show that patients with liver disease required a larger than average dose of tubocurarine to obtain adequate muscle relaxation. This finding was confirmed ten years later by EL-HAKIM and BARAKA (1963) and was attributed to the raised gamma globulin levels in such patients. Since then several other authors have attempted to correlate dosage requirements of neuromuscular blocking drugs in man with plasma protein fractions. In some of these studies, the dose necessary to produce muscle relaxation and the measurement of the plasma protein fractions were determined on different occasions. The results of such studies suggested a positive correlation between tubocurarine dosage and gamma globulin (STOVNER et al., 1971a) whereas gallamine (STOVNER et al., 1971b) and alcuronium (STOVNER et al., 1971a) requirements showed a positive correlation with the albumin fraction. On the other hand, pancuronium dosage requirement could not be correlated with any protein fraction (STOVNER et al., 1971b). Unfortunately, equilibrium dialysis of the plasma was not performed in any of these studies and they can only be considered to provide very tenuous evidence for protein binding. Many other factors are probably involved.

A more direct approach was made by SKIVINGTON (1972) who used an electrophoretic technique to separate the protein fractions in plasma obtained from patients paralysed with known amounts of neuromuscular blocking drugs. He found that dimethyltubocurarine was bound mainly by gamma globulin, whereas gallamine moved mainly with the beta globulin. Unfortunately, most of the drug was lost during electrophoresis because of the combined effect of dilution by the buffer wash and the electric current, so that it was not possible to calculate the amount of drug bound as a percentage of the administered dose.

The percentage of drug which becomes bound to protein can, however, be calculated when equilibrium dialysis of the plasma is performed. Such measurements have been made for four of the competitive neuromuscular blocking drugs, namely tubocurarine, dimethyltubocurarine, AH 8165 and stercuronium. The results are shown in the third column of Table 3 together with the concentrations of the drugs. In all these experiments the substances, which had been labelled with tritium, were added to the plasma in vitro and then dialysed against Sorenson's buffer or 0.9% sodium chloride solution. The greatest adsorption appears to occur with dimethyltubocurarine where 70% was bound to human plasma proteins (DAL SANTO, 1964). In the case of tubocurarine, 30% (COHEN et al., 1967) and 45—50% (ALADJEMOFF et al., 1958; GHONEIM et al., 1973) has been reported to be bound to plasma proteins. The amount of tubocurarine bound increased with a rise in pH (COHEN et al., 1965).

Table 4. Comparison of potency of competitive neuromuscular blocking drugs. Dose in μmol/kg to cause 90% block of indirectly elicited twitches. (The numbers in brackets give the dose in μg/kg obtained from the published data)

Species	Tubocurarine	Gallamine	Alcuronium	Pancuronium	Dacuronium	N,N'-dimethylconessine	Stercuronium	AH 8165
Cat	0.38 (a, d) (300)	0.67 (a) (600)	0.036 (a) (30)	0.05 (a) (40)	1.4 (f) (1000)	1.0 (c) (600)	0.98 (a) (500)	0.33 (g) (200)
	0.48 (c) (370)	0.96 (c) (860)		0.04 (d) (30)			0.98 (f) (500)	0.83 (f) (500)
	0.65 (i) (500)	0.50 (i) (450)						
	mean 0.47	mean 0.71		mean 0.045			mean 0.98	mean 0.58
Dog	0.65 (a) (500)	0.67 (a) (600)		0.025 (a) (20)			0.98 (a) (500)	0.08 (g) (50)
	0.38 (i) (300)							
	mean 0.51							
Monkey	0.38 (i) (300)					0.5 (c) (300)		0.17 (g) (100)
Man	0.26 (h) (200)	1.12 (h) (1000)		0.05 (h, j) (40)	2.8 (h) (2000)	0.5 (c) (300)		0.42 (k) (250)
	0.19 (i) (150)	2.0 (p) (1780)		0.06 (p) (50)				
	0.40 (p) (310)							
	mean 0.28	mean 1.56		mean 0.055				

(a) WIERIKS (1972); (b) PATON and ZAMIS (1952); (c) BUSFIELD et al. (1968); (d) BONTA and GOORISSEN (1968); (e) MUSHIN et al. (1949); (f) MARSHALL (1973a); (g) TYERS (personal communication); (h) SMITH (1975); (i) ZAIMIS (1953); (j) KATZ (1971); (k) BLOGG et al. (1973); (l) BRITTAIN and TYERS (1973); (m) VERNER (1963); (n) WALTS and DILLON (1968); (o) NORMAN and KATZ (1971); (p) DONLON et al. (1974).

Protein binding is much less important in the case of AH 8165 and stercuronium. Only 10% of AH 8165 was bound by rat plasma and 17% by human plasma (TYERS, personal communication). With stercuronium the binding was negligible (HESPE and WIERIKS, 1971). Measurement of plasma protein binding has not been performed for the remaining drugs listed in Table 3.

E. Factors Affecting Duration of Action in Animals and Man

I. Species Variation

1. Potency

A great number of authors have studied competitive neuromuscular blocking drugs in a variety of species. Table 4, however, gives the doses of eight of these drugs which produce comparable neuromuscular block in four species—cat, dog, monkey, and man. The data have been selected because they permit calculation of the dose which causes 90% blockade.

In Table 5 the potency of the individual neuromuscular blocking drugs is compared to that of tubocurarine. The calculations are based on the mean values in μmol/kg given in Table 4. It can be seen that the potency does not vary significantly between species. In cat, dog, and man dacuronium is the least potent of these drugs, whereas alcuronium and pancuronium are much more potent than tubocurarine.

Table 5. Potency of competitive neuromuscular blocking drugs compared with tubocurarine

Drug	Potency ratio[a]		
	Cat	Dog	Man
Tubocurarine	1	1	1
Gallamine	0.6	1	0.2
Alcuronium	11.4	36	—
Pancuronium	10.4	26	5
Dacuronium	0.3	—	0.09
N,N'-dimethylconessine	0.5	—	0.5
Stercuronium	0.5	0.7	—
AH 8165	0.8	6.4	0.2

Mean values taken from Table 4 for doses which produce 90% block.

[a] Potency ratio $= \dfrac{\text{dose tubocurarine in μmol/kg}}{\text{dose of x in μmol/kg}}$

2. Duration of Action

When the duration of action of these drugs is compared, considerable species differences are found. This is shown in Table 6 for the doses which cause a 90% block in cat, dog, and man. (A few quantitative results are available for the monkey and these are also included.) It can be seen that tubocurarine and gallamine have a comparable duration of action in all three species; in contrast the steroid neuromuscular block-

Table 6. Duration of action of competitive neuromuscular blocking drugs

Drug	Time (min) from injection of dose causing 90% block until 50% recovery of indirectly elicited twitch			
	Cat	Dog	Monkey	Man
Tubocurarine	20 (a) 30—50 (b)	20—40 (a)	—	35 (i)
Gallamine	20—30 (b) 12 (a)	15 (a)	—	20 (c) 23 (i)
Alcuronium	30 (a)	15 (a)	—	—
Pancuronium	9 (a)	10 (a)	—	36 (j) 37 (e)
Dacuronium	—	—	—	30 (j)
N,N'-dimethylconessine	5—20 (b)	—	60 (b)	33 (h)
Stercuronium	3— 4 (a) 15—20 (b)	5 (a)	—	—
AH 8165	2— 3 (d)	3—4 (d)	7 (g)	comparable (f) to pancuronium

(a) WIERIKS (1972); (b) BUSFIELD et al. (1968); (c) MUSHIN et al. (1949); (d) TYERS (1975); (e) KATZ (1971); (f) BLOGG et al. (1973); (g) BRITTAIN and TYERS (1973); (h) VERNER (1963); (i) WALTS and DILLON (1968); (j) NORMAN and KATZ (1971).

ing drugs are short-lasting in the cat and the dog (5 to 10 min) but have a similar duration of action to tubocurarine (approximately 30 min) in man and the monkey.

It has long been considered that the cat closely resembles man in its sensitivity and response to neuromuscular blocking drugs (PATON and ZAIMIS, 1952). Now, however, there is an exception to this rule, since the duration of action of the newly-introduced steroid neuromuscular blocking drugs is quite different in these two species. BIGGS et al. (1964) found that dipyrandium chloride had a short duration of action, comparable to that of suxamethonium, when administered to the cat, rabbit and chicken. In the rhesus monkey, however, the drug's duration of action was similar to that of tubocurarine. Dipyrandium was the first steroid neuromuscular blocking drug to be given a clinical trial and MUSHIN and MAPLESON (1964) found that its duration of action in man was also as long as that of tubocurarine. Two further examples of similarity between man and monkey as far as the duration of action of neuromuscular blocking drugs is concerned are provided by (1) isoquinolinium bis-quaternary compounds, BW 252 C 64 and BW 403 C 65 (HUGHES, 1972) and (2) NN'-dimethylconessine—a bis-quaternary steroid closely related to stercuronium (BUSFIELD et al., 1968). Conessine derivatives were found to remain longer in the blood of the monkey than the cat, and this was reflected in the duration of the neuromuscular block.

Thus as far as the duration of action of steroid neuromuscular blocking drugs is concerned, the results obtained using the monkey appear to be the best indication of the likely duration of action in man. There is, at present, no definitive explanation for the much shorter action of these drugs in the cat, dog, rabbit, and rat but it is relevant to consider factors which might be important.

It is usually assumed that the action of competitive neuromuscular blocking drugs is related to the concentration of the drug at the end-plate receptors, and that this concentration is determined by the plasma concentration of the drug. This assumption has recently been confirmed in man for tubocurarine using a sensitive radioimmunoassay technique. There was a highly significant inverse correlation between the serum concentration of tubocurarine and twitch tension (MATTEO et al., 1974) (see Fig. 10). From this follows a second assumption that the duration of the neuromuscular blocking action should be related to the half-life of the drug in the plasma.

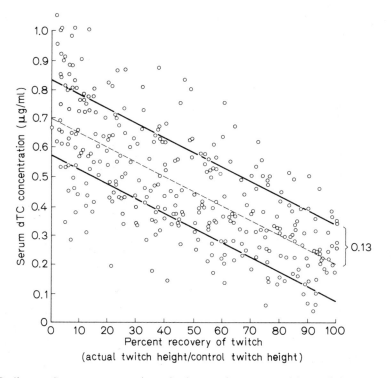

Fig. 10. Ordinate—Serum concentration of tubocurarine measured by radioimmunoassay, following intravenous injection of 0.3 or 0.6 mg/kg into anaesthetised patients. Abscissa: The percentage recovery of the indirectly elicited twitch of the adductor muscle of the thumb. The open circles represent 347 determinations in 48 patients. The regression line ± standard error of the mean was calculated from the pooled data from all the patients. There was a highly significant correlation between serum concentration of tubocurarine and twitch tension. The mean concentration at 50% recovery of the twitch was 0.45 ± 0.13 µg/ml. Complete recovery had occurred at a serum concentration of 0.20 ± 0.13 µg/ml. From MATTEO et. al., 1974

II. Biotransformation in the Liver

As we have seen in the preceding sections, the competitive neuromuscular blocking drugs, with the exception of AH 8165 and pancuronium, are not metabolised in the liver, thus biotransformation is unlikely to be an important factor.

III. Renal and Biliary Excretion

The question which remains to be answered is whether the rate of removal of the drug from the plasma is determined solely by renal and biliary excretion or whether other mechanisms are involved.

COHEN et al. (1967) studied the plasma concentration of tubocurarine in dogs following a single intravenous injection of 0.3 mg/kg. Nephrectomy produced little change in the plasma concentration during the first 20 min after the injection (see Fig. 11). Similar conclusions were reached for stercuronium from experiments in rats with renal artery ligation (HESPE and WIERIKS, 1971). The decline in the plasma concentration of tubocurarine and stercuronium in the first 20 min after administration is not, therefore, determined by the rate of elimination of these drugs from the body by the kidney.

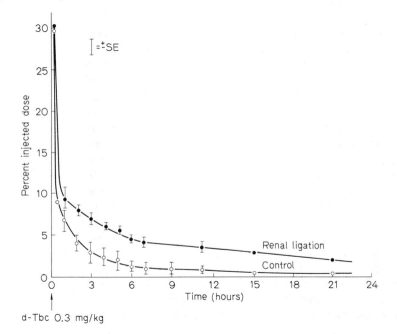

Fig. 11. Dogs; anaesthetized with pentobarbitone sodium (30 mg/kg). Mean values of concentration of ³H-tubocurarine in plasma following a single intravenous injection of 300 µg/kg. In the first 30 min after injection the fall in plasma concentration of tubocurarine is rapid and similar in both the control dogs (five) and in the dogs with ligated renal pedicles (seven). During the following hours, the decline in the plasma concentration in the nephrectomised animals was significantly slower. From COHEN et al. (1967)

This conclusion has important clinical implications. Provided that low doses are administered, the competitive neuromuscular blocking drugs can be used safely in patients with renal failure (McINTYRE and GAIN, 1971; DUVALDESTIN and VOURC'H, 1974). Tubocurarine has a slight advantage over the other drugs because as much as 15% of an injected dose can be eliminated in the bile in the absence of renal function (COHEN et al., 1967) (see Fig. 12).

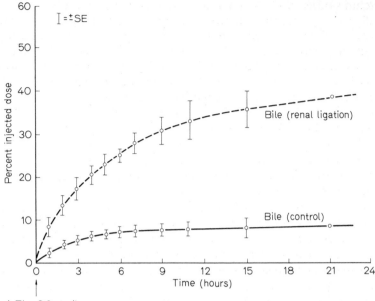

Fig. 12. Dog; anaesthetised with pentobarbitone sodium (30 mg/kg). Increased excretion of tubo-curarine in the bile following bilateral renal ligation. Mean values of concentration of ^{3}H-tubocurarine in plasma measured by scintillation counting following a single intravenous injec-tion of 300 μg/kg. In the eight control animals, only 5.9% (± 1.8) of the injected dose appeared as tritium in the bile within three hours, while in four animals with ligated renal pedicles, 15.6% (± 3.6) was recovered in the bile in a similar time. From Cohen et al. (1967)

In the case of the four drugs which are excreted into the bile (tubocurarine, stercuronium, AH 8165 and pancuronium), their duration of action could possibly be related to the rate of biliary excretion. However, it has been shown that ligation of the bile duct does not affect the plasma concentration of tubocurarine (Cohen et al., 1967) or stercuronium (Hespe and Wieriks, 1971) during the first 20 min following a single intravenous injection of the drug. Over the next hour, biliary excretion was an important route of elimination but this occurred too slowly to be of major impor-tance in terminating the blocking action of the drugs.

IV. Redistribution

1. Binding in Extracellular Compartment

Marsh (1952) was the first to suggest that the duration of action of tubocurarine, after a single injection, depends mainly upon the rate of redistribution of the drug from the circulation into various tissues within the extracellular compartment, and upon its binding to plasma proteins. This redistribution has since been extensively studied in dogs and in man by Cohen et al. (1965, 1967, 1968). Their results show that distribution of tubocurarine within the vascular system is confined to the plasma and that the drug does not enter the red blood cells. Equilibrium dialysis indicated that approximately one-third of the drug is protein bound (see Table 3). The unbound drug rapidly redistributes throughout the extracellular water compartment and the process is essentially completed within 15 to 20 min. By the end of the first hour the plasma contains approximately 10% of the injected dose, while distribution of the drug to the tissue compartments and urinary and biliary elimination continue. During the final phase of vascular redistribution the plasma concentration decays further and by the sixth hour only traces of tubocurarine are to be found.

Similar results have been obtained with gallamine (DAL SANTO, 1964), pancuronium (AGOSTON et al., 1973a and b) and stercuronium (HESPE and WIERIKS, 1971) in both animals and man. Thus it can be concluded that the process of redistribution within the extracellular compartment is the most important factor determining the half-life of these drugs in the plasma in the early moments after injection and consequently redistribution determines their duration of action.

It is relevant to consider which tissues are involved in the process of redistribution. Whole body autoradiography in the rat has shown that organs such as the spleen, liver, lungs and the heart temporarily remove tubocurarine from the circulation (COHEN et al., 1968). High concentrations of radioactivity were found in all these tissues soon after an intravenous injection of labelled tubocurarine, while the plasma concentration was falling rapidly. In the case of stercuronium similar results were obtained except that the distribution was less widespread and the drug became concentrated mainly in the liver and the kidneys (HESPE and WIERIKS, 1971).

Possible specific binding sites for these cationic drugs within the extracellular compartment and at the end-plate region are the acidic mucopolysaccharides (CHAGAS, 1962). These substances are a group of 2-amino-2-deoxyhexose-containing polysaccharides which are usually found in close combination with protein. They are characterised by an abundance of negative charges and their ability to form salts and to bind cations. Eight principal substances have been isolated, namely chondroitin, chondroitin-4-sulphate, chondroitin-6-sulphate, dermatin sulphate, heparin, heparin sulphate, hyaluronic acid and keratin sulphate. The term "mucopolysaccharide" was originally used to denote the close association of these substances with viscous secretions; however, as they are now known to exist in all mammalian tissues as well as in the fluids by which they are bathed, the term "glycosaminoglycans" has now been introduced (KENNEDY, 1973). However, the more familiar term, mucopolysaccharide, will be used here.

In skeletal muscle the mucopolysaccharides are an important constituent of the basement membrane which envelops the outside of the muscle fibre (COUTEAUX, 1972). In the junctional region, the presynaptic and postsynaptic membranes are separated at all points by a layer of mucopolysaccharides. Because of the considerable infolding of the muscle membrane at the junctional region, a high concentration of mucopolysaccharides has been demonstrated there (ZACHS and BLUMBERG, 1961).

The mucopolysaccharides, by virtue of their negative charges, could provide nonspecific binding sites for the cationic quaternary ammonium compounds, both on the muscle membrane and more generally within the extracellular compartment. Such non-specific binding could be an important factor in explaining the rapid redistribution of these drugs after an intravenous injection.

Some indirect evidence suggests that such binding may occur; CHAGAS (1962) has shown that there is some correlation between the mucopolysaccharide content and the amount of tubocurarine bound in various tissues in the dog. CHEYMOL et al. (1955a and b) also obtained data which indicated that tubocurarine could interact with these macro-molecules. They demonstrated that heparin antagonised the effect of tubocurarine in rabbit muscle. A similar interaction between stercuronium and heparin was shown in the isolated rat diaphragm preparation (WIERIKS, 1972). Whole body autoradiography in rats using radioactively labelled drugs such as stercuronium (HESPE and WIERIKS, 1971), tubocurarine (COHEN et al., 1968) and AH 8165 (TYERS, 1975) has shown rapid concentration of radioactive material over regions containing cartilage, a tissue known to be rich in mucopolysaccharides. The binding of tubocurarine to bovine nasal septum preparations and more specifically to chondroitin sulphate has also been shown *in vitro* using equilibrium dialysis (OLSEN and RIKER, 1974).

2. Binding at End-Plate Region

The end-plate region of skeletal muscle is known to be rich in mucopolysaccharides (ZACHS and BLUMBERG, 1961; CHAGAS, 1962), presumably because these substances are constituents of the basement membrane. WASER and LÜTHI (1962) and WASER (1966) concluded from their results, based on contact-autoradiography, that the accumulation of tritium-labelled tubocurarine found at the end-plate region represented binding of the drug to acetylcholine receptors. COOKSON and PATON (1969), however, challenged this assumption and suggested that the results of WASER and his colleagues could be explained by the binding of the drug to the negatively charged mucopolysaccharides. This suggestion is supported by the fact that denervation, which is known to greatly enlarge the receptor area, did not alter the distribution of radioactivity in Waser's preparations (WASER, 1962; WASER and HADORN, 1961). Autoradiography shows that pancuronium is also concentrated at the end-plate region, and a similar explanation could apply in this case (WIERIKS, 1972).

It appears, therefore, that non-specific binding by mucopolysaccharides may form a significant distribution pool for tubocurarine and possibly for stercuronium and AH 8165. Unfortunately, the binding of other neuromuscular blocking drugs to mucopolysaccharides has not been studied, but it seems likely that this may be a property which all these drugs share.

The influence of other ionizable groups may also be important; in addition, changes in pH might be expected to alter such non-specific binding (see p. 462).

V. Termination of Action by Chemical Inactivation of the Drug

The search continues for a competitive neuromuscular blocking drug which has a short duration of action in man. As the duration of action of the existing drugs during the initial 20 min period after administration appears to be dependent on redistribution within the extracellular compartment, binding to plasma proteins and non-specific binding—all factors which cannot easily be altered—attempts have been made recently to approach this problem in an entirely different way by searching for drugs which can be inactivated in the body at the desired moment by another chemical compound. This is the case with *bis*-ammonium derivatives of diphenyl-disulphide, synthesised by KHROMOV-BORISOV et al. in 1969. The neuromuscular block produced by such substances can be abolished by either sodium sulphite or cysteine. One of the compounds used has the chemical formula

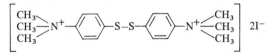

Another approach was made by GLOVER and YORKE (1971), using 1,1′-azobis (3-methyl-2-phenylbenzimidazolinium) dichloride, AH 10407. This was shown to be a competitive neuromuscular blocking drug in the cat, monkey and man having a duration of action of a few minutes only, due to its rapid degradation in the plasma by bicarbonate ions (BLOGG et al., 1975). Unfortunately, the fact that the short duration of action of this compound in the body is due to its chemical instability causes problems in its chemical development and pharmaceutical formulation.

F. Mechanism of Action at Neuromuscular Junction

In recent years an extensive and controversial body of literature has accumulated on the possibility that tubocurarine may have a pre-synaptic action (see HUBBARD and WILSON, 1973, for references). The controversy is related to the experimental difficulties involved in measuring transmitter output. With present methods, any small pre-synaptic effect of tubocurarine is difficult to demonstrate conclusively in the presence of its considerable action on the post-synaptic membrane where it acts as a competitive antagonist.

I. Evidence for Competitive Antagonism in vitro

A competitive antagonist may be regarded as a drug whose effect is receptor occlusion. When such a drug combines with the receptor no observable change is seen. However, when an agonist is added in the presence of the antagonist, the agonist is found to have less effect than it would exert alone. This is because it has access to only a part of the total receptor pool. The experimental analysis of competitive antagonism has been mainly based on the concept of the dose-ratio as defined by GADDUM et al. (1955). This is the ratio of the concentration of agonist required to produce a given response in the presence of the competitive antagonist to that required in its absence. The advantage of this method are (1) that the concentration of the drug in contact with the receptors does not need to be known (provided that proportionality with the concentration in the external fluid can be assumed) and (2) that the exact relation between receptor activation and the final response need not be specified (provided that this relationship is not affected by the antagonist) (GADDUM et al., 1955).

LANGLEY suggested in 1905 that curare and most other alkaloids produced their effects on muscle by combining with a "receptive substance" in the muscle and not by an action on endings, nor on the contractile substance. The nature of this action on the receptor was studied further in isolated muscle preparations by VAN MAANEN (1950), KIRSCHNER and STONE (1951) and ARIENS et al. (1956), using the contracture of frog rectus muscle as a measure of drug activity. Later, an elegant quantitative study by JENKINSON (1960) provided additional results consistent with the idea that tubocurarine acts by competing with depolarising drugs for the ACh receptor on a one-to-one basis. He used a direct method involving either extracellular or intracellular recording to measure the depolarisation produced in frog muscle by known concentrations of ACh or carbachol. The results could be fitted over a wide concentration range to the equations derived from Gaddum's theory of competitive inhibition.

Similar experiments have been performed *in vitro* using gallamine (LU, 1970), pancuronium (CHENG and WAUD, 1973; GOLDFINE, 1972), stercuronium (WIERIKS, 1972) and alcuronium (GOLDFINE, 1972). (See GINSBORG and JENKINSON's chapter for further discussion of the evidence obtained *in vitro* on the competitive mechanism of action of these drugs.)

There is evidence from recent experiments by KATZ and MILEDI (1973b) that tubocurarine does not modify the average size or time course of the acetylcholine induced fluctuation of membrane potential (acetylcholine "noise") but simply reduces the frequency. This suggests that the life-time of the channels opened by acetylcholine is unaltered, but that they are opened less frequently. This is compatible with an all-or-none occlusion of the receptors.

II. Evidence for Competitive Antagonism in vivo

1. Quantitative Studies

Under *in vivo* conditions, experimental proof of competitive antagonism is much more difficult to obtain. PATON and WAUD (1967) made the first attempt at a quantitative study, using gallamine and tubocurarine in anaesthetised cats and adopting a modification of the method developed by BURNS and PATON (1951) for extracellular recording (see p.432 for details of this method). In order to minimise complicating factors certain precautions were taken. Firstly, spinal cats were used to minimise any possible effects of anaesthesia on transmission. Secondly, the muscle was perfused via its artery at constant pressure with blood obtained from the carotid artery in order to prevent changes in blood flow to the muscle. Thirdly, urine flow was monitored and isotonic saline infused intravenously to maintain constant urine output and excretion of the drug. Using the tibialis and sartorius muscles PATON and WAUD measured the extent to which the end-plate depolarisation produced by suxamethonium, decamethonium, octamethonium and iodocholine was antagonised in the presence of neuromuscular block produced by tubocurarine or gallamine. It was found that the dose-response curve in the presence of the antagonists was not parallel to the control dose-response curve over the whole range of dosage of the agonists. At first sight, this might suggest that the antagonists were not acting competitively under these experimental conditions. However, the authors analysed the effect fully and concluded that it arose, not because of some interfering non-competitive process but because the antagonist was relatively firmly bound to the receptors. Thus during the relatively brief exposure to agonist, the equilibrium between the antagonist and the receptors was not significantly disturbed. They suggested that this state of quasi-equilibrium must be fairly common. It appears that at least for tubocurarine and gallamine, the neuromuscular block *in vivo*, as *in vitro*, is the result of competitive antagonism with ACh for the receptor. These *in vivo* experiments have not been repeated for the other competitive neuromuscular blocking drugs, nor has it been possible to make such direct tests of competitive antagonism for any of the neuromuscular blocking drugs in man.

2. Qualitative Studies

Because of the technical difficulties, it has become accepted practice to use a series of indirect tests to indicate whether a drug is interrupting neuromuscular transmission *in vivo* by competing with ACh for the receptors. These tests are based on the analysis by PATON and ZAIMIS (1952) of the differences between competitive and depolarising neuromuscular blocking drugs, and are listed below.

a) Response to Rapid Frequency of Stimulation

The response of a muscle to stimulation at a high frequency during a partial neuromuscular blockade gives a method for distinguishing between depolarising and competitive neuromuscular blocking drugs. In the case of a block caused by a depolarising drug, the resulting tetanus is well-sustained, whereas during the action of tubocurarine and other competitive antagonists the tetanic tension wanes during the period of rapid stimulation (ZAIMIS, 1953). The extent to which the tetanus fades varies from muscle to muscle and from drug to drug, and depends on the frequency of stimulation.

PATON and his colleagues (COOKSON and PATON, 1969; PATON and WAUD, 1967) have pointed out that the margin of safety for transmission will have a considerable influence on the results obtained in such a test. The term "margin of safety of neuromuscular transmission" was used to refer to the extent to which the synaptic mechanism could be interfered with before failure of transmission occurred. Under physiological conditions a quantity of transmitter in excess of that barely necessary for transmission of the impulse from nerve to muscle is released in response to a nerve action potential. It is not easy to determine acetylcholine release directly but the safety factor can be determined pharmacologically by measuring the extent to which a synthetic depolarising drug is antagonised by a dose of tubocurarine known to produce a certain degree of neuromuscular blockade.

Variations in the safety factor can be presumed to exist between different fibres in the same muscle. PATON and WAUD (1967) have shown that in a limb muscle such as the tibialis anterior of the cat, 75 to 80% of the receptors must be blocked by tubocurarine before even the most susceptible fibres fail to respond to infrequent nerve stimulation. This implies that in the most sensitive fibres, 4 to 5 times as much acetylcholine is released as is necessary for threshold action. At the most resistant junctions 90 to 95% of the receptors must be blocked before transmission fails. In the diaphragm, however, the safety factor is greater (WAUD and WAUD, 1972).

As the stimulus frequency is increased, so the margin of safety for transmission falls, presumably because the transmitter output per volley declines (COOKSON and PATON, 1969). Once partial blockade has been produced the effect of a procedure such as tetanic stimulation depends on the variation of safety factor between different fibres. If the variation is small, then small changes in the safety factor will have a large effect on the twitch response. On the other hand, if the variation is very large then a partial block will appear to be relatively insensitive to procedures which alter the safety factor. Both depolarising and competitive neuromuscular blocking drugs would be expected to alter the safety factor. In the case of depolarising drugs, slight depolarisation makes the fibre more excitable than normal, i.e. the safety factor has increased. On the other hand, deeply depolarised fibres become less excitable. Competitive neuromuscular blocking drugs should also reduce the safety factor, in this case by raising the threshold to ACh. In view of the complications introduced by variations in the safety factor it is not perhaps surprising that under clinical conditions, usually in the presence of many other drugs, the response to tetanic stimulation during partial blockade caused by a neuromuscular blocking drug often gives results whose interpretation in terms of depolarising or competitive mechanisms of action is difficult (see Chapter 5B).

If a muscle, in which partial blockade has been produced by a competitive neuromuscular blocking drug, is observed immediately after a period of tetanic stimulation, a short period in which the twitch increases is usually seen. The term post-tetanic decurarization is often used to describe this effect. Variations in the safety factor would be expected to influence post-tetanic decurarization also.

Despite these complications, experiments on laboratory animals under chloralose anaesthesia have shown that the response to tetanic stimulation fades rapidly and that post-tetanic decurarization occurs during partial blockade caused by all of the drugs listed in Table 1 (BIGGS et al., 1964; NORMAN et al., 1970; BUSFIELD et al., 1968; NORMAN and KATZ, 1971; FELDMAN and TYRRELL, 1970; BRITTAIN and TYERS, 1972). These results are identical to those obtained with tubocurarine.

b) Effect of Anticholinesterase Drugs Administered During Partial Blockade

If an anticholinesterase drug is administered during a partial blockade produced by a competitive antagonist, the block is antagonised and the twitch tension returns to normal. In contrast, the blockade produced by depolarising drugs is unaffected or increased by administration of an anticholinesterase drug (ZAIMIS, 1953). This effect was first demonstrated for the antagonism by physostigmine of the paralysis produced by tubocurarine (PAL, 1900).

Most of the experimental investigation of this phenomenon have been performed using tubocurarine as the competitive antagonist. It has been shown that anticholinesterases of the carbamate type (WHITE and STEDMAN, 1931; BACQ and BROWN, 1937; BÜLBRING and CHOU, 1947; BURGEN et al., 1949; HOLMSTEDT, 1951 and 1959) and anilinium ions (WESCOE et al., 1949; RIKER et al., 1949; RANDALL and LEHMAN, 1950; RANDALL, 1950; WESCOE and RIKER, 1951) are capable of exerting this anti-curare effect.

This anti-curare action can only be demonstrated over a limited range of concentrations of the anticholinesterase drug. If the inhibition of the enzyme is extensive and outlasts the action of tubocurarine, then a depolarising neuromuscular block will occur due to the excessive accumulation of acetylcholine (BURNS and PATON, 1951).

A further complication is introduced by the ability of the anticholinesterase drugs alone to cause repetitive firing of the muscle fibres with a resultant increase in the size of the indirectly elicited maximal twitch in all mammalian muscles (FENG and LI, 1941; ECCLES et al., 1942). Consequently, it is necessary to distinguish between antagonism of a neuromuscular blockade produced by an anticholinesterase drug because of recruitment of fibres on the one hand and an increase in muscle twitch because of repetitive firing in those fibres which were not paralysed by the blocking drug, on the other hand. The latter effect was recorded by BOWMAN (1962) in the cat. He injected neostigmine during a partial blockade induced by a depolarising neuro-muscular blocking drug (carbolonium bromide). The experimental records show clearly that the apparent antagonism of the blockade produced by the anticholines-terase drug was due to repetitive firing and was not due to recruitment of additional fibres. In the case of competitive blockade this effect can probably be ignored as tubocurarine and related drugs are able to depress repetitive firing, even at doses which are too small to cause neuromuscular block (VOLLE, 1967; KOJIMA and TAKA-GI, 1969; MASLAND and WIGTON, 1940).

It is widely accepted that the anticurare action of anticholinesterase drugs is due to inhibition of acetylcholinesterase which allows the accumulation of the transmit-ter in the synaptic gap. The main lines of evidence which support this theory are (a) that in a partially curarised muscle anticholinesterase drugs, particularly those of the carbamate type, increase the size of the end-plate potential and prolong its rise time and decay time (ECCLES et al., 1941, 1942; BOYD and MARTIN, 1956; BLABER and CHRIST, 1967), (b) there is a good correlation between anticholinesterase potency and anticurare action (BACQ and BROWN, 1937; BLASCHKO et al., 1949), (c) the time-course of the anticurare action of neostigmine correlated with the known time-course of decarbamylation of the enzyme (see Chapter 4C, p. 498), and finally (d) af-ter extensive inhibition of AChE the anticurare action of edrophonium and neostig-mine is abolished whereas a depolarising drug such as decamethonium continues to exert an anticurare action (HOBBIGER, 1952).

While there is general agreement that the anticholinesterase drugs cause accumu-lation of ACh in the synaptic gap, there is disagreement about the site or sites at which this additional ACh exerts its anticurare effect. Most workers subscribe to the view that the anticurare action of the carbamate and organophosphate anticholines-terase drugs is a post-synaptic effect and due to the increased concentration of ACh competing with the antagonist for the cholinoceptors. Recent experiments by KATZ and MILEDI (1973) have suggested one way in which inhibition of the cholinesterase enzyme may increase the effectiveness of ACh at the post-synaptic site. They re-corded ACh noise and miniature end-plate potentials with focal external electrodes and showed that neostigmine (3 µmol/l) had no effect on the ACh "noise" which reflects the duration of the molecular effect of acetylcholine but that it greatly pro-longed the miniature end-plate potentials which indicate that it influences the quan-tal effect of the transmitter. They suggested that after inhibition of ACh hydrolysis, the ACh molecules undergo repeated post-synaptic attachment, passing from recep-tor to receptor, making several successful collisions and sticking for a millisecond or so before finally escaping from the synaptic cleft.

The other possible explanation for the anti-curare action of the anticholinesterase drugs involves a pre-synaptic mechanism and this viewpoint has been discussed fully in Chapter 4C by HOBBIGER, p. 532. It must be pointed out that an increase in the ACh output from the nerve terminals would have exactly the same anticurare effect as that discussed above, i.e. it would tend to increase the size of the end-plate potential previously reduced by the competitive antagonist. This argument rests heavily on whether it can be shown conclusively that anticholinesterase drugs are able to increase the quantal content of the end-plate potential either by a direct pre-synaptic action or via a pre-synaptic action of the excess acetylcholine itself. (In the case of the organophosphate anticholinesterases, a direct action is unlikely as many of them do not possess either a tertiary or quaternary group.) The difficulties involved in the calculation of large quantal contents using the variance method are discussed fully by GINSBORG and JENKINSON in Chapter 3, p. 318. Because of the limited accuracy of the variance method, claims that a drug can alter quantal content must remain in doubt until more precise methods can be found.

Anticholinesterase drugs will antagonise the blockade induced by the following compounds:—dimethyltubocurarine (SWANSON et al., 1949; COLLIER, 1950), gallamine (MUSHIN et al., 1949), alcuronium (WASER and HARBECK, 1962; LUND and STOV-NER, 1962), dipyrandium (BIGGS et al., 1964), pancuronium (NORMAN et al., 1970; KATZ, 1971), dacuronium (FELDMAN and TYRRELL, 1970), NN'-dimethylconessine (BUSFIELD et al., 1968), stercuronium (WIERIKS, 1972) and AH 8165 (BRITTAIN and TYERS, 1972, 1973; BOLGER et al., 1972).

It appears that antagonism of a partial neuromuscular blockade by anticholines-terase drugs provides a reliable indication that the antagonist is acting in a competi-tive manner *in vivo*. This test, however, will only give predictable results if moderate doses of anticholinesterase drugs are used—doses which in themselves are too small to cause a depolarising neuromuscular blockade.

c) Response of Multiply-Innervated Fibres

In the mammal, most muscles contain only focally-innervated fibres which are sup-plied by branches of large-diameter α-motoneurones ending in discrete ("en plaque") end-plates (KRAUSE, 1863; HESS, 1961a and b). A few muscles, however, contain a proportion of multiply-innervated fibres supplied by many small-diameter myeli-nated γ-motoneurones which terminate on the surface of the fibre as clusters of small grape-like ("en grappe") bodies (TASAKI and MIZUTANI, 1944; COUTEAUX, 1953a and b). The extra-ocular muscles (GEREBTZOFF, 1959; KUPFER, 1960; HESS, 1962; HESS and PILAR, 1963; BACH-Y-RITA and ITO, 1966) and the striated muscle of the oeso-phagus (CSILLIK, 1965) are examples of mammalian muscles which contain a pre-dominance of multiply-innervated fibres.

In non-mammalian species, some muscles such as the anterior latissimus dorsi of the domestic fowl and the latissimus dorsi of the pigeon are composed almost entirely of multiply-innervated fibres (GINSBORG, 1960a and b). Other muscles, such as the posterior latissimus dorsi (GINSBORG and MACKAY, 1961; GINSBORG, 1960a and b) and the pectoral muscles of the domestic fowl consist entirely of focally-innervated fibres while others contain a mixture of fibres. Muscles with a predomi-nance of one fibre type are probably exceptions; it is more usual in birds and in reptiles for a muscle to consist of a mixture of both types of fibre as is found in the ileofibularis, rectus abdominis, gastrocnemius and semitendinosus muscles of the frog and the biventer cervicis, semispinalis cervicis, gastrocnemius and sartorius muscles of the fowl.

The focally-innervated and the multiply-innervated fibres differ markedly in their responses to acetylcholine and other depolarising drugs. In multiply-innervated fibres, the chemosensitive spots on the membrane are widely distributed over the

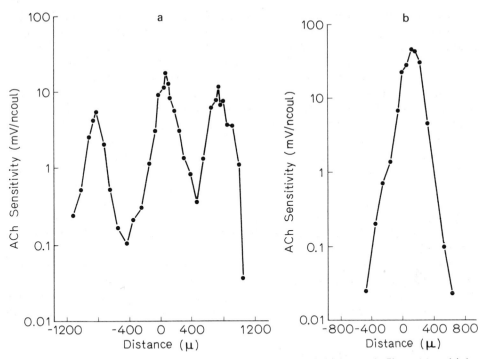

Fig. 13a and b. Acetylcholine sensitivity along the membrane of chick muscle fibres. (a) multiply-innervated anterior latissimus dorsi muscle; three distinct peaks of acetylcholine sensitivity averaging 790 μm apart were found. (b) focally-innervated posterior latissimus dorsi muscle with only one chemosensitive region. Figure prepared from FEDDE (1969)

membrane surface (FEDDE, 1969, see Fig. 13a). Consequently, the graded depolarisation produced by an injection of acetylcholine or any other depolarising drug may be sufficiently widespread to activate most of the contractile mechanism. This results in a prolonged shortening of the muscle—a contracture—which is not accompanied by propagated action potentials. In contrast, in a focally-innervated fibre, there is only one chemosensitive spot which occupies a very small proportion of the total fibre surface (FEDDE, 1969, see Fig. 13b). In these fibres, depolarising drugs produce a flaccid paralysis. Competitive neuromuscular blocking drugs cause a flaccid paralysis in both types of fibre in all species. BUTTLE and ZAIMIS (1949) suggested that the distinctive response of avian multiply-innervated muscle fibres to depolarising drugs provided a simple reliable test for distinguishing between these drugs and the competitive neuromuscular blocking drugs.

Using this test it has been shown that tubocurarine (BUTTLE and ZAIMIS, 1949), gallamine (BUSFIELD et al., 1968), dipyrandium (BIGGS et al., 1964), pancuronium (BUCKETT et al., 1968), NN'-dimethylconessine (BUSFIELD et al., 1968), stercuronium (WIERIKS, 1972) and AH 8165 (BRITTAIN and TYERS, 1972) all cause flaccid paralysis when injected intravenously into 3-day old chicks. These results thus support a competitive mode of action for all these drugs.

d) Response of Denervated Fibres

An increase in the chemosensitive area of the fibre membrane occurs after section of the motor nerve. In denervated mammalian muscle there is no accompanying increase in the sensitivity of the end-plate itself. Denervation has the same effect in frog muscle except that the end-plate zone always remains many times more sensitive than the rest of the membrane (MILEDI, 1960). Tritium—labelled bungarotoxin has proved a useful tool for demonstrating the spread of receptors along the membrane following section of the motor nerve (HARTZELL and FAMBROUGH, 1972). As a consequence of these changes, the sensitivity of the muscle to acetylcholine (GASSER and DALE, 1926; BROWN, 1937; ROSENBLUETH and LUCO, 1937; HARTZELL and FAMBROUGH, 1972) and to other depolarising drugs (ZAIMIS, 1951) increases.

Competitive neuromuscular blocking drugs would not be expected to have any significant effect on denervated muscle. However, a short lasting contracture has been claimed following the administration of drugs such as tubocurarine (McINTYRE et al., 1945; LUCO and SANCHEZ, 1959; BOWMAN and RAPER, 1964) and gallamine (BÜLBRING and DEPIERRE, 1949). It has been reported that gallamine, tubocurarine (RIKER and WESCOE, 1951; JONES and LAITY, 1964) and dimethyltubocurarine (PAYNE, 1961) also have a slight stimulant action on normal muscle and can cause an increase in the size of the indirectly elicited maximal twitch.

e) Interaction between Neuromuscular Blocking Drugs

The two types of neuromuscular blocking drugs are known to have a mutually antagonistic effect. Partial blockade by tubocurarine can be antagonised by decamethonium or suxamethonium Conversely, a depolarising blockade can be prevented or antagonised by injection of a small, sub-paralytic dose of a competitive neuromuscular blocking drug (PATON and ZAIMIS, 1952). In anaesthesia it is common practice when intubation is to be performed to preceed the injection of suxamethonium with a small dose of a competitive neuromuscular blocking drug in order to minimise the post-operative muscle pains associated with the depolarising drug. The presence of tubocurarine causes an increase in the threshold to suxamethonium and the dose of suxamethonium has to be increased by 50 to 70% to ensure adequate relaxation for intubation (SCHUH et al., 1974; CULLEN, 1971).

Consecutive applications of two competitive neuromuscular blocking drugs would be expected to have an additive effect and should produce a greater degree of neuromuscular block than either drug alone, and this effect has been demonstrated in several species by PATON and ZAIMIS (1952).

The interaction between two competitive neuromuscular blocking drugs, however, apparently depends on their relative potencies and on the kinetics of association and dissociation from the receptor. Using the isolated rat diaphragm preparation FERRY and MARSHALL (1973) have shown that hexamethonium (a quaternary ammonium compound with a weak competitive blocking action at the neuromuscular junction) can antagonise a neuromuscular blockade caused by tubocurarine; presynaptic actions were excluded as an explanation for this result. Recently, BLACKMAN et al. (1975) have extended these observations and shown that the action of a potent antagonist which dissociates slowly from the receptors, such as tubocurarine, pancuronium or alcuronium, can only be reversed by another competitive antagonist if the latter has a lower potency and rapid rate of dissociation from the receptors. Hexamethonium, gallamine, hyoscine and butylbromide have all been shown to produce this apparently anomalous interaction. The results of both groups of workers have been interpreted in terms of the hypothesis of STEPHENSON and GINSBORG (1969) which proposes that if an antagonist does not dissociate appreciably from the receptor in the time taken for the transmitter to achieve high occupancy of the receptors, then acetylcholine is excluded from a fraction of the receptors. Addition of a second antagonist with a low potency reduces the fraction of receptors occluded by tubocurarine and therefore the transmitter competes with the weak antagonist and gains access to more receptors. Consequently the blockade may be reversed.

The conditions necessary for this effect to occur are obviously very critical and depend principally on (1) the kinetics of occupation of the receptor by the transmitter and (2) the rate of dissociation of the slow but powerful antagonist. BLACKMAN et al. were able to alter the first of these factors by pre-treatment with an anticholinesterase drug. This prolonged the action of the transmitter and abolished the anticurare effect of hexamethonium. The second factor was found to vary in different species. For example, BLACKMAN et al. found that the anticurare effect of hexamethonium could not be demonstrated in toad sartorius muscle. As there is indirect evidence that the rate of dissociation of tubocurarine from the receptors is more rapid in amphibian muscle than in mammalian muscle (BERANEK and VYSKOCIL, 1967, 1968; LU, 1970) BLACKMAN et al. concluded that in the road, unlike the mammal, tubocurarine is able to dissociate significantly from the receptors during the short period of exposure to the transmitter.

III. Factors Affecting Neuromuscular Blocking Action

1. Sensitivity of Fast and Slow Fibres

a) Limb Muscles

The influence of the motor nerve is generally believed to be an important factor controlling the development of the chemosensitive area of the muscle membrane. This influence may be exerted by the release of some chemical substance (trophic factor, ECCLES, 1964) or via the control by the motor nerve of the mechanical activity of the muscle which in turn modifies the development of the receptors (JONES and VRBOVÀ, 1970; LOMO and ROSENTHAL, 1971). Consequently it might be expected that muscles with different types of innervation and functional activity would show differing patterns of acetylcholine sensitivity. This was shown to be the case in the rat's fast-contracting flexor longus digitorum muscle when compared with the slowly contracting soleus muscle (MILEDI et al., 1968). In this fast muscle, sensitivity to acetylcholine is restricted to the neuromuscular junction and to its immediate surroundings, while the soleus muscle exhibits a low, but clearly detectable sensitivity throughout the entire length of the muscle fibres. When the nerves to these two muscles were severed and the nerve formerly innervating the flexor longus digitorum was made to reinnervate the soleus, the cross-innervated soleus muscle acquired a pattern of acetylcholine sensitivity which closely remsembled that of the normal flexor longus digitorum muscle.

The sensitivity to antagonists which act on the acetylcholine receptor might also be expected to vary in different types of muscle. In normal adult cats the tibialis anterior muscle is usually more sensitive than the soleus muscle to depolarising neuromuscular blocking drugs. Conversely, the tibialis muscle is less sensitive than the soleus muscle to tubocurarine (JEWELL and ZAIMIS, 1954). Cross-union of the motor nerves to the tibialis and soleus muscles altered the mechanical properties of both muscles yet the response to depolarising neuromuscular blocking drugs was unaltered (MACLAGAN and VRBOVÀ, 1966 b). It was suggested that other factors, such as muscle atrophy and disuse were more important than the motoneurone in determining the pharmacological response to depolarising neuromuscular blocking drugs. Competitive neuromuscular blocking drugs were not included in this study but a reduced effectiveness of tubocurarine might be expected in any situation in which the sensitivity to depolarising drugs is increased. In fact, JEWELL and ZAIMIS (1954) had previously shown that disuse atrophy induced by tenotomy caused both a reduction in the sensitivity to tubocurarine and an increase in the sensitivity to depolarising drugs.

The different sensitivity of fast and slow muscles to tubocurarine does not extend to the other competitive neuromuscular blocking drugs. BONTA and GOORISSEN (1968) and MARSHALL (1973a) have shown that although the soleus muscle of the cat is more sensitive to tubocurarine than the tibialis muscle, when pancuronium (BONTA and GOORISSEN, 1968), AH 8165 or stercuronium (MARSHALL, 1973a) are used the opposite results are obtained. Dacuronium produced approximately equal degrees of block in both muscles. No explanation of these results is available at present.

b) Respiratory Muscles

PATON and ZAIMIS (1951) compared the degree of blockade of indirectly elicited twitches of the cat tibialis muscle with the reduction in spontaneous respiration following the intravenous administration of tubocurarine. They showed that respiration was still inadequate at a stage when the tibialis muscle had recovered almost completely. Similar results were obtained by BONTA and GOORISSEN (1968a). ALDERSON and MACLAGAN (1964) made a more direct assessment of the blockade in the respiratory muscles by recording evoked action potentials from the diaphragm and intercostal muscles and comparing them with indirectly elicited twitches of the tibialis muscle. Using both single stimuli and short bursts of tetanic stimulation at a frequency of 20/sec, they confirmed PATON and ZAIMIS, finding that the diaphragm was more sensitive to tubocurarine than the tibialis muscle but found that the difference in sensitivity between these two muscles could be considerably reduced by abolishing the temperature difference which normally exists in an anaesthetised cat between the warmer diaphragm muscle and the cooler limb muscles.

Quite different results were obtained by WAUD and WAUD (1972) who compared twitches of the diaphragm and of the tibialis muscle in the cat and at the same time measured the margin of safety of neuromuscular transmission by giving repeated test doses of suxamethonium during the period of blockade caused by tubocurarine (see p.452 for details of the method). The temperature of the muscles was not controlled in these experiments. They found that in the cat, the diaphragm recovered from the tubocurarine blockade *before* the tibialis muscle. Using isolated guinea-pig muscles, TAYLOR et al. (1964b) and LU (1970) also found that the diaphragm was less sensitive

to tubocurarine than the latissimus dorsi or serratus muscles. Lu (1970) also measured affinity constants of tubocurarine in the diaphragm and in the serratus anterior
and latissimus dorsi of the guinea-pig using a wide variety of agonists. The affinity of
the receptors for tubocurarine was similar in all three muscles so this cannot explain
the sensitivity differences.

The results obtained by WAUD and WAUD, TAYLOR et al. and Lu cannot be
reconciled with the results of PATON and ZAIMIS (1951), ALDERSON and MACLAGAN
(1954) or BONTA and GOORISSEN (1968). The techniques used in these experiments
were not strictly comparable; in particular TAYLOR et al. (1964a), WAUD and WAUD
(1972) and Lu (1970) administered repeated test doses of depolarising drugs in their
experiments. The other authors did not administer depolarising and competitive
drugs in the same experiment.

In anaesthetised patients the situation is much more complex. Many factors
probably contribute to the relative degree of paralysis in limb and respiratory muscles; among those suggested are the effects of general anaesthetics and of anoxia on
the respiratory centre, differences in the proportion of fast and slow fibres in the
muscles, differences in the rate of activity of the motor nerve to the muscles and
temperature differences between the limb and respiratory muscles. Under clinical
conditions respiration tends to be less affected by tubocurarine than the limb muscles but this difference in sensitivity is not very great (COLLIER et al., 1948; UNNA et
al., 1950; JOHANSEN et al., 1964). This has considerable clinical importance as respiration will invariably be depressed to some extent by a dose of neuromuscular
blocking drug which causes a significant paralysis of the limb or abdominal muscles.
There is extensive published literature on the search for a neuromuscular blocking
drug which would "spare" respiratory muscles. However, with the benefit of hind-
sight the futility of this search can be seen.

2. Effect of Temperature

BIGLAND et al. (1958) studied the effect of temperature on the action of tubocurarine
in the tibialis anterior muscle of the cat. They found that the blockade was smaller at
30° C than at 37° C. The blockade produced by depolarising neuromuscular blocking drugs, on the other hand, was affected in the opposite direction by a fall in muscle
temperature, both the magnitude of the blockade and its duration being increased
(BIGLAND et al., 1958). It was suggested that the repolarisation of the membrane
following the action of acetylcholine or any other depolarising drug was slowed by
cooling. Such an increase in the effectiveness of the transmitter could explain the
reduction in effectiveness of any competitive neuromuscular blocking drug. Similar
results were obtained in human leg muscles by CANNARD and ZAIMIS (1959), thus
confirming the clinical significance of this effect. HOLMES et al. (1951) studied the
action of tubocurarine in isolated rat diaphragm muscle at various temperatures.
They again found that a reduction of temperature from 40° C to 26° C reduced the
neuromuscular blocking action of tubocurarine. However, any further reduction in
temperature potentiated the action of tubocurarine. At about 10° C, neuromuscular
transmission failed in the absence of any drug. The only difference between the
results obtained in vivo and those obtained in vitro was that in the isolated muscle the
speed of onset and offset of the paralysis were dependant on the temperature. The

rate of action of the drug appeared to be determined by the rate of diffusion of the drug to and from the end-plate region. *In vivo*, however, BIGLAND et al. found that the duration of the blockade was almost unaffected by temperature, provided that large doses of tubocurarine, which produced cumulative effects, were avoided. This difference is not perhaps surprising as diffusion is less important in the *in vivo* preparation; the diffusion distance for tubocurarine from capillary blood to the extracellular fluid around the end-plate should be much shorter than the diffusion pathway in the *in vitro* preparation, where the drug has to diffuse from the bathing fluid.

3. Effect of Age

In 1955, STEAD reported that the neonate was much less sensitive to the action of tubocurarine than the adult patient. This was confirmed by LIM et al. (1964). However, CHURCHILL-DAVIDSON and WISE (1964) found that neonates and adults had a similar sensitivity to tubocurarine. WALTS and DILLON (1969) repeated these experiments and showed that the relative sensitivities of neonate and adult muscle were dependant on the method of calculating comparable doses for the different ages. When they used body surface area to calculate the doses, the newborn appeared to be much more sensitive than the adult. However, when they used body weight instead, their results showed a similar sensitivity for the two age groups. They also pointed out that the concentration of general anaesthetic needed to produce a given level of anaesthesia is different in neonates and in the adult and this would affect the sensitivity to neuromuscular blocking drugs.

Animals also show an age-dependant variation in sensitivity to neuromuscular blocking drugs. The muscles of young cats are very sensitive to tubocurarine and insensitive to depolarising drugs (MACLAGAN and VRBOVÀ, 1966a). In the case of the depolarising drugs the sensitivity has been shown to gradually increase as the animal matures (MANN and SALAFSKY, 1970).

In view of WALTS and DILLON's findings on the difficulty of choosing a suitable basis for the calculation of comparable doses for both the adult and neonate, a direct *in vitro* measurement of the change in sensitivity to neuromuscular blocking drugs during maturation is needed.

4. Effect of Acidosis

The experiments performed to investigate the effects of *metabolic* acidosis and alkalosis on the action of neuromuscular blocking drugs in various species have produced very conflicting results which may be due to the widely differing experimental conditions used (see Table 7). In contrast, in the case of *respiratory* acidosis (induced by breathing 5%, 10%, and 20% CO_2) and *respiratory* alkalosis (induced by hyperventilation) there is more agreement between the results obtained and a general trend emerges. Table 7 shows that in five separate tudies in the rabbit, cat and man respiratory acidosis potentiated the action of tubocurarine. With the other competitive neuromuscular blocking drugs, and also with suxamethonium and decamethonium, the effects were less marked, respiratory acidosis either antagonising their action or having no effect.

Table 7. Effect of acidosis and alkalosis on the action of neuromuscular blocking drugs

Agent	Author(s)	Preparation	Acidosis		Alkalosis	
			Respiratory	Metabolic[a]	Respiratory	Metabolic[b]
d-Tubocurarine	Kalow, 1954	frog rectus		potentiation		antagonism
	Payne, 1958, 1959, 1960	cat, sciatic-tibialis	potentiation	antagonism		potentiation
	Gamstorp and Vinnars, 1961	rabbit, sciatic-gastrocnemius	potentiation	potentiation	antagonism	antagonism
	Katz et al., 1963	cat, peroneal-tibialis				antagonism
	Hughes, 1970	cat, sciatic-gastrocnemius	potentiation	potentiation	antagonism	antagonism
	Coleman et al., 1966	man, ulnar-ring finger flexors	potentiation			
	Baraka, 1964	man, ulnar-ring finger flexors	potentiation		antagonism	
	Walts et al., 1967	man, ulnar-adductor pollicis			no effect	
Dimethyl-tubocurarine	Kalow, 1954	frog rectus		no effect		no effect
	Payne, 1958, 1959, 1960	cat, sciatic-tibialis	antagonism	antagonism		potentiation
	Gamstorp and Vinnars, 1961	rabbit, sciatic-gastrocnemius		no effect		no effect
	Katz et al., 1963	cat, peroneal-tibialis	no effect		no effect	potentiation
	Hughes, 1970	cat, sciatic-gastrocnemius	slight antagonism	slight antagonism	slight potentiation	slight potentiation
Gallamine	Payne, 1958, 1959	cat, sciatic-tibialis	antagonism		antagonism	
	Katz et al., 1963	cat, peroneal-tibialis				
	Hughes, 1970	cat, sciatic-gastrocnemius	antagonism	antagonism	potentiation	potentiation
	Walts et al., 1967	man, ulnar-adductor pollicis			potentiation	
Alcuronium	Coleman et al., 1966	man, ulnar-ring finger flexors	no effect			
Suxamethonium	Payne, 1958, 1959	cat, sciatic-tibialis	antagonism			potentiation
	Katz et al., 1963	cat, peroneal-tibialis	antagonism	no effect		no effect
	Hughes, 1970	cat, sciatic-gastrocnemius	antagonism		slight potentiation	
Decamethonium	Payne, 1958, 1959	cat, sciatic-tibialis	antagonism			antagonism
	Katz et al., 1963	cat, peroneal-tibialis				

[a] Metabolic acidosis produced by HCl infusion.
[b] Metabolic alkalosis produced by Na_2CO_3 infusion (Gamstorp and Vinnars, 1961; Katz et al., 1963; Hughes, 1970) or by $NaHCO_3$ (Payne, 1958, 1959) or by NaOH (Kalow, 1954).
Table modified and updated from Katz et al., 1963.

The opposite effects were obtained with respiratory alkalosis. In this case, the action of tubocurarine was antagonised in all experiments whereas the actions of dimethyltubocurarine, gallamine and suxamethonium were either slightly potentiated or unaltered.

Therefore, it is possible to conclude that the potency of tubocurarine is affected to a significant extent by both respiratory acidosis and alkalosis. The other neuromuscular blocking drugs of both competitive and depolarising types are affected to a lesser extent, if at all, and always in the opposite direction to the effect on tubocurarine.

It is assumed that in all these neuromuscular blocking drugs the quaternary nitrogen groups, having pK_a values of 13 or above, are completely ionized throughout the physiological pH range and could not contribute to the effects induced by either acidosis or alkalosis. KALOW (1954) put forward the hypothesis that the effects of acidosis and alkalosis on the potency of tubocurarine were the result of changes in the degree of ionization of hydroxyl groups. The molecule of tubocurarine, unlike that of the other neuromuscular blocking drugs, possesses two ionizable hydroxyl groups (Fig. 1). A fall in pH, within the physiological range, should reduce the degree of ionization of these hydroxyl groups (see Fig. 14). Using a method of spectrophotometric titration KALOW calculated pK_a values of 8.1 and 9.1 for the two hydroxyl groups. No such dissociation would occur with dimethyltubocurarine as the hydroxyl groups are methylated.

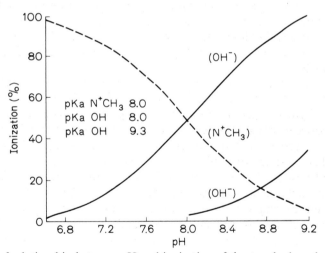

Fig. 14. Graph of relationship between pH and ionization of the two hydroxyl groups and the tertiary nitrogen group of tubocurarine. By kind permission of Dr. EVERETT of the Wellcome Research Laboratories

Later, when it was realised that tubocurarine had in fact a monoquaternary structure with an additional tertiary nitrogen group, EVERETT (personal communication) re-investigated the ionization of tubocurarine over a wide pH range. Ultraviolet and nuclear magnetic resonance methods for measuring the pK_a for the tertiary nitrogen group of tubocurarine gave a value of 8.0; the pK_a values for the two hydroxyl groups were 8.0 and 9.3 respectively, which were close to those previously obtained by KALOW. EVERETT considered that the increase in potency of tubocurarine when the pH is lowered is probably related to the protonation of the tertiary nitrogen and not to change in ionization of the hydroxyl groups. The relationship between pH and the degree of ionization of these three groups, i.e. the two hydroxyl groups and the tertiary nitrogen group, calculated from EVERETT's pK_a values for tubocurarine, is shown in Fig. 14. As pH is lowered, the degree of ionization of the tertiary nitrogen group increases whereas the ionization of both hydroxyl groups decreases. Within the physiological pH range one of the hydroxyl groups is relatively unaffected and can probably be ignored.

Exactly similar effects have been shown for two tertiary amines, eserine and nicotine. Eserine has a pK_a of 8.1 and as pH was reduced its inhibitory action on acetylcholinesterase (AChE) was found to increase in parallel with the increase in the degree of ionization of the tertiary nitrogen group (WILSON and BERGMAN, 1950). pH also affects nicotine-induced contractions of the isolated frog rectus abdominis muscle; on acidification of the bathing medium from pH 10 to pH 6.0 the ionization of nicotine's tertiary nitrogen group increased and this was accompanied by an increase in the potency of nicotine (MICHELSON and ZEIMAL, 1973). The results described above have been interpreted as indicating increased binding of tubocurarine and nicotine to the anionic sites of the acetylcholine receptor and of eserine to the enzyme AChE as the ionization of the tertiary nitrogen group increases during acidosis.

The question arises whether the change in pH during respiratory acidosis is large enough to explain the observed change in the potency of tubocurarine. KATZ et al. (1963) and HUGHES (1970) found that during respiratory acidosis the change in pH was less than 0.4 pH units. Unfortunately pH was not measured in most of the studies listed in Table 7.

Figure 14 shows that in the case of tubocurarine a reduction in pH from 7.4 to 7.0 would cause a 10% change in the ionization of both the tertiary nitrogen group and one of the hydroxyl groups. On theoretical grounds, because the graph of the relationship between pH and ionization of tubocurarine gives a line whose slope increases steeply above the "normal" pH of 7.4, an increase of 0.4 pH units above normal would be expected to produce a 20% change in ionization, i.e. twice as large an effect as that produced by a change of 0.4 pH units in the opposite direction. Thus it might be expected that alkalosis would cause a greater change in the magnitude of the tubocurarine blockade than acidosis. This was not supported by the results obtained by HUGHES (1970), who showed that acidosis had a significant effect on the blockade produced by tubocurarine whereas alkalosis had only a slight effect. No further information on this point is available at present.

Changes in ionization of the molecule would be expected to have numerous effects, including alterations in lipid solubility, renal excretion, plasma protein binding, and binding to the anionic site of the receptors and to the non-specific sites. Since pH changes affect the percentage ionization of the tertiary nitrogen group and the hydroxyl groups in opposite directions, the effect of such changes on the functions just mentioned will depend on which ion species in the tubocurarine molecule is the determining factor.

At present there is insufficient proof to distinguish between the two possibilities. There are three indirect pieces of evidence which should be considered in this context: BARAKA (1964) used a spectrophotometric assay method to show that the plasma concentration of tubocurarine was significantly higher in patients breathing 5% CO_2 than in another group of patients with respiratory alkalaemia. The higher plasma concentration of the drug was associated with prolonged neuromuscular block. This suggests that the redistribution and elimination of tubocurarine was altered by acidosis.

MEIJER and WEITERING (1970) showed that extraction of tubocurarine into octanol *in vitro* was reduced by lowering the pH from 8 to 6. The results are the opposite of what would be expected in terms of the dissociation of the hydroxyl groups of tubocurarine; as Fig. 14 shows, the hydroxyl groups are less dissociated at low pH and therefore an *increased* lipid solubility would be expected on this basis. MEIJER and WEITERING attempted to explain their anomalous results by suggesting that zwitterion formation occurred. However, these results could equally well be explained in terms of an increase in the dissociation of the tertiary nitrogen group as pH was reduced (Fig. 14).

Finally, the effect of pH on canine plasma protein binding of tubocurarine was studied by COHEN et al. (1965). They found that a fall in pH reduced plasma protein binding. This is most easily explained as a result of a reduction in dissociation of the hydroxyl groups. The interpretation of the results in these three studies is obviously difficult and controversial, and the relative importance of the two ion species in the tubocurarine molecule must remain unknown for the present. It is possible to conclude that ionization of the tertiary nitrogen and hydroxyl groups of tubocurarine are probably affected by pH changes within the physiological range, but it is a long jump from this observation to an explanation of the observed effect of either acidosis or alkalosis on the potency of tubocurarine *in vivo* in terms of a change in ionization of one or other of the ion species.

So far this discussion has been concerned primarily with tubocurarine, but it is an inescapable fact that the actions of dimethyltubocurarine, gallamine, suxamethonium and decamethonium can also be affected by acidosis and alkalosis, albeit to a lesser extent, and that when an effect occurs it is in the opposite direction to that observed with tubocurarine. The only ionizable groups these drugs possess are quaternary ammonium groups, which are always fully ionized. Therefore, changes in ionization cannot explain the modification of their activity *in vivo* by acidosis and alkalosis. The following alternative possibilities could be considered.

DEL CASTILLO et al. (1962), using the isolated toad muscle, found that when the pH of the medium was lowered to 4.0 there was a two-fold increase in the magnitude of the depolarisation produced by ionophoretically applied acetylcholine but that when the nerve was stimulated the resulting end-plate potentials were reduced to less than half their previous size. From this they concluded that a considerable reduction in the acetylcholine output from the nerve must have occurred.

Although this provides evidence linking pH changes with alteration in sensitivity to acetylcholine and in transmitter output, the experimental conditions were such that the conclusions drawn from these experiments are not applicable to *in vivo* situations. Firstly, the pH of 4.0 used in these experiments is completely outside the physiological range, and indeed is incompatible with life. Secondly, tubocurarine was present in the bathing fluid throughout the experiments in which end-plate potentials were measured. A fall in pH is known to increase the effectiveness of tubocurarine *in vitro* (KALOW, 1954) and this could explain the reduction in end-plate potential found in the experiments of DEL CASTILLO et al. Even if a change in the sensitivity of the post-synaptic membrane to acetylcholine or a change in the output of acetylcholine from the nerve terminals did occur within the physiological pH range, such effects would be expected to affect the potency of the two types of neuromuscular blocking drugs in opposite directions because these drugs have opposing mechanisms of action. [An analogy can be drawn with the effect of lowered muscle termperature, which increases the action of depolarising drugs but reduces the block caused by tubocurarine (BIGLAND et al., 1958).] However, as we have already seen, acidosis affects both depolarising and competitive neuromuscular blocking drugs in the same direction.

It seems more likely that the effect of acidosis on neuromuscular blocking drugs reflects some fundamental effect of pH on other parameters such as muscle blood flow, drug distribution, anionic charge on the receptors or muscle contractility. A change in any of these factors should theoretically have the same effect on the potency of both depolarising and competitive neuromuscular blocking drugs. In the case of tubocurarine, one can only suppose that these effects are overridden by the dominant effect of changes in ionization of the molecule.

G. Effects at Cholinergic Synapses in the Autonomic Nervous System

The action of neuromuscular blocking drugs is not entirely restricted to the acetylcholine receptors at the neuromuscular junction. In addition to their neuromuscular blocking activity many of these drugs are known to (1) block transmission at autonomic ganglia (LANGLEY and DICKINSON, 1899; BROWN and FELDBERG, 1936; CANNON and ROSENBLUETH, 1937) and (2) to mimic the action of atropine on the heart.

I. Actions on Autonomic Ganglia

BOWMAN and WEBB (1972) made a systematic comparison between the ganglionic effect of four neuromuscular blocking drugs (tubocurarine, benzoquinonium, gallamine, pancuronium) and that of two well known ganglion blocking drugs (hexamethonium and mecamylamine). The results showed that tubocurarine was a very potent ganglion blocking drug being, on a molar basis, about 5 times as potent as hexamethonium. Gallamine, on the other hand, had only weak ganglion blocking activity. Pancuronium was found to be about twice as potent as hexamethonium on a molar basis at a frequency of stimulation of 5 Hz. When a higher frequency was used (50 Hz) pancuronium appeared to be less potent than hexamethonium. Similar results at a higher frequency of stimulation were also obtained by BUCKETT et al. (1968).

These comparisons between ganglion and neuromuscular blocking potency provide much valuable information. However, in the clinical situation the important issue is whether ganglion blockade is likely to occur with concentrations of these drugs producing neuromuscular paralysis. On the basis of BOWMAN and WEBB's results, it would appear that only with tubocurarine does the ganglion blocking effect become clinically important. Indeed, there is evidence that tubocurarine can cause hypotension during anaesthesia (THOMAS, 1957; McDOWELL and CLARKE, 1969).

A similar comparison of ganglion and neuromuscular blocking activity in the cat was made for AH 8165, stercuronium and dacuronium by MARSHALL (1973 b). He compared the dose of each drug required to produce a 30% reduction of the response of the nictitating membrane when stimulated pre-ganglionically, with the dose required to achieve 30% reduction of the twitch of the tibialis muscle. The ratio was 16.7 for stercuronium, 8.5 for dacuronium and 3.8 for AH 8165. Therefore these drugs would not be expected to cause significant ganglion blockade at the doses used to produce neuromuscular block.

Although the activity of dimethyltubocurarine (COLLIER, 1950), alcuronium (WASER and HARBECK, 1962) and NN'-dimethylconessine (BUSFIELD et al., 1968) has not been studied as systematically as that of the other drugs, the workers mentioned above stated that the ganglion blocking activity of these drugs was very small at dose levels used to cause neuromuscular block.

II. Actions on the Heart

Many authors have reported that intravenous injections of gallamine (BOVET et al., 1949; JACOB and DEPIERRE, 1950), pancuronium (SAXENA and BONTA, 1970), dacuronium (NORMAN and KATZ, 1971) and AH 8165 (COLEMAN et al., 1973) cause tachycardia in man. The same effect occurs in anaesthetised cats (BOWMAN and WEBB, 1972; MARSHALL, 1973 b) and is thought to be due to an atropine-like action since it is greatly reduced by both atropine and bilateral vagotomy (BOWMAN and WEBB, 1972). It appears that the atropine-like action is limited to the cardiac acetylcholine receptors because the drugs do not antagonise the effect of acetyl-β-methyl choline on blood pressure (MARSHALL, 1973 b).

H. Histamine Release in Animals and Man

There is indirect evidence which suggests that paralysing doses of tubocurarine, suxamethonium and possibly pancuronium can cause histamine release in anaesthetised patients. The occurrence of urticaria, itching, hypotension and bronchoconstriction, and the development of erythema over the vein through which the drug is injected are all signs which indicate that histamine release has occurred, and these effects have been reported for tubocurarine in man (WHITACRE and FISCHER, 1945; COMROE and DRIPPS, 1946; SNIPER, 1952; SALEM et al., 1968; McDOWELL and CLARKE, 1969; BUSH, 1965). A second injection of a drug causing histamine release has a reduced effect, possibly due to the depletion of histamine stores in the mast cells. The speed of injection is also important, greater effects occuring at rapid injection rates, (MACINTOSH and PATON, 1949; PATON, 1959).

Histamine release has also been claimed in anaesthetised patients following the administration of suxamethonium (SMITH, 1957; FELLINI et al., 1963). In the case of alcuronium (LUND and STOVNER, 1962) and stercuronium (WIERIKS, 1972) there is no evidence that histamine release occurs with neuromuscular blocking doses in the common laboratory animals (i.e. the cat, rat, rabbit and dog) or in man. These results agree with the predictions based on the cat blood pressure and the human intradermal wheal tests (see below).

In the case of pancuronium, however, there are some discrepancies in the published results. Many authors have reported that pancuronium does not cause histamine release in man during clinical use (BAIRD and REID, 1967; CRUL, 1968; SELLICK, 1970; McDOWELL and CLARKE, 1969), and it has been safely used in asthmatics (NANA et al., 1972). It is also stated to be ineffective *in vitro*, failing to disrupt rat mast cells, and is inactive in both the cat blood pressure and the intradermal wheal test (BUCKETT and FRISK-HOLMBERG, 1970; BUCKETT et al., 1968). However, there are two reported cases of facial erythema, hypotension and severe bronchospasm following the injection of pancuronium (BUCKLAND and AVERY, 1973; HEATH, 1973). Both the patients were asthmatics and in one case the effectiveness of the drug in eliciting-bronchospasm could be correlated with the positive results of intradermal skin tests (BUCKLAND and AVERY, 1973), although skin testing was misleading in the other patient (HEATH, 1973). At present, therefore, the possibility that pancuronium may cause histamine release in anaesthetised patients must remain under discussion. However, there seems to be general agreement that the drug is ineffective as a histamine releasing agent in the common laboratory animals and in *in vitro* tests.

It should be possible to predict the likelihood of these untoward effects occuring in man. Logically, animal tissue would seem suitable for testing whether drugs cause histamine release, but such tests have not as yet proved very helpful. If given in sufficiently large concentrations, all of the competitive and depolarising neuromuscular blocking drugs are capable of releasing histamine from mast cells (see review by PATON, 1957). Tests used have involved the ability of the drug to disrupt rat mast cells (NORTON, 1954; FRISK-HOLMBERG and ÜVNAS, 1969), to produce bronchoconstriction in the guinea-pig (KONZETT and ROSSLER, 1940; BUCKETT et al., 1968); and perfusion of the isolated cat paw (BUCKETT and FRISK-HOLMBERG, 1970). The results of BUCKETT and FRISK-HOLMBERG showed that on the basis of these *in vitro* tests tubocurarine was the most active histamine releasing drug tested, followed in diminishing order of potency by dimethyltubocurarine, alcuronium, dacuronium and finally pancuronium. These authors concluded that the presence in the molecule of one or more free hydroxyl groups, whether primary, secondary or phenolic in nature, enhances its ability to cause histamine release. This would explain the high activity of tubocurarine and the lack of activity of pancuronium.

However, it should be stated that the concentrations necessary to liberate histamine *in vitro* are much larger than those found in the plasma during the administration of the same drug *in vivo* to produce a neuromuscular block. The minimal effective concentration in the *in vitro* experiments of BUCKETT et al. (1970) were in the millimolar range whereas the effective plasma concentration which produces a neuromuscular block is known to be a thousand times smaller—in the micromolar range (MATTEO et al., 1974; AGOSTON et al., 1973 b; KVISSELGARD and MOYA, 1961).

Another factor which complicates the application of results from *in vitro* experiments to conditions *in vivo* is that general anaesthetics are known to reduce the effectiveness of histamine liberators (MACINTOSH and PATON, 1949; KATZ, 1940). This may explain why many drugs which release histamine *in vitro* are ineffective under clinical conditions.

In attempts to obtain conclusive evidence for histamine release *in vivo*, efforts have been made to demonstrate a rise in plasma histamine levels following the administration of a neuromuscular blocking drug. WESTGATE and van BERGEN

(1962) are the only workers who have succeeded in measuring a rise in venous histamine content in anaesthetised patients using moderate intravenous doses of tubocurarine (0.44 mg/kg). Most of the other workers were able to measure a rise in plasma histamine only when very large doses of neuromuscular blocking drugs were used. ALAM et al. (1939) showed that in dogs considerable amounts of a histamine-like substance appeared in arterial blood after an intravenous injection of calabash curare and tubocurarine, but only doses as large as 100 mg were used. MONGAR and WHELAN (1953) infused 1 mg/min of tubocurarine for 5 min into the brachial artery in two conscious subjects without obtaining any increase in the concentration of histamine in the venous blood draining from the arm. Later in anaesthetised subjects they used close-arterial doses as high as 10 mg/min and only then were they able to measure a slight increase in plasma histamine. The difficulties of assaying the level of histamine in the plasma by simple methods and its rapid destruction probably account for the failures to detect a rise after moderate doses of tubocurarine. As direct measurement of histamine release *in vivo* has proved so disappointing, indirect tests have to be used to predict the effectiveness of a drug in producing histamine release in man under clinical conditions. PATON (1957) has suggested that two *in vivo* tests are particularly useful. These tests are (1) production of the triple response by intradermal injections into human skin and (2) the occurrence of a rapid fall in blood pressure, sometimes followed by a delayed depressor response, when the drug is injected intravenously into a cat anaesthetised with chloralose. Using these tests it has been shown by various workers that the following neuromuscular blocking drugs appear to cause histamine release *in vivo*—tubocurarine and its dimethyl ether and decamethonium (MACINTOSH and PATON, 1949), suxamethonium and gallamine (SNIPER, 1952), NN'-dimethylconessine (BUSFIELD et al., 1968) and AH 8165 (BRITTAIN and TYERS, 1973). Pancuronium (BUCKETT et al., 1968), alcuronium (LUND and STOVNER, 1962) and stercuronium (WIERIKS, 1972) do not cause histamine release in these tests.

J. Miscellaneous Drugs which Cause Muscle Paralysis

A very wide range of chemical substances can be shown to cause neuromuscular block in isolated muscle preparations if large enough concentrations are used (see GINSBORG and JENKINSON; Table 4, p. 290), but such concentrations are unlikely to be achieved *in vivo* in animals or man with most of these drugs. However, the general anaesthetics, barbiturates and certain other hypnotics and the antibiotics are known to effect neuromuscular transmission in doses which are used clinically.

I. General Anaesthetics

Muscle relaxation can be produced by volatile anaesthetics especially when administered in high concentration. This relaxation appears to be the result of their central action and not of a neuromuscular blockade. However, the general anaesthetics do have peripheral actions which are clinically important. Even under light anaesthesia with ether (PATON and ZAIMIS, 1951) or halothane (MILLER et al., 1972) the action of competitive neuromuscular blocking drugs is potentiated and the effect of depolarising drugs is reduced.

Experiments with muscles isolated from frog, cat and guinea-pig have shown that ether (KARIS et al., 1966, 1967; GISSEN et al., 1966) halothane (KARIS et al., 1967; WAUD et al., 1973) and ketamine (CRONNELLY et al., 1973) considerably reduce the depolarisation produced by ionophoretic or bath application of acetylcholine or carbachol. KARIS et al. (1966) found that the neuromuscular blockade induced by ether could not be antagonised by edrophonium or suxamethonium and concluded that ether was not acting as a competitive antagonist, but "altered the permeability-controlling mechanisms which are engaged subsequent to receptor site activation". Recent evidence to support this idea comes from the results of WAUD et al. (1973) who found that halothane did not alter the affinity of the receptors for tubocurarine or pancuronium. Secondly, measurements of acetylcholine-induced fluctuations of membrane potential (acetylcholine "noise") showed that ether reduced the voltage amplitude and shortened the underlying ionic pulse (see KATZ and MILEDI, 1973a). KATZ and MILEDI concluded that the average life-time of the ion channel was reduced by ether. In contrast, with a competitive inhibitor like tubocurarine, the life-time of the channel was unaffected but the molecular action occurred less frequently.

II. Barbiturate and Non-Barbiturate Hypnotic Drugs

In the rat, close-arterial injection of thiopentone causes an increase in the indirectly elicited twitch of the gastrocnemius-soleus muscle (QUILLIAM, 1955b). The same effect could be produced by adding hypnotic drugs to the fluid bathing isolated frog or rat muscle. This effect was thought to be due to a prolongation of the excitation-contraction mechanism. Higher concentrations of the barbiturates or of the non-barbiturate hypnotics, paraldehyde and methylpentynol, however, caused neuro-muscular block (QUILLIAM, 1955a and b). All of these drugs reduce the depolarisa-tion caused by acetylcholine and carbachol added to the bathing fluid (QUILLIAM, 1955a and b; PAYTON, 1966) or applied ionophoretically (ADAMS et al., 1970; SEY-AMA and NARAHASHI, 1975). This postsynaptic depressant action appears to be non-competitive in nature as the dose response curves become flattened in the presence of hypnotics and ecause anticholinesterase drugs are ineffective in antagonising the blockade (PAYTON, 1966).

Despite the universal finding that these drugs reduce the sensitivity to applied acetylcholine there is no agreement about their effects on the action of acetyl-choline released by the nerve ending. Miniature end-plate potentials have been reported to be reduced (THOMSON and TURKANIS, 1973) or unaffected (ADAMS et al., 1970). THOMSON and TURKANIS found that the end-plate potential was considerably increased by phcnobarbitone in a concentration of 200 µmol/l which was sufficient to reduce the sensitivity to ionophoretically applied acetylcholine. On the other hand, ADAMS et al. (1970) reported no change in end-plate potential with a comparable concentration of amylobarbitone or thiopentone. SEYAMA and NARA-HASHI (1975) demonstrated that the effect was dose dependent; with pentobarbitone in a concentration of 500 µmol/l the quantal content increased, presumably due to a presynaptic effect. The effect disappeared, however, at higher concentrations as the post-synaptic effect became dominant. In view of the various factors which contri-bute to the size and duration of the end-plate potential and miniature end-plate poten-tials the differences between the results are not so surprising. By means of the voltage clamp technique, known to improve the time resolution of the measurements and to avoid the complications introduced by the capacitance of the membrane, Adams (1974) has shown that higher concentrations of the barbiturates (5 mmol/l) reduce both the end-plate current itself and the miniature end-plate current. In particular the falling phase of the end-plate current was greatly accelerated; sodium current being more affected than the potassium current (Seyama and Narahashi, 1975). This is very similar to the action of atropine on the end-plate current (Beranek and Vyskocil, 1967; Magazanik and Vyskocil, 1969). Atropine is known to greatly reduce the noise which accompanies an Ach-induced potential change and to shorten the underlying elementary event (Katz and Miledi, 1973a) and it seems possible that the same mechanism may apply to the hypnotic drugs.

III. Local Anaesthetics

Under clinical conditions, local anaesthetics are unlikely to cause neuromuscular block on their own account. However, intravenous injection of procaine potentiates the action of neuromuscular blocking drugs (Ellis et al., 1953; Salgado, 1961). In animal experiments, however, procaine has been shown to cause neuromuscular block *in vivo* and *in vitro* (Harvey, 1939). In the rat diaphragm preparation a reduction in transmitter output was demonstrated by Straughan (1961) and Matthews and Quilliam (1964), and they suggested a pre-synaptic locus for the action of these drugs. However, Hirst and Wood (1971) have suggested that these results were due to the use of high frequency stimulation of the nerve which caused pre-junctional failure of transmission. Using low frequencies of stimulation Hirst and Wood found that procaine blocked neuromuscular transmission by reducing the sensitivity of the post-junctional membrane to acetylcholine. This is in agreement with earlier results obtained with microelectrode recording by del Castillo and Katz (1957). They found that procaine reduced the depolarisation caused by ionophoretic applications of acetylcholine or carbachol. In addition, procaine (Maeno, 1966) and xylocaine (Steinbach, 1968a) shortened the duration of the falling phase of the end-plate potential which was then followed by a greatly prolonged second phase. More recently it has been shown using voltage clamp techniques that the initial falling phase of the end-plate current is also accelerated by procaine. This is followed by a prolonged slow phase of current flow (Kordas, 1970; Deguchi and Narahashi, 1971; Maeno, 1966). The actions of local anaesthetics have been ascribed to separate effects on sodium and potassium conductances (Maeno, 1966; Maeno et al., 1971; Deguchi and Narahashi, 1971) or to a combination of the drug with the activated receptor so that the time-course of the activation produced by acetylcholine is altered (Steinbach, 1968a and b). The stability of the procaine-activated receptor complex appears to be dependant on the membrane potential (Kordas, 1970). Recent experiments using membrane noise analysis have shown that the ACh noise was substantially reduced by procaine, suggesting a decreased amplitude of the elementary potential change (Katz and Miledi, 1975). They suggested that the post-synaptic blocking action of procaine can be largely explained by the drastic shortening of the initial high intensity phase of the end-plate conductance change.

It can be seen that the effects of general and local anaesthetics, of barbiturates and atropine, have all been attributed to a change in the duration of the lifetime of the channels activated by acetylcholine. The general anaesthetics, atropine, the barbiturates and the local anaesthetics appear to cause the channels to stay open for a shorter time following activation by acetylcholine. On the other hand, aliphatic alcohols prolong the life-time of the channels. Among the mechanisms which have been suggested to explain these effects are a) change in the fluidity or dielectric constant of the lipid membrane (GAGE et al., 1975) or b) binding of the drug molecule into previously opened channels in such a way that the conductance is changed (ADAMS, 1974).

IV. Antibiotics

Antibiotics of the streptomycin group, as well as the tetracyclines and the polymyxins have all been reported to cause muscle paralysis under clinical conditions when the drug has been administered into the peritoneal cavity. Muscle paralysis has also been reported after systemic administration in a few unanaesthetised patients. Myasthenic patients may be particularly susceptible (HOKKANEN, 1964). However, the majority of cases have occured in patients under treatment with antibiotics who in addition received either a competitive neuromuscular blocking drug (FOGDALL and MILLER, 1974) or ether anaesthesia (CORRADO et al., 1959). The clinical incidence of antibiotic-induced paralysis has been well reviewed by PITTINGER et al. (1970).

Analysis of the mechanism of action of the antibiotics of the streptomycin type in animal experiments in vivo and in vitro has shown that they produce a flaccid paralysis which is associated with a reduction in the response to acetylcholine administered close-arterially (VITAL BRAZIL and CORRADO, 1957) or ionophoretically (ELMQVIST and JOSEFSSON, 1962; DRETCHEN et al., 1973). The action of streptomycin at the neuromuscular junction bears some resemblance to that of the competitive neuromuscular blocking drugs but there are certain fundamental differences. For example, tetanic stimulation during partial paralysis by streptomycin or neomycin is well maintained (VITAL BRAZIL and CORRADO, 1957); also neostigmine is only partially effective in antagonising the blockade (BEZZI et al., 1961; TANG and SCHROEDER, 1968). In addition, calcium salts produce a complete reversal of the blockade (VITAL BRAZIL and CORRADO, 1957; PITTINGER et al., 1958) in both animals and in man (PRIDGEN, 1956; JONES, 1959). It was suggested that the blocking action of the antibiotics resembles the action of magnesium ions (VITAL BRAZIL and CORRADO, 1957).

ELMQVIST and JOSEFSSON (1962) used microelectrode recording in isolated frog and rat muscles to study the blocking action of neomycin. They showed that the block was due to a reduction in the size of the end-plate potential. This was partly due to a decrease in the sensitivity of the post-junctional membrane to the depolarising action of acetylcholine. In addition, they suggested that neomycin might also reduce the output of transmitter in response to nerve stimulation as it was able to abolish the potassium-induced increase in miniature end-plate potential frequency. This effect could be reversed by increasing the concentration of calcium ions. Later, VITAL BRAZIL and PRADO-FRANCESCHI (1969) measured the release of acetylcholine from the isolated rat-diaphragm muscle using a bioassay method and confirmed that the release of transmitter was reduced by antibiotics, and that calcium salts abolished this effect.

Various mechanisms have been suggested to explain the action of the streptomycin group of antibiotics at the neuromuscular junction. The similarity of their action to that of magnesium ions and the antagonistic effect of calcium suggests competition with calcium ions at both pre- and post-synaptic sites.

In the case of the tetracyclines, which are known to chelate divalent metal ions, calcium binding is also likely.

Antibiotics of the polymyxin group also produce neuromuscular block but apparently by a different mechanism as calcium salts are ineffective in antagonising the paralysis and the compounds are not chelating agents (ADAMSON et al., 1960; FOGDALL and MILLER, 1974).

References

ADAMIČ, Š.: Accumulation of acetylcholine by the rat diaphragm. Biochem. Pharmacol. **19**, 2445—2451 (1970).

ADAMS, P. R.: The mechanism by which amylobarbitone and thiopentone block the end-plate response to nicotinic agonists. J. Physiol. (Lond.) **241**, 41—42 P (1974).

ADAMS, P. R., CASH, H. C., QUILLIAM, J. P.: Extrinsic and intrinsic acetylcholine and barbiturate effects on frog skeletal muscle. Brit. J. Pharmacol. **40**, 553 P (1970).

ADAMSON, R., MARSHALL, F. N., LONG, J. P.: Neuromuscular blocking properties of various polypeptide antibiotics. Proc. Soc. exp. Biol. (N.Y.) **105**, 494—497 (1960).

AGOSTON, S., KERSTEN, U. W., MEIJER, D. K. F.: The fate of pancuronium bromide in the cat. Acta anaesth. scand. **17**, 129—135 (1973a).

AGOSTON, S., VERMEER, G. A., KERSTEN, U. W., MEIJER, D. K. F.: The fate of pancuronium bromide in man. Acta anaesth. scand. **17**, 267—275 (1973b).

ALADJEMOFF, L., DIKSTEIN, S., SHAFRIR, E.: Binding of tubocurarine to plasma proteins. J. Pharmacol. exp. Ther. **123**, 43—47 (1958).

ALAM, M., ANREP, C. V., BARSOUM, G. S., TALOAT, M., WEININGER, E.: Liberation of histamine from the skeletal muscles by curare. J. Physiol. (Lond.) **95**, 148—158 (1939).

ALDERSON, A. M., MACLAGAN, J.: The action of decamethonium and tubocurarine on the respiratory and limb muscles of the cat. J. Physiol. (Lond.) **173**, 38—56 (1964).

ARIËNS, E. J., VAN ROSSUM, J. M., SIMONIS, A. M.: A theoretical basis of molecular pharmacology. Arzneimittel-Forsch. **6**, 282—293 (1956).

AUER, J., MELTZER, S. J.: The effect of ether inhalation upon the skeletal motor mechanism. J. Pharmacol. exp. Ther. **5**, 521—523 (1914).

BACH-Y-RITA, P., ITO, F.: In vivo studies on fast and slow muscle fibres in rat extraocular muscles. J. gen. Physiol. **49**, 1177—1198 (1966).

BACQ, Z. M., BROWN, G. L.: Pharmacological experiments on mammalian voluntary muscle in relation to the theory of chemical transmission. J. Physiol. (Lond.) **89**, 45—60 (1937).

BAIRD, W. L. M., REID, A. M.: The neuromuscular blocking properties of a new steroid compound, pancuronium bromide (A pilot study in man). Brit. J. Anaesth. **39**, 775—780 (1967).

BARAKA, A.: The influence of carbon dioxide on the neuromuscular block caused by tubocurarine chloride in the human subject. Brit. J. Anaesth. **36**, 272—278 (1964).

BARLOW, R. B.: Steric aspects of the chemistry and biochemistry of natural products. Biochemical Society Symposia No. 19, p. 46. Cambridge: Cambridge Univ. Press 1960.

BARNARD, E. A., WIECKOWSKI, J., CHIU, T. H.: Cholinergic receptor molecules and cholinesterase molecules at mouse skeletal muscle junctions. Nature (Lond.) **234**, 207—209 (1971).

BERANEK, R., VYSKOCIL, F.: The action of tubocurarine and atropine on the normal and denervated rat diaphragm. J. Physiol. (Lond.) **188**, 53—66 (1967).

BERANEK, R., VYSKOCIL, F.: The effect of atropine on the neuromuscular junction of the frog. J. Physiol. (Lond.) **195**, 493—503 (1968).

BEZZI, G., GESSA, G. L.: Influence of antibiotics on the neuromuscular transmission in mammals. Antibiot. and Chemother. **11**, 710—714 (1961).

BIGLAND, B., GOETZEE, B., MACLAGAN, J., ZAIMIS, E.: The effect of lowered muscle temperature on the action of neuromuscular blocking drugs. J. Physiol. (Lond.) **141**, 425—434 (1958).

BIGGS, R. S., DAVIS, M., WIEN, R.: Muscle-relaxant properties of a steroid *bis*-quaternary ammonium salt. Experientia (Basel) **20**, 119—121 (1964).

BISCOE, T. J.: The isometric contraction characteristics of cat intercostal muscle. J. Physiol. (Lond.) **164**, 189—199 (1962).

BLABER, L. C., CHRIST, D. D.: The action of facilitatory drugs on the isolated tenuissimus muscle of the cat. Int. J. Neuropharmacol. **6**, 473—484 (1967).

BLACKMAN, J. G., GAULDIE, R. W., MILNE, R. J.: Interaction of competitive antagonists. The anticurare action of hexamethonium and other antagonists at the skeletal neuromuscular junction. Brit. J. Pharmacol. **54**, 91—100 (1975).

BLASCHKO, H., BÜLBRING, E., CHOU, T. C.: Tubocurarine antagonism and inhibition of cholinesterase. Brit. J. Pharmacol. **4**, 29—32 (1949).

BLOGG, C. E., BRITTAIN, R. T., SIMPSON, B. R., TYERS, M. B.: AH 10407: a novel, short-acting, competitive neuromuscular blocking drug in animals and man. Brit. J. Pharmacol. **53**, 446 P (1975).

BOLGER, L., BRITTAIN, R. T., JACK, D., JACKSON, M. R., MARTIN, L. E., MILLS, J., POYNTER, D., TYERS, M. B.: Short lasting competitive neuromuscular blocking activity in a series of azobis-Arylimidazo-(1,2-*a*)-Pyridinium dihalides. Nature (Lond.) **238**, 354—355 (1972).

BONTA, I. L., GOORISSEN, E. M.: Different potency of pancuronium bromide in two types of skeletal muscle. Europ. J. Pharmacol. **4**, 303—308 (1968).

BOVET, D., BOVET-NITTI, F.: Succinylcholine chloride, curarising agent of short duration of action; pharmacodynamic activity and clinical applications. Sci. med. ital. **3**, 484 —513 (1955).

BOVET, D., COURVOISIER, S., DUCROT, R., HORCLOIS, R.: Propriétes curarisantes du di-iodoethylate de(quinoleyiloxy-*h*) 1,5-pentane. C.R. Acad. Sci. (Paris) **223**, 597—598 (1946).

BOVET, D., DEPIERRE, F., COURVOISIER, S., DE LESTRANGE, Y.: Recherches sur les poisons curarisants de synthèse: éther phénoliques à fonction ammonium quaternaire; action du triiodoéthylate de tri(diethylaminoéthoxy) benzéne. Arch. int. Pharmacodyn. **80**, 172—188 (1949).

BOWMAN, W. C.: Mechanisms of neuromuscular blockade. In: ELLIS, G. P., WEST, G. B. (Eds.): Progress in Medicinal Chemistry, Vol. 2, pp. 88—131. London: Butterworth 1962.

BOWMAN, W. C., RAPER, C.: Spontaneous fibrillary activity of denervated muscle. Nature (Lond.) **201**, 160—162 (1964).

BOWMAN, W. C., WEBB, S. N.: Neuromuscular blocking and ganglion blocking activities of some acetylcholine antagonists in the cat. J. Pharm. Pharmacol. **24**, 762—772 (1972).

BOYD, I. A., MARTIN, A. R.: The end-plate potential in mammalian muscle. J. Physiol. (Lond.) **132**, 74— 91 (1956).

BRITTAIN, R. T., TYERS, M. B.: AH 8165: a new short-acting competitive neuromuscular blocking drug. Brit. J. Pharmacol. **45**, 158 P—159 P (1972).

BRITTAIN, R. T., TYERS, M. B.: The pharmacology of AH 8165: a rapid-acting, short-lasting, competitive neuromuscular blocking drug. Brit. J. Anaesth. **45**, 837—843 (1973).

BROEN-CHRISTENSEN, C.: Distribution and biliary excretion of decamethonium in doubly nephrectomised rabbits. Acta pharmacol. (Kbh.) **23**, 275—286 (1965).

BROWN, G. L.: The action of acetylcholine on denervated mammalian and frog muscle. J. Physiol. (Lond.) **89**, 438—461 (1937).

BROWN, G. L., FELDBERG, W.: The action of potassium on the superior cervical ganglion of the cat. J. Physiol. (Lond.) **86**, 290—298 (1936).

BROWN, G. L., VON EULER, U. S.: The after effects of a tetanus on mammalian muscle. J. Physiol. (Lond.) **93**, 39—60 (1938).

BROWN, M. C., MATTHEWS, P. B. C.: The effect on a muscle twitch of the back-response of its motor nerve fibres. J. Physiol. (Lond.) **150**, 332—346 (1960).

BUCKETT, W. R., FRISK-HOLMBERG, M.: The use of neuromuscular blocking agents to investigate receptor structure requirements for histamine release. Brit. J. Pharmacol. **40**, 165 P (1970).

BUCKETT, W. R., MARJORIBANKS, E. B., MARWICK, F. A., MORTON, M. B.: The pharmacology of pancuronium bromide (ORG NA 97), a new potent steroidal neuromuscular blocking agent. Brit. J. Pharmacol. **32**, 671—682 (1968).

BUCKLAND, R. W., AVERY, A. F.: Histamine release following pancuronium: a case report. Brit. J. Anaesth. **45**, 518—521 (1973).

BÜLBRING, E., CHOU, T. C.: The relative activity of prostigmine homologues and other substances as antagonists to tubocurarine. Brit. J. Pharmacol. **2**, 8—22 (1947).

BÜLBRING, E., DEPIERRE, F.: The actions of synthetic curarizing compounds on skeletal muscle and sympathetic ganglia both normal and denervated. Brit. J. Pharmacol. **4**, 22—28 (1949).

BULLER, A. J., DORNHORST, A. C., EDWARDS, R., KERR, D., WHELAN, R. F.: Fast and slow muscles in mammals. Nature (Lond.) **183**, 1516—1517 (1959).

BULLER, A. J., ECCLES, J. C., ECCLES, R. M.: Differentiation of fast and slow muscles in the cat hind limb. J. Physiol. (Lond.) **158**, 399—416 (1960).

BULLER, A. J., RANATUNGA, K. M., SMITH, J.: Influence of temperature on the isometric myograms of cross-innervated mammalian fast twitch and slow twitch skeletal muscles. Nature (Lond.) **218**, 877—878 (1968).

BURGEN, A. S. V., KEELE, C. A., SLOME, D.: Pharmacological actions of tetra-ethyl-pyrophosphate and hexaethyltetraphosphate. J. Pharmacol. exp. Ther. **96**, 396—409 (1949).

BURNS, B. D., PATON, W. D. M.: Depolarisation of the motor end-plate by decamethonium and acetylcholine. J. Physiol. (Lond.) **115**, 41—73 (1951).

BUSFIELD, D., CHILD, K. J., CLARKE, A. J., DAVIS, B., DODDS, M. G.: Neuromuscular blocking activities of some steroidal mono and *bis*-quaternary ammonium compounds with special reference to NN′-dimethyl-conessine. Brit. J. Pharmacol. **32**, 609—623 (1968).

BUSH, G. H.: The clinical comparison with tubocurarine and diallylnortoxiferine in children. Brit. J. Anaesth. **37**, 540—543 (1965).

BUTTLE, G. A. H., ZAIMIS, E. J.: The action of decamethonium iodide in birds. J. Pharm. Pharmacol. **1**, 991—992 (1949).

CANNARD, T. H., ZAIMIS, E.: The effect of lowered muscle temperature on the action of neuromuscular blocking drugs in man. J. Physiol. (Lond.) **149**, 112—119 (1959).

CANNON, W. B., ROSENBLUETH, A.: The transmission of impulses through a sympathetic ganglion. Amer. J. Physiol. **119**, 221—235 (1937).

CHAGAS, C.: The fate of curare during curarization. In: DE REUCK, A. V. S. (Ed.): Curare and curare-like agents, pp. 2—10. Ciba Foundation Study Group No. 12. London: Churchill 1962.

CHEYMOL, J., BOURILLET, F., LEVASSORT, C.: Action anti-curarimétique de l'héparine et de l'héparinoides de synthèse chez le lapin. J. Physiol. (Paris) **47**, 132—136 (1955a).

CHEYMOL, J., BOURILLET, F., LEVASSORT, C.: Pouvoir anti-curarimétique de quelques molécules polysulfonées chez le lapin. Thérapie **10**, 616—624 (1955b).

CHURCHILL-DAVIDSON, H. C., WISE, R. P.: The response of the newborn infant to muscle relaxants. Canad. Anaesth. Soc. J. **11**, 1—6 (1964).

CLOSE, R.: Dynamic Properties of fast and slow skeletal muscles of the rat during development. J. Physiol. (Lond.) **173**, 74—95 (1964).

CODDING, P. W., JAMES, M. N. G.: The crystal and molecular structure of a potent neuromuscular blocking agent: *d*-tubocurarine dichloride pentahydrate. Acta Crystalogr. **29** B, 935—954 (1973).

COHEN, E. N.: Uptake, distribution, and elimination of the muscle relaxants. In: SCURR, C. F., FELDMAN, S. (Eds.): Scientific foundations of Anaesthesia, pp. 350—356. London: Heineman 1974.

COHEN, E. N., BREWER, B. H., SMITH, D.: The metabolism and elimination of *d*-tubocurarine-H^3. Anesthesiology **28**, 309—317 (1967).

COHEN, E. N., CORBASCIO, A., FLEISCHLI, G.: The distribution and fate of *d*-tubocurarine. J. Pharmacol. exp. Ther. **147**, 120—129 (1965).

COHEN, E. N., HOOD, N., GOLLING, R.: Use of whole body autoradiography for determination of uptake and distribution of labelled muscle relaxants in the rat. Anesthesiology **29**, 987—993 (1968).

COLEMAN, A. J., O'BRIEN, A., DOWNING, J. W., JEAL, D. E., MOYES, D. G., LEARY, W. P.: AH 8165: a new non-depolarizing muscle relaxant. Anaesthesia **28**, 262—267 (1973).

COLEMAN, A. J., RIPLEY, S. M., SLIOM, O. M., KNOWLES, S. L.: Influence of carbon dioxide on the neuromuscular blocking properties of tubocurarine chloride and Diallyl-nor-Toxiferine dichloride (Alloferin Roche) in man. In: Curare, pp. 98—105. Basel: Schwabe and Co. 1966.

COLLIER, H. O. J.: Pharmacology of D-0,0-dimethyl tubocurarine iodide in relation to its clinical use. Brit. med. J. **1950** I, 1293—1295.

COLLIER, H. O. J., PARIS, S. K., WOOLF, L. I.: Pharmacological activities in different rodent species of D-tubocurarine chloride and the di-methyl ether of D-tubocurarine iodide. Nature (Lond.) **161**, 817—819 (1948).

COMROE, J. H., DRIPPS, R. D.: The histamine-like action of curare and tubocurarine injected intracutaneously and intra-arterially in man. Anesthesiology **7**, 260—262 (1946).

COOKSON, J. C., PATON, W. D. M.: Mechanisms of neuromuscular block. A review article. Anaesthesia **24**, 395—416 (1969).

COOPER, S., ECCLES, J. C.: The isometric responses of mammalian muscles. J. Physiol. (Lond.) **69**, 377—385 (1930).

CORRADO, A. P., RAMOS, A. O., DE ESCOBAR, C. T.: Neuromuscular blockade by neomycin, potentiation by ether analgesia and D-tubocurarine and antagonism by calcium and neostigmine. Arch. int. Pharmacodyn. **121**, 380—394 (1959).

COUTEAUX, R.: Le système moteur a "petites" fibres nerveuses et la contraction "lente" contribution à son identification histologique sur le muscle de la grenouille. C.R. Ass. Anat. **39**, 264—269 (1953 a).

COUTEAUX, R.: Particularités histochimiques des zones d'insertion du muscle strié. C.R. Soc. Biol. (Paris) **147**, 1974—1976 (1953 b).

COUTEAUX, R.: Structure and cytochemical characteristics of the neuromuscular junction. In: CHEYMOL, J. (Ed.): International encyclopedia of pharmacology and therapeutics. Neuromuscular blocking and stimulating agents, Vol. 1. London: Pergamon Press 1972.

CREESE, R., ENGLAND, J. M.: Decamethonium in depolarised muscle and the effects of tubocurarine. J. Physiol. (Lond.) **210**, 345—361 (1970).

CREESE, R., MACLAGAN, J.: Entry of decamethonium in rat muscle studied by autoradiography. J. Physiol. (Lond.) **210**, 363—386 (1970).

CREESE, R., TAYLOR, D. B., CASE, R.: Labelled decamethonium in denervated skeletal muscle. J. Pharm. exp. Ther. **176**, 418—422 (1971).

CREESE, R., TAYLOR, D. B., TILTON, B.: The influence of curare on the uptake of a neuromuscular blocking agent labelled with radioactive iodine. J. Pharm. exp. Ther. **139**, 8—17 (1963).

CRONNELLY, R., DRETCHEN, K. L., SOKOLL, M. D., LONG, J. P.: Ketamine: myoneural activity and interaction with neuromuscular blocking agents. Europ. J. Pharmacol. **22**, 17—22 (1973).

CRUL, J. F.: Studies on new steroid relaxants. In: BOULTON, T. B. et al. (Eds.): Progress in anaesthesiology. Proceedings of the fourth World Congress of Anaesthesiologists London 1968, pp. 418—424. Amsterdam: Excepta Medica Foundation 1970.

CSILLIK, B.: Functional structure of the post-synaptic membrane in the myoneural junction. Budapest: Akademiai Kiado 1965.

CULLEN, D. J.: The effect of pretreatment with nondepolarising muscle relaxants on the neuromuscular blocking action of succinylcholine. Anesthesiology **35**, 572—578 (1971).

DAWSON, G. D., MERTON, P. A.: "Recurrent" discharges from motoneurones. In: Abstracts of Communications. XX th International Physiological Congress, Brussells, pp. 221—222 (1956).

DEGUCHI, J., NARAHASHI, T.: Effects of procaine on ionic conductances of end-plate membranes. J. Pharm. exp. Ther. **176**, 423—433 (1971).

DEL CASTILLO, J., KATZ, B.: A study of curare action with an electrical micromethod. Proc. roy. Soc. B **146**, 339—356 (1957).

DEL CASTILLO, J., NELSON, T. E., JR., SANCHEZ, V.: Mechanism of the increased acetylcholine sensitivity of skeletal muscle in low pH solutions. J. cell. comp. Physiol. **59**, 35—44 (1962).

DAL SANTO, G.: Kinetics of distribution of radioactive-labelled muscle relaxants. Anesthesiology **25**, 788—800 (1964).

DONLON, J. V., ALI, H. H., SAVARESE, J. J.: A new approach to the study of four non-depolarising relaxants in man. Anesth. Analg. Curr. Res. **53**, 934—938 (1974).

DRETCHEN, K. L., SOKOLL, M. D., GERGIS, S. D., LONG, J. P.: Relative effects of Streptomycin on motor nerve terminal and end plate. Europ. J. Pharmacol. **22**, 10—16 (1973).

DUNDEE, J. W., GRAY, T. C.: Resistance to D-tubocurarine chloride in the presence of liver damage. Lancet **1953 II**, 16—17.

DUVALDESTIN, P., VOURC'H, G.: Problèmes posés par l'anésthesie dans les transplantations rénales (a propos de 104 observations). Anesth. Analg. Réanim. **31**, 333—359 (1974).

EBERSTEIN, A., GOODGOLD, J.: Slow and fast twitch fibres in human skeletal muscle. Amer. J. Physiol. **215**, 535—541 (1968).

ECCLES, J. C.: The physiology of synapses. Berlin-Göttingen-Heidelberg: Springer 1964.

ECCLES, J. C., KATZ, B., KUFFLER, S. W.: Electric potential changes accompanying neuromuscular transmission. Biology Symp. **3**, 349—370 (1941).

ECCLES, J. C., KATZ, B., KUFFLER, S. W.: Effect of eserine on neuromuscular transmission. J. Neurophysiol. **5**, 211—230 (1942).

EL-HAKIM, E., BARAKA, A.: D-tubocurarine in liver disease. Kasr-El-Aini. J. Surg. **4**, 99—101 (1963).

ELLIS, C. H., WNUCK, A. L., DE BEER, E. J., FOLDES, F. F.: Modifying actions of procaine on the myoneural blocking actions of succinylcholine, decamethonium and D-tubocurarine in dogs and cats. Amer. J. Physiol. **174**, 277—282 (1953).

ELMQVIST, D., JOSEFSSON, J. O.: The nature of the neuromuscular block produced by neomycine. Acta physiol. scand. **54**, 105—110 (1962).

EPSTEIN, R. A., JACKSON, S. H.: Repetitive muscle depolarisation from single indirect stimulation in anaesthetized man. J. Appl. Physiol. **28**, 407—410 (1970).

EVERETT, A. J., LOWE, L. A., WILKINSON, S.: Revision of the structures of (+)-tubocurarine chloride and (+)-chondrocurine. J. chem. Soc. **D**, 1020—1021 (1970).

FATT, P.: The electromotive action of acetylcholine at the motor end-plate. J. Physiol. (Lond.) **111**, 408—422 (1950).

FEDDE, M. R.: Electrical properties and acetylcholine sensitivity of singly and multiply innervated avian muscle fibers. J. gen. Physiol. **53**, 624—637 (1969).

FELDMAN, S. A., COHEN, E. N., GOLLING, R. C.: The excretion of gallamine in the dog. Anesthesiology **30**, 593—598 (1969).

FELDMAN, S. A., TYRRELL, M. F.: A new steroid muscle relaxant. Dacuronium—NB.68 (Organon). Anaesthesia **25**, 349—355 (1970).

FELDMAN, S. A.: Muscle relaxants: major problems in anaesthesia, pp. 92—93. London: W. B. Saunders & Co. Ltd. 1973.

FELLINI, A. A., BERNSTEIN, R. L., ZANDER, H. L.: Bronchospasm due to suxamethonium. Brit. J. Anesth. **35**, 657—659 (1963).

FENG, T. P., LI, T. H.: Studies on the neuromuscular junction. XXIII. A new aspect of the phenomena of eserine potentiation and post-tetanic facilitation in mammalian muscle. Chin. J. Physiol. **16**, 37—56 (1941).

FERRY, C. B., MARSHALL, A. R.: An anti-curare effect of hexamethonium at the mammalian neuromuscular junction. Brit. J. Pharmacol. **47**, 353—362 (1973).

FOGDALL, R. P., MILLER, R. D.: Prolongation of a pancuronium-induced neuromuscular blockade by polymyxin B. Anesthesiology **40**, 84—87 (1974).

FRISK-HOLMBERG, M., UVNÄS, B.: The mechanism of histamine release from isolated rat peritoneal mast cells induced by D-tubocurarine. Acta physiol. scand. **76**, 335—339 (1969).

GADDUM, J. H., HAMEED, K. A., HATHWAY, D. E., STEPHENS, F. F.: Quantitative studies of antagonists for 5-hydroxytryptamine. Quart. J. exp. physiol. **40**, 49—74 (1955).

GAGE, P. W., McBURNEY, R. N., SCHNEIDER, G. J.: Effects of some aliphatic alcohols on the conductance change caused by a quantum of acetylcholine at the toad end-plate. J. Physiol. (Lond.) **244**, 409—429 (1975).

GAMSTORP, I., VINNARS, E.: Studies in neuromuscular transmission: influence of changes in blood pH and carbon dioxide tension on the effect of tubocurarine and dimethyltubocurarine. Acta physiol. scand. **53**, 160—173 (1961).

GASSER, H. S., DALE, H. H.: The pharmacology of denervated muscle. II. Some phenomena of antagonism and the formation of lactic acid in chemical contracture. J. Pharmacol. exp. Ther. **28**, 290—315 (1926).

GEREBTZOFF, M. A.: Cholinesterases: a histochemical contribution to the solution of some functional problems. London: Pergamon Press 1959.

GHONEIM, M. M., KRAMER, E., BANNOW, R., PANDYA, H., ROUTH, J. I.: Binding of D-tubocurarine to plasma proteins in normal man and in patients with hepatic or renal disease. Anesthesiology **39**, 410—415 (1973).

GINSBORG, B. L.: Spontaneous activity in muscle fibres of the chick. J. Physiol. (Lond.) **150**, 707—717 (1960a).

GINSBORG, B. L.: Some properties of avian skeletal muscle fibres with multiple neuromuscular junctions. J. Physiol. (Lond.) **154**, 581—598 (1960b).

GINSBORG, B. L., MACKAY, D.: A histochemical demonstration of two types of motor innervation in avian skeletal muscle. Bibl. anat. (Basel) **2**, 174—181 (1961).

GLOVER, E. E., YORKE, M. J.: Cyclic quaternary ammonium salts. Part IX. 1,1'-Azoimidazo (1,2-*a*)-pyridinium salts. J. chem. Soc. **C**, 3280—3285 (1971).

GISSEN, A. J., KARIS, J. H., NASTUK, W. L.: Effect of halothane on neuromuscular transmission. J. Amer. med. Ass. **197**, 770—774 (1966).

GOLDFINE, C.: Dissociation constants of competitive antagonists at the mammalian neuromuscular junction. Ph.D. Thesis. University of London (1972).

GORDON, G., PHILLIPS, C. G.: Slow and rapid components in a flexor muscle. Quart. J. exp. physiol. **38**, 35—45 (1953).

GRIFFITH, H. R., JOHNSON, G. E.: The use of curare in general anaesthesia. Anesthesiology **3**, 418—420 (1942).

HALL-CRAGGS, E. C. B.: The contraction times and enzyme activity of two rabbit laryngeal muscles. J. Anat. (Lond.) **102**, 241—255 (1968).

HARTZELL, H. C., FAMBROUGH, D. M.: Acetylcholine receptors: distribution and extrajunctional density in rat diaphragm after denervation correlated with acetylcholine sensitivity. J. gen. Physiol. **60**, 248—262 (1972).

HARVEY, A. M.: The actions of procaine on neuro-muscular transmission. Bull. Johns Hopk. Hosp. **65**, 223—238 (1939).

HEATH, M. L.: Bronchospasm in an asthmatic patient following pancuronium. Anaesthesia **28**, 437—440 (1973).

HESPE, W., WIERIKS, J.: Metabolic fate of the short-acting peripheral neuromuscular blocking agent stercuronium in the rat, as related to its action. Biochem. Pharmacol. **20**, 1213—1224 (1971).

HESS, A.: Structural differences of fast and slow extrafusal muscle fibres and their nerve endings in chickens. J. Physiol. (Lond.) **157**, 221—231 (1961 a).

HESS, A.: Structural differences of fast and slow extrafusal muscle fibres and their nerve endings in frogs, chickens and guinea-pigs. Anat. Rec. **139**, 237—245 (1961 b).

HESS, A.: Further morphological observations of "end plaque" and "en grappe" nerve endings on mammalian extrafusal muscle fibres with the cholinesterase technique. Rev. canad. Biol. **21**, 241—248 (1962).

HESS, A., PILAR, G.: Slow fibres in the extraocular muscles of the cat. J. Physiol. (Lond.) **169**, 780—798 (1963).

HILL, A. V.: The influence of temperature on the tension developed in an isometric twitch. Proc. roy. Soc. B **138**, 339—348 (1951).

HIRST, G. D. S., WOOD, D. R.: On the neuromuscular paralysis produced by procaine. Brit. J. Pharmacol. **41**, 94—104 (1971).

HOKKANEN, E.: Antibiotics in myasthenia gravis. Brit. med. J. **1964 I**, 1111—1112.

HOBBIGER, F.: The mechanism of anticurare action of certain neostigmine analogues. Brit. J. Pharmacol. **7**, 223—236 (1952).

HOLMSTEDT, B.: Synthesis and pharmacology of dimethyl-amidoethoxyphosphoryl cyanide (Tabun) together with a description of some allied anticholinesterase compounds containing the N-P bond. Acta physiol. scand. **25**, Suppl. **90**, 1—120 (1951).

HOLMSTEDT, B.: Pharmacology of organophosphorus cholinesterase inhibitors. Pharmacol. Rev. **11**, 567—688 (1959).

HOLMES, P. E. B., JENDEN, D. J., TAYLOR, D. B.: The analysis of the mode of action of curare on neuromuscular transmission; the effects of temperature changes. J. Pharmacol. exp. Ther. **103**, 382—402 (1951).

HUBBARD, J. I., WILSON, D. F.: Neuromuscular transmission in a mammalian preparation in the absence of blocking drugs and the effect of D-tubocurarine. J. Physiol. (Lond.) **228**, 307—325 (1973).

HUGHES, J. R., MORELL, R. M.: Posttetanic changes in human neuromuscular system. J. appl. Physiol. **11**, 51—57 (1957).

HUGHES, R.: The influence of changes in acid-base balance on neuromuscular blockade in cats. Brit. J. Anaesth. **42**, 658—668 (1970).

HUGHES, R.: Evaluation of the neuromuscular blocking properties and side effects of the two isoquinolinium bisquaternary compounds (BW 252 C 64 and BW 403 C 65). Brit. J. Anaesth. **44**, 27—41 (1972).

HUMPHREY, P. P. A.: Saturation effects in the uptake of decamethonium in skeletal muscle. Brit. J. Pharmacol. **39**, 219 P—220 P (1970).

HUNT, R., TAVEAU, R.: On physiological action of certain choline derivatives and new methods for detecting choline. Brit. med. J. **1906** II, 1788—1791.

JACOB, J., DEPIERRE, F.: Récherches sur l'action ganglionaire paralysante des curarisantes de la serie des éthers phénoliques de la triéthylcholine. Arch. int. Pharmacodyn. **83**, 1—14 (1950).

JENDEN, D. J., KAMIJO, K., TAYLOR, D. B.: The action of decamethonium on the isolated rabbit lumbrical muscle. J. Pharmacol. exp. Ther. **111**, 229—240 (1954).

JENKINSON, D. H.: The antagonism between tubocurarine and substances which depolarise the motor end-plate. J. Physiol. (Lond.) **152**, 309—324 (1960).

JEWELL, B. R., WILKIE, D. R.: An analysis of the mechanical components in frog's striated muscle. J. Physiol. (Lond.) **143**, 515—540 (1958).

JEWELL, P. A., ZAIMIS, E.: Changes at the neuromuscular junction of red and white muscle fibres in the cat induced by disuse atrophy and by hypertrophy. J. Physiol. (Lond.) **124**, 429—442 (1954).

JOHANSEN, S. H., JORGENSEN, M., NOLBREH, S.: Effect of tubocurarine on respiratory and non-respiratory muscle power in man. J. appl. Physiol. **19**, 990—994 (1964).

JONES, J. J., LAITY, J. L. H.: A note on a unusual effect of gallamine and tubocurarine. Brit. J. Pharmacol. **24**, 360—364 (1965).

JONES, R., VRBOVÀ, G.: Effect of muscle activity on denervation hypersensitivity. J. Physiol. (Lond.) **210**, 144—145 P (1970).

JONES, W. P. G.: Calcium treatment for ineffective respiration resulting from administration of neomycin. J. Amer. med. Ass. **170**, 943—944 (1959).

KALOW, W.: The influence of pH on the ionization and biological activity of D-tubocurarine. J. Pharmacol. exp. Ther. **110**, 433—442 (1954).

KARIS, J. H., GISSEN, A. J., NASTUK, W. L.: Mode of action of diethylether in blocking neuromuscular transmission. Anesthesiology **27**, 42—51 (1966).

KARIS, J. H., GISSEN, A. J., NASTUK, W. L.: The effect of volatile anaesthetic agents on neuromuscular transmission. Anesthesiology **28**, 128—134 (1967).

KATZ, B., MILEDI, R.: The effect of atropine on acetylcholine action at the neuromuscular junction. Proc. roy. Soc. B **184**, 221—226 (1973 a).

KATZ, B., MILEDI, R.: The binding of acetylcholine to receptors and its removal from the synaptic cleft. J. Physiol. (Lond.) **231**, 549—574 (1973 b).

KATZ, B., MILEDI, R.: The effect of procaine on the action of acetylcholine at the neuromuscular junction. J. Physiol. (Lond.) **249**, 269—284 (1975).

KATZ, G.: The action of anaesthesia on the histamine release in anaphylactic shock. Amer. J. Physiol. **129**, 735—743 (1940).

KATZ, R. L.: Clinical neuromuscular pharmacology of pancuronium. Anesthesiology **34**, 550—556 (1971).

KATZ, R. L., NGAI, S. H., PAPPER, E. M.: The effect of alkalosis on the action of neuromuscular blocking agents. Anesthesiology **24**, 18—22 (1963).

KENNEDY, J. F.: The chemistry of the acidic mucopolysaccharides (Glycosaminoglycans). Biochem. Soc. Transact. **1**, 807—813 (1973).

KHROMOV-BORISOV, N. V., GMIRO, V. E., MAGAZANIK, L. G.: Removal of a curare-like effect by direct inactivation of the myorelaxant molecule by disruption of the disulphide bond. Dokl. Akad. Nauk SSSR, old Biol. **186**, 236—239 (1969).

KING, H.: Curare alkaloids. I. Tubocurarine. J. chem. Soc. **2**, 1381—1383 (1935).

KIRSCHNER, L. B., STONE, W. E.: Action of inhibitors at the myoneural junction. J. gen. Physiol. **34**, 821—834 (1951).

KOELLE, G. B.: Neuromuscular blocking agents. In: GOODMAN, L. S., GILMAN, A. (Eds.): The pharmacological basis of therapeutics, pp. 601—619. London: Macmillan 1970.

KOJIMA, M., TAKAGI, H.: Effects of some anti-cholinergic drugs on antidromic activity in the rat phrenic nerve-diaphragm preparation. Europ. J. Pharmacol. **5**, 161—167 (1969).

Konzett, H. H., Rossler, R.: Versuchsanordnung zu Untersuchungen an der Bronchialmuskulatur. Naunyn-Schmiedebergs Arch. exp. Path. Pharmak. **195**, 71—74 (1940).

Kordas, M.: The effect of procaine on neuromuscular transmission. J. Physiol. (Lond.) **209**, 689—699 (1970).

Krause, W.: Über die Endigung der Muskelnerven. Z. rationelle Med. **18**, 136—160 (1863).

Kvisselgard, N., Moya, F.: Estimation of succinylcholine blood levels. Acta anaesth. scand. **5**, 1—11 (1961).

Kupfer, C.: Motor innervation of extra-ocular muscles. J. Physiol. (Lond.) **153**, 522—526 (1960).

Langley, J. N.: On the reactions of cells and of nerve-endings to certain poisons, chiefly as regards the reaction of striated muscle to nicotine and to curari. J. Physiol. (Lond.) **33**, 374—413 (1905).

Langley, J. N., Dickinson, W. L.: On the local paralysis of peripheral ganglia and on the connection of different classes of nerve fibres with them. Proc. roy. Soc. **46**, 423—431 (1889).

Lim, H. S., Davenport, H. T., Robson, J. G.: The response of infants and children to muscle relaxants. Anesthesiology **25**, 161—167 (1964).

Lindqvist, C.: Contraction properties of cat facial muscles. Acta physiol. scand. **89**, 482—490 (1973).

Lomo, T., Rosenthal, J.: Development of acetylcholine sensitivity in muscle following blockage of nerve impulses. J. Physiol. (Lond.) **216**, 52 P (1971).

Lu, T. C.: Affinity of curare-like compounds and their potency in blocking neuromuscular transmission. J. Pharmacol. exp. Ther. **174**, 560—566 (1970).

Luco, J. V., Sanchez, P.: The effect of adrenaline and noradrenaline on the activity of denervated skeletal muscle. Antagonism between curare and adrenaline-like substances. In: Bovet, D., Bovet-Nitti, F., Marcini-Bettolo, G. B. (Eds.): Curare and curare-like agents, pp. 405—408. Amsterdam: Elsevier 1959.

Lund, I., Stovner, J.: Experimental and clinical experiences with a new muscle relaxant Ro 4-3816. Acta anaesth. scand. **6**, 85—97 (1962).

Lüthi, U., Waser, P. G.: Verteilung und Metabolismus von ^{14}C-Decamethonium in Katzen. Arch. int. Pharmacodyn. **156**, 319—347 (1965).

Lüthi, U.: Verteilung und Metabolismus von curarisierenden Substanzen. In: Curare, pp. 501—510. Basel: Schwabe and Co. 1966.

MacIntosh, F. C., Paton, W. D. M.: The liberation of histamine by certain organic bases. J. Physiol. (Lond.) **109**, 190—219 (1949).

Mackay, D., Taylor, D. B.: Uptake of ^{3}H-labelled polymethylene bis-quaternary ammonium ions by mouse isolated diaphragm. Europ. J. Pharmacol. **9**, 195—206 (1970).

Maclagan, J.: A comparison of the responses of the tenuissimus muscle to neuromuscular blocking drugs in vivo and in vitro. Brit. J. Pharmacol. **18**, 204—216 (1962).

Maclagan, J., Creese, R.: Uptake of ^{3}H-decamethonium in cat muscle fibres. Vth International Congress on Pharmacology. San Francisco, July 1972.

Maclagan, J., Vrbovà, G.: A study of the increased sensitivity of denervated and re-innervated muscle to depolarising drugs. J. Physiol. (Lond.) **182**, 131—143 (1966 a).

Maclagan, J., Vrbovà, G.: The importance of peripheral changes in determining the sensitivity of striated muscle to depolarising drugs. J. Physiol. (Lond.) **184**, 618—630 (1966 b).

Maclagan, J., Zaimis, E.: The effect of muscle temperature on twitch and tetanus in the cat. J. Physiol. (Lond.) **137**, 89—90 P (1957).

Maeno, T.: Analysis of sodium and potassium conductances in the procaine end-plate potential. J. Physiol. (Lond.) **183**, 592—606 (1966).

Maeno, T., Edwards, C., Hashimura, S.: Difference in effects on end-plate potentials between procaine and lidocaine as revealed by voltage-clamp experiments. J. Neurophysiol. **34**, 32—46 (1971).

Magazanik, L. G., Vyskocil, F.: Different action of atropine and some analogues on the end-plate potentials and induced acetylcholine potentials. Experienta (Basel) **25**, 618—619 (1969).

Magladery, J. W., McDougal, D. B.: Electrophysiological studies of nerve and reflex activity in normal man. I. Identification of certain reflexes in the electromyogram and the conduction velocity of peripheral nerve fibres. Bull. Johns Hopk. Hosp. **86**, 265—290 (1950).

MAGLADERY, J. W., PORTER, W. E., PARK, A. M., TEASDALL, R. D.: Electrophysiological studies of nerve and reflex activity in normal man; (2)-neurone reflex and identification of certain action potentials from spinal roots and cord. Bull Johns Hopk. Hosp. **88**, 499—519 (1951).

MANN, W. S., SALAFSKY, B.: Development of the differential response to succinylcholine in the fast and slow twitch skeletal muscle of the kitten. J. Physiol. (Lond.) **210**, 581—592 (1970).

MARSDEN, C. D., MEADOWS, J. C.: The effect of adrenaline on the contraction of human muscle. J. Physiol. (Lond.) **207**, 429—448 (1970).

MARSH, D. F.: The distribution, metabolism and excretion of D-tubocurarine chloride and related compounds in man and other animals. J. Pharmacol. exp. Ther. **105**, 299—316 (1952).

MARSHALL, I. G.: The effects of three short-acting neuromuscular blocking agents on fast- and slow-contracting muscles of the cat. Europ. J. Pharmacol. **21**, 299—304 (1973a).

MARSHALL, I. G.: The ganglion blocking and vagolytic actions of three short-acting neuromuscular blocking drugs in the cat. J. Pharm. Pharmacol. **25**, 530—536 (1973b).

MARTENSSON, A., SKOGLUND, C. R.: Contraction properties of intrinsic laryngeal muscles. Acta physiol. scand. **60**, 318—336 (1964).

MASLAND, R. L., WIGTON, R. S.: Nerve activity accompanying fasciculations produced by prostigmine. J. Neurophysiol. **3**, 269—275 (1940).

MATTEO, R. S., SPECTOR, S., HOROWITZ, P. E.: Relation of serum D-tubocurarine concentration to neuromuscular blockade in man. Anesthesiology **41**, 440—444 (1974).

MATTHEWS, E. K., QUILLIAM, J. P.: Effects of central depressant drugs upon acetylcholine release. Brit. J. Pharmacol. **22**, 415—440 (1964).

McDOWELL, S. A., CLARKE, R. S. J.: A clinical comparison of pancuronium with D-tubocurarine. Anaesthesia **24**, 581—590 (1969).

McINTYRE, A. R., KING, R. E., DUNN, A. L.: Electrical activity of denervated mammalian skeletal muscle as influenced by D-tubocurarine. J. Neurophysiol. **8**, 297—307 (1945).

McINTYRE, J. W. R., GAIN, E. A.: Initial experience during the clinical use of pancuronium bromide. Anesth. Analg. Curr. Res. **50**, 813—823 (1971).

McISAAC, R. J.: The uptake of hexamethonium—C^{14} by kidney slinces. J. Pharmacol. exp. Ther. **150**, 92—98 (1965).

McISAAC, R. J.: The binding of organic bases to kidney cortex slices. J. Pharmacol. exp. Ther. **168**, 6—12 (1969).

McLEOD, J. G., WRAY, S. H.: An experimental study of the F-wave in the baboon. J. Neurol. Neurosurg. Psychiat. **29**, 196—200 (1966).

MEIJER, D. K. F., WEITERING, J. G.: Curare-like agents: relation between lipid solubility and transport into bile in perfused rat liver. Europ. J. Pharmacol. **10**, 283—289 (1970).

MERTON, P. A.: Contractions of muscle produced by synchronous and asynchronous motor volleys. J. Physiol. (Lond.) **112**, 6P (1950).

MERTON, P. A.: Interaction between muscle fibres in a twitch. J. Physiol. (Lond.) **124**, 311—324 (1954).

MICHELSON, M. J., ZEIMAL, E. V.: Acetylcholine. An approach to the molecular mechanism of action. London: Pergamon 1973.

MILEDI, R.: The acetylcholine sensitivity of frog muscle fibres after complete or partial denervation. J. Physiol. (Lond.) **151**, 1—23 (1960).

MILEDI, R.: Induction of receptors. In: MONGAR, J. L., DE REUCK, A. V. S. (Eds.): Ciba foundation symposium on enzymes and drug action, pp. 220—235. London: J. & A. Churchill 1962.

MILEDI, R., STEFANI, E., ZELENA, J.: Neural control of acetylcholine-sensitivity in rat muscle fibres. Nature (Lond.) **220**, 497—498 (1968).

MILLER, R. D., WAY, W. L., DOLAN, W. M., STEVENS, W. C., EGER, E. I.: The dependence of pancuronium and D-tubocurarine induced neuromuscular blockade on alveolar concentrations of halothane and forane. Anesthesiology **37**, 573—581 (1972).

MONGAR, J. L., WHELAN, R. F.: Histamine release by adrenalin and D-tubocurarine in the human subject. J. Physiol. (Lond.) **120**, 146—154 (1953).

MUSHIN, W. W., MAPLESON, W. W.: Relaxant action in man of dipyrandium chloride (M & B 9105A). Brit. J. Anaesth. **36**, 761—768 (1964).

MUSHIN, W. W., WIEN, R., MASON, D. F. J., LANGSTON, G. T.: Curare-like actions of *tri*-(diethyl-aminoethoxy)-benzene triethyliodide. Lancet **1949 I**, 726—728.

NANA, A., CARDAN, E., LEITERSDORFER, T.: Pancuronium bromide, its use in asthmatics and patients with liver disease. Anaesthesia 27, 154—158 (1972).

NORMAN, J., KATZ, R. L., SEED, R. F.: The neuromuscular blocking action of pancuronium in man during anaesthesia. Brit. J. Anaesth. 42, 702—710 (1970).

NORMAN, J., KATZ, R. L.: Some effects of the steroidal muscle relaxant, dacuronium bromide in anaesthetized patients. Brit. J. Anaesth. 43, 313—319 (1971).

NORTON, S.: Quantitative determination of mast cell fragmentation by compound 48/80. Brit. J. Pharmacol. 9, 494—497 (1954).

OLSEN, G. D., RIKER, W. F.: Binding of D-tubocurarine by cartilage. Fed. Proc. 33, 513 (1974).

PATON, W. D. M.: Histamine release by compounds of simple chemical structure. Pharmacol. Rev. 9, 269—328 (1957).

PATON, W. D. M.: The effects of muscle relaxants other than muscular relaxation. Anesthesiology 20, 453—463 (1959).

PATON, W. D. M., RANG, H. P.: The uptake of atropine and related drugs by intestinal smooth muscle of the guinea-pig in relation to acetylcholine receptors. Proc. roy. Soc. B 163, 1—44 (1965).

PATON, W. D. M., WAUD, D. R.: The margin of safety of neuromuscular transmission. J. Physiol. (Lond.) 191, 59—90 (1967).

PATON, W. D. M., ZAIMIS, E.: The pharmacological actions of polymethylene bistrimethyl-ammonium salts. Brit. J. Pharmacol. 4, 381—400 (1949).

PATON, W. D. M., ZAIMIS, E.: The action of D-tubocurarine and of decamethonium on respiratory and other muscles in the cat. J. Physiol. (Lond.) 112, 311—331 (1951).

PATON, W. D. M., ZAIMIS, E.: The methonium compounds. Pharmacol. Rev. 4, 219—253 (1952).

PAYNE, J. P.: The influence of carbon dioxide on the neuromuscular blocking activity of relaxant drugs in the cat. Brit. J. Anaesth. 30, 206—216 (1958).

PAYNE, J. P.: Changes in neuromuscular blocking activity of tubocurarine and dimethyl tubocurarine induced by the administration of carbon dioxide. Acta anaesth. scand. 3, 53—58 (1959).

PAYNE, J. P.: The influence of changes in blood pH on the neuromuscular blocking properties of D-tubocurarine and dimethyl tubocurarine in the cat. Acta anaesth. scand. 4, 83—90 (1960).

PAYNE, J. P.: The initial transient stimulating action of neuromuscular blocking agents in the cat. Brit. J. Anaesth. 33, 285—288 (1961).

PAYTON, B. W.: Use of the frog neuromuscular junction for assessing the action of drugs affecting synaptic transmission. Brit. J. Pharmacol. 28, 35—43 (1966).

PITTINGER, C. B., LONG, J. P., MILLER, J. R.: The neuromuscular blocking action of neomycin: a concern of the anesthesiologist. Anesth. Analg. Curr. Res. 37, 276—282 (1958).

PITTINGER, C. B., ERYASA, Y., ADAMSON, R.: Antibiotic-induced paralysis. Anesth. Analg. Curr. Res. 49, 487—501 (1970).

POINTER, D. J., WILFORD, J. G., BISHOP, D. C.: Crystal structure of a novel curariform agent. Nature (Lond.) 239, 332—333 (1972).

POTTER, L. T.: Synthesis, storage and release of [^{14}C] acetylcholine in isolated rat diaphragm muscles. J. Physiol. (Lond.) 206, 145—166 (1970).

PRIDGEN, J. E.: Respiratory arrest thought to be due to intraperitoneal neomycin. Surgery 40, 571—574 (1956).

QUILLIAM, J. P.: The action of hypnotic drugs on skeletal muscle. Brit. J. Pharmacol. 10, 133—140 (1955a).

QUILLIAM, J. P.: The action of thiopentone sodium on skeletal muscle. Brit. J. Pharmacol. 10, 141—146 (1955b).

RANDALL, L. O.: Anticurare action of phenolic quaternary ammonium salts. J. Pharmacol. exp. Ther. 100, 83—93 (1950).

RANDALL, L. O., LEHMANN, G.: Pharmacological properties of some neostigmine analogs. J. Pharmacol. exp. Ther. 99, 16—32 (1950).

RENKIN, E. M.: Permeability of frog skeletal muscle to choline. J. gen. Physiol. 44, 1159—1164 (1961).

RIKER, W. F., WESCOE, W. C., BROTHERS, M. J.: Studies on the interrelationships of certain cholinergic compounds. II. The effects of β-acetoxy phenyltrimethylammonium methylsulphate on neuromuscular transmission. J. Pharmacol. exp. Ther. 97, 208—221 (1949).

RIKER, W. F., WESCOE, W. C.: The pharmacology of Flaxedil with observations on certain analogs. Ann. N.Y. Acad. Sci. **54**, 373—394 (1951).

ROSENBLUETH, A., LUCO, J. V.: A study of denervated mammalian skeletal muscle. Amer. J. Physiol. **120**, 781—797 (1937).

SALEM, M. R., KIM, Y., ELETR, A. A.: Histamine release following I.V. injection of D-tubocurarine. Anesthesiology **29**, 380—382 (1968).

SALGADO, A. S.: Potentiation of succinylcholine by procaine. Anesthesiology **22**, 897—899 (1961).

SAVAGE, D. S., CAMERON, A. F., FERGUSON, G., HANNAWAY, C., MACKAY, I. R.: Molecular structure of pancuronium bromide ($3\alpha,17\beta$-diacetoxy-$2\beta,16\beta$-dipiperidino-5α-androstane dimethobromide) a neuromuscular blocking agent. Crystal and molecular structure of the water: methylene solvate. J. chem. Soc. B, 410—415 (1971).

SAXENA, P. R., BONTA, I. L.: Mechanism of selective cardiac vagolytic action of pancuronium bromide. Specific blockade of cardiac muscarinic receptors. Europ. J. Pharmacol. **11**, 332—341 (1970).

SCHANKER, L. S.: Concentrative transfer of an organic cation from blood into bile. Biochem. Pharmacol. **11**, 253—254 (1962a).

SCHANKER, L. S.: Passage of drugs across body membranes. Pharmacol. Rev. **14**, 501—530 (1962b).

SCHANKER, L. S.: Transport of drugs. In: HOKIN, L. E. (Ed.): Metabolic pathways, Vol. 6, pp. 543—571. New York: Academic Press 1972.

SCHUH, F. T., VIGUERA, M. G., TERRY, R. N.: The effect of a subthreshold dose of D-tubocurarine on the neuromuscular blocking action of succinylcholine in anesthetized man. Acta anaesth. scand. **18**, 71—78 (1974).

SELLICK, B. A.: Pancuronium bromide. Clinical experience of a new muscle relaxant. In: BOULTON, T. B. et al. (Eds.): Progress in anaesthesiology. Proceedings of the fourth World Congress of Anaesthesiologists London 1968, pp. 1144—1147. Amsterdam: Excepta Medica Foundation 1970.

SEYAMA, I., NARAHASHI, T.: Mechanism of blockade of neuromuscular transmission by pentobarbital. J. Pharmacol. exp. Ther. **192**, 95—103 (1975).

SKIVINGTON, M. A.: Protein binding of three tritiated muscle relaxants. Brit. J. Anaesth. **44**, 1030—1034 (1972).

SMITH, N. L.: Histamine release by suxamethonium. Anaesthesia **12**, 293—298 (1957).

SNIPER, W.: The estimation and comparison of histamine release by muscle relaxants in man. Brit. J. Anaesth. **24**, 232—237 (1952).

SOBELL, H. M., SAKORE, T. D., TAVALE, S. S., CANEPA, F. G., PAULING, P., PETCHER, T. J.: Stereochemistry of a curare alkaloid: 0,0′,N-Trimethyl-D-Tubocurarine. Proc. nat. Acad. Sci. (Wash.) **69**, 2212—2215 (1972).

STEAD, A. L.: Response of newborn infants to muscle relaxants. Brit. J. Anaesth. **27**, 124—130 (1955).

STEINBACH, A. B.: Alteration by xylocaine (lidocaine) and its derivatives of the time course of the end-plate potential. J. gen. Physiol. **52**, 144—161 (1968a).

STEINBACH, A. B.: A kinetic model for the action of xylocaine on receptors for acetylcholine. J. gen. Physiol. **52**, 162—180 (1968b).

STEPHENSON, R. P., GINSBORG, B. L.: Potentiation by an antagonist. Nature (Lond.) **222**, 790—791 (1969).

STOVNER, J., THEODORSEN, L., BJELKE, E.: Sensitivity to tubocurarine and alcuronium with special reference to plasma protein patterns. Brit. J. Anaesth. **43**, 385—391 (1971a).

STOVNER, J., THEODORSEN, L., BJELKE, E.: Sensitivity to gallamine and pancuronium with special reference to serum proteins. Brit. J. Anaesth. **43**, 953—958 (1971b).

STRAUGHAN, D. W.: The action of procaine at the neuromuscular junction. J. Pharm. Pharmacol. **13**, 49—52 (1961).

SWANSON, E. E., HENDERSON, F. G., CHEN, K. K.: Dimethylether of D-tubocurarine iodide. J. Lab. clin. Med. **34**, 516—523 (1949).

TANG, A. H., SCHROEDER, L. A.: The effect of linomycin on neuromuscular transmission. Toxicol. appl. Pharmacol. **12**, 44—47 (1968).

TASAKI, I., MIZUTANI, K.: Comparitive studies on the activities of the muscle evoked by two kinds of motor nerve fibres. Jap. J. med. Sci. Biol. **10**, 237—244 (1944).

TAYLOR, D. B., CREESE, R., SCHOLES, N. W.: Effect of curare concentration, temperature, and potassium ion concentration on the rate of uptake of a neuromuscular blocking agent labelled with radioactive iodine. J. Pharmacol. exp. Ther. **144**, 293—300 (1964a).

TAYLOR, D. B., CREESE, R., NEDERGAARD, O. A., CASE, R.: Labelled depolarizing drugs in normal and denervated muscle. Nature (Lond.) **208**, 901—902 (1965).

TAYLOR, D. B., PRIOR, R. D., BEVAN, J. A.: The relative sensitivity of diaphragm and other muscles of the guinea-pig to neuromuscular blocking agents. J. Pharmacol. exp. Ther. **143**, 187—191 (1964b).

THOMAS, E. T.: The effect of tubocurarine chloride on the blood pressure of anaesthetised patients. Lancet **1957** II, 772—773.

THOMSON, T. D., TURKANIS, S. A.: Barbiturate-induced transmitter release at a frog neuromuscular junction. Brit. J. Pharmacol. **48**, 48—58 (1973).

TOCHINO, Y., SCHANKER, L. S.: Active transport of biologic amine compounds by the rabbit choroid plexus. Pharmacologist **6**, 177 (1964).

TOCHINO, Y., SCHANKER, L. S.: Active transport of quaternary ammonium compounds by the choroid plexus in vitro. Amer. J. Physiol. **208**, 666—673 (1965).

TYERS, M. B.: Pharmacological studies on new short-acting competitive neuromuscular blocking drugs. PhD Thesis, C.N.A.A. (1975).

UNNA, K. R., PELIKAN, E. W., MACFARLANE, D. W., CAZORT, R. J., SADOVE, M. S., NELSON, J. T., DRUCKER, A. P.: Evaluation of curarizing drugs in man. I. Potency, duration of action, and effects of vital capacity of D-tubocurarine, dimethyltubocurarine and decamethylene-bis-(trimethylammonium bromide). J. Pharmacol. exp. Ther. **98**, 318—329 (1950).

VAN MAANEN, E. F.: The antagonism between acetylcholine and the curare alkaloids D-tubocurarine, c-curarine-I, c-toxiferine II and β-erythroidine in the rectus abdominis of the frog. J. Pharmacol. exp. Ther. **99**, 255—264 (1950).

VERNER, I. R.: Some problems in the clinical evaluation of relaxant drugs in man, with special reference to a new competitive agent. Communication to the section of anaesthetics, Royal Society of Medicine April 5th 1963.

VITAL BRAZIL, O., CORRADO, A. P.: The curariform action of streptomycin. J. Pharmacol. exp. Ther. **120**, 452—459 (1957).

VITAL BRAZIL, O., PRADO-FRANCESCHI, J.: The neuromuscular blocking action of gentamycin. Arch. int. Pharmacodyn. **179**, 65—67 (1969).

VOLLE, R.: Blockade by hexamethonium of drug induced neuromuscular facilitation. Arch. int. Pharmacodyn. **167**, 1—8 (1967).

WALTS, L. F., DILLON, J. B.: Durations of action of D-tubocurarine and gallamine. Anesthesiology **29**, 499—504 (1968).

WALTS, L. F., DILLON, J. B.: The response of newborns to succinylcholine and D-tubocurarine. Anesthesiology **31**, 35—38 (1969).

WALTS, L. F., LEBOWITZ, M., DILLON, J. B.: The effects of ventilation on the action of D-tubocurarine and gallamine. Brit. J. Anaesth. **39**, 845—850 (1967).

WASER, P. G.: Relation between enzymes and cholinergic receptors. In: MONGAR, J. L., DE-REUCK, A. V. S. (Eds.): Ciba foundation symposium on enzymes and drug action, pp. 206—217. London: Churchill 1962.

WASER, P. G.: Autoradiographic investigations of cholinergic and other receptors in the motor endplate. Advan. Drug. Res. **2**, 81—120 (1965).

WASER, P. G., HADORN, I.: Relations of cholinergic receptors to acetylcholinesterase of end-plates in denervated muscle. Bibl. anat. (Basel) **2**, 155—160 (1961).

WASER, P. G., HARBECK, P.: Pharmakologie und klinische Anwendung des kurzkauerndian muskel relaxans Diallyl-nor-Toxiferin. Anaesthetist **11**, 33—37 (1962).

WASER, P. G., LÜTHI, U.: Autoradiographische Lokalisation von ^{14}C-Calebassen-Curarine-I und ^{14}C-Decamethonium in der motorischen Endplatte. Arch. int. Pharmacodyn. **112**, 272—296 (1957).

WASER, P. G., LÜTHI, U.: On C^{14}-curare fixation in end-plates. Helv. physiol. pharmacol. Acta **20**, 237—251 (1962).

WASER, P. G., SCHMID, H., SCHMID, K.: Resorbtion, Verteilung und Ausscheidung von Radio-Calebassen-Curarin bei Katzen. Arch. int. Pharmacodyn. **961**, 386—405 (1954).

WAUD, B. E., CHENG, M. C., WAUD, D. R.: Comparison of drug receptor dissociation constants at the mammalian neuromuscular junction in the presence and absence of halothane. J. Pharmacol. exp. Ther. **187**, 40—46 (1973).

WAUD, B. E., WAUD, D. R.: The margin of safety of neuromuscular transmission in the muscle of the diaphragm. Anesthesiology **37**, 417—422 (1972).

WESCOE, W. C., RIKER, W. F., BROTHERS, M. J.: Studies on the interrelationship of certain cholinergic compounds. I. The pharmacology of 3-acetoxy phenyltrimethylammonium methylsulphate. J. Pharmacol. exp. Ther. **97**, 190—207 (1949).

WESCOE, W. C., RIKER, W. F.: The pharmacology of anti-curare agents. Ann. N.Y. Acad. Sci. **54**, 438—455 (1951).

WESTGATE, H. D., VAN BERGEN, F. H.: Changes in histamine blood levels following D-tubocurarine administration. Canad. Anaesth. Soc. J. **9**, 497—503 (1962).

WHITE, A. C., STEDMAN, E.: On the physostigmine-like action of certain synthetic urethanes. J. Pharmacol. exp. Ther. **41**, 259—288 (1931).

WHITACRE, R. J., FISCHER, A. J.: Clinical observations on the use of curare in anesthesia. Anesthesiology **6**, 124—130 (1945).

WIERIKS, J.: Farmacologisch onderzoek van MYC 1080 (Stercuronium), Een niewe kortwerkende motorische-eindplaatremmer. PH. D. THESIS, Rotterdam, University of Rotterdam (1972).

WILSON, I. B., BERGMAN, F.: Studies on cholinesterase. VII. The active surface of acetylcholine esterase derived from effect of pH on inhibitors. J. biol. Chem. **185**, 479—489 (1950).

ZACHS, S. I., BLUMBERG, J. M.: Observations on the fine structure and cytochemistry of mouse and human intercostal neuromuscular junctions. J. biophys. biochem. Cytol. **10**, 517—528 (1961).

ZAIMIS, E.: The action of decamethonium on normal and denervated mammalian muscle. J. Physiol. (Lond.) **112**, 176—190 (1951).

ZAIMIS, E.: Motor end-plate differences as a determining factor in the mode of action of neuromuscular blocking substances. J. Physiol. (Lond.) **122**, 238—251 (1953).

Pharmacology of Anticholinesterase Drugs

F. Hobbiger

A. Introduction

The transmission of nerve impulses at the neuromuscular junction involves the following consecutive events

1) arrival of an impulse at the nerve terminal,

2) release of acetylcholine (ACh) from the nerve terminal into the synaptic cleft,

3) transient occupation by ACh of receptors (cholinoceptors) at the surface of the postsynaptic membrane, leading to a nonspecific increase in membrane permeability which gives rise to the end-plate potential (e.p.p.),

4) initiation by the e.p.p., on attaining a critical amplitude of 10 to 20 mV, of a propagated muscle action potential which triggers a contraction of the muscle fibre,

5) termination of the action of ACh on the postsynaptic membrane by its removal from the synaptic cleft.

For the junction to meet physiological requirements it must be able to transmit impulses at a rate of approximately 10 to 30 Hz and for this it is necessary that the postsynaptic action of ACh is speedily terminated. Acetylcholinesterase (acetylcholine acetylhydrolase; E.C. 3.1.1.7; AChE), a constituent of the membranes forming the synaptic cleft, plays an essential role in the removal of ACh from the synaptic cleft by hydrolysing ACh to give choline and acetic acid. In the concentrations found at the neuromuscular junction, the hydrolysis products are inert, i.e. they neither mimic nor antagonize the postsynaptic action of ACh. Two facts indicate that AChE plays a critical part in the function of the neuromuscular junction. First, inhibition of AChE profoundly modifies neuromuscular transmission. This can be shown by electrophysiological analyses, by studies of the response of the muscle to nerve stimulation and by observations on muscular activity in the intact animal in the absence of applied nerve stimulation. Secondly, although normally there is no cellular uptake of ACh, as determined by analyses of perfusates of a muscle *in vivo* or of the bathing fluid surrounding an isolated nerve-muscle preparation, such uptake occurs when AChE is inhibited (see also MacIntosh and Collier, this volume, p. 117).

The decision on whether an effect on neuromuscular transmission is or is not due to inhibition of AChE is by no means always as simple as is often thought. Many substances are only capable of inhibiting AChE *in vitro* in concentrations or under conditions never obtained *in vivo* and thus AChE inhibition plays no part in their actions *in vivo*. Furthermore, even if a substance is shown to be capable of inhibiting AChE *in vitro* under conditions which might be applicable *in vivo*, it does not necessarily follow that the action *in vivo* is solely or largely due to inhibition of

AChE, since it is possible to mimic the consequences of AChE inhibition in a variety of ways. In this chapter the term anticholinesterase is used for those substances on which wide, although by no means uniform, agreement exists that their actions at the neuromuscular junction are at least largely the result of AChE inhibition. Typical representatives of this group of substances are carbamates such as physostigmine (eserine), neostigmine and pyridostigmine; substances closely related to carbamates such as ambenonium, an aminoalkylamide; organophosphates such as TEPP (tetra-ethyl pyrophosphate), DFP (diisopropylphosphorofluoridate; dyflos), paraoxon (die-thyl-4-nitrophenylphosphate), sarin (*isopropyl* methylphosphonofluoridate), or ta-bun (ethyl-N-dimethyl phosphoramidocyanidate) and the organophosphate insecti-cides. Effects at the neuromuscular junction comparable to those following the ad-ministration of the anticholinesterases mentioned are obtained with 3- and 4-hydroxyanilinium ions such as edrophonium (3-hydroxyphenyldimethylethyl-ammonium). However, it is much more difficult to show satisfactorily that the in *vivo* action of these substances, referred to in the text as anilinium ions, is the result of AChE inhibition than is the case with anticholinesterases of the carba-mate and organophosphate type. Therefore, without prejudging the issue, in this chapter the term anticholinesterase will not be used in conjunction with anilinium ions but they will be referred to separately.

Studies on anticholinesterases and anilinium ions have been carried out in many laboratories over a considerable period. Consequently, the number of papers pub-lished on the subject is enormous even when, as in this chapter, the field is narrowed to those aspects which are mainly pharmacological and concern the neuromuscular junction. Individual contributions to our knowledge before the 1960's have been collated in an extensive and thorough review by Werner and Kuperman (1963). Progress since then has been reviewed by Thesleff and Quastel (1965), Karczmar (1967), and Riker and Okamoto (1969). In addition, excellent comprehensive reviews have been written by Koelle and Gilman (1949), Holmstedt (1959) and Bowman and Webb (1972). In this chapter, therefore, no attempt was made at an extensive survey of the published literature on the classical actions of anticholinesterases. Instead the subject is covered on a broad basis with an emphasis on why it is sometimes difficult to be sure that an action at the neuromuscular junction is due to AChE inhibition. For this, some knowledge of the localisation and properties of AChE and of the essential features of the kinetics of AChE inhibition and the meaning of measurements of AChE inhibition is important. To this end a brief account of these basic aspects precedes a more detailed presentation of the actions of anticholinesterases and anilinium ions at the neuromuscular junction.

Much of the pioneer work on the physiology of neuromuscular transmission has been carried out on amphibian neuromuscular junctions (see Katz, 1966, 1969; Hubbard, 1970) but the number of truly pharmacological studies on the action of anticholinesterase drugs upon them is very limited and there has been no important contribution in this respect for quite some time. This chapter, therefore, deals with the actions of anticholinesterases at mammalian neuromuscular junctions and the data on amphibian muscle are summarised briefly in Appendix I. The Appendix also gives reasons why the widely adopted practice of using data obtained in the frog for interpreting results obtained in mammals is questionable. For a more detailed ac-count of the actions of anticholinesterase drugs on amphibian muscle the reviews by

WERNER and KUPERMAN (1963) and BOWMAN and WEBB (1972) which also give information on the actions of anticholinesterases on avian neuromuscular junctions should be consulted.

A final introductory comment on the mammalian neuromuscular junction itself is necessary (see also BOWDEN and DUCHEN, this volume, p. 27). Mammalian muscle fibres may be innervated focally, with the nerve terminals forming discrete ("en plaque") end-plates or multiply, with the nerve terminals forming small grape-like ("en grappe") end-plates (TIEGS, 1953). Most mammalian muscles contain only focally innervated muscle fibres and the actions of anticholinesterases and anilinium ions discussed in this chapter are those arising from an action at such sites. For results of studies of the actions of anticholinesterases at the neuromuscular junctions of multiply innervated fibres, the reviews by WERNER and KUPERMAN (1963) and BOWMAN and WEBB (1972) should be consulted.

B. Morphology and Function of Acetylcholinesterase (AChE)

I. Localization of AChE at the Motor End-Plate

That acetylcholinesterase is a component of the neuromuscular junction is readily demonstrated. Sections of muscle containing motor end-plates are incubated with a substrate for AChE which on hydrolysis by the enzyme yields a product that is itself coloured or by interacting with another substance produces a visible end product. When such sections are examined under a light microscope the end product (stain) can be seen to be concentrated at the motor end-plate whereas little of it is present in adjacent parts of the muscle (Fig. 1 a).

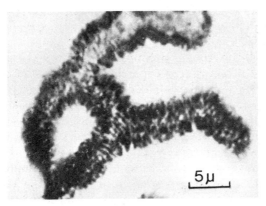

Fig. 1a. Histochemical staining of a motor end-plate in mouse intercostal muscle. Tissue sections fixed with formalin are incubated for 45 min at pH 4.7 with acetylthiocholine and $CuSO_4$. The stain is produced by the reaction of $CuSO_4$ with thiocholine (formed during the hydrolysis of acetylthiocholine by cholinesterases) to give Cu-thiocholine, and the subsequent conversion of Cu-thiocholine to CuS by H_2S. Although AChE and ChE are both present at motor end-plates and hydrolyse acetylthiocholine, the stain is predominantly the result of the action of AChE. Magnification × 1500. (From COUTEAUX and TAXI, 1952)

The ideal substrate for histochemical studies of AChE would be an ester which is hydrolysed by AChE alone. No such substrate exists and the substrates which are used are hydrolysed not only by AChE but also by at least one other type of esterase. The substrate which in the earlier studies has given the most useful information is acetylthiocholine, introduced by Koelle and Friedenwald (1949). In addition to AChE, one other enzyme found at the motor end-plate can hydrolyse both ACh and acetylthiocholine but as far as is known plays no role under physiological conditions in the hydrolysis of ACh released from the nerve terminals (Hawkins and Gunter, 1946; Heffron, 1972). This enzyme is nowadays called cholinesterase (acylcholine acyl-hydrolase; E.C. 3.1.1.8; ChE; see Section D IX). Its contribution to staining in histochemical studies of AChE can be largely eliminated by incubating the sections with the anticholinesterase DFP which inhibits ChE more readily than AChE and thus, when used for a short period, in low concentrations, e.g. 0.1 μmol/l, gives a fairly selective inhibition of ChE. Most of the substrates used are non-choline esters. Esterases other than AChE and ChE also contribute to the hydrolysis of the non-choline esters and information on AChE is usually obtained by comparing the differences in staining between sections treated with substrate, sections treated before addition of substrate with DFP to eliminate ChE and sections treated before addition of substrate with the anticholinesterase physostigmine which inhibits both AChE and ChE.

To pinpoint sites of AChE activity within the motor end-plate, the histochemical techniques have been modified to produce a stain which is easily located by electron microscopy.

Detailed information on the histochemical localisation of AChE is beyond the scope of this chapter and for this the reader is referred to the reviews by Koelle (1963b) and Koelle et al. (1967), the paper by Csillik and Knyihár (1968) and the references given therein.

Considerable information has been gained from the histochemical investigations. At the myoblast stage AChE is initially distributed diffusely throughout the cell but when the nerve terminal establishes functional contact with the muscle fibre, the enzyme becomes concentrated at the motor end-plate and to a much smaller extent at the musculo-tendinous junction (Kupfer and Koelle, 1951). Two morphological features characterise the motor end-plate. Firstly the axonal membrane of the nerve terminal (presynaptic membrane) indents the sarcoplasmic membrane (postsynaptic membrane; subneural apparatus) to form a synaptic gutter. Secondly, the sarco-plasmic membrane has deep secondary folds into which the axonal membrane does not enter (Andersson-Cedergren, 1959).

Histochemical studies show that the stain resulting from the hydrolysis of a substrate by AChE is more dense in the depth of the secondary sarcoplasmic mem-brane folds than in the vicinity of the presynaptic membrane (Fig. 1b; Barnett, 1962; Koelle, 1963b; Eränko and Teräväinen, 1967; Koelle et al., 1968; Csillik and Knyihár, 1968). This finding has led to the widely accepted conclusion that AChE is predominantly associated with the postsynaptic membrane.

The disadvantage of histochemical studies is that they do not locate the enzyme itself but the product of the hydrolysis of the substrate. Diffusion of the product away from the enzyme, together with factors which affect its site of deposition can lead to erroneous conclusions on the number of enzyme sites and their exact loca-tion. To obtain reliable quantitative information on AChE and its location, the enzyme itself must be located. This can be achieved by exposing the tissue to [³H]-

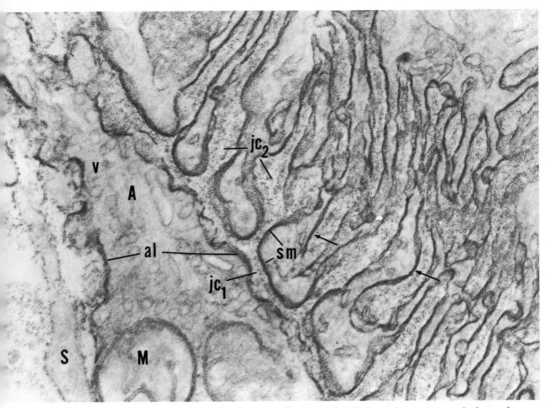

Fig. 1b. Electron microscopic histochemical localization of AChE at the motor end-plate of mouse intercostal muscle by the gold-thiolacetic method. Hydrolysis of acetyl disulfide by cholinesterases yields perthiolacetic acid which on reacting with a gold salt forms gold sulfide. Although both AChE and ChE hydrolyse acetyl disulfide the former is thought to contribute most to hydrolysis. The figure is a high magnification ($\times 63000$) view of the junctional complex, showing the axonal terminal (A) containing mitochondria (M) and numerous synaptic vesicles (v), the junctional cleft (jc), and junctional folds of the sarcolemma (sm). The electron-dense granules, 4 to 5 nm in diameter, consist of gold sulfide. The axolemma (al) exhibits marked enzymic activity both on the surface facing the primary junctional cleft (jc_1) and at the surface facing the teloglial Schwann cell sheath (S) (the axonal terminal is somewhat separated from the Schwann cell in this micrograph). Where the plane of section is perpendicular to the sarcolemma (arrows), the particles form a dense line about 12 to 14 nm in thickness. A few particles are also present in the primary (jc_1) and secondary (jc_2) junctional clefts possibly indicating some diffusion of the reaction product. (From KOELLE, 1971)

or $[^{32}P]$-DFP which combines with AChE to form labelled di*iso*propylphosphoryl-AChE (see Section C I), under conditions where the labelling of other esterases is excluded. Phosphorylation of AChE by DFP is irreversible and thus the number of enzyme sites and their location can be determined by a combination of electron microscopy and autoradiography. Studies of this type have been carried out by SALPETER (1967, 1969) and showed that at motor end-plates in mouse sternomastoid muscle 85% of AChE was located at the postsynaptic membrane and 10 to 15% was associated with the presynaptic membrane. Since the relationship between the surface areas of the pre- und post-synaptic membrane is about 1:10, the concentration of AChE in the two membranes is comparable. These results bring into question the widely held view that the role of AChE at the motor end-plate is solely to terminate the transmitter action of ACh. The enzyme could also be important in protecting the nerve terminals from the action of ACh.

II. Hydrolysis of ACh

Our knowledge of the active site(s) of mammalian AChE and its action on ACh is largely derived from *in vitro* studies on AChE in lysed erythrocytes and brain homogenates. These studies have shown that AChE seems to differ very little between species and between sites in the same species. The most important aspects of these studies are briefly summarised below (for details see Cohen and Oosterbaan, 1963):

Hydrolysis of ACh by AChE involves the sequence of reactions

$$
EH + ACh \longrightarrow EH.ACh \rightleftharpoons E.\underset{\substack{\| \\ O}}{C}{-}CH_3 \xrightarrow{+H_2O} EH \tag{1}
$$

$$
\searrow \qquad\qquad \searrow
$$

$$
\text{Choline} \qquad\qquad CH_3{-}COOH
$$

where EH is the protonated species of AChE and $E.\underset{\substack{\| \\ O}}{C}{-}CH_3$ is acetylated AChE.

The rate at which AChE hydrolyses ACh in low concentration increases with the substrate concentration until a concentration of approximately 3 mmol/l is reached and the K_M of ACh is 5×10^{-4}. Higher concentrations of ACh impede the deacylation of acetylated AChE and at concentrations above 3 mmol/l the rate of hydrolysis is inversely related to substrate concentration. Thus a bell-shaped curve is obtained when rate of hydrolysis is plotted against the logarithm of the substrate (ACh) concentration (Fig. 2). The rate of hydrolysis of ACh is also dependent upon pH, the optimum pH being 8.25, and upon the medium in the vicinity of the active site. For example, inorganic ions are capable of increasing or reducing activity depending on their concentration. Furthermore the rate of hydrolysis increases with temperature. These factors must influence to some extent the results obtained in studies of the actions of anticholinesterases carried out under different experimental conditions, but on the whole little notice has been taken of their influence.

Studies on human erythrocyte AChE suggest that a single AChE molecule consists of six subunits, each with one active site (Wright and Plummer, 1973). The turnover of ACh by AChE under conditions where the enzyme is saturated with and only marginally inhibited by substrate has been calculated to be of the order of 1.6 to 3.5×10^5 molecules ACh. min^{-1}: active enzyme site (subunit)$^{-1}$ (Berry, 1951; Cohen et al., 1955). For simplicity the terms AChE or AChE site will be used subsequently instead of the term subunit of the AChE molecule.

In the terminals of motor neurones ACh is stored in vesicles with a diameter of about 50 nm. Individual vesicles release their ACh content, known as a quantum of ACh, into the synaptic cleft at random intervals. The average width of the synaptic cleft is 50 nm. The ACh thus released gives rise to a miniature end-plate potential (m.e.p.p.) at the postsynaptic membrane. The m.e.p.p. has an amplitude of 0.5 to

1.5 mV and is a localised event which does not lead to a propagated muscle action potential. On the arrival of a nerve impulse the ACh content of about 300 vesicles (i.e. 300 quanta of ACh) is released, and this gives rise to the e.p.p. (BOYD and MARTIN, 1956b; HUBBARD et al., 1969b; BLABER, 1972). POTTER (1970) measured the ACh content in the rat isolated nerve-diaphragm preparation and from this and data on the number of motor end-plates in the preparation and the likely volume of the nerve terminals, calculated that the concentration of ACh in a single vesicle was 0.5 to 1 mol/l, i.e. one vesicle containing 4000 to 9000 molecules of ACh. He also measured the amounts of ACh released by 360 stimuli in the presence of neostigmine during stimulation of the phrenic nerve at frequencies of 1 to 20 Hz. The release of ACh amounted to 3.5 to 7×10^{-18} mol of ACh per motor end-plate per nerve impulse. If we divide this figure by the number of quanta of ACh (approximately 300) released by each nerve impulse the concentration of ACh in a single vesicle is of the order of 0.75 to 1.5 mol/l. Direct determination of the ACh content of vesicles, by bioassay for example, would give more reliable information but has as yet not been carried out. Studies on vesicles prepared from rat brain, which might be expected to resemble closely vesicles in motor nerve terminals, gave an ACh content of 1500 molecules per vesicle (WHITTAKER, 1965). The figures based on the data obtained by POTTER (1970) are thus likely to be over-estimates. However, even if we accept WHITTAKER's figure it is apparent that in spite of any dilution which might occur in the interval between the release of ACh from the nerve terminals and the time of its peak postsynaptic action, the initial concentration of ACh at postsynaptic cholinoceptors is likely to be in a range which according to *in vitro* studies inhibits its own enzymic hydrolysis to some extent (see Fig. 2).

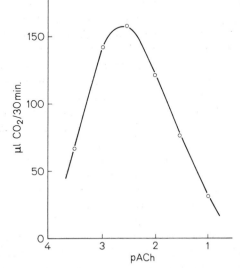

Fig. 2. Relationship between the rate of hydrolysis of ACh by AChE and the concentration of ACh. The data were obtained by the manometric (Warburg) method with haemolysed cow erythrocytes (100 μl) as the source of enzyme. Ordinate: rate of enzymic hydrolysis, expressed in μl CO_2/30 min. Abscissa: negative log of ACh concentration. (From AUGUSTINSSON, 1948)

Another factor which must be important for the hydrolysis of ACh at motor end-plates is the number of AChE sites and their concentration relative to that of cholinoceptors. As mentioned before, the number of AChE sites can be determined with labelled DFP. The number of cholinoceptors can be found by using α-bungarotoxin, which combines selectively and in a fairly stable manner with the cholinoceptors. Such studies have shown that in the mouse diaphragm the number of AChE sites per motor end-plate, determined by the binding of $[^{32}P]$- or $[^{3}H]$-DFP, is 2 to 3×10^7 (Waser and Reller, 1965; Barnard et al., 1971b), and the number of cholinoceptors, determined by the binding of ^{3}H-α bungarotoxin, is 3×10^7 (Barnard et al., 1971b). In the rat diaphragm the number of AChE sites, determined by the binding of $[^{32}P]$- or $[^{3}H]$-DFP, is 4.6×10^7 (Barnard et al., 1971a) and that of cholinoceptors, determined by the binding of $[^{131}I]$ or $[^{125}I]$-α-bungarotoxin, is 4 to 5×10^7 (Miledi and Potter, 1971; Fambrough and Hartzell, 1972). Barnard et al. (1971a) also showed that in a given species the number of AChE sites at individual motor end-plates of the same type of muscle is fairly constant but that there are twice as many sites at end-plates in white muscle as in red muscle.

These findings suggest that there are at least 10 AChE sites and 10 cholinoceptors available for each molecule of ACh released by a single nerve impulse. Thus, even if ACh initially reaches only 10% of the total postsynaptic area and its concentration is initially so high that it inhibits its own hydrolysis to some extent, AChE should still be able to lower the concentration of ACh at the cholinoceptors markedly within a millisecond, provided cholinoceptors and AChE sites are evenly distributed and the rates of hydrolysis determined *in vitro* apply. Furthermore, even if as many as 90% of the AChE sites are inhibited, there should still be sufficient uninhibited enzyme left for hydrolysis to proceed at a rate which prevents the accumulation of ACh released at random or by nerve impulses at low rates of nerve stimulation. While showing that AChE is certainly capable of playing a primary role in the hydrolysis of ACh at motor end-plates these calculations do not offer conclusive proof. The consequence of slowing down the hydrolysis of ACh should be a prolongation of both the m.e.p.p. and e.p.p., if AChE really has a primary and not a secondary role in removing ACh from the synaptic cleft. Information on this is given by studies of the consequences of inhibition of AChE on the time-course of the postsynaptic depolarisation produced by graded amounts of ACh released from nerve terminals, using intracellular recording in order to obtain a true measure of events at an individual motor end-plate. Such studies have been carried out on the rat isolated nerve-diaphragm preparation by Kuba and Tomita (1971) who stimulated the nerve terminals with graded currents in the presence of tetrodotoxin which by blocking channels for sodium transport restricts stimulation to the nerve terminals and prevents contraction of muscle fibres. In the absence of an anticholinesterase the amplitude of end-plate depolarisation was found to be proportional to the current applied whereas the half-decay times remained constant. When the anticholinesterase neostigmine was added to the preparation in a concentration sufficient to produce extensive inhibition of AChE according to *in vitro* data (3 μmol/l, i.e. 1 μg/ml), the magnitude of the end-plate depolarisation produced by a given current was increased and in addition the half-decay time was no longer constant but increased exponentially relative to the magnitude of the end-plate depolarisation. For example, in the presence of neostigmine, the half-decay time of an end-plate depolarisation with an amplitude of 20 mV was

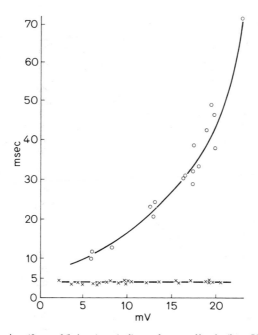

Fig. 3. Effect of neostigmine (3 μmol/l, i.e. 1 μg/ml) on the amplitude (in mV) and half-decay time (in msec) of e.p.p.s triggered by application of graded pulses to the nerve terminal in the rat isolated nerve-diaphragm preparation bathed in oxygenated Krebs solution containing 1 μg tetrodotoxin/ml. Crosses represent results in the absence of neostigmine and open circles results obtained in its presence. (From KUBA and TOMITA, 1971)

approximately ten times longer than that of the controls (see Fig. 3). These studies clearly support the view that AChE has a primary role in terminating the postsynaptic action of ACh but there must be some doubt as to whether the results are quantitatively fully applicable under different experimental conditions. When tubocurarine is used to prevent the initiation of the muscle action potential, it is found that neostigmine, 3 μmol/l, prolongs the half-decay time of the e.p.p. at mammalian motor end-plates elicited by nerve stimulation only 2 to 3 times, as assessed from intracellular recordings (BOYD and MARTIN, 1956b; BLABER and CHRIST, 1967). It is also known that at motor end-plates in frog muscle neostigmine markedly prolongs the e.p.p. when the extracellular sodium concentration is low (FATT and KATZ, 1951; KORDAS, 1968). This work has not been repeated for mammalian muscle, but indicates that the presence of tetrodotoxin in the experiments of KUBA and TOMITA (1971) might have reduced the rate of sodium flux at the motor end-plate and that this exaggerated the effect of AChE inhibition on the half-decay time of end-plate depolarisations.

Neostigmine, in a concentration of 3 μmol/l increases the size of m.e.p.p.s 2 to 3 fold, as shown by studies on the cat isolated tenuissimus nerve-muscle preparation (BOYD and MARTIN, 1956a; BLABER and CHRIST, 1967). In studies on the rat isolated nerve-diaphragm preparation, HALL and KELLY (1971) showed that 3 μmol/l neostigmine doubled the half-decay time of m.e.p.p.s and that the same effect was obtained when the diaphragm was treated with collagenase, which renders AChE soluble and thus reduces its concentration at the motor end-plate. When collagenase-treated diaphragms were exposed to neostigmine a 30% increase only in the half-decay time of the m.e.p.p. was seen.

Several conclusions can be drawn from these findings. AChE indeed plays a primary role in the removal of ACh from the synaptic cleft and limits both the intensity and duration of its postsynaptic action. Since in the absence of an anticholinesterase the half-decay time of end-plate depolarisations is independent of the number of vesicles which release their ACh content into the synaptic cleft (Kuba and Tomita, 1971), each vesicle which contributes to the e.p.p. produced by a nerve impulse appears to release its ACh content into an area which contains more than enough AChE to prevent diffusion of the ester in an effective concentration to neighbouring areas affected by ACh released from other vesicles. Even when AChE is extensively inhibited, diffusion of ACh together with hydrolysis by uninhibited enzyme is still sufficient to terminate the postsynaptic action of ACh so that it does not accumulate, provided nerve stimulation proceeds at a low rate. The results of Kuba and Tomita might overestimate the effect of AChE inhibition but a 2 to 3 fold prolongation of the half-decay time of the e.p.p. would still be sufficient to lead to an accumulation of ACh at the postsynaptic site not only at high rates of nerve stimulation (50 or 100 Hz) but also at physiological rates (about 10 to 30 Hz).

It is widely assumed that inhibition of AChE necessarily leads to an increase in the amplitude and duration of the e.p.p. As shown by Blaber and Christ (1967) and Blaber (1972) neostigmine, ambenonium and edrophonium, in a certain range of concentrations, and in the presence of tubocurarine can increase the amplitude of the e.p.p. without affecting its time-course. The question therefore arises whether this effect is due to an increase in the quantal release of ACh by a direct action rather than by inhibition of AChE. There are no detailed studies on the relationship between graded levels of AChE inhibition and their effect on the e.p.p. In view of the high concentration of AChE at motor end-plates it is possible that lower levels of AChE inhibition only affect the early part of the e.p.p., giving rise to an increase in the amplitude of the e.p.p. and perhaps in the duration of the peak depolarisation without any effect on the duration of the e.p.p. This would still mean that the area of distribution of ACh is increased and consequently could allow ACh to reach nerve terminals and by an action there increase the quantal release of ACh. In the case of edrophonium and other anilinium ions it is also possible that, for kinetic reasons, the inhibition of AChE relative to that produced by anticholinesterases has a more pronounced effect on the amplitude of the e.p.p. than on its duration (see Section C I). Until there is evidence against these views it seems premature to conclude that if a substance in certain concentrations exerts neuromuscular actions but affects only the amplitude but not the duration of the e.p.p. that these actions are not a consequence of AChE inhibition.

Diffusion of ACh away from cholinoceptors undoubtedly is an essential contributory factor in the termination of its transmitter action but calculations aimed to show that this process might suffice on its own (Ogston, 1955; Eccles and Jaeger, 1958) fail to take into consideration the existence of cholinoceptors in the pathway of diffusion and their progressive saturation with ACh.

C. Inhibition of AChE

It is difficult to determine the exact level of inhibition of AChE *in vivo* and its time-course. Furthermore, the location of the AChE sites which are inhibited is more important than their total number. An understanding of the kinetics of inhibition by different substances and of the meaning of measurements of inhibition is essential to the proper interpretation of experimental results.

I. Kinetics of Inhibition of AChE

The active site of AChE consists of an anionic (negatively charged) site and an esteratic site which must be in a protonated form to be active. Inhibition of the hydrolysis of ACh by AChE [see reaction (1)] can be accomplished either by revers-ible occupation of the active site of the enzyme by another substance or by acylation of its esteratic site. The principal kinetic features of these two types of inhibition are well established and for detailed accounts on them the reader is referred to the reviews by DAVIES and GREEN (1958), O'BRIEN (1960), HEATH (1961), COHEN and OOSTERBAAN (1963), HEILBRONN (1967) and ALDRIGE and REINER (1972).

Reversible Inhibition. Substances producing this type of inhibition interact with the enzyme in a truly reversible manner

$$EH + I \rightleftharpoons EH.I \tag{2}$$

where I is the inhibitor and ACh competes with it. Under the experimental condi-tions used *in vitro* an equilibrium between EH, I and ACh is established quickly (Fig. 4). Consequently the level of enzyme inhibition obtained with a given concen-tration of I is inversely related to the concentration of ACh and inhibition is readily reversed by dilution. *In vivo*, inhibition initially will be for a very short period of time non-competitive and thus greater than expected from *in vitro* data on inhibition.

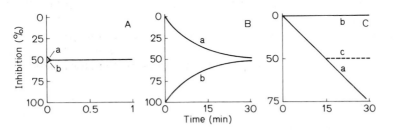

Fig. 4A–C. Inhibition of AChE by (A) edrophonium and other anilinium ions, (B) carbamates such as neostigmine or physostigmine and (C) organophosphates such as TEPP, paraoxon or DFP. In (A) and (B): (a) represents inhibition if ACh is added to the enzyme jointly with or before the inhibitor; (b) represents inhibition if the inhibitor is added to the enzyme several minutes before the addition of ACh. The horizontal line represents the equilibrium state, which is shifted downwards when the concentration of ACh is decreased. The opposite applies when inhibitor concentration is decreased. For (C): (a) inhibition in the absence of ACh; (b) ACh added before the inhibitor; (c) ACh added to enzyme 15 min after inhibitor. Ordinate: % inhibition. Abscissa: time in min

Consequently its effect on the amplitude of the e.p.p. and possibly on the duration of the peak depolarisation could be greater than the effect on the duration of the e.p.p.

No useful quantitative information can be obtained on AChE inhibition *in vivo* by measurements of the enzyme activity of tissues removed after the administration of a reversible inhibitor because of the ease with which inhibition is reversed by dilution and by substrate. On the other hand, a good correlation between the concentrations at which closely related reversible inhibitors produce equal degrees of inhibition *in vitro* and the doses which give comparable effects *in vivo*, is consistent with the view that such substances can act by virtue of AChE inhibition.

Reversible inhibitors of AChE which are relevant in the context of this chapter are the halides of 3- and 4-hydroxyphenyltrialkylammonium. They are referred to as anilinium ions. A typical representative of them is edrophonium (3-hydroxyphenyl-dimethylethylammonium) which has been used in pharmacological studies to a much greater extent than the other anilinium ions. The concentration of edrophonium which inhibits by 50% AChE (of human erythrocytes) in the presence of 0.03 mol/l substrate is 16 µmol/l (4 µg/ml) (HOBBIGER, 1952). Under non-competitive conditions 0.16 µmol/l would give approximately the same inhibition.

Inhibition by Acylation. Acetylcholinesterase not only hydrolyses ACh [see reaction (1)] but also interacts with carbamates and organophosphates in an analogous manner forming carbamylated and phosphorylated AChE, respectively. The deacylation (so-called spontaneous reactivation) of acetylated AChE at 37° C takes less than 0.1 msec (COHEN et al., 1955). With carbamylated and phosphorylated AChE the deacylation reaction is very much slower and until it has taken place the enzyme cannot hydrolyse ACh, i.e. it is inhibited.

Carbamates which have been studied in greatest detail and which in the absence of ACh inhibit AChE in concentrations below 0.1 µmol/l, have the general structure

$$R_3-O-\underset{\underset{O}{\|}}{C}-N\underset{R_2}{\overset{R_1}{<}}$$

where R_1 is H or an alkyl group, R_2 an alkyl group and R_3 usually an aromatic group with a tertiary or quaternary nitrogen.

Typical representatives of this type of carbamate are physostigmine, a monomethyl-carbamate ($R_1 = H$; $R_2 = CH_3$), and neostigmine and pyridostigmine, two dimethyl-carbamates (R_1 and $R_2 = CH_3$).

The deacylation of carbamylated AChE, i.e. the rate of spontaneous reactivation,

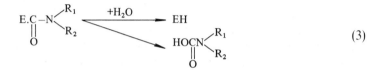

$$(3)$$

is determined by R_1 and R_2 and thus is identical for all carbamates which form the same type of carbamylated AChE. As shown by REINER and ALDRIDGE (1967), using bovine erythrocyte AChE, at pH 8 and 25° C, 50% of monomethylcarbamyl-AChE

($R_1 = H$; $R_2 = CH_3$; formed by physostigmine) undergoes spontaneous reactivation in 30 min. The corresponding value for dimethylcarbamyl-AChE (R_1 and $R_2 = CH_3$; formed by neostigmine and pyridostigmine) is 57 min. The rate of spontaneous reactivation is also dependent on pH, and is halved by lowering the pH from 8 to 7.

An analysis of the individual steps of the reaction between AChE and carbamates shows that rates of formation of the carbamylated enzyme from the enzyme-carbamate complex are very similar for different carbamates; thus the affinity of a carbamate for the enzyme plays the most important part in determining the relative anticholinesterase potency of carbamates which form the same type of carbamylated AChE (O'BRIEN, 1967). Carbamates with exceptionally high anticholinesterase potency have been obtained by joining two molecules of neostigmine, linking the C_5 ring carbons with an O-$(CH_2)_3$-O group (compound 3113 CT; FUNKE et al., 1954), or joining the carbamyl nitrogens of two molecules of neostigmine or pyridostigmine with a polymethylene bridge (BC compounds; also called *bis*neostigmines and *bis*pyridostigmines; KRAUPP et al., 1955). The compound 3113 CT forms dimethylcarbamyl-AChE and with BC compounds the ensuing type of carbamylated AChE is characterised by a rate of spontaneous reactivation which is only 1 to 3% of that of dimethylcarbamyl-AChE (WILSON et al., 1961). In both cases marked inhibition of AChE in the absence of ACh can be obtained with concentrations below 1 nmol/l.

ACh competes with carbamates for AChE but does not affect decarbamylation. Thus, when AChE is incubated with a carbamate and ACh is added subsequently, the level of inhibition progressively declines at a rate dependent on the type of carbamylated enzyme involved until an equilibrium is reached between carbamylation and decarbamylation. The reverse, progressive inhibition until the equilibrium is reached, occurs if a carbamate is added to the enzyme after ACh (Fig. 4). In both situations, as with reversible inhibition, the level of the equilibrium is a function of the concentrations of ACh and carbamate. The level of inhibition obtained in an individual experiment varies according to which time interval, after addition of ACh to the enzyme, is chosen for recording enzyme activity and the order in which ACh and carbamate are added to the enzyme if measurements involve periods before an equilibrium is reached.

In vivo the rates of decarbamylation are too slow to enable the ACh released by a single nerve impulse to affect the level of enzyme inhibition but if a nerve is stimulated for more than several minutes at high frequencies some reversal of inhibition should occur even if the carbamate is still present at the site. As in the case of reversible inhibitors, the inhibition produced *in vivo* by mono- and di-methylcarbamates, the most widely studied carbamates, cannot be determined by assay of the AChE activity of tissues removed subsequent to their administration because of spontaneous reactivation under the assay conditions. A point also worthwhile mentioning in this context is that the enzyme-carbamate complex which precedes carbamylation (O'BRIEN, 1967) itself represents inhibition and thus can contribute to the effects seen *in vivo* in the early stages after the administration of a carbamate.

If carbamates produce their effects *in vivo* by AChE inhibition it is unlikely that with different carbamates the anticholinesterase potencies *in vitro* will be linearly related to the doses which are equiactive *in vivo*, unless the volumes of distribution *in vivo* and concentration: time profiles at neuromuscular junctions are very similar and differences between rates of spontaneous reactivation of the carbamylated AChEs involved are not too great.

A number of substances which are not carbamates but aminoalkylamides have *in vitro* an anticholinesterase potency approaching or even exceeding that of neostigmine. The exact mechanism by which they inhibit AChE is not known but since the nature and time-course of their action *in vivo* closely resemble those of mono- and dimethylcarbamates, their actions are best considered with those of the carbamates. The aminoalkylamide whose effect on neuromuscular transmission has been studied most widely is ambenonium (Mytelase; WIN 8077) (Lands et al., 1958).

For a detailed account of the relationship between the structure of carbamates and the inhibition of AChE the reader is referred to the review by Long (1963) which also deals with inhibitors of AChE which are neither carbamates nor organophosphates.

Organophosphates which act as anticholinesterases either inhibit AChE in their own right or in the case of the so-called organophosphate insecticides become inhibitors as the result of their metabolism by hepatic enzymes (see Mounter, 1963; DuBois, 1963). The former and the active metabolite of the latter have the general structure

where R_1 represents a variety of groups which may be linked to the phosphorus either directly or through oxygen, nitrogen or sulphur, R_2 is usually an alkoxygroup and X is an acyl radicle (Holmstedt, 1959, 1963).

The most widely studied organophosphates are the dialkylphosphates. They are anticholinesterases in their own right, have an alkoxygroup in the R_1 and R_2 position and comprise

dimethylphosphates (R_1 and $R_2 = OCH_3$), e.g. methylparaoxon (dimethyl-4-nitrophenylphosphate),

diethylphosphates (R_1 and $R_2 = OC_2H_5$), e.g. TEPP (tetraethyl pyrophosphate) and paraoxon (diethyl-4-nitrophenylphosphate), and

diisopropylphosphates (R_1 and $R_2 = OC_3H_7$), e.g. DFP (diisopropyl phosphorofluoridate; dyflos).

Two widely used organophosphate insecticides which must be metabolised before they act as anticholinesterase and whose active metabolite is a dialkylphosphate are

parathion (diethyl-4-nitrophenyl phosphorothioate), the active metabolite of which is the oxygen analogue paraoxon) and

malathion (dimethyl-S-(1,2-dicarboxymethyl) phosphorodithioate), the active metabolite of which is also the oxygen analogue ($\overset{\parallel}{\underset{O}{P}}$ instead of $\overset{\parallel}{\underset{S}{P}}$).

Other organophosphates which have been studied in detail and which are anticholinesterases in their own right are

sarin (*isopropyl* methylphosphonofluoridate; $R_1 = OC_3H_7$, $R_2 = CH_3$) and tabun [ethyl-N-dimethyl phosphoramidocyanidate; $R_1 = OC_2H_5$, $R_2 = N(CH_3)_2$].

The reaction between AChE and organophosphates which are anticholinesterases in their own right or the active metabolites of organophosphate insecticides is analogous to the hydrolysis of ACh [see reaction (1)]. It yields phosphorylated AChE. The fate of phosphorylated AChE is more complex than that of acetylated or carbamylated AChE, both of which only undergo hydrolysis by water to give the active enzyme (spontaneous reactivation). Phosphorylated AChE is subject to two reactions

$$\text{spontaneous reactivation} \quad \text{E.P} \overset{R_1}{\underset{\overset{\|}{O}}{\diagdown}} R_2 \quad \xrightarrow{+H_2O} \quad \text{EH} + \text{HO-P} \overset{R_1}{\underset{\overset{\|}{O}}{\diagdown}} R_2 \tag{4}$$

and

$$\text{ageing process} \quad \text{E.P} \overset{R_1}{\underset{\overset{\|}{O}}{\diagdown}} R_2 \quad \xrightarrow{+H_2O} \quad \text{E.P} \overset{OH}{\underset{\overset{\|}{O}}{\diagdown}} R_2 + R_1H \tag{5}$$

(R$_1$ is an alkoxy group)

which occur concurrently but proceed at greatly differing rates with individual types of phosphorylated AChE. The rates of spontaneous reactivation and ageing are similar *in vivo* to those obtained at 37° C and pH 7—7.5 *in vitro*. Typical values are shown in Table 1.

In the absence of enzymes capable of inactivating anticholinesterases of the organophosphate type (see MOUNTER, 1963) the time-course of phosphorylation of AChE *in vitro* follows first order kinetics (Fig. 4). An exception to this are organophosphates which form dimethylphosphoryl-AChE. In their case spontaneous reactivation is sufficiently fast (see Table 1) to cause a deviation of the time-course of inhibi-

Table 1. Spontaneous reactivation and ageing of various types of phosphorylated AChE

	Time in hours for 50%	
	spontaneous reactivation	ageing
Dimethylphosphoryl—AChE	1.2—2 [1, 2]	7 [7]
Diethylphosphoryl—AChE	44—64 [2—6]	41 [6]
Di*iso*propylphosphoryl—AChE	no measurable	4 [6]
*Iso*propyl methylphosphonyl—AChE	spontaneous	3 [8]
Phosphorylated AChE formed by tabun	reactivation	14 [9]

References

1. ALDRIDGE (1953), pH 7.8, rabbit erythrocytes.
2. VANDEKAR and HEATH (1957), *in vivo*, rat erythrocytes.
3. BURGEN and HOBBIGER (1951), pH 7.4, human erythrocytes.
4. HOBBIGER (1951), pH 7.4, human and guinea pig erythrocytes.
5. BLABER and CREASEY (1960), pH 7.4 and *in vivo*, sheep erythrocytes.
6. HOBBIGER (1956), pH 7.4, bovine erythrocytes.
7. HOBBIGER (1968), pH 7.4, human erythrocytes.
8. DAVIES and GREEN (1956), pH 7.4, human erythrocytes.
9. HEILBRONN (1963), pH 7.4, human erythrocytes.
Values for other types of phosphorylated AChE have been catalogued by ALDRIDGE and REINER (1972).

tion from first order kinetics under experimental conditions generally used in inhibi-tion studies.

The rate of formation of phosphorylated AChE is fast relative to the rate of formation of the enzyme-organophosphate complex and thus the affinity of the organophosphate for the enzyme is the most important factor determining anticho-linesterase potency. Acetylcholine competes with organophosphates for AChE and thus reduces the rate of phosphorylation.

Many organophosphates are speedily metabolised to inert products by enzymes such as phosphoryl phosphatases (Mounter, 1963). The phosphatases are present in the liver and other organs and also in blood, and when crude enzyme preparations, such as lysed erythrocytes, are used for *in vitro* studies on inhibition the presence of these enzymes can modify the time-course of inhibition. *In vivo* the rate of inactiva-tion is not constant for different organophosphates and the volume of distribution can also vary. Therefore, the rates of phosphorylation of AChE obtained with differ-ent organophosphates *in vitro* are unlikely to be an accurate guide to the doses required to produce equal effects *in vivo*.

However, organophosphates such as DFP, sarin and tabun which inhibit AChE irreversibly, and diethylphosphates such as TEPP and paraoxon, are suitable for studying the correlation between the number of AChE sites inhibited *in vivo* and the effects produced, provided precautions are taken to minimize spontaneous reactiva-tion of diethylphosphoryl-AChE during preparation of the tissue and while assess-ment of AChE activity is being carried out.

Certain types of phosphorylated AChE, provided they have not undergone age-ing, can be dephosphorylated, i.e. reactivated, by nucleophilic substances such as pralidoxime (N-methylpyridinium-2-aldoxime) and *bis*quaternary pyridinium aldo-ximes, e.g. TMB-4 (N,N-trimethylene *bis*(pyridinium-4-aldoxime) and obidoxime (N,N-oxydimethylene *bis*(pyridinium-4-aldoxime) in concentrations which are ob-tainable *in vivo* (see Hobbiger, 1963, 1968; Ellin and Wills, 1964). The active form of the oximes is the anion and reactivation proceeds as follows

$$\text{E.P}\underset{\overset{\|}{O}}{\overset{R_1}{\underset{R_2}{<}}} + \text{RCHNO}^- \longrightarrow \text{E} + \text{RCHNOP}\underset{\overset{\|}{O}}{\overset{R_1}{\underset{R_2}{<}}} \tag{6}$$

where RCHNO$^-$ is the oxime anion.

The rate of reactivation by oximes depends on the type of phosphorylated AChE. It is highest with dialkylphosphoryl-AChEs (diethylphosphoryl-AChE > dimethyl-phosphoryl-AChE > di*iso*propylphosphoryl-AChE) and *iso*propyl methylphospho-nyl AChE. The rate of reactivation is much slower with the phosphorylated AChE formed by tabun and no reactivation can be obtained if AChE is inhibited by organophosphates such as the methylfluorophosphorylcholines (Enander, 1958) or OMPA (octamethylpyrophosphortetramide; Kewitz, 1975).

Rates of reactivation *in vitro* by pralidoxime follow first order kinetics but the phosphorylated oximes formed by TMB-4 and by obidoxime, rephosphorylate to some extent AChE and this leads to a curtailment of reactivation with time. Rephos-phorylation is prevented by the presence of ACh and under such conditions TMB-4 is approximately twenty times more potent as a reactivator of a given type of dialkylphosphoryl-AChE than is pralidoxime (HOBBIGER et al., 1960). This difference is less for other types of phosphorylated AChE (see HOBBIGER, 1963). Results with obidoxime are very similar to those obtained with TMB-4 (HOBBIGER and VOJVODIĆ, 1966).

The aged forms of all types of phosphorylated AChE cannot be reactivated by oximes (HOBBIGER, 1963).

For a detailed account of the relationship between the structure of organophosphates and the inhibition of AChE the reader is referred to the reviews by HOLMSTEDT (1959, 1963).

II. Measurements of the in vivo Inhibition of AChE

Since the kinetics of AChE inhibition differ between groups of inhibitors, there is no universally applicable *in vitro* method for obtaining values of relative anticholinesterase potency which would reflect the relative activity *in vivo*, even if the actions are solely due to AChE inhibition. Only when the kinetics of inhibition are identical in all respects and the substances have the same volume of distribution and concentration: time profile at the neuromuscular junction, can studies of relative anticholinesterase potency *in vitro* provide information which would help decide whether actions *in vivo* can be the result of AChE inhibition. This is also true for studies comparing anticholinesterase potency *in vitro* with relative activity in isolated muscle preparations.

The most conclusive evidence that an effect at the neuromuscular junction *in vivo* and in isolated muscle preparations is the consequence of AChE inhibition is a correlation between the enzyme inhibition and its time-course, as determined by assay of the AChE activity of tissues, and the pharmacological effect and its time-course. The reversal of inhibition by dilution and substrate precludes this type of study with reversible inhibitors such as edrophonium and with mono- or di-methylcarbamates. On the whole, the view is taken that neuromuscular effects arise from AChE inhibition if in the absence of substrate a substance inhibits AChE *in vitro* in concentrations which are likely to be obtained *in vivo*, intensifies and prolongs the action of exogenous ACh, and itself has actions which can be explained by a prolongation of the action of ACh released from nerve terminals (see KOELLE, 1963a; HOBBIGER, 1964). The prototype of such a substance is the alkaloid physostigmine (eserine) which has played a unique role in the elucidation of neuromuscular transmission. An analysis of the role of the various groups of the physostigmine molecule in the inhibition of AChE has led to the synthesis of many potent anticholinesterases (STEDMAN and BARGER, 1925; STEDMAN, 1926; AESCHLIMANN and REINERT, 1931; KOELLE and GILMAN, 1949; LONG, 1963; HOLMSTEDT, 1972).

Inhibition of AChE at motor end-plates and its relation to the actions of anticholinesterases can be investigated with organophosphates like DFP which inhibit AChE irreversibly, or with diethylphosphates such as TEPP or paraoxon, provided spontaneous reactivation of diethylphosphoryl-AChE is negligible under the experimental conditions. The difficulty here lies in obtaining values for inhibition which are applicable to those AChE sites which ACh encounters after its release from nerve terminals. In many studies inhibition has been determined by measuring the AChE activity of homogenates of muscles treated with DFP or a diethylphosphate and expressing the result as a percentage of the AChE activity of homogenates from control muscles. Doubt about the general validity of such measurements has arisen because of results obtained in experiments with quaternary anticholinesterases. In 1959, McIsaac and Koelle showed that in equiactive doses the quaternary anticholinesterase phospholine (diethyl-S-(2-trimethylammoniumethyl) phosphorothioate; echothiophate), which forms diethylphosphoryl-AChE, produced much less inhibition of AChE in the superior cervical ganglion of the cat than was obtained with its tertiary analogue. From these results and similar findings in earlier studies on the central nervous system (Burgen and Chipman, 1952; Koelle and Steiner, 1956) it was concluded that cholinergic synapses have two fractions of AChE; a surface-located fraction which is readily accessible to ACh released from nerve terminals and to quaternary anticholinesterases, and a second fraction which is located intracellularly, and does not participate in the hydrolysis of ACh released from nerve terminals and is not affected by quaternary anticholinesterases (McIsaac and Koelle, 1959; see Koelle, 1963b). As proposed by Koelle and his co-workers the two fractions of AChE are now generally described as *functional* and *reserve* AChE, respectively. The AChE activity of tissue homogenates represents the combined activity of functional and reserve AChE and is called *total* AChE activity.

Obviously information on the inhibition of functional AChE would be more useful than information on the inhibition of total AChE. To measure functional AChE activity the assumption is made that a quaternary substrate for AChE which reaches the synaptic cleft by diffusion gains access only to those AChE sites which are reached by ACh released from the nerve terminals. Therefore, functional AChE activity is determined by incubating intact tissue, such as a rat isolated diaphragm in a medium containing a quaternary substrate for AChE. The rate of uptake of the substrate by the tissue or the rate of appearance of a metabolite of the substrate in the incubation medium are then determined and taken as a measure of functional

Table 2. Measurement of Functional AChE activity. The rat isolated diaphragm is incubated in a medium containing a quaternary substrate for AChE and enzyme activity is determined from the rate of disappearance of substrate from the medium or the rate of appearance of the enzymic metabolite in the medium

Substrate in Medium	Measurement	Authors
ACh, 0.125 mmol/l or less	Rate of uptake of ACh by the diaphragm determined by bioassay on anticholinesterase treated frog rectus preparation	Fleisher et al. (1960)
1 μmol/l ACh or 5 μmol/l acetyl-β-methylcholine[a] with a ^{14}C-choline label	Rate of uptake of the labelled substrate by the diaphragm determined by scintillation counting	Mittag et al. (1971)
1 mmol/l acetylthiocholine	Rate of appearance of the enzymic metabolite thiocholine, determined colourimetrically by the method of Ellman et al. (1961)	Lancaster (1972)

[a] Acetyl-β-methylcholine is a selective substrate for AChE. Ach and acetylthiocholine are hydrolysed by AChE and ChE but at concentrations of 1 mmol/l and less the contribution of ChE to their hydrolysis at motor end-plates is well below 10% and from a practical point of view the two esters are selective substrates for AChE.

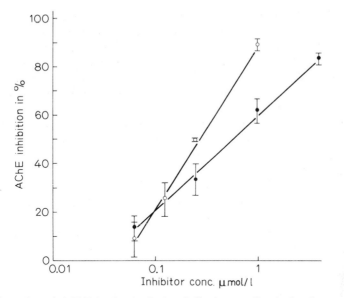

Fig. 5. Inhibition of total AChE in the rat isolated diaphragm. Rat isolated nerve-diaphragm preparations were incubated for 20 min at 37° C in Tyrode solution containing the quaternary anticholinesterase pinacolyl-S-(2-trimethylammoniumethyl) methylphosphonothioate (●) or its tertiary derivative (○) in the concentrations shown. Results are presented as means ±S.E.M.($n = 4$). (From LANCASTER, 1973)

AChE activity (see Table 2). Inhibition of functional AChE in tissues which have previously been treated with an anticholinesterase is calculated in the same way as that of total AChE and represents the ratio $a/b \times 100\%$, where a is the AChE activity of a tissue from an animal treated with an anticholinesterase, and b that from a control animal.

From studies of functional AChE MITTAG et al. (1971) concluded that in the rat diaphragm only 20% of the total number of AChE sites at motor end-plates are functional AChE sites and the K_M of ACh for functional AChE is 1.05×10^{-3}, i.e. about double the values observed with muscle homogenates. An even higher K_M value for ACh, 3.1×10^{-3}, was obtained in studies of the functional AChE at motor end-plates in muscle membranes isolated from the rat tibialis anterior muscle (NAMBA and GROB, 1968).

Before accepting that this method does in fact determine functional AChE, we must consider some pertinent evidence.

A situation identical to that used for measuring functional AChE exists when in the rat isolated nerve-diaphragm preparation we add ACh to the bathing fluid and study its effect on twitch tension. If ACh can penetrate in an effective concentration into the synaptic cleft of the muscle fibres it will reduce twitch tension by persistent depolarisation of the end-plate areas. The experimental data (HOBBIGER and HEFFRON, unpublished) show that concentrations of ACh which will reduce twitch tension are very similar to those of choline necessary to produce the same effect. Inhibition of AChE, however, markedly increases the effectiveness of ACh only. This suggests that in normal muscle ACh does not diffuse into the entire synaptic cleft but is completely hydrolysed at its outer region so that effective penetration to cholino-ceptors can only occur when AChE is inhibited.

LANCASTER (1972, 1973) in studies of the inhibition of AChE, determined on homogenates, found that in the rat isolated nerve-diaphragm preparation the addition to the bathing fluid of a quaternary anticholinesterase [pinacolyl-S-(2-trimethyl-ammoniumethyl) methylphosphonothioate] which forms a very stable phosphory-lated AChE, produced an inhibition of AChE which followed first order kinetics. Furthermore, it was found that when graded concentrations of the quaternary anti-cholinesterase were added to the bathing fluid for a fixed period, the level of inhibition increased steadily with the anticholinesterase concentration, i.e. did not remain constant over any range of the latter (Fig. 5). Therefore, functional and reserve AChE are not in two separate compartments. That ACh behaves like a quaternary anticho-linesterase and is likely to reach all AChE sites when sufficient AChE is inhibited, is indicated by the findings of POTTER (1970) and ADAMIČ (1970). These authors showed that in the rat diaphragm treated with an anticholinesterase, ACh, added to the incubation medium, is taken up by the nerve terminals and muscle fibres, whereas no such uptake occurs in control preparations.

Finally, there is evidence that the access of quaternary substances to the synaptic cleft is restricted. In his studies on the rat isolated nerve-diaphragm preparation, LANCASTER (1973) observed that when the quaternary anticholinesterase and its tertiary analogue were added in equal concentrations to the bathing fluid for a fixed period, the former produced less inhibition of AChE although the reverse applied to rates of phosphorylation of erythrocyte AChE. The most likely site at which diffu-sion of the quaternary anticholinesterase into the synaptic cleft is impeded is at the layer of serosa cells covering the muscle.

These findings suggest that in determinations of functional AChE there is impeded entry of substrate into the motor end-plate and a gradient in substrate concentration from the outer to the inner parts of the synaptic cleft. In normal muscle the gradient is steep but this is reduced when AChE is inhibited. Thus in normal muscle the contribution made by individual enzyme sites to substrate hy-drolysis is not constant but progressively decreases towards the centre of the synap-tic cleft, and when AChE is inhibited more enzyme sites are involved than in a control tissue. Therefore, the percentage inhibition calculated from functional AChE measurements, as opposed to total AChE measurements, is not a measure of the percentage of AChE sites inhibited and is best referred to as the percentage reduction of functional AChE activity.

Measurements of total AChE and of functional AChE activity can give useful information if interpreted correctly, and data on their inhibition will be referred to in the survey of the actions of anticholinesterases and of anilinium ions. The main limitation of total AChE measurements appears to be that in the case of quaternary inhibitors they will underestimate the level of enzyme inhibition at those AChE sites which ACh released from nerve terminals actually encounters. The factors determin-ing functional AChE activity seem to be the same as those which determine the removal of ACh released from nerve terminals and the percentage inhibition of functional AChE activity thus should be equivalent to the percentage reduction in the rate of removal (by hydrolysis and diffusion) from the postsynaptic membrane of

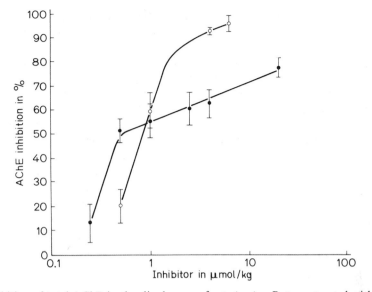

Fig. 6. Inhibition of total AChE in the diaphragm of rats *in vivo*. Rats pretreated with atropine were injected subcutaneously with the quaternary anticholinesterase pinacolyl-S-(2-trimethylammoniumethyl) methylphosphonothioate (●) or its tertiary derivative (○) in the doses shown. The figure shows the levels of AChE inhibition 30 min after injection of the anticholinesterase drugs, presented as means ± S.E.M. (*n* = 3 or more). (From LANCASTER, 1972)

ACh released from nerve terminals. Furthermore, data on the functional AChE activity should be equally valid with quaternary and non-quaternary anticholinesterases. However, AChE at the periphery of the synaptic cleft seems to be mainly responsible for functional AChE activity and anticholinesterases will also reach this area before they get to the more central parts of the synaptic cleft. This could mean that an assessment of the inhibition of functional AChE activity could overestimate the percentage reduction in the rate of removal of ACh released from nerve terminals.

A question which still remains to be answered is whether the accessibility of AChE at different sites of the motor end-plate is the same *in vivo* as in isolated muscle preparations. As shown by LANCASTER (1972, 1973) in the rat isolated nerve-diaphragm preparation a quaternary anticholinesterase can gain access to all AChE sites suggesting that there are no fixed compartments of functional and reserve AChE. Studies *in vivo* (LANCASTER, 1972) however showed that only approximately 50 to 60% of the AChE sites in the rat diaphragm are reached easily by a quaternary anticholinesterase (see Fig. 6). If this is applicable to other neuromuscular junctions also, then measurements of functional AChE activity might to some extent be misleading as to the consequences of AChE inhibition on the removal of ACh released from nerve terminals *in vivo*. The same might apply to the transfer to *in vivo* situations of results obtained on isolated muscle preparations in general.

The validity of conclusions drawn from studies of AChE inhibition might also depend on whether the enzyme is in fact located mainly at motor end-plates. According to studies by Buckley and Nowell (1966) this is the case in the rat diaphragm where 85% of the enzyme is at the motor end-plate. However, according to Namba and Grob (1968) in rat tibialis anterior muscle this applies only to 20%. All measurements on AChE inhibition referred to later, have been carried out on diaphragm preparations and thus it seems that conclusions drawn from them are not affected by Namba and Grob's findings.

D. Actions of Anticholinesterases of the Carbamate and Organophosphate Type and of Anilinium Ions

Anticholinesterases of the carbamate and organophosphate type have a number of characteristic actions at the neuromuscular junction. In the absence of nerve stimulation they produce spontaneous fasciculations of the muscle fibres and with large doses muscle weakness or complete neuromuscular block. In the muscle stimulated through its nerve the effects depend on the frequency of stimulation; at low frequencies, the twitch tension is potentiated due to repetitive firing of the muscle fibres; at high rates of stimulation the muscle is unable to maintain a tetanic contraction.

The actions of these substances are not confined to the neuromuscular junction but also involve autonomic ganglia and effector cells (smooth muscle, glands and heart muscle) innervated by postganglionic cholinergic fibres. The actions of acetylcholine at the ganglionic synapse and at the neuromuscular junction have been termed "nicotinic", while all the actions resulting from acetylcholine liberated at the postganglionic cholinergic nerve fibres are known as "muscarinic". Both terms were introduced by Dale in 1914. Muscarine-like effects include: slowing of the heart rate, weakening of the heart contraction, dilatation of peripheral vessels, fall in blood pressure, constriction of the pupil, increased tone and movements of the gastrointestinal tract, constriction of the bronchi, contraction of the urinary bladder, secretion of tears, saliva, pancreatic, gastric and intestinal juice, and increased bronchial secretion. With lipid-soluble anticholinesterases central nervous system actions are also produced (see Machne and Unna, 1963).

When AChE is extensively inhibited, death ensues. The primary cause of death is respiratory failure, generally arising from central impairment of respiration, combined with bronchoconstriction, bronchosecretion and failure of neuromuscular transmission. The relative importance of these factors varies with the species of animal and the distribution (lipid-solubility) of the anticholinesterase (Candole et al., 1953; Schaumann, 1959).

Anilinium ions such as edrophonium produce effects at the neuromuscular junction comparable with those obtained with anticholinesterases of the carbamate and organophosphate type. However, high doses of anilinium ions, while having marked effects at the neuromuscular junction tend to produce only weak muscarinic symptoms (Randall and Lehmann, 1950; Randall, 1950; McFarlane et al., 1950; Hobbiger, 1952).

1. Twitch Potentiation

Anticholinesterases of the carbamate and organophosphate type potentiate the tension developed by skeletal muscles in response to submaximal or maximal indirect

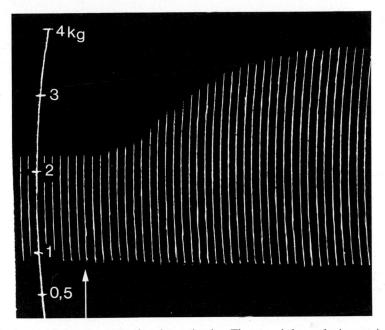

Fig. 7. Spinal cat; twitch potentiation by physostigmine. The record shows the isometric contractions of the gastrocnemius muscle in response to supramaximal stimulation of the sciatic nerve at 0.1 Hz. The arrow shows the point at which 0.2 mg (0,5 µmol/)/kg of physostigmine (eserine) was injected intravenously. (From BROWN et al., 1936)

stimulation at low frequencies both *in vivo* and in isolated muscle preparations (Fig. 7; see KOELLE and GILMAN, 1949; WERNER and KUPERMAN, 1963).

Normally a single supramaximal stimulus, applied to a nerve, elicits at each individual motor end-plate a single cnd-plate potential (e.p.p.) which in turn triggers a short-lasting contraction of the muscle fibre by means of a propagated muscle action potential. Muscle action potentials in individual muscle fibres are fairly synchronous and the response of the whole muscle to a single indirect stimulus is a twitch. About forty years ago BROWN et al. (1936) and BROWN (1937a) demonstrated in cats that following the intravenous administration of physostigmine, a single indirect stimulus produces a short burst of muscle action potentials (repetitive) and consequently the muscle responds as if stimulated at a high frequency. This explains the increase in twitch tension (the so-called twitch potentiation). The same results are obtained with other anticholinesterases of the carbamate or organophosphate type (see Fig. 11; KOELLE and GILMAN, 1949; WERNER and KUPERMAN, 1963).

Studies of the actions of neostigmine (MASLAND and WIGTON, 1940) and physostigmine (FENG and LI, 1941) in cats showed that twitch potentiation was also associated with repetitive antidromic nerve action potentials (Fig. 8). Furthermore, MASLAND and WIGTON found that doses of tubocurarine which in the absence of neostigmine had no effect on twitch responses abolished both twitch potentiation and repetitive antidromic nerve action potentials. Close-arterial injections of ACh were also found to elicit repetitive antidromic nerve action potentials. From these findings

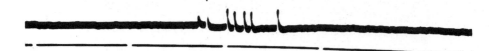

Fig. 8. Action potentials recorded from a few fibres of the anterior root of a cat subsequent to the application of a single stimulus to the sciatic nerve. The anterior root was sectioned near the cord and 0.25 mg (0.8 µmol) neostigmine were injected intravenously before the nerve was stimulated. The record shows an initial small stimulus artifact followed by the nerve action potential triggered by the stimulus and then a series of nerve action potentials in a single nerve fibre. Time base: 0.05 sec. (From MASLAND and WIGTON, 1940)

it was concluded that neostigmine, by inhibiting AChE, allowed ACh access to nerve terminals from whence it triggered repetitive antidromic nerve action potentials. They also implied, but did not state so directly, that this was the real cause of twitch potentiation.

ECCLES et al. (1942) studying the action of physostigmine in cats, found that following its administration repetitive muscle action potentials were sometimes present without concomitant repetitive antidromic nerve action potentials, whereas the e.p.p., recorded with surface electrodes, was always markedly prolonged. From these findings they concluded that the prolongation of the e.p.p. was mainly responsible for triggering repetitive muscle action potentials, although there was, in their opinion, no doubt that an antidromic nerve action potential sometimes preceded a muscle action potential.

Whether twitch potentiation is the result of a prolongation of the e.p.p. or of an action of ACh on the nerve terminal can be decided by studying the temporal relationship between antidromic nerve action potentials and repetitive muscle action potentials of an individual motor unit. A method suitable for providing such information is the so-called matched pair technique. This technique was developed by RIKER et al. (1959a and b), WERNER (1960a and b, 1961) and STANDAERT (1963, 1964) with the object of investigating the site and mechanism of action of anilinium ions.

The principal features of the matched pair technique when applied to the soleus muscle (Fig. 9; see RIKER and OKAMOTO, 1969) will now be described. The soleus muscle of a cat is exposed, then a ventral root, usually L7, is cut close to the spinal cord. The part of the root which is distal to the cut is sub-divided into fine filaments and a filament that contains only one motor axon which innervates surface muscle fibres, is prepared by careful dissection. The nerve fibre is stimulated via an electrode placed at the filament or more distally and action potentials are recorded with electrodes placed at the filament and the end-plate region of the motor unit, the neurone of which is contained in the filament. The soleus muscle is a red muscle which has the advantage over white muscle, such as the tibialis anterior, that repetitive antidromic nerve action potentials are also produced by nerve stimulation at high frequencies in the absence of an anticholinesterase. Thus motor units innervating surface muscle fibres can be located easily. Results comparable to those on the soleus muscle are obtained when the same technique is applied to the gastrocnemius or flexor digitorum longus muscles (WERNER, 1960a, 1961).

Studies in which the matched pair technique has been used have shown that following the close-arterial administration of anticholinesterases such as physostig-

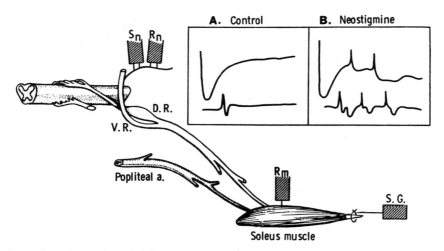

Fig. 9A and B. Illustration of the matched pair technique for simultaneous recording of action potentials in a single motor axon and the muscle fibres innervated by it. S_n and R_n are stimulating and recording electrodes, respectively. Both are placed on a fine ventral root (V.R.) filament containing a motor axon which innervates surface located muscle fibres from which action potentials are recorded with a microelectrode (R_m). S.G.: strain gauge for recording muscle tension; D.R.: dorsal root; Popliteal a.: popliteal artery. The two inserts show the nerve action potential (upper trace) and muscle action potential (lower trace) records obtained before (A) and after (B) the injection of neostigmine into the popliteal artery. The nerve action potential records have been shifted to the left to allow for conduction time from the point of initiation of antidromic nerve action potentials to the recording electrode R_n (2.4 msec). (From RIKER and OKAMOTO, 1969)

mine, neostigmine or DFP and usually also of anilinium ions, a single orthodromic stimulus produces repetitive antidromic nerve action potentials and repetitive muscle action potentials bearing a fixed temporal relationship with one another (Fig. 9; see WERNER and KUPERMAN, 1963; RIKER and OKAMOTO, 1969). That these nerve action potentials are not ephaptic responses generated in the nerve by muscle action currents, which as shown in normal muscle (LLOYD, 1942; BROWN and MATTHEWS, 1960), will re-excite the muscle, can be illustrated in several ways. They occur after a latent period which is longer than that associated with ephaptic responses (WERNER, 1961); they are abolished by low doses of tubocurarine, 5 µg/kg given intravenously, which have no effect on ephaptic nerve action potentials and on twitch tension in control muscles (WERNER, 1961), and they are unaffected under conditions which abolish the ephaptic response, i.e. when a submaximal stimulus is applied to a muscle via the motor nerve (BLABER and BOWMAN, 1963a). Judging by the time elapsing between the application of the orthodromic stimulus and their appearance, ephaptic nerve action potentials probably originate in some myelinated part of the intramuscular nerve branches (WERNER, 1960b). On the other hand, repetitive antidromic nerve action potentials following an orthodromic stimulus in animals treated with an anticholinesterase of the carbamate or organophosphate type or an anilinium ion appear to have their origin at or near the nerve terminal since they also occur when the orthodromic stimulus is applied focally at motor end-plates (WERNER, 1961). When allowance is made for the conduction time of impulses from the nerve termin-

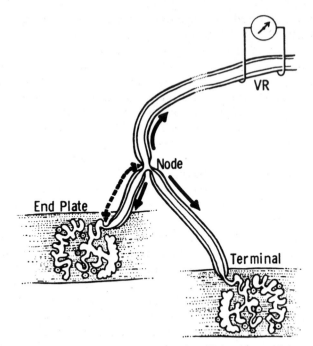

Fig. 10. Diagram showing how anticholinesterases and anilinium ions might produce repetitive antidromic nerve action potentials and, by an axon reflex, repetitive muscle action potentials. Following the arrival of an orthodromic impulse at the nerve terminals depolarisation of the first node of Ranvier occurs at one of these terminals. This gives rise to an antidromic nerve action potential (upward arrow) and to an invasion by an action potential of the nerve terminals (downwards arrows) and consequently a muscle action potential. The process then repeats itself. (From RIKER and OKAMOTO, 1969)

als to the root filament from which the antidromic nerve action potentials are recorded, it is found that a nerve action potential precedes each muscle action potential and thus muscle action potentials cannot be the cause but must be the consequence of nerve action potentials (see WERNER and KUPERMAN, 1963; RIKER and OKAMOTO, 1969). To explain this, WERNER (1960a and b, 1961) put forward the hypothesis that anticholinesterases of the carbamate and organophosphate type and anilinium ions augment the after-potentials at nerve terminals following their invasion by an orthodromic stimulus. The augmented negative after-potentials outlast the refractory period of neighbouring myelinated parts of the axon and thus generate antidromic impulses. This is, WERNER claimed, assisted by a lowering of the excitability at the first node of Ranvier. One or more nerve terminals act as triggering point(s), probably in turn, and the antidromic activity initiated by them is conducted centripetally in the neurone and also as an axon reflex to the other nerve terminals (Fig. 10), thus giving rise to a synchronised stimulation of the individual muscle fibres of a motor unit.

   With some anilinium ions the coupling between repetitive muscle action potentials and repetitive antidromic nerve action potentials is not consistent. For example, in some experiments following the administration of 3-hydroxyphenylmethyldiethylammonium or 3-hydroxyphenyltriethylammonium, an orthodromic stimulus produces repetitive muscle action potentials without repetitive antidromic nerve action potentials (RIKER et al., 1959a; WERNER, 1960a). In such cases repetitive antidromic nerve action potentials could be recorded following a brief period of nerve stimulation at high frequencies or when a dose of physostigmine (0.1 to 0.2 µg/kg), which did not produce twitch potentiation, was given close-arterially (WERNER, 1960a). The opposite, i.e. suppression of repetitive antidromic nerve action potentials in experiments in which repetitive muscle action potentials and repetitive antidromic nerve action potentials were previously coupled, was obtained in cats with doses of pentobarbitone above those required for adequate anaesthesia, and with cyclopropane and procaine (RIKER et al., 1959a).

That repetitive antidromic nerve action potentials can be recorded in the absence of repetitive muscle action potentials could be explained as the consequence of decreased excitability of the nerve terminal if, for example, an enhanced positive after-potential is present at the critical time. The presence of repetitive muscle action potentials without repetitive antidromic nerve action potentials was thought by RIKER et al. (1959a) to be attributable to the fact that muscle action potentials could be more easily triggered from the first node of Ranvier than repetitive antidromic nerve action potentials. It is rather difficult to accept this view. A marginal depression in the excitability of consecutive Ranvier nodes seems a more attractive proposition. This could account for the effects of pentobarbitone, cyclopropane and procaine but at present no evidence exists which could explain the effect of 3-hydroxyphenylmethyldiethylammonium or 3-hydroxyphenyltriethylammonium in similar terms. Perhaps these substances have more complex actions than anilinium ions such as edrophonium which consistently produce coupled repetitive muscle action potentials and repetitive antidromic nerve action potentials. Most experiments with anilinium ions seem to have been carried out with fixed dose levels. Studies of the effects produced by graded doses might give further useful information on why repetitive muscle action potentials are sometimes not coupled with repetitive antidromic nerve action potentials.

In spite of the difficulties in interpreting the results obtained with some anilinium ions the evidence provided by the matched pair technique suggests that it is the nerve terminals which trigger the repetitive muscle action potentials by an axon reflex, and that the repetitive muscle action potentials thus generated are the cause of twitch potentiation (by anticholinesterases and anilinium ions). It is plausible that the axon reflex might be a consequence of changes in the time-course and magnitude of the negative after-potentials in the nerve terminals (WERNER, 1960a and b, 1961). This view is supported by the studies of HUBBARD and SCHMIDT (1961) and HUBBARD et al. (1965). These authors determined the threshold for focal stimulation of nerve terminals in the rat isolated nerve-diaphragm preparation at various intervals after arrival of an orthodromic impulse initiated by stimulation of the phrenic nerve. The addition of neostigmine to the bathing fluid produced changes in the threshold from which it could be concluded that both the intensity and duration of the negative after-potential were increased.

Results similar to those observed using the matched pair technique have been obtained on isolated nerve-muscle preparations with cut muscle fibres. This type of preparation was introduced by BARSTAD (1962); in the isolated phrenic nerve-diaphragm the muscle fibres are cut on both sides in the vicinity of the motor end-plate so that no muscle action potential can be triggered by the e.p.p. Electrodes placed on the nerve and intracellularly, record nerve action potentials and e.p.p.s, respectively. Using this preparation BARSTAD observed that when neostigmine, 3 μmol/l, or DFP, 10 μmol/l, were added to the bathing fluid, an orthodromic nerve impulse produced repetitive antidromic nerve action potentials as in preparations with intact muscle fibres. In later experiments the same result was obtained with physostigmine (BARSTAD and LILLEHEIL, 1968). RANDIĆ and STRAUGHAN (1964) confirmed these findings and also reported that repetitive antidromic nerve action potentials were obtained even when the end-plate region was extensively depolarised. These experiments are open to critisism on the grounds that the resting potential, probably through potassium leakage from the cuts, was sometimes as low as 20 to 30 mV. BLABER (1970, 1972, 1973) adapted Barstad's method to the cat isolated tenuissimus muscle which behaves pharmacologically like the cat tibialis anterior muscle (MACLAGAN, 1962). On this preparation which had a much more satisfactory resting potential Blaber observed that when edrophonium, 0.1 μmol/l, was added to the bathing fluid, an orthodromic nerve impulse produced repetitive muscle action potentials and antidromic nerve action potentials in five out of twelve experiments.

Before attempting to interpret these results we must consider some of the conditions under which they were obtained. In the rat isolated nerve-diaphragm cutting the muscle fibres causes a conduction block in the phrenic nerve. Although this wears off gradually repetitive antidromic nerve action potentials are never as marked after recovery as in preparations with intact muscle fibres. Lowering the potassium concentration in the bathing fluid speeds up recovery and intensifies the effect of anticholinesterases (RANDIĆ and STRAUGHAN, 1964). In the cat isolated tenuissimus muscle with cut muscle fibres repetitive antidromic nerve action potentials can only be recorded when the potassium concentration in the bathing fluid is low (BLABER, 1972). Furthermore, when a stimulus is applied to the nerve an e.p.p. can be recorded only from some end-plates in both preparations (BARSTAD and LILLEHEIL, 1968; BLABER, 1972). This and the paucity of repetitive antidromic nerve action potentials must mean that repetitive antidromic nerve action potentials are generated only at a few motor end-plates. It could be argued, therefore, that in isolated muscle preparations with cut muscle fibres the situation is so artificial that observations on them shed no light on the situation *in vivo* or even in isolated muscle preparations with intact muscle fibres. However, it is also possible that these preparations are abnormal only in that their nerve terminals are less efficient in triggering antidromic nerve action potentials and that the conclusions arrived at by the authors using the technique are generally applicable. In other words, the studies on the isolated muscle preparations with cut muscle fibres like the studies on single motor units (matched pair technique) implicate the nerve terminals as the main site for triggering repetitive muscle action potentials and thus causing twitch potentiation.

Twitch potentiation is abolished by low doses of tubocurarine which have no effect on normal twitch tension, by ether (BROWN et al., 1936) and by lignocaine (LOWNDES and JOHNSON, 1971). Both groups of authors showed that antagonism of twitch potentiation was associated with a return of normal muscle action potentials and in addition LOWNDES and JOHNSON (1971) found that repetitive antidromic nerve action potentials were abolished at the same time. Tubocurarine, ether and

Table 3. Relationship between inhibition of total AChE and effects produced by paraoxon, 0.1 µmol/l, on the rat isolated nerve-diaphragm preparation. (After BARNES and DUFF, 1953)

Time after adding paraoxon (min)	Condition of diaphragm	Calculated % activity of total AChE
6	Beginning of twitch potentiation[a]	42
18	Tetanic fade[b]	8
20	End of twitch potentiation[a]	5
60	50% inhibition of twitch tension by 5 µmol/l acetylcholine[c]	0.1

[a] Rate of stimulation 0.13 Hz
[b] Stimulation at 50 Hz for 5 sec.
[c] In the absence of paraxon 2—3mmol/l acetylcholine is required for this effect.

lignocaine thus act at the site where the antidromic nerve action potentials originate, i.e. at nerve terminals, but it does not follow from this that they have a common mechanism of action.

The question which arises now is, how do anticholinesterases of the carbamate and organophosphate type and anilinium ions alter the behaviour of nerve terminals and affect the threshold of excitability at the most distal node of Ranvier, so that the terminals act as impulse generators subsequent to the arrival of an orthodromic nerve impulse? In principle there are two possibilities which could operate either singly or in conjunction. These are (1) inhibition of AChE which allows ACh to gain access to nerve terminals, and (2) a direct action on nerve terminals.

Measurements of the inhibition of total AChE (i.e. the percentage inhibition of the total number of AChE sites at the neuromuscular junction; see Section C II), and calculations based on them gave the following information on the relationship between twitch potentiation and inhibition of AChE. BARNES and DUFF (1953) added paraoxon to the bathing fluid of the rat isolated nerve-diaphragm preparation and recorded its effect on the twitch tension evoked by supramaximal indirect stimulation. After thirty minutes they measured the level of inhibition of total AChE and by making the assumption, since proved correct (LANCASTER, 1973), that the rate of inhibition followed first order kinetics, they calculated that the inhibition of total AChE at the time when twitch potentiation began was approximately 60% (Table 3). Using the same preparation MEER and MEETER (1956) found that twitch potentiation by DFP was associated with at least 80% inhibition of total AChE. MITTAG et al. (1971) measured inhibition of functional AChE activity (i.e. the percentage reduction in the rate of hydrolysis of ACh by intact tissue; see Section C II) in the rat isolated nerve-diaphragm preparation and obtained the following results. In a concentration which potentiated twitch tension by 164% phospholine inhibited functional AChE activity by 91% and with DFP in a concentration which potentiated twitch tension by 275%, the extent of inhibition was 88%. The twitch potentiation by DFP was reversed by pralidoxime, a reactivator of the phosphorylated AChE formed by DFP, and when the oxime had restored normal twitch tension, inhibition of functional AChE activity was reduced to 35%.

A

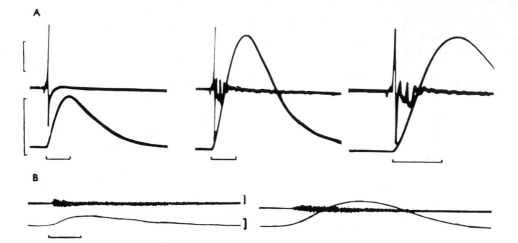

B

Fig. 11 A and B. Potentiation by neostigmine of the responses of the cat tibialis anterior muscle to nerve stimulation and injected ACh. The experiment was performed under chloralose anaesthesia. The upper records (A) show muscle action potentials (recorded with a concentric needle electrode) and below them twitch responses (recorded with a strain gauge), triggered by supramaximal nerve stimulation. The lower records (B) show muscle action potentials and below them muscle contractions produced by close-arterial injection of 1 μg acetylcholine. Neostigmine, 150 μg (0.5 μmol), was injected intravenously between the first and second records of A and B. The calibrations for muscle action potentials are 5 and 0.4 mV and for muscle tension 1 and 0.1 kg in A and B, respectively. The horizontal time scales indicate periods of 0.02 and 0.2 sec in A and B, respectively. (From BLABER, 1963)

Comparable data for physostigmine and neostigmine, cannot be obtained since the types of carbamylated AChE formed by them are not sufficiently stable to permit assay of the inhibition produced *in vivo* (see Section C I). However, there is considerable indirect evidence that inhibition of AChE caused by them is associated with the twitch potentiation. In doses (concentrations) which affect twitch tension the anticholinesterases of the carbamate type potentiate muscle responses to close-arterial injections of ACh (Fig. 11; BROWN et al., 1936; BLABER, 1963), protect AChE *in vivo* against phosphorylation by anticholinesterases of the organophosphate type (KOSTER, 1946; KOELLE, 1957), produce effects on other cholinergic synapses (see KOELLE and GILMAN, 1949; HOLMSTEDT, 1959) and in higher concentrations protect ACh released from nerve terminals against hydrolysis by AChE (DALE et al., 1936).

In the case of edrophonium, MITTAG et al. (1971) in their studies on the rat isolated nerve-diaphragm preparation observed that a concentration which increased twitch tension by 188% inhibited functional AChE activity by 77% and also markedly protected AChE against phosphorylation by DFP. Furthermore, KUPERMAN et al. (1961) showed in the cat gastrocnemius muscle that with 3- and 4-hydroxyanilinium ions the relationship between graded doses and the extent of twitch potentiation was the same as with neostigmine (Fig. 12). A good correlation was also found between the doses required to give 50% of the maximum obtainable twitch potentiation and the concentrations which produced 50% inhibition of human erythrocyte AChE *in vitro* (Table 4). With unsubstituted anilinium ions and those of their deriva-

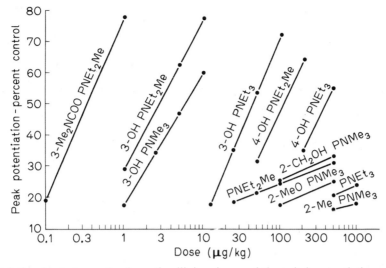

Fig. 12. Relationship between the dose of anilinium ions and the twitch potentiation produced. The experiments were performed in cats (under chloralose anaesthesia) which had been pretreated with atropine. The ordinate gives the maximum increase in twitch tension observed on the gastrocnemius muscle, stimulated indirectly with supramaximal stimuli at a rate of 0.2 Hz. All test substances were injected into the popliteal artery and each point in the figure represents the mean of 4 to 12 (average 7) individual observations. The chemical structure of the substances which are referred to in an abbreviated form is given in Appendix II. (From KUPERMAN et al., 1961)

tives which had a hydroxyl or other group in the 2-position, the increase in twitch tension obtained by increasing the dose was small (Fig. 12) and the correlation between twitch potentiating potency and anticholinesterase potency *in vitro* poor (Table 4). It seems unlikely, therefore, that these compounds could exert actions at the neuromuscular junction predominantly by AChE inhibition and for this reason they are not considered in this chapter. BLABER (1963) observed that edrophonium, in a dose which produced twitch potentiation, did not increase the effect of a close-arterial injection of ACh in the cat tibialis anterior muscle. For ACh released from nerve terminals the inhibition of AChE by edrophonium is initially non-competitive (see Section C I) whereas with ACh diffusing into the synaptic cleft after a close-arterial injection, there is much more time available for reversal of inhibition by ACh. Thus the level of enzyme inhibition is likely to differ in the two situations and this could account for Blaber's finding.

Since inhibition of AChE will prolong the postsynaptic action of ACh, studies of the relationship between e.p.p. and twitch potentiation also should provide useful information on the role of AChE inhibition.

However, studies of the e.p.p. present certain difficulties. The e.p.p. itself can only be recorded if the muscle action potential triggered by it is eliminated. This can be done with tubocurarine, and the effects of substances on the amplitude and duration of the e.p.p. in the presence of tubocurarine are often used as evidence on whether a substance acts by AChE inhibition. However, effects on the e.p.p. in the presence of

Table 4. Relationship between twitch potentiation and anticholinesterase potency obtained with anilinium ions. (After KUPERMAN et al., 1961)

	Twitch potentiation		Anticholin-esterase activity (K_I)
	Mean threshold dose $\pm$ S.E. giving potentiation (µg/kg)	Dose giving 50% of maximal potentiation (µg/kg)	(mol/l)
3-Me$_2$NCOO PNEt$_2$Me	0.08± 0.6	0.3	2.04×10^{-8}
3-OH PNEt$_2$Me	0.67± 0.9	2.5	1.03×10^{-7}
3-OH PNMe$_3$	1.31± 1.1	5.7	4.26×10^{-7}
3-OH PNEt$_3$	14 ± 3.2	40	1.59×10^{-6}
4-OH PNEt$_2$Me	32 ± 4.6	113	5.44×10^{-6}
4-OH PNEt$_3$	119 ±10.9	374	2.30×10^{-5}
2-CH$_2$OH PNMe$_3$	28 ± 4.3	—	1.20×10^{-5}
PNEt$_2$Me	36 ± 4.8	—	1.05×10^{-5}
2-MeO PNMe$_3$	78 ± 5.8	—	6.03×10^{-6}
PNEt$_3$	214 ±12.2	—	5.21×10^{-5}
2-Me PNME$_3$	291 ±15.6	—	5.19×10^{-5}

Experiments were carried out in cats under chloralose anaesthesia. The table shows effects on the twitch tension of the gastrocnemius muscle following injection of the test substances into the popliteal artery. K_I is the dissociation constant of the enzyme-inhibitor complex calculated from the inhibition of AChE of haemolysed human erythrocytes, with 4 mmol/l ACh as substrate. The chemical structure of the substances which are referred to in an abbreviated form is given in Appendix II.

tubocurarine do not necessarily correspond in all respects to those obtained in its absence.

The muscle action potential can be eliminated without the use of tubocurarine if a pair of stimuli is applied to a nerve and the second stimulus is so timed that the peak of its postsynaptic effect falls within the refractory period of the muscle, the e.p.p. triggered by the second stimulus is not obscured by a propagated muscle action potential. Studies of this type in cats by ECCLES et al. (1941) showed that physostigmine, in a dose of 0.6 mg/kg which produced marked twitch potentiation, increased the duration of the e.p.p. In these studies the e.p.p. was recorded extracellularly and thus represents the sum of potential changes at a number of motor end-plates. For this reason there is a second negative component of the e.p.p. which is never seen with intracellular recordings from single motor end-plates. Studies on isolated muscle preparations in which the muscle action potential was eliminated with either tetrodotoxin or by cutting the muscle fibres at both sides of the motor end-plate have also been performed. This approach was used to study the effect on the intracellularly recorded e.p.p. of anticholinesterases and edrophonium in concentrations known to produce twitch potentiation. In the rat isolated nerve-diaphragm treated with tetrodotoxin, 3 µmol/l neostigmine markedly increased the amplitude and duration of e.p.p.s of 20 mV or more, triggered by nerve terminal stimulation (Fig. 3; KUBA and TOMITA, 1971). In the rat isolated nerve-diaphragm with cut muscle fibres BARSTAD and LILLEHEIL (1968) found that neostigmine, physostigmine and DFP, in concentrations which gave rise to repetitive antidromic nerve action

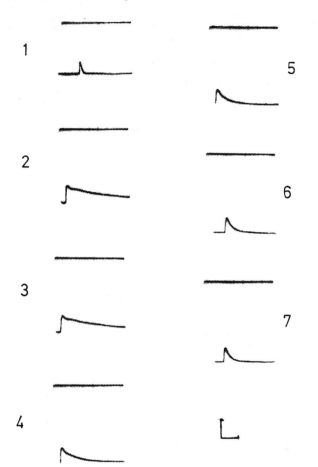

Fig. 13. Effect of DFP on the e.p.p. in the rat isolated nerve-diaphragm preparation with cut muscle fibres bathed in Tyrode solution at 37° C. 1: Control e.p.p. 2: e.p.p. after 15 min exposure of the preparation to 4 µg (0.02 µmol) DFP/ml. 3: e.p.p. at 30 min, after removing DFP from the bathing fluid. 4 to 7: e.p.p.s recorded after the addition of obidoxime 80 µg (0.2 µmol)/ml to the bathing fluid. Recordings were made 2.5, 5, 10 and 16 min after adding obidoxime, respectively. Records 2 to 7 were all obtained on the same motor end-plate. The e.p.p. was recorded with an intracellular electrode and the calibrations are 10 mV and 4 msec. (From BARSTAD and LILLE-HEIL 1968)

potentials following the application of a single stimulus to the phrenic nerve, increased both the amplitude and the duration of the e.p.p. The effect of DFP was fully reversed by obidoxime, a reactivator of the di*iso*propylphosphoryl-AChE formed by DFP (Fig. 13). In the cat isolated tenuissimus muscle preparation with cut muscle fibres, BLABER (1972) showed that edrophonium produced a concentration-dependent effect. In a concentration of 0.1 µmol/l the drug increased the amplitude of the e.p.p. without affecting its time-course; with concentrations of 1 µmol/l and higher, however, not only was the amplitude of the e.p.p. increased but also its rise-time and half-decay time were both prolonged.

Measurements of AChE inhibition at motor end-plates, experiments providing indirect evidence of inhibition, studies of the correlation between anticholinesterase and twitch potentiating potencies, and studies of the e.p.p. are all consistent with the view that anticholinesterases of the carbamate and organophosphate type produce twitch potentiation by the inhibition of AChE. In the case of anilinium ions the close correlation between anticholinesterase and twitch potentiating potencies supports the view that they too cause twitch potentiation by AChE inhibition. Consistent with this hypothesis are studies of the effect of edrophonium on functional AChE activity. On the other hand, repetitive antidromic nerve action potentials can be produced under conditions where only the amplitude and not the duration of the e.p.p. is changed. As already pointed out (see Section B II) we do not know what the relationship between different levels of AChE inhibition and the effects on the e.p.p. is; furthermore, inhibition of AChE caused by reversible inhibitors is not comparable to that produced by acylating anticholinesterases and it is possible that at least in lower concentrations the former affect the amplitude of the e.p.p. more than its duration. Until more is known about this it seems premature to postulate that twitch potentiation by anilinium ions cannot be the consequence of AChE inhibition.

The hypothesis that a direct action on nerve terminals accounts for twitch potentiation has first been put forward by Riker and his coworkers (see RIKER et al., 1959 b; RIKER and OKAMOTO, 1969) using the following stated or implied reasoning: 1) anilinium ions produce twitch potentiation in doses which are thought not to inhibit AChE *in vivo* on the basis of *in vitro* measurements of anticholinesterase potency; 2) anilinium ions produce far less intense muscarinic symptoms than anticholinesterases of the carbamate and organophosphate type; 3) anticholinesterases of the carbamate and organophosphate type produce twitch potentiation like anilinium ions, and quaternary carbamates share with anilinium ions the property of exerting, in appropriate doses, a postsynaptic ACh-like action when injected close-arterially. Thus there is no reason why evidence of AChE inhibition *in vivo* by quaternary carbamates should be relevant as to the mechanism by which twitch potentiation is produced; and 4) acetylcholine injected close-arterially cannot reproduce satisfactorily the effects of anticholinesterases of the carbamate and organophosphate type and of anilinium ions. Much of the argument therefore rests on the interpretation of the data obtained with anilinium ions. As pointed out before evidence against the view that inhibition of AChE is the mechanism by which the anilinium ions exert their actions at the neuromuscular junction is by no means as conclusive as is sometimes made out, if due consideration is given to all the experimental evidence and to the kinetics of inhibition. Any direct action of anilinium ions on nerve terminals, if such an action exists, is likely to be the result of an interaction with a receptor. Anilinium ions are quaternary ammonium compounds and thus they might act on a presynaptic cholinoceptor. There is no correlation between the twitch potentiating potency of individual anilinium ions and their agonist activity on postsynaptic cholinoceptors at motor end-plates and marked neuromuscular effects can be obtained with only negligible effects at other cholinergic synapses (RANDALL and LEHMANN, 1950; RANDALL, 1950). Thus if the presynaptic receptor is a cholinoceptor its properties must differ considerably from those of known cholinoceptors. Alternatively the hydroxyl group could be of importance for a presynaptic action. This too seems unlikely since anilinium ions with substituent groups other than hydroxyl groups are also very potent in affecting neuromuscular transmission (RAN-DALL and LEHMANN, 1950; RANDALL, 1950). All this seems to speak against a direct presynaptic action of anilinium ions. On the other hand, twitch potentiation is produced by substances such as tetraethyl ammonium (TEA) whose mechanism of action is unlikely to be the result of inhibition of AChE (see RIKER and OKAMOTO, 1969). It seems reasonable, therefore, not to reject entirely a direct presynaptic action as a cause of twitch potentiation by anilinium ions but to consider it as an unproven alternative to AChE inhibition. If anilinium ions have a direct presynaptic action, inhibition of AChE could contribute to it and the relative importance of the two mechanisms might be dose (concentration) dependent. If we accept this, then we must also keep an open mind as to the possibility that with those anticholinesterases of the carbamate and organophosphate type which are quaternary substances, a direct action on nerve terminals could contribute to twitch potentiation particularly in its early phase.

A question which we now have to answer is, how inhibition of AChE might alter the negative after-potentials in nerve terminals and the excitability of the first node of Ranvier so that an orthodromic impulse might generate repetitive nerve action potentials at the nerve terminals. BOWMAN and WEBB (1972) pointed out that the increase in amplitude and duration of the e.p.p. caused by AChE inhibition could affect the nerve terminals ephaptically. The observation of RANDIĆ and STRAUGHAN (1964) that in the rat isolated nerve-diaphragm with cut muscle fibres an orthodromic stimulus still produces repetitive antidromic nerve action potentials when the motor end-plate is extensively depolarised and muscle action potentials are absent does not support BOWMAN and WEBB's suggestion.

An alternate mechanism is an action of ACh on the nerve terminals against which they are normally protected by AChE. MASLAND and WIGTON (1940) injected ACh into the popliteal artery of cats and found that it produced repetitive antidromic nerve action potentials in the sciatic nerve. In 1966 RIKER analysed this action of ACh, using the matched pair technique. He found that when ACh was injected into the popliteal artery during indirect stimulation of the soleus muscle at 2 Hz, there was a shortlasting neuromuscular block followed by twitch potentiation. During the period of twitch potentiation repetitive antidromic nerve action potentials coupled with repetitive muscle action potentials were recorded. The temporal relationship between the two was such that an antidromic nerve action potential preceded each muscle action potential. This result was obtained in 4 out of 5 cats. Although the possibility cannot be excluded that in these experiments and in those of MASLAND and WIGTON (1940) choline might account at least in part for the findings, subsequent studies on the same preparation by CITRIN (1968) strengthen the view that ACh itself is responsible for the antidromic nerve action potentials. Citrin showed that neostigmine in a dose too small to have any effect on its own, greatly enhanced the effectiveness of ACh in eliciting repetitive antidromic nerve action potentials and twitch potentiation at low rates of nerve stimulation.

In the experiments of RIKER (1966) antidromic nerve action potentials were not seen during the period when the postsynaptic action of ACh was at its height. Similarly BARSTAD (1962) observed that in the rat isolated nerve-diaphragm with cut muscle fibres and treated with DFP, ACh in a concentration of 3 μmol/l arrested repetitive antidromic nerve action potentials. These findings are consistent with the view (Riker, 1966) that initiation of antidromic nerve action potentials by ACh is by a presynaptic action and that if the concentration of ACh at presynaptic sites is too high, the terminals cease to trigger antidromic nerve action potentials possibly because of the excessive depolarisation at the first node of Ranvier.

Further evidence that ACh is able to act presynaptically is provided by experiments of Hubbard et al. (1965) on the rat isolated nerve-diaphragm preparation, treated with neostigmine and bathed in a solution containing a high concentration of magnesium ions. They found that ACh lowered the threshold of excitability of the nerve terminals to focal stimulation, but unlike electrical stimulation it did not raise the frequency of the m.e.p.p.s. From these and related findings the authors concluded that ACh did not depolarise the nerve terminals to any significant extent but lowered the level of polarisation at the first node of Ranvier. Consistent with this are observations on the cat isolated tenuissimus muscle preparation by Blaber and Christ (1967). They found that ACh in a concentration of 1 μmol/l and higher only marginally increased the frequency of m.e.p.p.s.

The action of ACh at the postsynaptic membrane increases the concentration of potassium ions in the synaptic cleft, and high concentrations of potassium, injected close-arterially, initiate repetitive antidromic nerve action potentials and twitch potentiation (Citrin, 1967). However, extensive depolarisation of the motor end-plates, probably through an action of potassium ions, does not initiate repetitive antidromic nerve action potentials in the rat isolated nerve-diaphragm with cut muscle fibres (Randić and Straughan, 1964). This seems to exclude any major role of potassium ions in twitch potentiation.

Summarising the present position concerning twitch potentiation by anticholinesterases of the carbamate and organophosphate type and by anilinium ions, the following two points appear to be the most important. Firstly, twitch potentiation seems to be largely the consequence of changes occurring in nerve terminals (and the first node of Ranvier) so that subsequent to the arrival of an orthodromic impulse they initiate repetitive e.p.p.s in individual motor units by an axon reflex; ephaptic nerve stimulation by muscle currents and initiation of repetitive muscle action potentials by the e.p.p. itself are unlikely to play more than a subsidiary role. Secondly, the axon reflex can only be a consequence of a presynaptic action of ACh (as the result of AChE inhibition) in the case of anticholinesterases of the organophosphate type. All experimental evidence is consistent with the view that this also applies to anticholinesterases of the carbamate type. In the case of anilinium ions the experimental data on the whole are consistent with AChE inhibition being the mode of action but a direct action on nerve terminals cannot be excluded entirely. If this is so a direct action could contribute to some extent to twitch potentiation by quaternary anticholinesterases. An ephaptic effect of the end-plate current and increase of the concentration of potassium ions in the synaptic cleft as a result of the postsynaptic action of ACh are unlikely to play any major part in the initiation of the axon reflex.

Aspects so far not discussed are *the rate of onset and the duration of twitch potentiation.* When anticholinesterases of the carbamate or organophosphate type are given to animals intravenously in submaximally effective doses twitch potentiation is of gradual onset and often reaches a maximum after 2 to 5 min. This conforms to the expected time-course of inhibition of AChE as judged by the kinetics of inhibition and the likely time: concentration profile of the anticholinesterases at the neuromuscular junction. Anticholinesterases which are mono- or di-methylcarbamates, like physostigmine and neostigmine, produce *in vitro* a near maximum inhibition of AChE by carbamylation in about 5 min (WILSON, 1955). With anticholinesterases of the organophosphate type such as TEPP, paraoxon, DFP or sarin, inhibition of AChE is in principle that of a first order reaction. However, hydrolysis by phosphoryl phosphatases (MOUNTER, 1963; DuBOIS, 1963) speedily inactivates these organophosphates and so arrests inhibition. Exceptions are organophosphates which are not subject to enzymic degradation, e.g. the dialkylphosphoryl analogues of neostigmine (the so-called phosphostigmines; BURGEN and HOBBIGER, 1951). With them inhibition of AChE can progress over a longer period of time and correspondingly it takes longer for a maximum effect on twitch tension to be obtained.

In isolated muscle preparations the concentration of phosphoryl phosphatases is low and anticholinesterases of the organophosphate type which are subject to hydrolysis by phosphoryl phosphatases increase progressively, in submaximally effective concentrations, the twitch tension over a much longer period of time than they do *in vivo*.

The duration of twitch potentiation *in vivo* by anticholinesterases of the carbamate and organophosphate type is dose dependent for the range of doses which produce a submaximal peak effect. Furthermore, under these conditions, there is also a correlation between the stability of the acylated AChE involved (see Section C I) and the duration of twitch potentiation. For example, with neostigmine in doses which give a submaximal peak effect, twitch tension can be potentiated for 30 min to 1 hr. However, with higher doses, particularly of anticholinesterases of the organophosphate type, the duration of twitch potentiation becomes inversely related to the dose and after a transient phase of twitch potentiation, twitch tension usually returns to control levels or even falls below it.

Results on the rat isolated nerve-diaphragm preparation are similar to those obtained *in vivo*. BARNES and DUFF (1953) showed that when paraoxon was added to the bathing fluid in a final concentration of 0.4 μmol/l, the twitch response was only transiently potentiated and soon returned towards control levels. When the bathing fluid then was changed and paraoxon added to it again in a final concentration of 0.4 μmol/l twitch tension was unaffected. BARNES and DUFF measured the level of total AChE activity at 30 min after adding paraoxon to the bathing fluid. Assuming that the rate of inhibition followed first order kinetics, a view supported by the studies of LANCASTER (1973), they calculated that twitch potentiation started when the inhibition of total AChE was approximately 60% and at the time when twitch tension returned to normal in spite of the continued presence of the anticholinesterase it amounted to 95% (Table 3). MEER and MEETER (1956) using DFP instead of paraoxon, found that twitch potentiation started when total AChE was inhibited by about 80% and at a time when twitch tension had returned to normal in spite of the continued presence of DFP in the bathing fluid, the inhibition was nearly 100%.

Twitch potentiation, therefore, only occurs over a limited range of AChE inhibition. The reason for this could be an excessive action of ACh at nerve terminals or at the postsynaptic membrane, or both. Results obtained by BARSTAD (1962) implicate the nerve terminals. He found that in the rat isolated nerve-diaphragm ACh arrested repetitive antidromic nerve action potentials elicited by orthodromic stimulation subsequent to treatment of the preparation with DFP. Experiments by CHENNELS et al. (1949) might also be interpreted as indicating that an excessive presynaptic action of ACh leads to an arrest of repetitive antidromic nerve action potentials and thus terminates twitch potentiation. These authors injected cats intravenously with TEPP in doses which produced only a transient twitch potentiation. By recording muscle action potentials from the quadriceps muscle they found that the return of normal twitch tension was associated with a return of normal muscle action potentials. On the other hand, there is evidence which implicates the postsynaptic site. DOUGLAS and PATON (1954) injected cats intravenously with doses of TEPP which according to CHENNELS et al. (1949) produce only transient twitch potentiation. Recording with an external electrode from the end-plate region of the gracilis muscle they found that TEPP produced a sustained depolarisation which developed gradually and was intensified by nerve stimulation and antagonised by tubocurarine. The same results were obtained by MEETER (1958). Using a concentration of DFP which produced only transient twitch potentiation, and a moving fluid electrode he noted that DFP produced a sustained depolarisation at the motor end-plate region when the nerve was stimulated at 0.5 Hz. Both depolarisation and inhibition of AChE were reversed by pralidoxime. Finally, BARSTAD and LILLEHEIL (1968) showed that in the rat isolated nerve-diaphragm with cut muscle fibres treated with an anticholinesterase, the decline of the e.p.p. was prolonged to such an extent that summation of e.p.p.s occurred when the nerve was stimulated at 0.2 Hz.

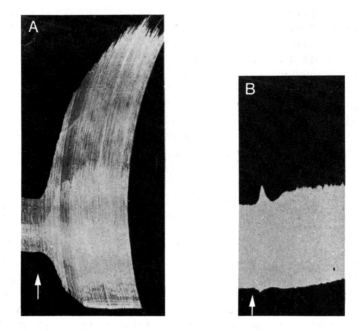

Fig. 14. Dependence of twitch potentiation by neostigmine on the rate of nerve stimulation. The experiments were carried out on the rat isolated nerve-diaphragm preparation, suspended in Tyrode solution at 37° C and stimulated indirectly at rates of 0.1 (experiment A) and 5 (experiment B) Hz. The arrows indicate the addition of neostigmine to the Tyrode solution in a final concentration of 0.1 µmol/l (0.03 µg/ml). (From WALTHER, 1969)

If an excess of ACh at the nerve terminals or at the postsynaptic site, or at both, is the cause of the absence of twitch potentiation at high levels of AChE inhibition then the degree and duration of twitch potentiation obtained with a given concentration of an anticholinesterase should also be inversely related to the frequency of nerve stimulation. This is indeed the case as shown in studies on the rat isolated nerve-diaphragm preparation (Fig. 14; MEER and MEETER, 1956; WALTHER, 1969).

Observations on the time-course of twitch potentiation and the results of other studies further substantiate the conclusion that the twitch potentiation by anticholinesterases of the organophosphate type can only be the result of AChE inhibition. These observations provide no evidence for a direct action of quaternary anticholinesterases of the carbamate type being of importance *in vivo* and thus they too probably cause twitch potentiation mainly, if not solely, by AChE inhibition.

The onset of twitch potentiation by anilinium ions *in vivo* is so fast that a peak effect is obtained in under one minute and the duration of the effect is only a few minutes. Furthermore, when twitch tension has returned to normal following a dose of an anilinium ion, a second equal dose will reproduce the effect of the first dose. However, in the rat isolated nerve-diaphragm preparation a failure of higher concentrations of anilinium ions to produce a sustained effect on twitch tension has been noted (HOBBIGER, 1952).

II. Fasciculations

In the absence of applied nerve stimulation the anticholinesterases of the carbamate type (MASLAND and WIGTON, 1940; FENG and LI, 1941; ECCLES et al., 1942; BLABER and GOODE, 1968) and the organophosphate type (MODELL et al., 1946; RIKER and WESCOE, 1946; MEER and MEETER, 1956) and edrophonium (BLABER and GOODE, 1968) and other anilinium ions (RIKER et al., 1957) produce fasciculations, which may be defined as intermittent synchronised contractions of muscle fibres constituting a motor unit (Fig. 15). Such fasciculations may be seen in conscious animals, in animals anaesthetised with chloralose, and in isolated nerve-muscle preparations. They are always found to be associated with repetitive antidromic nerve action potentials and both fasciculations and antidromic nerve action potentials may be abolished by low doses of tubocurarine which have no effect on twitch tension (see RIKER and OKAMOTO, 1969).

In the cat isolated tenuissimus muscle preparation concentrations of neostigmine, ambenonium and edrophonium which produce fasciculations not only increase the frequency of m.e.p.p.s (which indicates involvement of the nerve terminals) but also their amplitude and duration (BOYD and MARTIN, 1956a; BLABER and CHRIST, 1967). In the cat, a dose of TEPP which produces fasciculations causes the gradual development of a maintained depolarisation at the motor end-plates in the gracilis muscle in the absence of nerve stimulation (DOUGLAS and PATON, 1954). Finally, the duration of fasciculations *in vivo* is proportional to the duration of AChE inhibition, and with anticholinesterases of the organophosphate type reactivation of the phosphorylated AChE by an oxime causes fasciculations to cease (HOLMES and ROBINS, 1955).

As in the case of twitch potentiation, fasciculations only occur within a limited range of inhibition of total AChE, disappearing when inhibition exceeds 95%

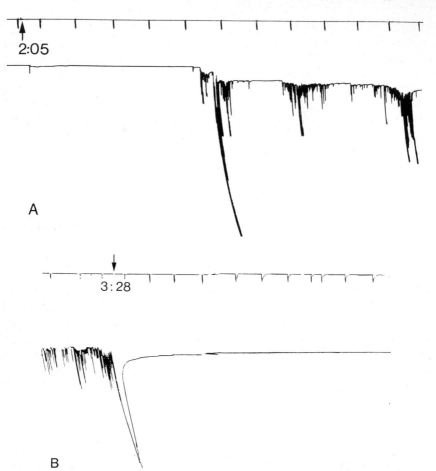

Fig. 15 A and B. Fasciculations produced by DFP and their termination by ACh. The experiments were carried out in dogs under dial anaesthesia and both records show the tension in the gastrocnemius-soleus muscle group, recorded with a torsion wire myograph. (A) The effect of DFP, 1 mg (5 μmol)/kg injected close—arterially at the arrow (↑). (B) Tracing commences 18 min after the injection of DFP, 0.4 mg/kg, and illustrates the termination of its action by ACh, 25 μg/kg, injected at the arrow (↓). Both DFP and ACh were given close-arterially. Time marker: 30 sec intervals. (From Riker and Wescoe, 1946)

(Barnes and Duff, 1953). When cats are injected with a dose of DFP which produces fasciculations, a subsequent close-arterial injection of ACh, in a dose which has little postsynaptic action, greatly reduces the fasciculations (Fig. 15; Riker and Wescoe, 1946). Similarly in the rat isolated nerve-diaphragm preparation ACh added to the bathing fluid arrests antidromic nerve action potentials (Barstad, 1962).

These findings indicate that fasciculations like twitch potentiation are caused by axon reflexes originating at a presynaptic site. Since nerve stimulation is not involved and there is no evidence that the nerve terminals themselves can be depolarised sufficiently to act as stimulus generators in their own right the site at which the axon reflex is most likely to originate is the first node of Ranvier.

In the case of anticholinesterases of the carbamate and organophosphate type the evidence points to the initiation of the axon reflex being the result of the inhibition of AChE, which allows ACh released at random in the absence of nerve stimulation to gain access to the first node of Ranvier and to depolarise it. This action of ACh is self-limiting when inhibition of AChE becomes too extensive. In the case of edrophonium, the only anilinium ion studied in detail in this context, the results are consistent with AChE inhibition being at least partly responsible for the fasciculations produced, but the possibility that a direct presynaptic ACh-like action of edrophonium might be involved cannot be excluded.

In conscious animals efferent impulses in individual motor neurones probably enhance fasciculations since a period of nerve stimulation is followed by an increased rate of fasciculation (BLABER, unpublished).

III. Tetanic Fade

Mammalian muscle normally responds to indirect stimulation at frequencies of 20 Hz or higher, applied for short periods, with a sustained increase in tension. Following the administration of an anticholinesterase of the carbamate type (BACQ and BROWN, 1937; BLABER and BOWMAN, 1963b) or organophosphate type (BURGEN and HOBBIGER, 1951; BARNES and DUFF, 1953) or of edrophonium (BLABER and BOWMAN, 1963b), in appropriate doses (concentrations), the response to such stimulation consists of a rapid increase in tension followed at once by partial or complete relaxation while stimulation is maintained (Fig. 16). The extent of this relaxation, the so-called tetanic fade, is dose (concentration) dependent and it can be antagonised by tubocurarine (BLABER and BOWMAN, 1963b).

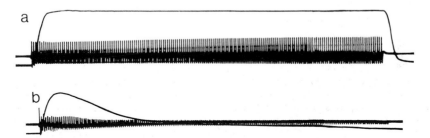

Fig. 16 a and b. Tetanic fade produced by neostigmine in the gastrocnemius muscle of the cat anaesthetised with chloralose. Each of the two records shows the muscle tension recorded with a strain gauge (smooth line) and muscle action potentials recorded from belly-tendon leads, during a period of nerve stimulation at a rate of 100 Hz. (a) control responses, (b) the record obtained 5 min after injection of 10 µg (0.03 µmol) neostigmine into the popliteal artery. (From BLABER and BOWMAN, 1963 b)

Detailed investigations have only been undertaken with anticholinesterases of the carbamate and organophosphate type. These studies have shown that the tetanic fade produced by these anticholinesterases is associated with marked inhibition of AChE. BARNES and DUFF (1953) found that in the rat isolated nerve-diaphragm preparation, stimulated indirectly at a frequency of 50 Hz for 5 sec, paraoxon produces a complete tetanic fade when the inhibition of total AChE amounts to 95%.

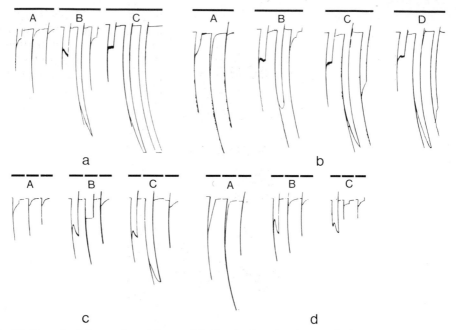

Fig. 17. Tetanic fade produced by anticholinesterases in the rat isolated nerve-diaphragm preparation, suspended in Tyrode solution at 37° C, and its reversal by removal of the anticholinesterases from the organ bath. Each panel shows responses of the muscle to nerve stimulation for 5 sec at a rate of 25, 50, and 100 Hz. Individual anticholinesterases were added to the organ bath for 1 hour and in the case of neostigmine and dimethylphosphostigmine panel A shows the responses of the muscle at this time. All other panels illustrate responses of the muscle following removal of the anticholinesterase from the organ bath.

	Anticholinesterase	Time in min after removal of anti-cholinesterase from organ bath	Type of acylated AChE formed
(a)	neostigmine	B: 10, C: 30	dimethylcarbamyl — AChE
(b)	dimethylphosphostigmine	B: 10, C: 20, D: 40	dimethylphosphoryl — AChE
(c)	diethylphosphostigmine	A: 10, B: 50, C: 90	diethylphosphoryl — AChE
(d)	di*iso*propylphosphostigmine		di*iso*propylphosphoryl — AChE

The rate of spontaneous reactivation of the acylated AChEs is: dimethylcarbamyl—AChE > dimethylphosphoryl—AChE > diethylphosphoryl—AChE ≫ di*iso*propylphosphoryl—AChE (see Section C 1 and Table 1). Results obtained with TEPP were comparable to those with diethylphosphostigmine and results obtained with DFP and di*sec*butylphosphostigmine were comparable to those with di*iso*propylphosphostigmine. (From Burgen and Hobbiger, 1951)

Such a level of inhibition is considerably greater than that associated with threshold twitch potentiation (Table 3). In the mouse isolated nerve-diaphragm preparation, stimulated indirectly at a frequency of 120 Hz, DFP produces a tetanic fade when the level of inhibition of total AChE is 80% or more but when the frequency of stimulation is 60 Hz a similar degree of fade occurs only when inhibition of total AChE exceeds 95% (Barnard et al., 1971 b).

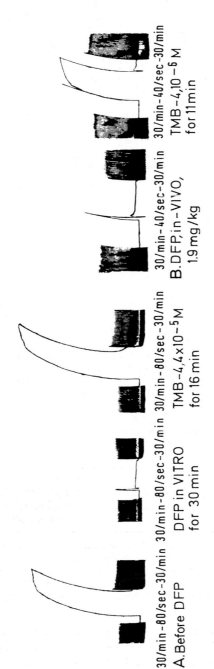

Fig. 18 A and B. Tetanic fade produced in the rat diaphragm by DFP *in vivo* and in the isolated muscle preparation (in Tyrode solution at 37° C), and its reversal by the oxime TMB-4. (A) The effect of DFP, 10 μmol/l (2 μg/ml) on the isolated muscle preparation and its reversal by TMB-4, 50 μmol/l (20 μg/ml). (B) Isolated muscle preparation from an atropinised rat injected subcutaneously with 1.9 mg (10 μmol) DFP/kg; TMB-4 added to the organ bath. (From FLEISHER et al., 1960)

In the rat isolated nerve-diaphragm preparation the removal of anticholinesterases of the carbamate or organophosphate type from the bathing fluid after tetanic fade has been elicited is followed by a gradual return of a sustained muscle
contraction in response to indirect stimulation provided the acylated AChE undergoes spontaneous reactivation. The rates of recovery are: (1) inversely related to the
frequency of indirect stimulation, (2) very similar for anticholinesterases which form
the same type of acylated AChE and (3) proportional to the rate of spontaneous
reactivation of the acylated AChE present (see Section C I) (BURGEN and HOBBIGER,
1951). This is illustrated in Fig. 17.

The tetanic fade produced by the organophosphate anticholinesterases TEPP,
DFP and sarin in the rat diaphragm, during indirect stimulation at frequencies of 40
to 100 Hz, can be completely reversed both *in vivo* and in isolated nerve-muscle
preparations by oximes (BERRY and LOVATT EVANS, 1951; HOLMES and ROBINS,
1955; FLEISHER et al., 1960). This is illustrated in Fig. 18. BERRY and LOVATT EVANS
(1951) and FLEISHER et al. (1960) measured the total AChE activity of the rat diaphragm and observed that with a frequency of indirect stimulation of 80 to 100 Hz
the tetanic fade was associated with AChE inhibition in excess of 90% and that when
a normal tetanic response was restored by an oxime the level of AChE activity had
risen at most by 6%. However, studies of functional AChE activity performed by
FLEISHER et al. (1960) showed that at a frequency of indirect stimulation of 80 Hz the
oxime-induced reversal of the tetanic fade produced by DFP was paralleled by a
decrease in the level of inhibition from 90% to 64%. The oxime used in these studies
was TMB-4. Similar results were obtained by MEER and WOLTHUIS (1965). In studies
of the tetanic fade produced in the rat isolated nerve-diaphragm preparation by
sarin, tabun and DFP these authors observed that reversal of tetanic fade by the
oxime pralidoxime was associated with a 14 to 20% increase in functional AChE
activity when the frequency of indirect stimulation was 100 Hz and a 40% increase at
a stimulation rate of 200 Hz.

These experiments indicate that at any given frequency of indirect stimulation
there is only a small difference between the levels of AChE inhibition at which tetanic
tension is fully maintained and that at which tetanic fade is complete (and that this
critical range is dependent on the frequency of stimulation). To study this in more
detail HOBBIGER and HEFFRON(unpublished) carried out the following experiments.
The rat isolated nerve-diaphragm preparation was incubated with 0.18 µmol/l paraoxon. Five min later, when there was a complete tetanic fade during indirect stimulation for 10 sec at frequencies of 50 and 100 Hz, the bathing fluid was exchanged
with paraoxon-free bathing fluid. The diethylphosphoryl-AChE formed by paraoxon
undergoes slow spontaneous reactivation (see Section C I) and the gradual recovery
of the tetanic response following removal of paraoxon from the bathing fluid was
recorded. Changes in sensitivity of the diaphragm to ACh during the recovery of the
tetanic response were also determined by assaying the concentration of ACh which
on addition to the bathing fluid produced in 5 min a 50% reduction in twitch tension
(frequency of stimulation 0.2 Hz). In a second series of experiments, preparations
were incubated for 5 min with concentrations of DFP ranging from 3.6 to 18 µmol/l
to produce irreversible inhibition of AChE. Following removal of DFP from the
bathing fluid the sensitivity of individual preparations to ACh was determined as
already described and subsequent to this the level of functional AChE activity, as

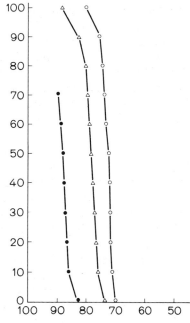

Fig. 19. Relationship between tetanic fade and inhibition of functional AChE activity in the rat isolated nerve-diaphragm preparation, suspended in Tyrode solution at 37° C. Ordinate: Per cent reduction in muscle tension at the end of a 10 sec period of nerve stimulation at a rate of 20 (●), 50 (△) and 100 (○) Hz, expressed as per cent of controls. Abscissa: per cent inhibition of functional AChE activity. For experimental details see text. (From Hobbiger and Heffron, unpublished Fig.)

reflected by the rate of uptake of ACh (50 μmol/l; 1 ml/100 mg tissue) by the intact diaphragm. Using the relationship between the sensitivity of the diaphragm to ACh and inhibition of functional AChE activity in the DFP treated diaphragms and assuming that equal changes in sensitivity to ACh produced by paraoxon and DFP reflect equal changes in functional AChE activity, the inhibition of functional AChE activity associated with different levels of tetanic fade during recovery of preparations from exposure to paraoxon was calculated. As can be seen from Fig. 19 which shows the result of these calculations, the tetanic tension declined by 50% over a period of 10 seconds with rates of indirect stimulation of 20, 50, and 100 Hz when the inhibition of functional AChE activity amounted to 87%, 77% and 72%, respectively. Furthermore, the difference between the level of inhibition at which the tetanic fade was just perceptible and that at which the tetanic fade was complete was relatively narrow (73 to 88% and 70 to 78% for rates of stimulation of 50 and 100 Hz, respectively).

If we consider all the information obtained in studies on the tetanic fade produced by anticholinesterases of the carbamate and organophosphate type and referred to above, there can be no doubt that AChE inhibition is the cause of tetanic fade. The level of enzyme inhibition at which the tetanic fade occurs lies in the upper part of the range associated with twitch potentiation. Under these conditions the e.p.p. is prolonged (see Section D I). Consequently at high frequencies of nerve stimulation summation of consecutive e.p.p.s will occur and the neuromuscular junction will be blocked by depolarisation of the postsynaptic membrane. The tetanic fade produced by edrophonium is undoubtedly attributable to the same mechanism.

Observations by Burns and Paton (1951) are consistent with this interpretation. In studies on the gracilis muscle in cats they found that subsequent to the administration of neostigmine or physostigmine indirect stimulation for 5 to 10 sec at frequencies of 70 to 690 Hz produced an end-plate negativity which outlasted considerably the stimulation period. Furthermore, $100\,\mu g$ of ACh injected close-arterially subsequent to the administration of physostigmine, rendered the end-plate electrically inexcitable. These effects of neostigmine and physostigmine disappeared when an anodal current of $50\,\mu A$ was applied to the end-plate region and were also abolished by tubocurarine.

Although the experimental evidence suggests that a depolarisation block at the postsynaptic site as a consequence of AChE inhibition is the cause of the tetanic fade, the possibility that other factors might contribute to it should not be overlooked. Briscoe (1938) in studies of the response of the quadriceps muscle in cats to indirect stimulation at high frequencies noted that the first effect of physostigmine was to cause a notch in the record of the muscle response, i.e. the initial increase in muscle tension was followed by a very transient fall and then a further increase in tension. The same can be seen in some of the muscle responses illustrated in Fig. 18. Blaber and Bowman (1963 b) in studies on cats observed that when a nerve was stimulated at high frequencies following the administration of neostigmine, ambenonium or edrophonium, antidromic nerve action potentials were present during the initial period of stimulation. Low doses of tubocurarine which act presynaptically (see Section D I), and which do not block neuromuscular transmission, abolished both the antidromic nerve action potentials and the notch in the muscle response. The major component of the tetanic fade, however, was only antagonised by higher doses of tubocurarine which compete with ACh for postsynaptic cholinoceptors. From these findings Blaber and Bowman concluded that the major cause of the tetanic fade was a depolarisation block at the postsynaptic site, but that partial extinction of orthodromic stimuli by antidromic nerve action potentials contributed to its early phases.

In conscious animals the frequency of impulses in motor neurones during muscular activity ranges from 9 to 110 Hz, with a mean of 50 Hz (Adrian and Bronk, 1928, 1929; Krnjević and Miledi, 1958). Since the anticholinesterases of the carbamate and organophosphate type impair the ability of the neuromuscular junction to respond normally to high frequency stimulation, one would expect muscular weakness to be one of the symptoms produced by these substances in conscious animals. This is indeed the case.

IV. Anticurare Action

The ability of an anticholinesterase to antagonise neuromuscular block was first demonstrated by Pal (1900) and Rothberger (1901). They observed that in rabbits, cats and dogs physostigmine restored spontaneous respiration and responses of muscles to nerve stimulation after these had been abolished by curare. Subsequent work has shown that certain aspects of the anticurare action might depend on the frequency of nerve stimulation. It is thus best to separate a discussion of the anticurare action at low frequencies of nerve stimulation from that at high frequencies of nerve stimulation.

1. Anticurare Action at Frequencies of Nerve Stimulation which Normally Produce Twitch Responses

Tubocurarine is a competitive antagonist of ACh for the postsynaptic cholinoceptors and thus reduces the amplitude of the e.p.p. When the concentration of tubocurarine at a motor end-plate is such that the e.p.p. no longer reaches the critical amplitude (10 to 20 mV) required to trigger a propagated muscle action potential, a nerve impulse fails to elicit a contraction of the muscle fibre, i.e. there is a neuromuscular block (ECCLES et al., 1941, 1942). The extent of the neuromuscular block is proportional to the number of motor end-plates which have ceased to transmit impulses.

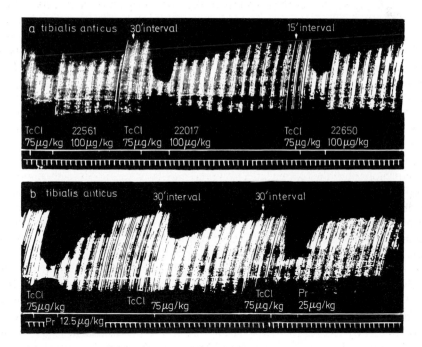

Fig. 20. Anticurare action of neostigmine and three anilinium ions (Ro 2—2017, 2—2561, and 2—2650). The experiment was performed in a dog which had been treated with atropine. The animal weighed 10 kg and was anaesthetised with dial-urethane. The records show twitch responses of the tibialis anterior muscle in response to maximal nerve stimulation at a rate of 0.12 Hz. Tubocurarine (TcCl), anilinium ions and neostigmine (Pr) were injected into the femoral vein in the doses shown. Neostigmine was given in doses of 12.5 and 25 μg (40 and 80 nmol)/kg. Ro 2-2561 is 3-OH phenyltrimethylammonium and Ro 2-2017 and Ro 2-2650 are its 3-acetoxy and 3-benzoxy derivatives, respectively. They were each given in a dose of 100 μg/kg which corresponds to 0.3, 0.3 and 0.5 μmol/kg, respectively. Ro 2-2017 is speedily hydrolysed *in vivo* to Ro 2-2561 (HOBBIGER, 1952). (FROM RANDALL and LEHMANN, 1950)

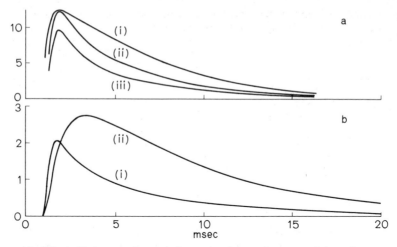

Fig. 21 a and b. Effect of tubocurarine and physostigmine on the e.p.p. of the soleus muscle in the cat. (a) Two successive e.p.p.s are evoked, the first and second being separated by 1.6 msec. i: normal muscle; ii and iii: after successive doses of tubocurarine. (b) e.p.p. produced by single nerve volley in same experiment. i: after a dose of tubocurarine, ii: after doses of tubocurarine and physostigmine; the rate of rise is slower than in (i) because of deeper curarisation. Ordinate: percentage of maximum spike potential. Abscissa: time from nerve stimulus. (From Eccles et al., 1941)

All anticholinesterases of the carbamate type antagonise the action of tubocurarine (Fig. 20; White and Stedman, 1931; Bacq and Brown, 1937; Bülbring and Chou, 1947; Koelle and Gilman, 1949). This is also true of anticholinesterases of the organophosphate type (Hunt, 1947; Burgen et al., 1949; Chennels et al., 1949; Holmstedt, 1951, 1959) and of the anilinium ions (Fig. 20; Wescoe et al., 1949; Riker et al., 1949; Randall and Lehmann, 1950; Randall, 1950; Wescoe and Riker, 1951).

Studies of the mechanism responsible for the anticurare action of the anticholinesterases have largely involved the carbamates and it has become widely accepted that their anticurare action is due to the inhibition of AChE which allows ACh to accumulate and therefore compete more effectively with tubocurarine for postsynaptic cholinoceptors. The evidence for this interpretation will now be considered. Eccles et al. (1941, 1942) using extracellular recording observed that in the soleus muscle of the cat physostigmine given after tubocurarine raised the amplitude of the e.p.p. and prolonged its rise- and decay-time (Fig. 21). This is exactly what might be expected if inhibition of AChE enables ACh to compete effectively with tubocurarine for the postsynaptic cholinoceptors. Results similar to those of Eccles et al. were obtained by Boyd and Martin (1956 b) and Blaber and Christ (1967) with 0.3 μmol/l and 0.1 to 1 μmol/l neostigmine, respectively, using the cat isolated tenuissimus muscle preparation. In these experiments the e.p.p. was recorded intracellularly.

Additional evidence on the role of AChE inhibition in the anticurare action is provided by comparisons between anticholinesterase potency *in vitro* and anticurare potency. Bacq and Brown (1937) compared the anticholinesterase potency of physostigmine and five related substances with their anticurare potency on the gastroc-

Table 5. Relationship between the anticholinesterase and anticurare potencies of 12 anticholinesterases of the carbamate type. (After BLASCHKO et al., 1949)

	Anticurare potency	Anticholinesterase potency
Neostigmine (RNMe$_3$)[a]	7.60	7.4
3392 (RNMe$_2$Et)	8.19	8.0
3393 (RNMeEt$_2$)	8.57	8.2
S208 (RNEt$_3$)	6.59	7.4
Miotine HCl	7.85	6.4
Physostigmine	7.21	7.1
No. 38	6.23	7.1
Nu 1250	7.26	7.4
Nu 1197	7.31	6.9
Nu 683	5.44	6.2
5130	5.26	6.4
5220/5 (RNMe$_2$OH)	4.77	4.5

[a] $R = -(CH_3)_2N.CO_2C_6H_4$.

Anticurare potency was determined on the rat isolated nerve-diaphragm preparation; the figures given are the negative logarithms of the molar concentrations of the carbamates which antagonised the effect of 3 µmol/l tubocurarine to such an extent that it produced only a 20% reduction in twitch tension.

Anticholinesterase potency was determined with the Warburg method at 38° C, using homogenates of the dog caudate nucleus as enzyme source and 6 mmol/l ACh as substrate. The figures given represent the negative logarithms of the molar concentrations of the carbamates which when added together with ACh to the enzyme reduced the hydrolysis of ACh by 50% during a 30 min period commencing 3 minutes after the addition of the substrate and carbamate to the enzyme. Although the enzyme preparation used contains some ChE in addition to AChE, this had a negligible effect on the results obtained. — The structure of the carbamates listed is shown in Appendix II.

nemius muscle of the cat; BÜLBRING and CHOU (1947) did a similar comparison using neostigmine and 4 related carbamates as well as physostigmine on the rat isolated nerve-diaphragm preparation and on the gastrocnemius muscle in the cat. BLASCHKO et al. (1949) determined the anticholinesterase potency of neostigmine and 11 other carbamates and evaluated their anticurare potency on the rat isolated nerve-diaphragm preparation (Table 5). In all these experiments a good correlation between anticholinesterase and anticurare potency was observed although anticholinesterase potency varied up to 1000 fold between substances. These experiments might be criticised because the degree of ionisation and thus the rates of diffusion into the diaphragm are not constant for all the substances tested and on the whole several carbamates were administered in the same experiment at intervals which did not allow for complete decarbamylation of AChE. However, it seems unlikely that these limitations affected the results to the extent of markedly distorting the true correlation between anticholinesterase and anticurare potency.

All these findings are certainly consistent with the view that inhibition of AChE accounts largely if not solely for the anticurare action of anticholinesterases of the carbamate type. Increased competition of ACh with tubocurarine for the postsynaptic cholinoceptors as the result of AChE inhibition, however, is not the only mechanism by which an e.p.p. which is reduced by tubocurarine can be raised to its critical height. For example, the same effect can be achieved by increasing the ACh output of nerve terminals, i.e. increasing the quantal release of ACh. In this context experiments by BLABER and CHRIST (1967) are relevant. They recorded e.p.p.s in the presence of tubocurarine and m.e.p.p.s in its absence in the cat isolated tenuissimus muscle preparation. It was observed that neostigmine, 0.1 to 1 µmol/l, and ambenonium, 0.01 to 0.1 µmol/l, increased the amplitude and prolonged the rise- and decay-time of both the e.p.p. and the m.e.p.p. On the other hand, neostigmine, 0.01 µmol/l, and ambenonium, 0.0001 to 0.001 µmol/l, increased the amplitude of the e.p.p. without affecting its time-course and had no effect on the m.e.p.p.

Published work on the anticurare action of neostigmine has largely been carried out with doses (concentrations) of neostigmine which are likely to give peak concentrations of at least 0.1 µmol/l at motor end-plates. According to the results of BLABER and CHRIST, the anticurare action under these conditions might be explained by an increased competition of ACh with tubocurarine for the postsynaptic cholinoceptors as the result of AChE inhibition, although other factors might also be involved. Difficulties in interpreting the mechanism of the anticurare action arise from the results obtained with concentrations of neostigmine and ambenonium below 0.1 µmol/l and 0.01 µmol/l, respectively. Since in the presence of tubocurarine such concentrations only raise the amplitude of the e.p.p. without changing its time-course and in the absence of tubocurarine have no effect on the m.e.p.p., BLABER and CHRIST concluded that neostigmine and ambenonium increased the quantal release of ACh through a direct action on nerve terminals and that this was an important feature of their anticurare action.

The conclusion that neostigmine and ambenonium might cause an increased quantal release of ACh by a direct action on nerve terminals is open to doubt. The duration of the anticurare action of neostigmine *in vivo* (Fig. 20) is consistent with the time-course of decarbamylation and much longer than would be expected to result from the reversible action of a monoquaternary substance. Furthermore, the anticholinesterase potency of ambenonium is approximately 6 times greater than that of neostigmine (LANDS et al., 1958) and their relative potency in raising the e.p.p. in the presence of tubocurarine seems to be of the same magnitude (BLABER and CHRIST, 1967). These observations certainly are more consistent with the view that inhibition of AChE which allows access of ACh to the nerve terminals is responsible for increasing the quantal release of ACh rather than a direct action of ambenonium and neostigmine at the nerve terminals. Studies of the effects of a range of doses of anticholinesterases of the organophosphate type on the e.p.p. in the presence of tubocurarine would allow determination of the level of AChE inhibition at motor end-plates and might clarify the situation. Until such information is available the following interpretation of the mechanism of the anticurare action of anticholinesterases of the carbamate type and related substances such as ambenonium seems justified. With the doses (concentrations) which have been most widely used inhibition of AChE, allowing ACh to compete more effectively with tubocurarine for the postsynaptic cholinoceptors, is undoubtedly very important. Increased quantal release of ACh might contribute to this and indeed might be the sole mechanism responsible for the anticurare action in the lower range of doses (concentrations) required to antagonise the action of tubocurarine. Experimental data suggest that the increase in the quantal release of ACh is a result of AChE inhibition allowing

ACh access to nerve terminals rather than being caused by a direct action of the anticholinesterases.

There are no detailed studies of the action of anticholinesterases of the organophosphate type on the e.p.p. in the presence of tubocurarine. Most of the organophosphates do not possess a tertiary or quaternary nitrogen and therefore it is difficult to see how their anticurare action could involve any mechanism other than inhibition of AChE. That AChE inhibition is involved is supported by the finding that both the anticurare action of these compounds and their inhibition of AChE develop gradually (BURGEN et al., 1949).

The anticurare action of edrophonium and other anilinium ions is very much quicker in onset than that of anticholinesterases of the carbamate or organophosphate type and lasts only a few minutes *in vivo* (Fig. 20). BLABER and CHRIST (1967) in their studies on the cat isolated tenuissimus muscle which involved recording e.p.p.s in the presence of tubocurarine and m.e.p.p.s in its absence, observed that edrophonium in concentrations of 1 to 10 µmol/l raised the amplitude of the e.p.p. and increased its rise- and decay-time without affecting m.e.p.p.s. At concentrations of 0.1 to 1 µmol/l only the amplitude of the e.p.p. was raised. From data obtained in subsequent studies on the cat isolated tenuissimus muscle with cut muscle fibres, BLABER (1972) calculated by the method described in Appendix III that the increase in the amplitude of the e.p.p. obtained with 0.1 µmol/l edrophonium in the presence of tubocurarine was due to an increase in the quantal release of ACh. A number of published data on the anticurare action of edrophonium were obtained with doses which according to the results of BLABER and CHRIST (1967) might only have given rise to an increase in the amplitude of the e.p.p. without affecting its time-course. The case for an increased quantal release of ACh being an essential component of their anticurare action, therefore, is stronger with anilinium ions than with neostigmine and ambenonium. However, as pointed out when discussing twitch potentiation (see Section D I) edrophonium's prolongation of e.p.p.s might not be as good an index of AChE inhibition (relevant to ACh released from the nerve terminals) as that by the anticholinesterases. Furthermore, until it is shown that in the presence of tubocurarine inhibition of AChE itself does not raise the quantal content of the e.p.p. we are not in a position to decide whether anilinium ions increase the quantal release of ACh as a result of inhibition of AChE which allows ACh access to nerve terminals or through a direct action on nerve terminals. Supporting this cautious approach are results by WILSON and QUAN (1958) and STANDAERT (1959) which are consistent with the view that inhibition of AChE is important for the anticurare action of anilinium ions. WILSON and QUAN (1958) found that the anticholinesterase potency of anilinium ions was proportional to the ionisation of the hydroxyl group and subsequently STANDAERT (1959) observed that the anticurare action of the phenolate ions was much greater than that of the undissociated bases.

The observation by HOBBIGER (1952) that in cats extensive inhibition of AChE abolishes the anticurare action of edrophonium but not that of decamethonium is interesting in this context. Similarly, BOWMAN (1958) and BLABER and BOWMAN (1962) found that neuromuscular block produced by benzoquinonium, a potent inhibitor of AChE which differs from anticholinesterases such as neostigmine by having also a marked tubocurarine-like action (HOPPE et al., 1955; CHRIST and BLABER, 1968; see Section D VI) can be antagonised at least partly by decamethonium, but not by edrophonium or neostigmine. These findings are consistent with the view that the anticurare action of edrophonium and neostigmine is solely the result of AChE inhibition or if the two substances do act directly on nerve terminals that their site(s) of action there is shared by ACh.

Since neostigmine affects the excitability of nerve terminals following the arrival of an orthodromic impulse in a manner consistent with an increase in the amplitude and duration of the negative after-potential (Hubbard and Schmidt, 1961) it is tempting to suggest that this could be responsible for increasing the quantal release of ACh. However, tubocurarine has an opposite effect on the negative after-potential to that of neostigmine (Hubbard and Schmidt, 1961) and also suppresses repetitive antidromic nerve action potentials (and thus twitch potentiation) which are thought to be triggered by an effect of anticholinesterases and anilinium ions on the negative after-potential. Therefore, for anticholinesterases and anilinium ions to increase the quantal release of ACh in the presence of tubocurarine by an effect on the negative after-potential the following conditions would have to apply: 1) tubocurarine only reducing and not fully antagonising the effect of the anticholinesterases and anilinium ions on the negative after-potential and 2) this reduction being sufficient to prevent initiation of repetitive antidromic nerve action potentials either on its own or in conjunction with an effect of tubocurarine on the first node of Ranvier, which also is thought to play an essential role in the initiation of repetitive antidromic nerve action potentials.

2. Anticurare Action at Frequencies of Nerve Stimulation which Normally Produce a Sustained Contraction of Muscles

When the nerve is stimulated for short periods at frequencies above 20 Hz a sustained contraction of the muscle is normally produced. In the presence of tubocurarine the muscle loses this ability and we see an initial contraction followed at once by relaxation, i.e. a tetanic fade. Studies on the rat isolated nerve-diaphragm preparation and isolated human intercostal muscle, under steady state conditions for tubocurarine, show that the fade is associated with a progressive reduction (fall off) in the amplitude of consecutive e.p.p.s (Lilleheil and Naess, 1961; Thesleff, 1966; Hubbard et al., 1969b). Fade also occurs under conditions where there is very little or no fall off in the amplitude of consecutive e.p.p.s in the absence of tubocurarine and appears not to be paralleled by a decrease in the sensitivity of the postsynaptic membrane to ACh (Hutter, 1952; Liley, 1956a). Lilleheil and Naess (1961), Thesleff (1966) and Hubbard et al. (1969b), therefore, concluded that the progressive reduction in the amplitude of consecutive e.p.p.s produced by tubocurarine during short periods of nerve stimulation at high frequencies was due to a progressive reduction in the quantal release of ACh by a presynaptic action of tubocurarine and that this action in conjunction with the competition between tubocurarine and ACh at the postsynaptic cholinoceptors accounted for the tetanic fade.

In order to obtain more information on the presynaptic action of tubocurarine Hubbard et al. (1969b) and Blaber (1970, 1972, 1973) recorded the e.p.p.s produced during short periods of nerve stimulation at 100 and 200 Hz in the rat isolated nerve-diaphragm and cat isolated tenuissimus muscle preparations with cut muscle fibres. From measurements of these e.p.p.s (see Appendix III) they calculated that tubocurarine reduced the rate of refilling of the ACh store in nerve terminals and that this led to its partial depletion. According to these calculations tubocurarine actually increases the fractional release of ACh but this action is not sufficient to compensate fully for the depletion of the ACh store. The action of tubocurarine on the quantal release of ACh is proportional to the rate of nerve stimulation but here is no evidence to support the view that it contributes to neuromuscular block at low rates of nerve stimulation.

In the cat isolated tenuissimus muscle preparation edrophonium, 0.1 μmol/l, reverses the reduction by tubocurarine in the rate of refilling of the ACh store in nerve terminals (BLABER, 1972). It is not known whether this is true of the anticholinesterases of the carbamate and organophosphate type. If it is, the mechanisms by which they and anilinium ions can antagonise a tubocurarine-induced tetanic fade would consist of: 1) the mechanisms which are responsible for the anticurare action at low rates of nerve stimulation, and 2) reversal of the tubocurarine-induced reduction in the rate of refilling of the ACh store in nerve terminals. If the muscle is stimulated indirectly at high frequencies subsequent to the administration of an anticholinesterase or anilinium ion and of tubocurarine, mechanism (2) alone should be able to prevent a tetanic fade.

The view that progressive reduction in the quantal release of ACh contributes essentially to the tetanic fade produced by tubocurarine has not remained unchallenged although at present there appears to be no satisfactory alternative explanation. AUERBACH and BETZ (1971) reported that in the rat isolated nerve-diaphragm, cutting the muscle fibres close to the motor end-plates, as was done in the experiments of HUBBARD et al. (1969 b) and BLABER (1970, 1972, 1973), reduced the space constant so that junctional signals were distorted by the cable properties of the muscle fibres when microelectrodes were more than 100 to 200 μm from the motor end-plates. When they made allowance for this, tubocurarine seemed to have no significant effect on the quantal release of ACh.

BLABER (1973) pointed out that the artifact induced by cutting of the muscle fibres certainly could not apply to his studies since e.p.p.s had a rise time of less than 1 msec which meant that the microelectrodes must have been located within 20 μm of end-plates.

Contradicting a presynaptic action of tubocurarine which reduces the quantal release of ACh at high rates of nerve stimulation, are also the results of bioassays of the ACh output from nerve terminals. In these studies isolated muscle preparations, usually a rat nerve-diaphragm, are treated with concentrations of anticholinesterases which produce near complete inhibition of AChE. The amount of ACh which appears in the bathing fluid after a fixed period of nerve stimulation is then determined by bioassay. Using this method KRNJEVIĆ and MITCHELL (1961), CHEYMOL et al. (1962) and CHANG et al. (1967) could not find any reduction in the ACh output of the nerve terminals by tubocurarine. Only BEANI et al. (1964) reported such a reduction. If anticholinesterases behave like edrophonium and prevent tubocurarine from reducing the quantal release of ACh then it is not surprising that the studies referred to do not provide evidence for a reduction of the quantal release of ACh by tubocurarine.

Studies of the anticurare action at high rates of nerve stimulation are undoubtedly of greater relevance for man than those at low rates of nerve stimulation and the paucity of such information, therefore, is regrettable. Another point worth mentioning in this context is that the anticholinesterases of the carbamate and organophosphate type and the anilinium ions can effectively antagonise neuromuscular block produced by a limited range of doses (concentrations) of tubocurarine only (Maanen, 1952; Kuperman and Okamoto, 1964). Furthermore, if inhibition of AChE is extensive and outlasts the action of tubocurarine, a neuromuscular block by depolarisation of the motor end-plates will follow an initial reversal of the neuromuscular block produced by tubocurarine.

V. Reversal of the Symptoms of Myasthenia Gravis

Myasthenia gravis is a chronic disease in man, characterised by weakness and abnormal fatigability of skeletal muscles, particularly those innervated by the cranial nerves. The term disease is probably a misnomer since as judged by clinical features and results of laboratory investigations, myasthenia gravis is probably a syndrome rather than a disease with a single cause (Johns and McQuillen, 1966). *In vivo* the muscles of myasthenic patients respond to nerve stimulation at various frequencies like muscles of control subjects injected with a dose of tubocurarine large enough to produce a partial neuromuscular block (Grob et al., 1956). This similarity also extends to the action of anticholinesterases of the carbamate and organophosphate type in the two situations. These substances not only antagonise the neuromuscular block produced by tubocurarine but also markedly alleviate or even abolish completely the muscular symptoms in most patients with myasthenia gravis (Glaser, 1966). This was first noted by Remen (1932) and independently by Walker (1934) in myasthenic patients to whom they administered neostigmine and physostigmine, respectively. In subsequent studies Walker (1935) found that neostigmine was therapeutically superior to physostigmine. In the 1950's a variety of anticholinesterases of the carbamate and organophosphate type such as pyridostigmine, ambenonium, demecarium (BC-48; a bisneostigmine where the carbamyl nitrogens of two neostigmine molecules are joined by a $[CH_2]_{10}$ group), distigmine (hexamarium; BC-51; a bispyridostigmine where the carbamyl nitrogens of the two pyridostigmine molecules are joined by a $[CH_2]_6$ group), DFP, TEPP, OMPA (octamethyl pyrophosphortetramide), phospholine and sarin were tested and found also to produce a good therapeutic effect (see Grob, 1963). Treatment of myasthenia gravis nowadays, however, appears to be largely limited to the use of neostigmine, pyridostigmine or ambenonium which are shorter acting than the other anticholinesterases mentioned and thus have the advantage of being less likely to give rise to over-dosage through accumulation and of allowing better control of fluctuations in the severity of symptoms.

Histological studies have shown that there are marked morphological differences between the motor end-plates in muscles of myasthenic patients and those in muscles of healthy people (Bergman et al., 1971; Engel and Santa, 1971). In muscles of myasthenic patients the size of the motor end-plates is smaller than normal. The nerve fibre is extended in length and gives rise to multiple small terminals of reduced size. The postsynaptic membrane is extremely simplified in that secondary synaptic clefts are sparse, shallow and abnormally wide. In addition, there are marked deviations from normal in the Schwann cells and in muscle capillaries. On the basis of these changes alone one would not be surprised to find that neuromuscular transmission in myasthenic patients differs from that in healthy people.

Valuable information on the nature of the impairment of neuromuscular transmission in myasthenia gravis has been obtained in studies which ELMQVIST et al. (1964) and LAMBERT and ELMQVIST (1971) carried out on intercostal muscles obtained from patients with the disease (myasthenic muscles) and healthy subjects (control muscles). In these studies on the isolated muscles the following observations were made. Carbachol and decamethonium, added to the bathing fluid in near maximally effective concentrations only, produced identical levels of depolarisation in myasthenic and control muscles. From this the authors concluded that the postsynaptic membrane was not the site at which neuromuscular transmission was impaired in myasthenic muscle. Studies of the m.e.p.p. then showed that the amplitude of m.e.p.p.s at motor end-plates of myasthenic muscles was only 0.2 ± 0.11 mV whereas that at motor end-plates of control muscles was 0.98 ± 0.3 mV. On the other hand, the frequency of m.e.p.p.s in the two types of muscle was very similar and the same applied to the rate of increase in the frequency of m.e.p.p.s obtained by raising the concentration of potassium in the bathing fluid to 20 mmol/l. The e.p.p. at motor end-plates of myasthenic muscle was found to be markedly reduced in size but values for the quantal content of the e.p.p. and the number of quanta (vesicles) in the nerve terminals, calculated from e.p.p. recordings (see Appendix III), were very similar to normal values. This is supported by the observation of ENGEL and SANTA (1971) that the density of vesicles in nerve terminals in myasthenic muscle is very similar to that in normal nerve terminals.

These findings suggest that the important lesion in myasthenia gravis is a marked reduction in the ACh content of the vesicles. As a consequence the amplitude of the e.p.p. is reduced, being close to the critical level at some motor end-plates and even below it at others (THESLEFF, 1966). This could account for the muscle weakness observed.

When isolated preparations of myasthenic intercostal muscle are stimulated indirectly at frequencies of 40 Hz or more, i.e. at rates corresponding to the frequency of nerve impulses during muscle activity, it is found that there is an initial rapid fall off in the amplitude of consecutive e.p.p.s (ELMQVIST et al., 1964; THESLEFF, 1966). This fall off increases the number of motor end-plates with a subthreshold e.p.p. Consequently, when a nerve is stimulated *in vivo* at 50 Hz the compound muscle action potential in muscles of myasthenic patients rapidly declines in size (GROB et al., 1956) and in the case of an isolated muscle preparation a myasthenic muscle loses its ability to respond with a sustained increase in tension when stimulated indirectly at high frequencies (Fig. 22). *In vivo* and in the absence of nerve stimulation an increase in the fatigability of muscles is observed.

The ACh content of the vesicles in the nerve terminals of myasthenic muscle cannot be raised by adding choline to the bathing fluid of isolated myasthenic intercostal muscle preparations, and unlike in normal nerve-muscle preparations exposed to hemicholinium it is not reduced by nerve stimulation at high frequencies (ELMQVIST et al., 1964; THESLEFF, 1966). From these observations the authors concluded that an impairment of choline uptake by the nerve terminals could not be a major causative factor in myasthenia gravis. The experimental findings also appear to rule out the possibility that there is a deficiency in choline acetyltransferase. It is

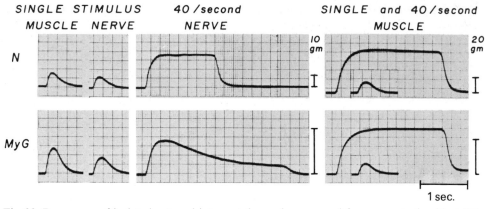

Fig. 22. Responses of isolated external intercostal muscles removed from a control subject (N) and a patient with myasthenia gravis (MyG) to indirect (nerve) and direct (muscle) stimulation, at 32 to 33° C. Muscle tension was recorded with a strain gauge. (From LAMBERT and ELMQVIST, 1971)

tempting, therefore, to consider that a reduction in the ACh content of the vesicles might arise from a deficiency in the synthesis of vesiculin, the protein which is probably important for the storage of ACh in the vesicles (WHITTAKER, 1966).

In view of the marked morphological difference between the motor end-plates in myasthenic muscles and those in normal muscles it is rather surprising that studies on isolated intercostal muscle preparations should suggest that impairment of neuromuscular transmission in patients with myasthenia gravis arises solely from a deficiency in the storage of ACh in the vesicles. However, studies on isolated muscle preparations do not necessarily give information on all aspects which are important *in vivo*. This also seems to apply to studies on myasthenic muscles. GROB (1971) using a steel wire electrode of 0.1 mm diameter, recorded the electrical activity in the relaxed opponens pollicis muscle of normal subjects and of patients with severe generalised myasthenia gravis. In both groups he observed negative potentials of about 20 μV which closely resembled m.e.p.p.s in rise- and decay-time and continued for hours at a frequency of 45 to 50 Hz. The close-arterial injection of ACh, 0.02 to 2 mg, markedly increased the amplitude and frequency of these "m.e.p.p.s". When ACh was injected repeatedly the dose required for a threshold effect progressively increased. The only difference between control and myasthenic subjects was that in the myasthenic subjects the threshold dose at which ACh affected the "m.e.p.p.s" was higher and that the decrease in the effectiveness of ACh on repeated administration was greater. From these findings GROB (1971) concluded that the postsynaptic membrane of motor end-plates in myasthenic muscle is less sensitive to ACh than that of normal end-plates and is also more readily desensitised by ACh. It seems that this conclusion might not be fully justified since vascular lesions in the vicinity of motor end-plates could at least partly account for the findings. On the other hand, the observations on "m.e.p.p.s" seem to be important. There can be little doubt that these "m.e.p.p.s" were initiated from nerve terminals but it is difficult to understand why the "m.e.p.p.s" in normal and myasthenic muscle were of comparable amplitude if the basic lesion in myasthenia gravis is a reduction in the ACh content of vesicles.

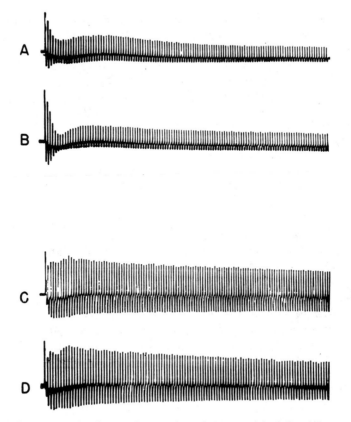

Fig. 23 A—D. Effect of neostigmine on the muscle action potential of the abductor digiti quinti muscle in a patient with myasthenia gravis, at a high rate of nerve stimulation. The muscle action potential was recorded via 7 mm silver discs attached with bentonite — KCl paste to the skin over the belly and tendon of the muscle. The ulnar nerve was stimulated percutaneously just above the elbow with supramaximal rectangular pulses of 0.15 msec duration. (A), (B), (C), and (D): muscle action potentials triggered by 121 nerve stimuli applied at a rate of 50 Hz. The interval between A and B was 5 sec, as was that between C and D. C and D were recorded after the injection of 2 mg (7 μmol) neostigmine into the brachial artery. (From GROB et al., 1956)

It is interesting to note that in earlier work on isolated intercostal muscle from myasthenic patients, the amplitude of m.e.p.p.s was also found to be in the normal range (DAHLBÄCK et al., 1961). Obviously much more work is needed before we will arrive at a full understanding of the nature of the impairment of the transmission of nerve impulses at motor end-plates in myasthenic muscle. In such work a consideration of the correlation between the morphology of the motor end-plates and the results of electrophysiological and pharmacological studies in the same muscles might be advantageous.

Anticholinesterases of the carbamate and organophosphate type restore effective transmission of nerve impulses at motor end-plates in patients with myasthenia gravis (Fig. 23). There are no studies on the action of these anticholinesterases on isolated muscle preparations obtained from myasthenic patients, but studies in man

(Grob et al., 1956; Grob and Johns, 1958a and b; Grob, 1963) have shown the following. In doses required for a therapeutic effect, the various anticholinesterases potentiate the action of injected ACh at motor end-plates and have a duration of action which is related to the duration of AChE inhibition. In the case of anticholinesterases of the organophosphate type which form a reactivatable phosphorylated AChE the therapeutic effect is abolished by pralidoxime and TMB-4, when given in doses which reactivate the phosphorylated AChE. Furthermore, in his studies on the opponens pollicis muscle, Grob (1971) found that neostigmine increased the amplitude and duration of the "m.e.p.p.s" in myasthenic muscles in the same way as in the muscles of control subjects who had previously been given tubocurarine. These findings are consistent with the view that the various anticholinesterases reduce or abolish the symptoms of myasthenia gravis either entirely or mainly by inhibition of AChE. This would intensify the postsynaptic action of ACh and possibly increase the quantal release of ACh.

Excessive inhibition of AChE leads to neuromuscular block by depolarisation and thus the dose range over which anticholinesterases reverse the symptoms of myasthenia gravis is limited and with an over-dose the patient will show the same symptoms as in the absence of treatment and may even by worse off than before treatment (Grob, 1963).

The symptoms of myasthenia gravis can also be reduced or abolished by edrophonium, but the effect of a single dose lasts for a few minutes only. Edrophonium, therefore, is of no therapeutic value but it is useful in the diagnosis of myasthenia gravis and may be used to decide whether muscular weakness in patients treated with neostigmine or other anticholinesterases is due to under- or over-dosage (Westerberg et al., 1951; Osserman and Kaplan, 1953; Osserman and Genkins, 1966; Foldes and Glaser, 1971). The mechanism by which edrophonium exerts its antimyasthenia action is likely to be the same as that which accounts for its anticurare action at low rates of nerve stimulation, i.e. probably an inhibition of AChE (which enhances the postsynaptic action of ACh and possibly increases the quantal release of ACh) to which an increased quantal release of ACh by a direct action on the nerve terminals might contribute. The only experimental evidence available on the mode of action of edrophonium is the finding that its beneficial effect in myasthenia is associated with potentiation of the action of injected ACh (Grob et al., 1956). This indicates that AChE inhibition might be more important than a direct action.

The treatment of myasthenic patients is purely symptomatic and not curative, and generally must be continued throughout the patient's life. The consequences of such prolonged treatment itself are not known but certain results might be relevant. Roberts and Thesleff (1969) observed that when rats were injected subcutaneously twice daily with 1 mg (3 μmol) neostigmine/kg for 5 to 7 days, the m.e.p.p.s and e.p.p.s at motor end-plates in the diaphragm and tail muscles were reduced in amplitude. From this and an analysis of e.p.p. records (see Appendix III) they concluded that the ACh content of vesicles and the fraction of the vesicles (quanta of ACh) in the nerve terminals released by a nerve impulse were both reduced. These studies were extended by Chang et al. (1973) who injected rats subcutaneously for 7 days twice daily with 0.1 mg neostigmine/kg. They observed that the ACh content of the diaphragm, determined by bioassay, was unchanged but the quantal release of ACh during stimulation of the phrenic nerve at 100 Hz, also determined by bioassay, was reduced by about 50%. They also determined the number of cholinoceptors at motor end-plates in the diaphragm by measuring the binding of [³H]acetyl α-bungarotoxin and found it to be reduced from 2.1×10^7 (the value in controls) to 1.2×10^7 molecules per motor end-plate. If treatment with neostigmine and other anticholinesterases has similar consequences in man, treatment with anticholinesterases might at least in part defeat its own object in due course and could be responsible for the progressive reduction in the effectiveness of treatment, seen in some patients and usually interpreted as a progression of the disease. Furthermore, it is possible that at least some of the experimental results obtained in the studies of myasthenia gravis, including those on isolated intercostal muscle, were affected by the treatment the patients had received and thus might be misleading, at least quantitatively if not qualitatively.

VI. Selectivity of Action

As discussed earlier (see Sections D I and D IV), the mechanism by which anticholinesterases of the carbamate type and anilinium ions produce twitch potentiation and exert an anticurare action might involve in addition to AChE inhibition a direct (? ACh-like) presynaptic action but it seems unlikely that a direct action is important *in vivo*. In addition, there is no evidence supporting the view that under any experimental conditions a direct presynaptic action could be part of the action of those anticholinesterases of the organophosphate type which have been studied in the greatest detail, i.e. with TEPP, paraoxon, DFP or sarin.

In view of the structural similarity between the active site of AChE and cholinoceptors, the anticholinesterases of the carbamate and organophosphate type and the anilinium ions might also exert a direct action on the postsynaptic cholinoceptors at the neuromuscular junction. Here they could act either as agonists, partial agonists or antagonists and thus exert an ACh-like, limited ACh-like or tubocurarine-like action, respectively.

If a substance possesses an ACh-like action on postsynaptic cholinoceptors at motor end-plates it produces a dose-dependent contraction of rapid onset and short duration in innervated muscle and a contracture in denervated muscle. In this way an ACh-like postsynaptic action has been demonstrated with neostigmine (Fig. 24; RIKER and WESCOE, 1946) and very large doses of sarin and DFP (GROBLEWSKI et al., 1956). However, studies on the cat isolated tenuissimus muscle preparation have shown that the concentrations of neostigmine required to produce motor end-plate depolarisation, are very much higher than those which in the presence of tubocurarine markedly increase the amplitude and prolong the time-course of the e.p.p. (BLABER and CHRIST, 1967).

The anilinium ions also exert an ACh-like postsynaptic action when given close-arterially in appropriate doses (Fig. 24) but there is no correlation between their relative potency as regards this action and that for twitch potentiation or an anticurare action (RANDALL and LEHMANN, 1950). Furthermore, using the cat isolated tenuissimus muscle preparation BLABER and CHRIST (1967) and BLABER (1972) noted that as in the case of neostigmine a marked difference exists between the concentrations of edrophonium which depolarise the motor end-plate and those which increase the amplitude and prolong the time-course of the e.p.p. in the presence of

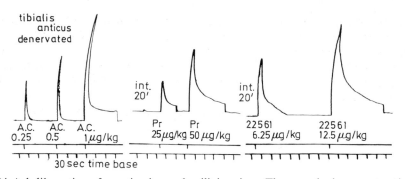

Fig. 24. Ach-like action of neostigmine and anilinium ions. The records show contractions of the denervated tibialis anterior muscle in the dog (anaesthetised with dial-urethane), produced by injection into a branch of the femoral artery of 0.25, 0.5, and 1 μg Ach (A.C.), 25 and 50 μg (0.08 and 0.16 μmol) neostigmine (Pr) and 6.25 and 12.5 μg (0.025 and 0.05 μmol) Ro 2-2561 (3-OH phenyltrimethylammonium). Muscle tension was recorded isotonically with a torsion wire myograph. (From RANDALL and LEHMANN, 1950)

tubocurarine or give rise to repetitive antidromic nerve action potentials following application of a single stimulus to the nerve.

There are no studies on mammalian muscle which suggest that anticholinesterases of the carbamate and organophosphate type or anilinium ions might possess a tubocurarine-like component of action *in vivo*. An exception appears to be ambenonium, an anticholinesterase related to the carbamates. In general

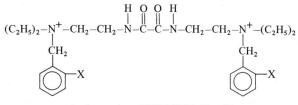

Ambenonium (WIN 8077): X = Cl
Methoxyambenonium (WIN 8078): X = OCH$_3$

the actions of this anticholinesterase are comparable with those of other anticholinesterases. However, in doses which are at least 10 times greater than those which markedly potentiate twitch tension and exert a good anticurare action, ambenonium also antagonises the neuromuscular block produced in cats by decamethonium (KARCZMAR, 1957; BLABER, 1960; BLABER and KARCZMAR, 1967). This is an action shared by tubocurarine. Structural alterations of the ambenonium molecule generally reduce its anticholinesterase potency (LANDS et al., 1958) and enhance the tubocurarine-like component of its action (BLABER and KARCZMAR, 1967). For example, with methoxyambenonium, a substance which has one seventh of the anticholinesterase potency of neostigmine (LANDS et al., 1958), the tubocurarine-like action is so dominant that a neuromuscular block is obtained without any initial twitch potentiation. An anticurare action is the only feature shared with ambenonium or neostigmine and other typical anticholinesterases. According to the studies of BLABER and

CHRIST (1967) on the cat isolated tenuissimus muscle preparation the anticurare action is due to a rise in the e.p.p. which with higher concentrations is associated with a prolongation of its rise- and decay-time. Thus the mechanism of the anticurare action of methoxyambenonium is the same as that of ambenonium and neostigmine and a tubocurarine-like action on nerve terminals accounts for the absence of twitch potentiation.

The actions of methoxyambenonium are shared by benzoquinonium and its analogues.

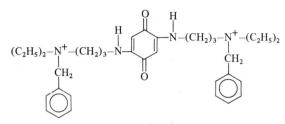

Benzoquinonium

The actions of benzoquinonium, which has one quarter of the anticholinesterase potency of neostigmine (HOPPE et al., 1955), have been studied in some detail with the following results. In cats, doses of benzoquinonium which in themselves have no effect on twitch tension prevent repetitive antidromic nerve action potentials from being triggered by an orthodromic nerve impulse following the injection of neostigmine, ambenonium or edrophonium. Thus benzoquinonium prevents these substances from producing twitch potentiation (BLABER and BOWMAN, 1963b). In higher doses benzoquinonium produces neuromuscular block at low rates of nerve stimulation by reducing the e.p.p. below its critical height (BLABER and CHRIST, 1967). When the amplitude of the e.p.p.s is reduced to an equal extent by benzoquinonium and tubocurarine, comparison reveals that the e.p.p. affected by benzoquinonium has a slower rise-time and longer duration. The reduction of the e.p.p. by benzoquinonium cannot be reversed by neostigmine, ambenonium or edrophonium (CHRIST and BLABER, 1968) and consequently these substances are unable to antagonise the neuromuscular block produced by benzoquinonium (BLABER and BOWMAN, 1962). On the other hand, benzoquinonium reverses the neuromuscular block produced by tubocurarine and in higher doses that produced by decamethonium (BLABER and BOWMAN, 1962). These findings are consistent with the interpretation that with benzoquinonium, as in the case of methoxyambenonium, a tubocurarine-like action is so pronounced that instead of twitch potentiation, a reduction in twitch tension is observed. However, the concomitant anticholinesterase action of the compound is unmasked by tubocurarine and thus it can reverse neuromuscular block produced by tubocurarine-like substances. Methoxyambenonium and benzoquinonium clearly should not be classified as anticholinesterases but as neuromuscular blocking agents.

Experimental evidence supports the view that in vivo ACh-like or tubocurarine-like actions on postsynaptic cholinoceptors at the motor end-plate are unlikely to be of any importance with those anticholinesterases of the carbamate and organophosphate type and anilinium ions which produce effects at the neuromuscular junction comparable to those first demonstrated with physostigmine, except perhaps when

they are given close-arterially. This selectivity of action does not necessarily apply
when these substances are used in high concentrations on isolated nerve-muscle
preparations and caution must be used when extrapolating from data obtained in
such experiments to the situation *in vivo*.

An interesting property of physostigmine has been demonstrated which might
intensify the neuromuscular actions arising from AChE inhibition. When the AChE
in rat brain slices is inhibited extensively by paraoxon or sarin, exogenous ACh gains
access to intracellular sites (which it normally does not reach) by an active uptake
mechanism which is inhibited by physostigmine (POLAK and MEEUWS, 1966; SCHUB-
ERTH and SUNDWALL, 1967). It is not known whether this also applies to the neuromuscular junction or whether physostigmine is unique in blocking the cellular uptake of ACh after AChE inhibition.

The anticholinesterases of the organophosphate type are not only inhibitors of
cholinesterases (AChE and ChE) but also of other esterases which in common with
them have a serine group at the active site of the enzyme (HEATH, 1961). The concentrations needed for inhibition of the other esterases are of an order which are unlikely to occur even with near lethal doses *in vivo*. However, under conditions where
an animal is protected by atropine and an oxime (see Section D VIII) and survives
very high doses of some anticholinesterases of the organophosphate type, concentrations of an order which give rise to inhibition of esterases other than cholinesterases
might arise. The same situation will prevail when isolated nerve-muscle preparations
are exposed to excessive concentrations.

The anticholinesterases of the organophosphate type pose an additional problem. PREUSSER (1967), FISCHER (1968, 1970) and ARIËNS et al. (1969) observed that
rats injected with near lethal doses of DFP, paraoxon or soman develop necrotic
lesions in the muscle at the motor end-plate region which can be prevented by
tubocurarine. In view of the widespread use of carbamate and organophosphate
insecticides which are converted *in vivo* into potent anticholinesterases (see DUBOIS,
1963) and human poisoning by them (QUINBY and DOORNINK, 1965; TOIVONEN et
al., 1965; DAVIES et al., 1967; HAYES, 1967; WOLFE et al., 1967; ROBERTS and WILSON,
1972), it seems important to establish whether these necrotic lesions are produced by
all anticholinesterases and insecticides; how and when they are repaired; and
whether they might lead to some impairment of muscle function which would escape
notice in acute experiments solely limited to testing effects on classical parameters of
neuromuscular transmission.

VII. Adaptation to Prolonged Inhibition of AChE

In conscious animals and in man the muscular symptoms produced by sublethal
doses of the anticholinesterases of the carbamate and organophosphate type consist
of fasciculations and muscle weakness. With anticholinesterases which are readily
inactivated *in vivo* the duration of these symptoms in animals surviving equiactive
doses, e.g. an LD_{50} dose given by injection, is inversely related to the rate of spontaneous reactivation of the acylated AChE (HOBBIGER, unpublished). The same relationship is found to apply to the intervals at which the different anticholinesterases
must be administered in order to maintain a therapeutic effect in patients with
myasthenia gravis.

Following administration of a single parenteral dose of an anticholinesterase no residual muscular symptoms are noticeable after 24 hrs, except when the acylated AChE does not undergo spontaneous reactivation, as in the case of di*iso*propyl-phosporyl-AChE which is formed by DFP. In such a situation the return of AChE activity depends solely on the synthesis of new enzyme which is relatively slow, and fasciculations and muscular weakness may be observed for several days, depending on the dose given. This is illustrated by results obtained by HUNT and RIKER (1947), who injected cats daily for several days with 1 mg (4 µmol) DFP/kg intravenously until fasciculations and muscle weakness became very marked. After the injections of DFP had been stopped fasciculations continued for 3 to 4 days and muscle weakness lasted on average for 7 days. The ability of the gastrocnemius muscle to respond with a sustained contraction when stimulated indirectly with submaximal stimuli at a frequency of 18.5 Hz returned to normal after 6 to 8 days. In these experiments inhibition of total AChE activity at the motor end-plates in the diaphragm was found to be 94% after the last injection of DFP and 6 days later it had fallen to approximately 50 per cent.

Organophosphate insecticides, while not effective anticholinesterases in their own right, are converted into anticholinesterases in the body. They are initially stored in body fats from which they are then slowly released. The conversion to anticholinesterases thus proceeds over a period of hours and sometimes days. Consequently, fasciculations and muscular weakness develop much more gradually and persist longer than when a single dose of the active metabolite is given. A typical example is the organophosphate insecticide parathion which *in vivo* is converted to the anticholinesterase paraoxon (GAGE, 1953; ERDMANN and LENDLE, 1958; DU-BOIS, 1963).

Since the muscular symptoms produced by a single dose of an anticholinesterase or an organophosphate insecticide can last for several days, the neuromuscular junction does not seem to be able to adapt itself quickly to AChE inhibition to any great extent. Some adaptation, however, does occur as shown by results obtained in several laboratories.

BUCKLEY and HEADING (1971) added neostigmine, 0.08 mg (0.25 µmol)/ml, to the drinking water of rats and then very gradually increased its concentration to 2.25 mg/ml. The only muscular symptoms observed were fasciculations, which only occurred during the first three days. On the other hand, rats which were given drinking water containing 0.5 mg/ml of neostigmine for 3 days, 1.0 mg/ml for the next 3 days and thereafter four times the original concentration, also showed fasciculations during the first 3 days but in addition exhibited marked muscle weakness throughout the whole period of the experiment. In earlier studies BUCKLEY and HEADING (1970) had observed that when neostigmine was added to the drinking water of rats for 4 weeks in a concentration of 0.25 to 1 mg/ml such rats, unlike controls, failed to show fasciculations when injected with 40 µg (0.12 µmol) neostig-mine/kg. This undoubtedly suggests adaptation but the published data are not suitable for any quantitative assessment of its extent to be made. MCPHILLIPS and COON (1966) in a follow-up of earlier observations by RIDER et al. (1952) studied the muscular symptoms produced in rats by prolonged administration of the organo-phosphate insecticide OMPA (which becomes an anticholinesterase after its metabo-lism *in vivo*, probably being converted to its N-oxide form) (CASIDA et al., 1954;

DUBOIS, 1963). The phosphorylated AChE formed by the active metabolite of
OMPA does not appear to undergo spontaneous reactivation and thus daily administration of OMPA produces a cumulative inhibition of AChE. In the experiments
carried out by MCPHILLIPS and COON rats were divided into two groups. The rats in
group I received a daily subcutaneous injection of 2.5 mg (9 µmol) OMPA/kg. All
died within 5 days, showing marked symptoms of AChE inhibition at all cholinergic
synapses before death. Inhibition of total AChE activity in the diaphragm at the time
of death was 80%. The rats in group II received daily doses of OMPA starting at
0.5 mg/kg with subsequent daily increases by 0.5 mg/kg until the fifth injection;
thereafter doses of 2.5 mg/kg were given daily for 9 weeks. Only 20% of these rats
died, mostly succumbing on the sixth day. At this time all the rats which survived
showed only mild fasciculations and increased excitability and no deaths occurred
after the sixth day. Inhibition of total AChE activity in the diaphragm of the survi-
vors progressively increased to 80% by the 20th day, then fell quite rapidly to 60% at
which level it remained for the following 5 weeks. Treatment with OMPA had no
effect on the rates of OMPA metabolism (i.e. both the conversion to the active
metabolite and its degradation to inert metabolites) and appeared to increase rather
than reduce the toxicity of an additional dose of OMPA, since at the end of the
experiment a dose of OMPA which killed control rats also killed the OMPA-treated
rats and did so in a shorter time.

A reduction of the intensity of muscular symptoms with time was observed in rats
receiving over a longer period daily doses of the organophosphate insecticides EPN
(ethyl-4-nitrophenyl phenylphosphonothioate; HODGE et al., 1954), systox (diethyl-
O-(2-ethylthioethyl) phosphorothioate; BARNES and DENZ, 1954), disyston (diethyl-
S-(2-ethylthioethyl) phosphorodithioate; BOMBINSKI and DUBOIS, 1958; BRODEUR
and DUBOIS, 1964; MCPHILLIPS, 1969), or delnev (2,3-p-dioxanedithiol-S,S-bis(diethyl phosphorodithioate; COOPER, 1962). In the studies with disyston it was observed also that the reduction in the intensity of muscular symptoms with time was
accompanied by a decrease in the intraperitoneal LD_{50}/kg of tubocurarine and decamethonium from 0.21 mg to 0.14 mg and 2.9 mg to 1.5 mg, respectively (MCPHIL-
LIPS, 1969).

In order to obtain more quantitative information on the adaptation of the neuromuscular junction to prolonged inhibition of AChE by an organophosphate which
in this case was an anticholinesterase in its own right, HOBBIGER, MITCHELSON and
VOJVODIĆ (unpublished) injected rats subcutaneously with 0.6 mg (2.5 µmol)DFP/kg
on 5 consecutive days each week, for 7 weeks. During the third week the rats showed
fasciculations following each injection but such an effect was not seen subsequently.
The treatment with DFP for 7weeks had no effect on the rate at which DFP was
hydrolysed by plasma or liver homogenates, and progressive inhibition of total
AChE activity in the diaphragm was observed amounting to 50% at the end of the
second week and reaching 60% at the end of the seventh week. The sensitvity of the
diaphragm to ACh, determined on the isolated nerve-diaphragm preparation by the
concentration of ACh required to reduce twitch tension by 50% when added to the
bathing fluid for 5 min increased 4-fold during the first 2 weeks and in the subsequent
5 weeks declined gradually to about two thirds of this value. Qualitatively comparable results were obtained with choline and carbachol but the increase in sensitivity to
these substances was less pronounced than that to ACh, amounting to approxi-

mately 25% at the end of the 7th week. When rats which had been treated with 0.6 mg DFP/kg for 7 weeks were injected subcutaneously on 5 consecutive days with 1.2 mg DFP/kg, marked fasciculations followed the third and subsequent two injections but all rats survived. Controls injected for 5 consecutive days with 1.2 mg DFP/kg showed fasciculations after the third, fourth and fifth injections and 60% of the animals died.

These experiments show that when DFP or organophosphate insecticides are administered daily to rats at certain dose levels, muscular symptoms arising from AChE inhibition decline with time. This adaptation is not due to an increased metabolism of the anticholinesterase as is illustrated by the results obtained with DFP and OMPA. It occurs at a time when the level of AChE inhibition at motor end-plates is either still increasing or constant. The studies with OMPA also show that the time-course of AChE inhibition is a crucial factor in the development of adaptation. When the progression of inhibition is sufficiently slow, rats show few or no muscular symptoms when the level of enzyme inhibition at motor end-plates is as high as that associated with marked muscular symptoms and death when inhibition is produced at a faster rate.

As far as the mechanism responsible for adaptation is concerned, the studies with DFP indicate that changes in sensitivity of the postsynaptic membrane to ACh are too small to account for it completely. As discussed earlier (see Section D V) repeated administration of neostigmine leads to a reduction in the quantal release of ACh and the number of postsynaptic cholinoceptors (ROBERTS and THESLEFF, 1969; CHANG et al., 1973). Such effects, if common to all anticholinesterases, could contribute to adaptation.

In adapted rats the LD_{50} of a further dose of the anticholinesterase which has caused the adaptation is at most only marginally raised in comparison with control rats. In quantitative terms the adaptation to prolonged AChE inhibition, therefore, is only small by comparison with the desensitisation of cholinoceptors to ACh obtainable in isolated muscle preparations with an ionophoretic application of ACh (AXELSSON and THESLEFF, 1958).

Adaptation only persists as long as AChE remains inhibited and when treatment with the anticholinesterase is discontinued the motor end-plate recovers from adaptation at a rate which parallels the rate of return of AChE activity (MCPHILLIPS and COON, 1966).

VIII. Antidotal Effects of Tubocurarine and Reactivators of Phosphorylated AChE; Selectivity of Action of Reactivators

One of the life threatening consequences of the administration of an anticholinesterase of the carbamate or organophosphate type is the impairment of neuromuscular transmission by prolonged depolarisation of the postsynaptic membrane through an excessive action of ACh released from nerve terminals. Tubocurarine competes as an antagonist with ACh for the postsynaptic cholinoceptors at motor end-plates and could be expected to raise the LD_{50} of anticholinesterases if neuromuscular block by depolarisation plays a causal role in death. This is indeed the case as shown by the results obtained by PARKES and SACRA (1954). They observed that in mice tubocurarine, injected before the anticholinesterase, raised the LD_{50} of neostigmine and of two quaternary anticholinesterases of the organophosphate type approximately 14-fold. With TEPP, the LD_{50} was raised only 4-fold. The antidotal action of tubocurarine on TEPP is less marked because this anticholinesterase is lipid-soluble and unlike the quaternary anticholinesterases also impairs respiration through inhibition of AChE at central sites (SCHAUMANN and JOB, 1958; SCHAUMANN, 1960). The data obtained in mice, however, are only qualitatively but not quantitatively applicable to other species since the extent to which inhibition of AChE at different cholinergic synapses contributes to death is species-dependent (CANDOLE et al., 1953). The antidotal action of tubocurarine is shared by other substances which act as competitive antagonists to ACh at the neuromuscular junction (WILLS, 1963).

Tubocurarine does not affect the level of AChE inhibition but exerts an antidotal action by reducing the consequences of AChE inhibition at motor end-plates. Repair of the biochemical lesion itself, i.e. reactivation of the inhibited AChE, would be a much more desirable form of antidotal treatment in all those cases where inhibition arises from acylation. Acylated AChEs which can be reactivated relatively easily include the various types of phosphorylated AChE formed by dialkylphosphates, e.g. TEPP, paraoxon and DFP, and by sarin, as long as they have not undergone ageing (see Section C I). The pyridinium aldoximes like pralidoxime, TMB-4 and obidoxime can be used to produce reactivation *in vivo*. The antidotal activity of these oximes is on the whole proportional to their reactivating potency, but even when the oximes are given before the organophosphate anticholinesterase the degree of protection obtained is usually only small except in the case of quaternary organophosphates. However, the antidotal action of the oximes can be increased markedly when they are given in combination with atropine (KEWITZ et al., 1956; HOBBIGER, 1957; HOBBIGER and SADLER, 1959; see HOBBIGER, 1963). The mechanism by which the oximes raise the LD_{50} is undoubtedly at least in part by reactivation of phosphorylated AChE at motor end-plates and the consequent improvement in neuromuscular transmission (see Section D III) but reactivation at other cholinergic synapses is also likely to contribute. Atropine is thought to enhance the antidotal action of oximes by protecting central and peripheral muscarinic cholinoceptors against an excessive action of ACh thus delaying death and allowing the oximes to produce a greater degree of reactivation (see HOBBIGER, 1963, 1968).

Although pyridinium aldoximes can reactivate certain types of phosphorylated AChE, it does not follow that at the neuromuscular junction reactivation might not be associated with other actions, some of which could mimic reactivation. Such associated actions might be of particular importance in studies on isolated nerve-muscle preparations where the oximes can be used in concentrations far above those which can be obtained *in vivo* without harmful side effects or when oximes are given by close-arterial injection. Oximes possess several actions which are unrelated to reactivation and generally only observed with very high doses (concentrations). In cats and on the rat isolated nerve-diaphragm preparation, oximes antagonise tubocurarine induced neuromuscular block to a limited extent and also enhance the neuromuscular blocking action of suxamethonium (WILLS et al., 1959; WISLICKI, 1960; FLEISHER et al., 1965). Given alone oximes produce neuromuscular block (HOLMES and ROBINS, 1955; HOBBIGER and SADLER, 1959). Finally, some antagonism of the neuromuscular block caused by anticholinesterases which form non-reactivatable types of phosphorylated AChE can also be obtained in the rat isolated nerve-diaphragm preparation but this effect is considerably less than that achieved on the neuromuscular block produced by those anticholinesterases which form reactivatable types of phosphorylated AChE (ENANDER, 1958; FREDRIKSSON and TIBBLING, 1959). All these effects are consequences of one or more of the following actions exerted by oximes at high doses (concentrations): (1) reversible inhibition of AChE (HOBBIGER, 1956; BERGNER and WAGLEY, 1958; HOBBIGER and SADLER, 1959); (2) a tubocurarine-like action at the postsynaptic membrane of motor end-plates (FLEISHER et al., 1965); and (3) an increase in the quantal release of ACh from motor nerve terminals in lower concentrations and a decrease in higher concentrations (GOYER, 1970). In vivo the half-life of oximes is short (see HOBBIGER, 1972) and if an action other than reactivation is responsible for an observed effect, the effect is short-lasting compared with that of the organophosphates. In isolated nerve-muscle preparations effects other than those arising from reactivation will be speedily reversed by removal of the oxime from the bathing fluid. Whether actions other than reactivation are involved can be tested by appropriate control experiments but in the past insufficient attention seems to have been paid to this. As far as the data which were obtained with oximes and which have been referred to in previous Sections are concerned there is no evidence that actions other than reactivation of phosphorylated AChE were involved to an extent which could invalidate the conclusions drawn from them.

IX. Inhibition of Cholinesterase (ChE)

The motor end-plates (in mammals) possess in addition to AChE a second type of esterase capable of hydrolysing ACh. This second enzyme is called cholinesterase (ChE; acylcholine acyl-hydrolase; E.C. 3.1.1.8.; often referred to in the past as pseudocholinesterase, butyrylcholinesterase, plasmacholinesterase or nonspecific cholinesterase). Cholinesterase, like AChE, is a structural component of the motor end-plate and histochemical studies have shown that although mainly associated with Schwann cells it is also present in the synaptic cleft; furthermore, its concentration is not uniform at all neuromuscular junctions, but higher at motor end-plates of the "en grappe" type than at those of the "en plaque" type (DENZ, 1953; HOLMSTEDT, 1957; HÄGGQVIST, 1960; CHRISTOFF et al., 1966; ERÄNKO and TERÄVÄINEN, 1967; BERRY and RUTLAND, 1971; CHOKROVERTY et al., 1971; DAVIS et al., 1972).

   The main difference between ChE and AChE is that quaternary substances, including ACh, have a lower affinity for ChE and that its esteratic site can accommodate bulkier groups of substrates and inhibitors. Furthermore, there are considerable differences in these respects between the ChEs of different species. The mechanisms of inhibition of ChE by different anticholinesterases are in principle the same as those described for AChE but the rate constants of individual steps in acylation and deacylation reactions differ for the two types of enzyme (see AUGUSTINSSON, 1963; COHEN and OOSTERBAAN, 1963; ALDRIDGE and REINER, 1972).

   With most anticholinesterases, except bisquaternary substances such as BW 284 C 51   [1,5-bis(4-allyldimethylammoniumphenyl) pentane-3-one diiodide], marked inhibition of AChE in vivo and in isolated nerve-muscle preparations is associated with at least some inhibition of ChE and particularly if the anticholinesterase is a non-quaternary organophosphate, inhibition of ChE is often greater than that of AChE (see HOLMSTEDT, 1959; AUGUSTINSSON, 1963). In extreme cases, e.g. with *iso*-OMPA (tetramono*iso*propyl pyrophosphortetramide) or mipafox (N,N'-di*iso*propylphosphorodiamidic fluoride), selective inhibition of ChE can be obtained but because of species differences in ChE the degree of selectivity of inhibition is markedly species-dependent (ALDRIDGE, 1953; AUSTIN and BERRY, 1953).

Selective inhibition of ChE produces no overt muscle symptoms *in vivo* (HAWKINS and GUNTER, 1946) and in the rat isolated nerve-diaphragm preparation has no effect on the muscle response to indirect stimulation at frequencies up to 100 Hz (HEFFRON, 1972).

Cholinesterase is of pharmacological importance because it hydrolyses the neuromuscular blocking agent suxamethonium (WHITTAKER and WIJESUNDERA, 1952) and thus plays an essential role in determining its duration of action. In man there are two important genetically controlled variants of ChE, referred to as usual and atypical ChE (KALOW and GENEST, 1957; KALOW and STARON, 1957). In subjects with only usual ChE (about 96% of the population) the intravenous injection of 10 to 30 mg suxamethonium produces neuromuscular block lasting for 3 to 5 min. Atypical ChE hydrolyses suxamethonium only at about 1% of the rate at which it is hydrolysed by the usual ChE (HOBBIGER and PECK, 1969) and in subjects possessing only atypical ChE (less than 1% of the population) a dose of 10 to 30 mg suxamethonium produces neuromuscular block lasting for several hours. The main reason for this long duration of action is that in man cholinesterase is present in high concentrations in plasma and in subjects with usual ChE a large proportion of the injected dose of suxamethonium is hydrolysed in the blood before reaching the

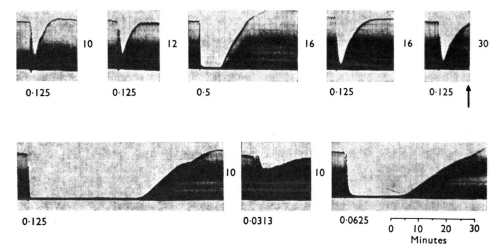

Fig. 25. Potentiation by *iso*-OMPA, 7.5 μmol (2.5 mg)/kg given intravenously, of the effect of intravenous suxamethonium on twitch tension in a cat weighing 1.9 kg and anaesthetised with pentobarbitone sodium. The records show responses of the soleus-gastrocnemius muscle group, recorded with a strain gauge, to supramaximal stimulation of the sciatic nerve at 0.2 Hz. The figures between the records denote the time (in min) elapsing between each, and figures below the records represent the doses of suxamethonium, in μmol/kg, injected (1 μmol of suxamethonium = 400 μg). *Iso*-OMPA, injected at the arrow, produced a selective 97% inhibition of ChE in blood. (From HOBBIGER and PECK, 1970)

motor end-plates. In subjects with atypical ChE only, little hydrolysis occurs in the blood (KALOW and GUNN, 1957; NEITLICH, 1966; LITWILLER, 1969). Extensive inhibition of ChE in a subject with the usual ChE prolongs the duration of action of suxamethonium and produces effects identical with those found in individuals with atypical ChE. The ChEs of the most widely used laboratory animals (dogs, cats, rats and mice) hydrolyse suxamethonium at a much lower rate than does the usual type of human ChE, little if any hydrolysis occuring in blood before the ester reaches the motor end-plates. However, in these species the neuromuscular blocking action of suxamethonium is also as shortlasting as in man, and is in fact markedly prolonged by selective inhibition of ChE (Fig. 25; BRÜCKE, 1956; KELEMEN and VOLLE, 1966; HOBBIGER and PECK, 1970). Thus enzymic hydrolysis of suxamethonium is clearly important. Studies in cats have shown that when suxamethonium is injected intravenously, hydrolysis by ChE in plasma is negligible (HOBBIGER and PECK, 1970) and temporary arrest of the blood flow through a muscle after neuromuscular block has reached a maximum has no effect on the time-course of the recovery of the response of the muscle to indirect stimulation (ARGENT et al., 1955). From these results we can conclude that in laboratory animals ChE at the neuromuscular junction itself plays an important role in terminating the action of suxamethonium.

One exceptional laboratory animal should be mentioned. Monkey ChE hydrolyses suxamethonium as fast as that of man and a considerable proportion of intravenously administered suxamethonium is hydrolysed before it reaches the motor endplate (PECK, 1972).

General Conclusions

The number of AChE sites at the mammalian motor end-plate greatly exceeds the number of ACh molecules released by a single nerve impulse and this ensures that under physiological conditions the concentration of ACh at the postsynaptic membrane approaches the "no effect" level within the rising phase of the e.p.p. even if, as seems likely, the primary area of contact of ACh is limited to no more than 10% of the area of the postsynaptic membrane. If we consider the distribution of AChE we find that the enzyme is present not only at the postsynaptic membrane but also at the presynaptic membrane and that its concentration at the two sites is similar. Much of the present controversy about the mode and site of action of anticholinesterases and anilinium ions is attributable to the widely accepted view that the role of AChE is confined to terminating the action of ACh at the postsynaptic membrane. The experimental evidence suggests that this is not the case and that when AChE is inhibited, ACh gains access to nerve terminals and exerts actions there. If we differentiate between actions arising at nerve terminals and at the postsynaptic membrane the various consequences of AChE inhibition can be grouped as follows.

Presynaptic Actions Arising from AChE Inhibition. These comprise *twitch potentiation* and *fasciculations*. In the case of twitch potentiation experimental evidence indicates that the following sequence of events is involved. By a presynaptic action ACh enhances and prolongs the negative after-potential in nerve terminals following an action potential and lowers the threshold of excitability at the first node of Ranvier. In consequence the nerve terminal triggers an antidromic nerve action potential which by an axon reflex invades the other nerve terminals of the same motor unit. The ACh released in this way from the nerve terminals triggers another muscle action potential and also sets up a further antidromic nerve action potential. This sequence of events continues for a limited period. As a consequence, stimulation of a nerve by a single stimulus initiates repetitive muscle action potentials and twitch tension is potentiated.

Fasciculations also appear to be presynaptic in origin. There is no evidence to suggest that ACh can depolarise a nerve terminal to such an extent that it might initiate on its own an antidromic nerve action potential which then invades other nerve terminals and produces a synchronised contraction of muscle fibres in individual motor units. It is more likely that fasciculations are triggered by ACh (released at random from nerve terminals) depolarising the first node of Ranvier. The subsequent sequence of events would be analogous so that initiated by the application of a single stimulus to the nerve.

Both twitch potentiation and fasciculations occur within a limited range of AChE inhibition only and when AChE inhibition reaches a high level, probably in excess of 90%, they cease. When this occurs the muscle responds to the application of a single stimulus to the nerve in the same way as before inhibition of AChE.

Postsynaptic Action Arising from AChE Inhibition. The effect of the inhibition of AChE at the postsynaptic membrane is to enhance and prolong the action of ACh there. This leads to neuromuscular block by depolarisation at high rates of nerve stimulation and largely accounts for the so-called *tetanic fade*. The extinction of orthodromic nerve action potentials by antidromic nerve action potentials (initiated by a presynaptic action of ACh) probably plays a contributory role in the initial part of the tetanic fade. The equivalent of the tetanic fade *in vivo* (in the absence of nerve stimulation) is *muscle weakness* and in the extreme case *muscle paralysis*.

Postsynaptic Consequences of AChE Inhibition to which a Presynaptic Action of AChE Might Make an Essential Contribution. These consist of *antagonism to tubocurarine* and other neuromuscular blocking substances with the same mode of action and *reversal of the symptoms of myasthenia gravis*. Although these two actions at higher effective dose levels can be explained satisfactorily in terms of enhancement of the intensity of the postsynaptic action of ACh as the result of AChE inhibition, we cannot exclude the possibility that an increase in the quantal release of ACh by a presynaptic action of ACh (as a consequence of AChE inhibition) contributes to and might even be predominantly responsible for the actions at lower effective dose levels. At high rates of nerve stimulation an additional factor seems to be involved. Under these conditions tubocurarine appears to reduce the quantal release of ACh. Edrophonium antagonises this action of tubocurarine. It is likely that the anticholinesterases have the same effect through their inhibition of AChE.

In the case of anticholinesterases of the organophosphate type the experimental data are not only consistent with the view that their actions at motor end-plates are entirely the consequence of AChE inhibition but they provide direct proof of this.

With those anticholinesterases of the carbamate type which have been studied in detail, i.e. neostigmine, and 3- or 4-hydroxyanilinium ions and substances derived from them, the position as to whether AChE inhibition accounts fully or at least mainly for their actions at motor end-plates is less certain if stringent criteria are applied. Two factors account for this. Firstly, the inhibition produced by these substances is not sufficiently stable to allow the study of the exact relationship between the level of enzyme inhibition and the intensity of an individual action and its time-course. In contrast to phosphorylated AChE where enzyme activity can be restored by oximes, there is no way of distinguishing clearly between actions arising from AChE inhibition and other actions. The second difficulty arises from observations on the e.p.p. With edrophonium repetitive antidromic nerve action potentials have been observed in the absence of changes in the e.p.p., and within a certain range of concentrations neostigmine, ambenonium and edrophonium raise the amplitude of the e.p.p. in the presence of tubocurarine without affecting its time-course. These observations might be interpreted as providing evidence that a direct presynaptic action of carbamates and reversible inhibitors of AChE is essential to the actions these substances exert except in the case of the tetanic fade. However, acceptance of this interpretation also implies acceptance of the view that ACh released from nerve terminals can gain access to presynaptic sites only when the inhibition of AChE is sufficient to produce a change in the e.p.p. and also that a change in the amplitude of the e.p.p. without a concomitant lengthening of its duration is not consistent with AChE inhibition. Neither of these two concepts can be considered to have been proven. Experiments with graded concentrations of appropriate anticholinesterases of the organophosphate type involving observation of the modification by oximes of the level of enzyme inhibition obtained would be most informative. Until such experiments have been carried out a direct presynaptic action cannot be considered as proven but it might be prudent not to exclude the possibility that such an action could be important to the actions of anticholinesterases of the carbamate type and substances closely related to them like ambenonium. However, a wide range of data, including pharmacokinetic considerations, are much more consistent with AChE inhibition being the mechanism responsible for the actions of such substances. The same applies to reversible inhibitors of AChE such as edrophonium. In their case indirect evidence pointing towards inhibition of AChE as the mechanism responsible for their actions is necessarily much more limited than in the case of anticholinesterases of the carbamate type since they produce the least stable form of enzyme inhibition and have a very short duration of action *in vivo*. This considerably limits the scope of experiments which might yield conclusive information on mechanisms of action.

There is no evidence to support the view that at the motor end-plate the actions of anticholinesterases such as physostigmine or neostigmine, when given in sublethal doses to animals, are modified to any significant extent by an ACh-like action on postsynaptic cholinoceptors or by a tubocurarine-like action. This undoubtedly applies to all other anticholinesterases which have the same qualitative actions. However, there are a vast number of substances which in sublethal doses will inhibit AChE *in vivo* and if their actions deviate from those of physostigmine and neostigmine this might be explicable in terms of an ACh-like action on postsynaptic cholinoceptors or a tubocurarine-like action. Examples of this are provided by methoxy-ambenonium and benzoquinonium.

Most studies on anticholinesterases have been concerned with effects obtained in acute experiments. However, anticholinesterases are given over long periods in the treatment of myasthenia gravis and in the case of organophosphorus insecticides there is a danger of chronic poisoning (i.e. chronic inhibition of AChE). Studies on the consequences of prolonged (chronic) inhibition of AChE are thus also very necessary. However, little information on the subject is available and the data which we do possess do not adequately cover long periods of AChE inhibition. The few existing data indicate that prolonged inhibition of AChE leads at motor end-plates to a limited degree of adaptation to the consequences of inhibition and that this is associated with a reduction in the quantal release of ACh. Changes also occur at the postsynaptic membrane, the significance of which in relation to the postsynaptic action of ACh is not known. Further studies in this field are undoubtedly needed and the information provided by them might well lead to a reappraisal of current methods used in the treatment of myasthenia gravis.

A final comment is necessary concerning ChE which like AChE is a structural constituent of the motor end-plate. Although quaternary anticholinesterases on the whole, inhibit AChE to a greater extent than ChE, the reverse is true of non-quaternary anticholinesterases. The acute inhibition of ChE has no obvious effects on neuromuscular transmission but it does give rise to a marked prolongation of the neuromuscular blocking action of suxamethonium in all mammals. The physiological function of ChE is unknown. This, however, does not mean that we can ignore the enzyme and the complete lack of information on the consequences of its prolonged inhibition is disquieting.

Acknowledgement. The author wishes to thank Dr. L. C. BLABER of Roche Products Ltd. for advice on the presentation of those parts of the text which deal with experiments involving electrophysiological techniques.

Appendix I. Studies on Frog Muscles

Some of the pioneer work on neuromuscular transmission has been and still is carried out in frogs and there can be no doubt about its importance. However, a survey of the literature shows that in these studies physostigmine and other anticholinesterases often were used only as tools for eliminating cholinesterases. Furthermore, the assumption was usually made that these substances were selective in their anticholinesterase action and that this action predominantly or solely led to a prolongation of the action of ACh at the postsynaptic membrane. Only a very limited number of studies were designed in such a way that they could shed some light on mode and site of action, effects of graded concentrations or differences between the actions of various anticholinesterases. The question also arises whether studies on frog neuromuscular junctions give information which is strictly applicable to mammalian neuromuscular junctions. It is highly unlikely that frog AChE is in all respects identical to mammalian AChE, particularly since the two enzymes have to operate effectively at very different temperatures. Studies of the relationship between inhibition and pharmacological actions, and comparative studies of the affinity of different anticholinesterase drugs for frog and mammalian AChE's and of the various rate constants for acylating anticholinesterases are important in this context. Hardly any conclusive studies of this type have been undertaken. It also remains to be established that the cholinoceptors themselves and their distribution relative to that of AChE are identical at frog and mammalian neuromuscular junctions. Finally, there are quantitative as well as qualitative differences between the actions of the anticholinesterases on the two types of neuromuscular junction. These might well arise from morphological differences between them. It therefore seems advisable to take the view that the actions of anticholinesterases on frog neuromuscular junctions are not necessarily qualitatively or quantitatively applicable to the actions of these substances on mammalian neuromuscular junctions and to resist the temptation of using data obtained in the frog for the interpretation of results obtained in mammals. The latter unfortunately is often done. Pertinent information on the actions of anticholinesterases and anilinium ions on frog neuromuscular junctions is summarized briefly below.

Anatomical Aspects

There are two types of muscle fibres in the frog. One type, the so-called twitch fibre type, has a focal innervation from large diameter alpha motor neurones and stimulation of the neurone produces an end-plate potential which triggers a propagated muscle action potential that is associated with a short-lasting muscle contraction (twitch). Muscle fibres of this type are the equivalent of the twitch fibres in mammals. The second type, the so-called tonus fibre type, is innervated by small diameter gamma motor neurones and in their case each muscle fibre is covered by a dense cluster of motor end-plates. Nerve impulses in gamma motor neurones evoke a graded, relatively long-lasting end-plate depolarisation which does not initiate a propagated muscle action potential (KUFFLER and VAUGHAN WILLIAMS, 1953a and b). The non-propagated depolarisation is associated with contraction of the muscle fibre in the area of depolarisation and since each muscle fibre has many motor end-plates, the contractile mechanism can be activated over most of the length of the muscle fibre. This type of contractile response is referred to as a contracture. Because the coupling between the contractile response and membrane depolarisation is sustained, the degree of contracture is a measure of the intensity of the action of ACh and thus can be used for its quantitative assay.

Each muscle contains a mixture of twitch and tonus fibres but their proportion varies between muscles (KUFFLER and VAUGHAN WILLIAMS, 1953b; CSILLIK, 1965). The sartorius muscle is almost entirely composed of twitch fibres. The same applies to the iliofibularis muscle where the tonus fibres form a separate compact bundle. The gastrocnemius muscle contains a sizeable proportion of tonus fibres and tonus fibres prevail over twitch fibres in the rectus abdominis muscle.

Cholinesterases

Motor end-plates in the rectus abdominis muscle contain two types of cholinesterase which qualitatively behave like the AChE and ChE of mammals, as shown by studies of the rate of hydrolysis of acetyl-, propionyl- and butyryl-choline and the effect of the selective inhibitors of mammalian AChE and ChE, compound 3313CT and DFP, respectively (JACOB and PECOT-DECHAVASSINE, 1958). These and earlier studies by the same authors indicate that only AChE and not ChE is likely to play a significant role in the termination of the transmitter action of ACh liberated from nerve terminals.

The cholinesterases are concentrated at the motor end-plates (Marney and Nachmansohn, 1938). Histochemical studies have shown that the concentration of AChE is lower at frog neuromuscular junctions than at mammalian ones and greater in twitch fibres than in tonus fibres; the reverse applies for ChE (Couteaux, 1958; Häggquist, 1960; Csillik, 1965).

There are no data on the relationship between levels of enzyme inhibition produced in twitch fibres by graded doses of anticholinesterases and the corresponding pharmacological actions of these substances. However, in the sartorius muscle physostigmine (40 µmol/l and higher concentrations) has been shown to reduce the ACh-hydrolysing capacity of the muscle below measurable levels while causing a marked prolongation of the end-plate potential (Eccles et al., 1942).

Actions of Anticholinesterases and Anilinium Ions

a) Muscles in which Twitch Fibres Predominate. Studies of the effects of anticholinesterases on twitch tension have given variable results. Brown (1937b) and Raventos (1937), recording twitch tension of the gastrocnemius muscle *in vivo*, and Cowan (1940), recording twitch tension in the isolated sartorius muscle, failed to obtain twitch potentiation with physostigmine. Feng (1937), however, noted that although physostigmine did not potentiate twitch tension if the nerve was stimulated at a rate of 1 Hz it did so at a rate of stimulation of 0.005 Hz. Cowan (1940) then observed that in satorius muscles obtained from frogs which had been kept for more than 40 hrs at 0—5° C (in contrast with muscles of frogs kept at more usual temperatures) physostigmine and neostigmine potentiated twitch tension, and Nastuk and Alexander (1954) reported that neostigmine and edrophonium consistently increased the twitch tension of the isolated sartorius muscle.

Physostigmine and edrophonium do not produce repetitive antidromic nerve action potentials following invasion of a nerve terminal by an othodromic impulse (Dun and Feng, 1940; Eccles et al., 1942; Katz, 1969). Thus the mechanism responsible for twitch potentiation in frog muscles cannot be the same as that in mammalian muscles. Physostigmine, neostigmine and related anticholinesterases of the carbamate type, edrophonium and 3-hydroxyphenyltrimethylammonium have all been reported to produce a limited number of propagated muscle action potentials following the arrival of a single orthodromic impulse at nerve terminals (Feng, 1940, 1941; Cowan, 1940; Eccles et al., 1942; Nastuk and Alexander, 1954). This could play a role in twitch potentiation but it remains to be shown that under conditions where twitch potentiation is absent, repetitive muscle action potentials are also absent. It is known that in frogs transmission initiated at neuromuscular junctions by a single indirect stimulus is incomplete (Kuffler, 1952); therefore one explanation for the twitch potention by anticholinesterases and anilinium ions could be that under certain experimental conditions these substances improve the effectiveness of transmission by the recruitment of fibres in which the transmitter action was previously below the threshold for initiating a propagated muscle action potential.

There is no report in the literature on any fasciculations being produced by anticholinesterases or anilinium ions.

Anticholinesterases and anilinium ions decrease the decay rate of the e.p.p. (Feng, 1940, 1941; Eccles et al., 1942; Nastuk and Alexander, 1954) and this is thought to be responsible for the repetitive propagated muscle action potentials (following arrival of a single orthodromic impulse at nerve terminals) seen after their administration.

Anticholinesterases have little effect on the frequency of m.e.p.p.s but increase their amplitude and slow their decay rate, as shown by FATT and KATZ (1952) in studies of neostigmine on the isolated sartorius muscle.

Neostigmine and edrophonium also have been shown to prolong the duration of action of ACh applied ionophoretically to motor end-plates in the isolated sartorius muscle. This action was obtained with concentrations which had no effect on the response to carbachol applied in the same way (KATZ and THESLEFF, 1957; CASTILLO and KATZ, 1957).

At rates of nerve stimulation which produce a sustained shortening of the muscle in the frog, the muscle response consists in principle of two components, a tetanic contraction of the twitch fibres and a more slowly developing contracture of the tonus fibres. By selecting a suitable frequency of nerve stimulation the two components can be partly separated as shown by COWAN (1938). Thus tension records can be obtained which show an initial increase in tension followed by some relaxation and then a second sustained rise in tension. The same result can be obtained with close-arterial injections of ACh (BROWN, 1937b). Physostigmine, neostigmine and other anticholinesterases of the carbamate type accentuate the relaxation and slightly enhance the secondary rise in tension during nerve stimulation (COWAN, 1938; FENG, 1941). The secondary rise in tension produced by injected ACh also is somewhat enhanced by physostigmine (BROWN, 1937b). The effect of anticholinesterases in reducing the ability of the muscle to sustain an increase in tension developed by the twitch fibres can be fully explained as the result of a prolongation of the end-plate potential, leading to progressive neuromuscular block by depolarisation (FENG, 1941). In curarised muscle anticholinesterases and anilinium ions exert an anticurare action by prolonging the rising phase of the e.p.p. and slowing its decay rate. This has been demonstrated with physostigmine, neostigmine, a variety of other anticholinesterases of the carbamate type, DFP and edrophonium and other anilinium ions (FENG, 1940, 1941; ECCLES et al., 1942; ECCLES and MACFARLANE, 1949; NASTUK and ALEXANDER, 1954).

All these findings are consistent with the view that anticholinesterases and anilinium ions produce their effects mainly if not solely by inhibition of AChE which in turn prolongs the duration of the action of ACh at the postsynaptic membrane. Unfortunately, there are no data on the relationship between AChE inhibition and intensity of effects, and there is a paucity of data on anticholinesterases of the organophosphate type which produce an inhibition which can be recorded accurately. The major discrepancy between results of studies on frog twitch fibres and those on mammalian muscle is that in frogs twitch potentiation is not a constant phenomenon and often occurs only under special conditions whereas it is an impressive feature in mammals. Studies in frogs are also complicated by the presence of tonus fibres which when activated complicate analyses.

b) Muscles in which Tonus Fibres Predominate. Anticholinesterases of the carbamate and organophosphate type and anilinium ions sensitize the rectus abdominis muscle to exogenous ACh and a muscle treated with such a substance is useful for the bioassay of low concentrations of ACh (CHANG and GADDUM, 1933; MACIN-TOSH, 1950). A detailed study showed that the degree of sensitisation (HOBBIGER, 1950, 1952) obtainable with individual anticholinesterases and anilinium ions varies because some anticholinesterases, e.g. physostigmine, also exert a tubocurar-ine-like action in higher concentrations. On the other hand neostigmine, edrophon-ium and some other anilinium ions have an ACh-like action at higher concentra-tions, in addition to sensitising the muscle. The organophosphate anticholinesterase DFP, in higher concentrations, produces a partly reversible sensitisation to ACh (COHEN and POSTHUMUS, 1955). Since in the case of mammalian AChE the phospho-rylation of AChE by DFP is totally irreversible, the authors concluded that sensitisa-tion by higher concentrations of DFP cannot be entirely the consequence of AChE inhibition. On the other hand, HOBBIGER (1952) observed that pretreatment of a rectus abdominis muscle with TEPP completely abolished the anticurare action of edrophonium and other anilinium ions. This indicates that anticholinesterases of the organophosphate type can be useful in giving information on the mode of action of other substances on the rectus abdominis muscle. SMITH et al. (1952) compared the extent of sensitisation to ACh of the rectus abdominis muscle by TEPP, neostigmine, physostigmine and edrophonium and three other anilinium ions with the level of AChE inhibition. They found that there was a good correlation between the two parameters. This is rather surprising since during the assay of inhibition considerable reversal of the inhibition by anilinium ions should have occurred if frog AChE is identical with or closely related to mammalian AChE. The studies of HOBBIGER (1952), SMITH et al. (1952) and NASTUK and ALEXANDER (1954) seem to exclude the possibility that factors other than AChE inhibition are involved in the anticurare action of edrophonium in the frog.

The ACh- and tubocurarine-like actions of anticholinesterases of the carbamate type particularly and of anilinium ions are also observed when they are present in higher concentrations at neuromuscular junctions in twitch fibres (ECCLES et al., 1942; NASTUK and ALEXANDER, 1954). These actions mask the effects on the e.p.p. arising from AChE inhibition. As a result the effect on the e.p.p. of some anticho-linesterases, eg. physostigmine and edrophonium, is maximal at a certain concentra-tion and does not level out as the concentration is increased but declines. With neostigmine this does not occur, unless very high concentrations are used.

The sensitisation of the rectus abdominis muscle by sarin can be reversed by pralidoxime (FLEISHER et al., 1958). This indicates that frog AChE qualitatively behaves like mammalian AChE, i.e. it undergoes phosphorylation when exposed to anticholinesterases of the organophosphate type. Studying the relationship between the rate of hydrolysis of ACh, determined on muscle homogenates, and the reversal of the sensitisation to ACh by sarin, the authors concluded that the reversal of sensitisation was much greater than would be expected from the reversal of inhibi-tion. This might be taken to indicate that at frog neuromuscular junctions, as at mammalian neuromuscular junctions, not all AChE sites play an equal role in the hydrolysis of ACh.

Appendix II. Anticholinesterases and Anilinium Ions Referred to in the Text

A. Organophosphates which are Anticholinesterases in their Own Right.

The chemical formula is based on the structure $\begin{array}{c} R_1 \\ R_2 \end{array} P \begin{array}{c} O \\ X \end{array}$ and the type of phosphorylated AChE formed is given by $\begin{array}{c} R_1 \\ R_2 \end{array} P \begin{array}{c} O \\ AChE \end{array}$.

Abbreviation or code used in text	Full chemical name. Other abbreviations or names	Chemical formula
Methylparaoxon	dimethyl-4-nitro-phenylphosphate (Paraoxon-Me)	$\begin{array}{c} CH_3O \\ CH_3O \end{array} P \begin{array}{c} O \\ O \end{array}$—⬡—$NO_2$
Paraoxon	diethyl-4-nitro-phenylphosphate (E 600)	$\begin{array}{c} C_2H_5O \\ C_2H_5O \end{array} P \begin{array}{c} O \\ O \end{array}$—⬡—$NO_2$
Phospholine	diethyl-S-(2-trimethyl-ammoniummethyl) phosphorothioate (echothiopate; 217 MI)	$\begin{array}{c} C_2H_5O \\ C_2H_5O \end{array} P \begin{array}{c} O \\ SCH_2CH_2N^+(CH_3)_3 \end{array}$ I^-
Tertiary analogue of phospholine	diethyl-S-(2-dimethyl-aminoethyl) phosphorothioate (218 AO)	$\begin{array}{c} C_2H_5O \\ C_2H_5O \end{array} P \begin{array}{c} O \\ SCH_2CH_2N(CH_3)_2 \end{array}$ $\frac{1}{2} \begin{array}{c} COOH^- \\ COOH \end{array}$
TEPP	tetraethyl pyrophosphate	$\begin{array}{c} C_2H_5O \\ C_2H_5O \end{array} P{-}O{-}P \begin{array}{c} OC_2H_5 \\ OC_2H_5 \end{array}$, with $\overset{\parallel}{O}$ and $\overset{\parallel}{O}$
DFP	diisopropyl phosphoro-fluoridate (dyflos)	$\begin{array}{c} i{-}C_3H_7O \\ i{-}C_3H_7O \end{array} P \begin{array}{c} O \\ F \end{array}$
Sarin	isopropyl methyl-phosphonofluoridate (GB)	$\begin{array}{c} i{-}C_3H_7O \\ H_3C \end{array} P \begin{array}{c} O \\ F \end{array}$
Soman	pinacolyl methyl-phosphonofluoridate	$(CH_3)_3C\overset{\underset{\mid}{CH_3}}{C}HO$, $\begin{array}{c} \\ H_3C \end{array} P \begin{array}{c} O \\ F \end{array}$
—	pinacolyl-S-(2-tri-methylammoniummethyl) methylphosphono-fluoridate [used by LANCASTER (1972, 1973)]	$(CH_3)_3C\overset{\underset{\mid}{CH_3}}{C}HO$, $\begin{array}{c} \\ H_3C \end{array} P \begin{array}{c} O \\ SCH_2CH_2N^+(CH_3)_3 \end{array}$ $CH_3SO_4^-$

Abbreviation or code used in text	Full chemical name. Other abbreviations or names	Chemical formula
—	pinacolyl-S-(2-di-methylaminoethyl) methylphosphono-fluoridate [used by Lancaster (1972, 1973)]	$(CH_3)_3CCHO$, CH_3 above; H_3C—P(=O)—$SCH_2CH_2N(CH_3)_2$ HCl^-
Tabun	ethyl-N-dimethyl-phosphor-amidocyanidate	$(CH_3)_2N$—P(=O)—; C_2H_5O, CN

Methylfluorophosphorylcholines

Methylfluorophosphorylcholine
$(R:(CH_3)_3N^+$—CH_2CH_2—O—$)$
Methylfluorophosphoryl-β-methylcholine
$(R:(CH_3)_3N^+$—CH_2CH—O—$)$
                                      $|$
                                   CH_3
Methylfluorophosphorylhomocholine
$(R:(CH_3)_3N^+$—$CH_2CH_2CH_2$—O—$)$
Methylfluorophosphorylcarbocholine
$(R:(CH_3)_3C$—CH_2CH_2—O—$)$

H_3C—P(=O)(R)(F) I^-

Phosphostigmines

Dimethylphosphostigmine
$(Ro\ 3\text{-}0412; R=OCH_3)$
Diethylphosphostigmine
$(Ro\ 3\text{-}0340; R=OC_2H_5)$
Diisopropylphosphostigmine
$(Ro\ 3\text{-}0411; R=OC_3H_7$—$i)$
Disecbutylphosphostigmine
$(Ro\ 3\text{-}0397; R=OC_4H_9$—$s)$

R—P(=O)(R)(O)—(phenyl)—$N^+(CH_3)_3$ $CH_3SO_4^-$

| iso-OMPA (selective inhibitor of ChE) | tetramonoisopropyl pyrophosphortetramide | i—C_3H_7NH, i—C_3H_7NH —P—O—P— (O)(O), NHC_3H_7—i, NHC_3H_7—i |
| Mipafox (selective inhibitor of ChE) | N,N′-diisopropyl-phosphorodiamidic fluoride (Isopestox; Pestox XV) | i—C_3H_7NH, i—C_3H_7NH —P(=O)(F) |

B. Organophosphate Insecticides which are Converted in vivo into Anticholinesterases

Abbreviation or code used in text	Full chemical name. Other abbreviations or names	Chemical formula
Malathion	dimethyl-S-(1,2-dicarbethoxyethyl phosphorodithioate (Thiophos; E 605)	CH_3O, CH_3O —P(=S)—$SCHCOOC_2H_5$ $|$ $CHCOOC_2H_5$

Abbreviation or code used in text	Full chemical name. Other abbreviations or names	Chemical formula
Parathion	diethyl-4-nitrophenyl phosphorothioate (Thiophos; E 605)	
Systox	diethyl-0-(2-ethylthioethyl) phosphorothioate (Demeton; E 1059)	
Disyston	diethyl-S-(2-ethylthioethyl) phosphorodithioate (Dithiosystox; Disystox; Bayer 19639)	
EPN	ethyl-4-nitrophenyl phenylphosphonothioate	
OMPA	octamethyl pyrophosphortetramide (Schradan)	
Delnev	2.3-p-dioxanedithiol-S,S-bis(diethyl phosphorodithioate) (Hercules AC-528)	

C. Anticholinesterases of the Carbamate Type

Official name, abbreviation or code used in text	Chemical formula	
Neostigmine		$CH_3SO_4^-$
Physostigmine (Eserine)		$^1/_2 HSO_4^-$

Official name, abbreviation or code used in text	Chemical formula	

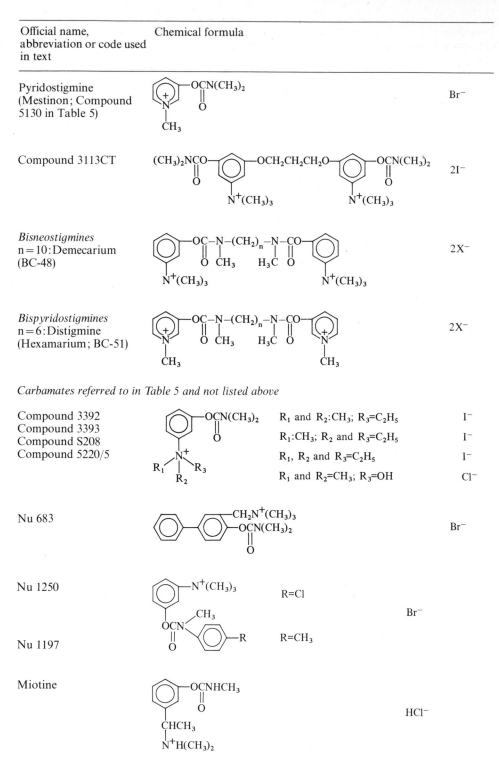

Pyridostigmine (Mestinon; Compound 5130 in Table 5)

Br^-

Compound 3113CT

$2I^-$

Bisneostigmines n = 10:Demecarium (BC-48)

$2X^-$

Bispyridostigmines n = 6:Distigmine (Hexamarium; BC-51)

$2X^-$

Carbamates referred to in Table 5 and not listed above

Compound 3392 R_1 and R_2:CH_3; R_3=C_2H_5 I^-
Compound 3393 R_1:CH_3; R_2 and R_3=C_2H_5 I^-
Compound S208 R_1, R_2 and R_3=C_2H_5 I^-
Compound 5220/5 R_1 and R_2=CH_3; R_3=OH Cl^-

Nu 683

Br^-

Nu 1250   R=Cl

                                                                       Br^-

Nu 1197   R=CH_3

Miotine

                                                                       HCl^-

Official name, abbreviation or code used in text	Chemical formula
Compound 38	(CH$_3$)$_2$NCO—[quinolinium ring N$^+$CH$_3$] CH$_3$SO$_4^-$
Ambenonium (Mytelase; WIN 8077; related to carbamates but not a carbamate)	(C$_2$H$_5$)$_2$N$^+$CH$_2$CH$_2$NHC—CNHCH$_2$CH$_2$N$^+$(C$_2$H$_5$)$_2$, CH$_2$ O O CH$_2$, two o-Cl-benzyl groups, 2X$^-$

D. Reversible Inhibitors

Name, abbreviation or code used in text	Full chemical name	Chemical formula
BW284C51	1,5-*bis*(4-allyldimethyl-ammoniumphenyl)pentane-3-one	CH$_2$CH$_2$CCH$_2$CH$_2$, O; two phenyl rings with N$^+$(CH$_3$)$_2$ CH$_2$CHCH$_2$; 2I$^-$
3-hydroxyanilinium ions e.g. edrophonium	3-hydroxyphenyl-dimethylethylammonium	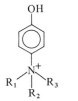 X$^-$ R$_1$, R$_2$ and R$_3$:CH$_3$ or C$_2$H$_5$
4-hydroxyanilinium ions		4-hydroxyphenyl structure with N$^+$R$_1$R$_2$R$_3$, X$^-$; R$_1$, R$_2$ and R$_3$:CH$_3$ or C$_2$H$_5$

Substances referred to in Table 4 and Fig. 14

Code	Full chemical name	
3-Me$_2$NCOOPNEt$_2$Me (This is as carbamate used as reference substance)	3-dimethylcarbamylphenyldiethylmethylammonium	
3-OHPNMe$_3$	3-hydroxyphenyltrimethylammonium	
3-OHPNEt$_2$Me	3-hydroxyphenyldiethylmethylammonium	
3-OHPNEt$_3$	3-hydroxyphenyltriethylammonium	
4-OHPNEt$_2$Me	4-hydroxyphenyldiethylmethylammonium	used as I$^-$
4-OHPNEt$_3$	4-hydroxyphenyltriethylammonium	
2-CH$_2$OHPNMe$_3$	2-hydroxymethylphenyltrimethylammonium	
2-MeOPNMe$_3$	2-methoxyphenyltrimethylammonium	
2-MePNMe$_3$	2-methylphenyltrimethylammonium	
PNEt$_2$Me	phenyldiethylmethylammonium	
PNEt$_3$	phenyltriethylammonium	
NMe$_3$Et	ethyltrimethylammonium	
NEt$_4$	tetraethylammonium	

Appendix III. An Outline of the Methods Used to Calculate the Quantal Content of the e.p.p. and the Rate of Refilling and Size of the ACh Store in Nerve Terminals

These calculations are based on e.p.p. recordings from isolated nerve-muscle preparations. To record e.p.p.s it is necessary to eliminate muscle action potentials. This can be accomplished by three methods: (1) reducing the calcium or raising the magnesium content of the bathing solution, or a combination of both; (2) the use of tubocurarine; or (3) cutting the muscle fibres close to the motor end-plate on both sides. It is highly unlikely that method (1) (LILEY, 1956b; HUBBARD, 1961; HUBBARD and WILLIS, 1968) can give results which would be conclusive as regards individual aspects of the mechanism of action of anticholinesterases and anilinium ions. Method (2) can be criticised because under the conditions used to obtain the appropriate e.p.p. records, i.e. at high rates of nerve stimulation, tubocurarine reduces the quantal release of ACh from nerve terminals (HUBBARD et al., 1969b; GALINDO, 1971; HUBBARD and WILSON, 1973; BLABER, 1973). Results obtained in experiments which involve the use of tubocurarine, therefore, cannot give information on the quantal release of ACh. This information, however, can be obtained in experiments on isolated nerve-muscle preparations with cut muscle fibres [method(3)]. Suitable preparations of this type can be obtained from the rat diaphragm (BARSTAD, 1962; BARSTAD and LILLEHEIL, 1968) or the tenuissimus muscle of the cat (BLABER, 1970).

In order to obtain by methods (2) or (3) the e.p.p. records required for the calculations, a train of 40 to 100 stimuli is applied to the nerve usually at a rate of 100 to 200 Hz. E.p.p.s are then analysed by the method used initially by ELMQVIST and QUASTEL (1965) in studies on human isolated intercostal muscle treated with tubocurarine.

To calculate the quantal content (number of quanta of ACh) of the e.p.p. the quantal size, i.e. the depolarisation produced by a single quantum of ACh (the amount of ACh released from one vesicle) must first be found. The value for the quantal size *(q)* is obtained by the equation

$$q = V/\bar{X}$$

where V is the variance of the 20th and subsequent e.p.p.s produced by the train of stimuli and $\bar{X}$ is the mean amplitude (height) of these e.p.p.s. The validity of this approach is confirmed by the finding that the calculated value of q is the same as that obtained by direct measurements of m.e.p.p.s (ELMQVIST and QUASTEL, 1965; HUBBARD and WILSON, 1973).

Having obtained the value for q the mean quantal content (m) of the e.p.p. can be calculated by using the equation

$$m = \text{amplitude of the e.p.p.}/q$$

where the amplitude of the e.p.p. is corrected for non-linear summation (MARTIN, 1966) and the e.p.p. on which calculations are based is the first e.p.p. produced by the train of stimuli.

In preparations treated with tubocurarine the record produced by a train of stimuli shows a marked progressive decline of the first 10 to 15 e.p.p.s. This decline is linear for the first 5 e.p.p.s and proportional to the rate of nerve stimulation (ELMQVIST and QUASTEL, 1965; BLABER, 1970). It can be described by the equation

$$d = m_x - 1/p + n \text{ (BLABER, 1970)}$$

where d represents the cumulative quantal contents of $(x-1)$ e.p.p.s, m_x is the quantal content of the xth e.p.p., p is the fractional release of quanta from the store in nerve terminals, and n is the number of quanta in the store. If the values of d for each of the first five e.p.p.s are plotted against the appropriate values of m_x the intercept on the y axis is n and the slope is $-1/p$.

Subsequent to the first 10 to 15 e.p.p.s the amplitude of the remaining 25 to 85 e.p.p.s is fairly constant in the rat isolated diaphragm and cat isolated tenuissimus muscle with cut muscle fibres (HUBBARD et al., 1969b; BLABER, 1970). In human isolated intercostal muscle there is a further decline although at a much slower rate than initially (ELMQVIST and QUASTEL, 1965).

For details of the calculations and the concepts on which they are based the reader is referred to the publications by ELMQVIST and QUASTEL (1965), MARTIN (1966), HUBBARD et al. (1969a) and BLABER (1970).

References

ADAMIČ, Š.: Accumulation of acetylcholine by the rat diaphragm. Biochem. Pharmacol. **19**, 2445—2451 (1970).

ADRIAN, E. D., BRONK, D. W.: The discharge of impulses in motor nerve fibres. Part I. Impulses in single fibres of the phrenic nerve. J. Physiol. (Lond.) **66**, 81 −101 (1928).

ADRIAN, E. D., BRONK, D. W.: The discharge of impulses in motor nerve fibres. Part II. The frequency of discharge in reflex and voluntary contractions. J. Physiol. (Lond.) **67**, 119—151 (1929).

AESCHLIMANN, J. A., REINERT, M.: Pharmacological action of some analogues of physostigmine. J. Pharmacol. exp. Ther. **43**, 413—444 (1931).

ALDRIDGE, W. N.: The inhibition of erythrocyte cholinesterase by triesters of phosphoric acid: 3. The nature of the inhibitory process. Biochem. J. **54**, 442—448 (1953).

ALDRIDGE, W. N., REINER, E.: Enzyme inhibitors as substrates. In: NEUBERGER, A., TATUM, E. L. (Eds.): North-Holland Research Monographs Frontiers of Biology, Vol. 26. Amsterdam: North-Holland Publ. Comp. 1972.

ANDERSSON-CEDERGREN, E.: Ultrastructure of motor endplate and sarcoplasmic components of mouse skeletal muscle fibre as revealed by three-dimensional reconstructions from serial sections. J. ultrastruct. Res., Suppl **1**, 1—191 (1959).

ARGENT, D. E., DINNICK, O. P., HOBBIGER, F.: Prolonged apnoea after suxamethonium in man. Brit. J. Anaesth. **27**, 24—30 (1955).

ARIËNS, A. TH., MEETER, E., WOLTHUIS, O. L., BENTHEIM, R. M. J. VAN: Reversible necrosis at the endplate region in striated muscles of the rat poisoned with cholinesterase inhibitors. Experientia (Basel) **25**, 57—59 (1969).

AUERBACH, A., BETZ, W.: Does curare affect transmitter release? J. Physiol. (Lond.) **213**, 691—705 (1971).

AUGUSTINSSON, K.-B.: Cholinesterases. A study in comparative enzymology. Acta physiol. scand. **15**, Suppl. **52**, 1—182 (1948).

Augustinsson, K.-B.: Classification and comparative enzymology of the cholinesterases and methods for their determination. In: Koelle, G. B. (Ed.): Handbuch der experimentellen Pharmakologie, Ergänzungswerk XV, Cholinesterases and Anticholinesterase Agents, pp. 89—128. Berlin-Göttingen-Heidelberg: Springer 1963.

Austin, L., Berry, W. K.: Two selective inhibitors of cholinesterase. Biochem. J. **54**, 695—700 (1953).

Axelsson, J., Thesleff, S.: The desensitizing effect of acetylcholine on the mammalian motor end-plate. Acta physiol. scand. **43**, 15—26 (1958).

Bacq, Z. M., Brown, G. L.: Pharmacological experiments on mammalian voluntary muscle in relation to the theory of chemical transmission. J. Physiol. (Lond.) **89**, 45—60 (1937).

Barnard, E. A., Rymaszewska, T., Wieckowski, J.: Cholinesterases at individual neuromuscular junctions. In: Triggle, D. J., Moran, J. F., Barnard, E. A. (Eds.): Cholinergic Ligand Interactions, pp. 175—200. New York: Academic Press 1971a.

Barnard, E. A., Wieckowski, J., Chiu, T. H.: Cholinergic receptor molecules and cholinesterase molecules at mouse skeletal muscle junctions. Nature (Lond.) **234**, 207—209 (1971b).

Barnes, J. M., Denz, F. A.: The reaction of rats to diets containing octamethyl pyrophosphoramide (Schradan) and 0,0-diethyl-S-ethyl mercaptoethyl thiophosphate (Systox). Brit. J. industr. Med. **11**, 11—19 (1954).

Barnes, J. M., Duff, J. I.: The role of cholinesterase at the myoneural junction. Brit. J. Pharmacol. **8**, 334—339 (1953).

Barnett, R. J.: The fine structural localization of acetylcholinesterase at the myoneural junction. J. Cell Biol. **12**, 247—262 (1962).

Barstad, J. A. B.: Presynaptic effect of the neuromuscular transmitter. Experientia (Basel) **18**, 579—582 (1962).

Barstad, J. A. B., Lilleheil, G.: Transversally cut diaphragm preparation from rat. Arch. int. Pharmacodyn. **175**, 373—390 (1968).

Beani, L., Bianchi, C., Ledda, F.: The effect of tubocurarine on acetylcholine release from motor nerve terminals. J. Physiol. (Lond.) **174**, 172—183 (1964).

Bergman, R. A., Johns, R. J., Afifi, A. K.: Ultrastructural alterations in muscle from patients with myasthenia gravis and Eaton-Lambert syndrome. Ann. N.Y. Acad. Sci. **183**, 88—122 (1971).

Bergner, A. D., Wagley, P. F.: An effect of pyridine-2-aldoxime methiodide (2-PAM) on cholinesterase at motor end-plates. Proc. Soc. exp. Biol. (N.Y.) **97**, 90—92 (1958).

Berry, W. K.: The turnover number of cholinesterase. Biochem. J. **49**, 615—620 (1951).

Berry, W. K., Lovatt Evans, C.: Cholinesterase and neuromuscular block. J. Physiol. (Lond.) **115**, 46P—47P (1951).

Berry, W. K., Rutland, J. P.: Choline ester hydrolases in diaphragm muscle. Biochem. Pharmacol. **20**, 669—682 (1971).

Blaber, L. C.: The antagonism of muscle relaxants by ambenonium and methoxyambenonium in the cat. Brit. J. Pharmacol. **15**, 476—484 (1960).

Blaber, L. C.: Facilitation of neuromuscular transmission by anticholinesterase drugs. Brit. J. Pharmacol. **20**, 63—73 (1963).

Blaber, L. C.: The effect of facilitatory concentrations of decamethonium on the storage and release of transmitter at the neuromuscular junction of the cat. J. Pharmacol. exp. Ther. **175**, 664—672 (1970).

Blaber, L. C.: The mechanism of the facilitatory action of edrophonium in cat skeletal muscle. Brit. J. Pharmacol. **46**, 498—507 (1972).

Blaber, L. C.: The prejunctional actions of some non-depolarising blocking drugs. Brit. J. Pharmacol. **47**, 109—116 (1973).

Blaber, L. C., Bowman, W. C.: The interaction between benzoquinonium and anticholinesterases in skeletal muscle. Arch. int. Pharmacodyn. **138**, 90—104 (1962).

Blaber, L. C., Bowman, W. C.: The effects of some drugs on the repetitive discharges produced in nerve and muscle by anticholinesterases. Int. J. Neuropharmacol. **2**, 1—16 (1963a).

Blaber, L. C., Bowman, W. C.: Studies on the repetitive discharges evoked in motor nerve and skeletal muscle after injection of anticholinesterase drugs. Brit. J. Pharmacol. **20**, 326—344 (1963b).

Blaber, L. C., Christ, D. D.: The action of facilitatory drugs on the isolated tenuissimus muscle of the cat. Int. J. Neuropharmacol. **6**, 473—484 (1967).

BLABER, L. C., CREASEY, N. H.: The mode of recovery of cholinesterase activity *in vivo* after organo-phosphorus poisoning. I. Erythrocyte cholinesterase. Biochem. J. **77**, 591—596 (1960).

BLABER, L. C., GOODE, J. W.: A comparison of the action of facilitatory and depolarizing drugs at the mammalian motor nerve terminal. Int. J. Neuropharmacol. **7**, 429—440 (1968).

BLABER, L. C., KARCZMAR, A. G.: Multiple cholinoceptive and related sites at the neuromuscular junction. Ann. N.Y. Acad. Sci. **144**, 571—583 (1967).

BLASCHKO, H., BÜLBRING, E., CHOU, T. C.: Tubocurarine antagonism and inhibition of cholinesterase. Brit. J. Pharmacol. **4**, 29—32 (1949).

BOMBINSKI, T. J., DUBOIS, K. P.: Toxicity and mechanism of action of "di-syston". Arch. Ind. Hlth. **17**, 192—197 (1958).

BOWMAN, W. C.: The neuromuscular blocking action of benzoquinonium chloride in the cat and in the hen. Brit. J. Pharmacol. **13**, 521—530 (1958).

BOWMAN, W. C., WEBB, S. N.: Acetylcholine and anticholinesterase drugs. International Encyclopaedia of Pharmacology and Therapeutics. Section 14, Volume 2, J. Cheymol, Ed., pp. 427—502. Oxford: Pergamon Press 1972.

BOYD, I. A., MARTIN, A. R.: Spontaneous subthreshold activity at mammalian neuromuscular junctions. J. Physiol. (Lond.) **132**, 61—73 (1956a).

BOYD, I. A., MARTIN, A. R.: The endplate potential in mammalian muscle. J. Physiol. (Lond.) **132**, 74—91 (1956b).

BRISCOE, G.: Changes in muscle contraction curves produced by drugs of the eserine and curarine groups. J. Physiol. (Lond.) **93**, 194—205 (1938).

BRODEUR, J., DUBOIS, K. P.: Studies on the mechanism of acquired tolerance by rats to 0,0-diethyl S-2-(ethylthio)ethyl phosphorodithioate (Di-Syston). Arch. int. Pharmacodyn. **149**, 560—570 (1964).

BROWN, G. L.: Action potentials of normal mammalian muscle. Effects of acetylcholine and eserine. J. Physiol. (Lond.) **89**, 220—237 (1937a).

BROWN, G. L.: The actions of acetylcholine on denervated mammalian and frog's muscle. J. Physiol. (Lond.) **89**, 438—461 (1937b).

BROWN, G. L., DALE, H. H., FELDBERG, W.: Reactions of the normal mammalian muscle to acetylcholine and to eserine. J. Physiol. (Lond.) **87**, 394—424 (1936).

BROWN, M. C., MATTHEWS, P. B. C.: The effect on a muscle twitch of the back response of its motor nerve. J. Physiol. (Lond.) **150**, 332—346 (1960).

BRÜCKE, F.: Dicholinesters of α-ω-dicarboxylic acids and related substances. Pharmacol. Rev. **8**, 265—335 (1956).

BUCKLEY, G. A., HEADING, C. E.: Tolerance to neostigmine. Brit. J. Pharmacol. **40**, 590P—591P (1970).

BUCKLEY, G. A., HEADING, C. E.: The effects of prolonged neostigmine treatment. J. Physiol. (Lond.) **219**, 6P—7P (1971).

BUCKLEY, G. A., NOWELL, P. T.: Micro-colorimetric determination of cholinesterase activity of motor endplates in the rat diaphragm. J. Pharm. Pharmacol. **18**, 146S—150S (1966).

BÜLBRING, E., CHOU, T.: The relative activity of prostigmine homologues and other substances as antagonists to tubocurarine. Brit. J. Pharmacol. **2**, 8—22 (1947).

BURGEN, A. S. V., CHIPMAN, L. M.: Location of cholinesterase in central nervous system. Quart. J. Exper. Physiol. **37**, 61—74 (1952).

BURGEN, A. S. V., HOBBIGER, F.: Inhibition of cholinesterase by alkylphosphates and alkylphenol-phosphates. Brit. J. Pharmacol. **6**, 593—605 (1951).

BURGEN, A. S. V., KEELE, C. A., SLOME, D.: Pharmacological actions of tetraethylpyrophosphate and hexaethyltetraphosphate. J. Pharmacol. exp. Ther. **96**, 396—409 (1949).

BURNS, B. D., PATON, W. D. M.: Depolarisation of the motor end-plate by decamethonium and acetylcholine. J. Physiol. (Lond.) **115**, 41—73 (1951).

CANDOLE, C. A. DE, DOUGLAS, W. W., LOVATT EVANS, C., HOLMES, R., SPENCER, K. E. V., TORRANCE, R. W., WILSON, K. M.: The failure of respiration in death by anticholinesterase poisoning. Brit. J. Pharmacol. **8**, 466—475 (1953).

CASIDA, J. E., ALLEN, T. C., STAHMANN, M. A.: Mammalian conversion of octamethyl-pyrophosphoramide to a toxic phosphoramide-N-oxide. J. biol. Chem. **210**, 607—616 (1954).

CASTILLO, J. DEL, KATZ, B.: A comparison of acetylcholine and stable depolarizing agents. Proc. roy. Soc. B **146**, 362—368 (1957).

CHANG, C. C., CHEN, T. F., CHUANG, S.-T.: Influence of chronic neostigmine treatment on the number of acetylcholine receptors and the release of acetylcholine from the rat diaphragm. J. Physiol. (Lond.) 230, 613—618 (1973).

CHANG, C. C., CHENG, H. C., CHEN, T. F.: Does d-tubocurarine inhibit the release of acetylcholine from motor nerve endings? Jap. J. Physiol. 17, 505—515 (1967).

CHANG, H. C., GADDUM, J. H.: Choline esters in tissue extracts. J. Physiol. (Lond.) 79, 255—285 (1933).

CHENNELS, M., FLOYD, W. F., WRIGHT, S.: Action of condensed alkyl phosphates on the nerve-muscle preparation and the central nervous system of the cat. J. Physiol. (Lond.) 108, 375—397 (1949).

CHEYMOL, J., BOURILLET, F., OGURA, Y.: Action de quelques paralysants neuromusculaires sur la libération de l'acétylcholine au niveau des terminaisons nerveuses motrices. Arch. int. Pharmacodyn. 139, 187—197 (1962).

CHOKROVERTY, S., PARAMESWAR, K. S., CO, C.: Nonspecific esterases in the myoneural junction of human striated muscle. J. Histochem. Cytochem. 19, 798—800 (1971).

CHRIST, D. D., BLABER, L. C.: The actions of benzoquinonium in the isolated cat tenuissimus muscle. J. Pharmacol. exp. Ther. 160, 159—165 (1968).

CHRISTOFF, N., ANDERSON, P. J., SLOTWINER, P., SONG, S. K.: Electrophoretic and histochemical evaluation of anticholinesterase drugs. Ann. N.Y. Acad. Sci. 135, 150—162 (1966).

CITRIN, G.: Actions of KCl on the neuromuscular junction. Fed. Proc. 26, 512 (1967).

CITRIN, G.: Interaction of anticholinesterases and acetylcholine (ACh) on mammalian motor nerve terminals (M.N.T.). Fed. Proc. 27, 407 (1968).

COHEN, J. A., OOSTERBAAN, R. A.: The active site of acetylcholinesterase and related esterases and its reactivity towards substrates and inhibitors. In: KOELLE, G. B. (Ed.): Handbuch der experimentellen Pharmakologie, Ergänzungswerk XV. Cholinesterases and Anticholinesterase Agents, pp. 299—373. Berlin-Göttingen-Heidelberg: Springer 1963.

COHEN, J. A., OOSTERBAAN, R. A., WARRINGA, M. G. P. J.: The turnover number of ali-esterase, pseudo- and true-cholinesterase and the combination of these enzymes with diisopropylfluorophosphate. Biochim. biophys. Acta (Amst.) 18, 228—235 (1955).

COHEN, J. A., POSTHUMUS, C. H.: The mechanism of action of anti-cholinesterases. Acta physiol. pharmacol. neerl. 4, 17—36 (1955).

COOPER, F. A.: Delnav 2:3-p dioxane S-bis-(0,0-diethyl dithiophosphate) as an ixocide. Vet. Rec. 74, 103—112 (1962).

COUTEAUX, R.: Morphological and cytochemical observations on the post-synaptic membrane at motor end-plates and ganglionic synapses. Exp. Cell. Res., Suppl. 5, 294—322 (1958).

COUTEAUX, R., TAXI, J.: Recherches histochimiques sue la distribution des activités cholinestérasiques au niveau de la synapse myoneurale. Arch. Anat. micro. Morph. exp. 41, 352—392 (1952).

COWAN, S. L.: The action of eserine-like and curare-like substances on the responses of frog's nerve-muscle preparations to repetitive stimulation. J. Physiol. (Lond.) 93, 215—262 (1938).

COWAN, S. L.: The actions of eserine-like compounds upon frog's nerve-muscle preparations, and conditions in which a single shock can evoke an augmented muscular response. Proc. roy. Soc. B 129, 356—391 (1940).

CSILLIK, B.: Functional structure of the post-synaptic membrane in the myoneural junction. Budapest: Akademiai Kiado 1965.

CSILLIK, B., KNYIHÁR, E.: On the effect of motor nerve degeneration on the fine-structural localization of esterases in the mammalian motor end-plate. J. Cell Sci. 3, 529—538 (1968).

DAHLBÄCK, O., ELMQVIST, D., JOHNS, T. R., RADNER, S., THESLEFF, S.: An electrophysiologic study of the neuromuscular junction in myasthenia gravis. J. Physiol. (Lond.) 156, 336—343 (1961).

DALE, H. H., FELDBERG, W., VOGT, M.: Release of acetylcholine at voluntary motor nerve-endings. J. Physiol. (Lond.) 86, 353—380 (1936).

DAVIES, D. R., GREEN, A. L.: The kinetics of reactivation, by oximes, of cholinesterase inhibited by organophosphorus compounds. Biochem. J. 63, 529—535 (1956).

DAVIES, D. R., GREEN, A. L.: The mechanism of hydrolysis by cholinesterase and related enzymes. In: NORD, F. F. (Ed.): Advanc. Enzymol., Vol. 20, pp. 283—318. New York: Interscience Publishers Inc. 1958.

DAVIES,J.E., DAVIS,J.H., FRAZIER,D.E., MANN,J.B., REICH,G.A., TOCCI,P.M.: Disturbances of metabolism in organophosphate poisoning. Industr. Med. Surg. **36**, 58—62 (1967).
DAVIS,D.A., WASSERKRUG,H.L., HEYMAN,I.A., PADMANABHAN, K.C., SELIGMAN,G.A., PLAPIN-GER,R.E., SELIGMAN,A.M.: Comparison of ultrastructural cholinesterase demonstration in the motor end-plate with α-acetylthiol-m-toluenediazonium ion and 3-acetoxy-5-indolediazonium ion. J. Histochem. Cytochem. **20**, 161—172 (1972).
DENZ,F.A.: On the histochemistry of the myoneural junction. Brit. J. exp. Path. **34**, 329—339 (1953).
DOUGLAS,W.W., PATON,W.D.M.: The mechanism of motor end-plate depolarization due to a cholinesterase-inhibiting drug. J. Physiol. (Lond.) **124**, 325—344 (1954).
DUBOIS,K.P.: Toxicological evaluation of the anticholinesterase agents. In: KOELLE,G.B. (Ed.): Handbuch der experimentellen Pharmakologie, Ergänzungswerk XV. Cholinesterases and Anticholinesterase Agents, pp.833—859. Berlin: Springer-Verlag 1963.
DUN,F.T., FENG,T.P.: Studies on the neuromuscular junction. XX. The site of origin of the junctional after discharge in muscles treated with guanidine, barium or eserine. Chin. J. Physiol. **15**, 433—444 (1940).
ECCLES,J.C., JAEGER,J.C.: The relationship between the mode of operation and the dimensions of the junctional region at synapses and motor endorgans. Proc. roy. Soc. B **148**, 38—56 (1958).
ECCLES,J.C., KATZ,B., KUFFLER,S.W.: Electric potential changes accompanying neuromuscular transmission. Biol. Symp. **3**, 349—370 (1941).
ECCLES,J.C., KATZ,B., KUFFLER,S.W.: Effect of eserine on neuromuscular transmission. J. Neurophysiol. **5**, 211—230 (1942).
ECCLES,J.C., MacFARLANE,W.V.: Actions of anti, -cholinesterases of endplate potential of frog muscle. J. Neurophysiol. **12**, 59—80 (1949).
ELLIN,R.I., WILLS,J.H.: Oximes antagonistic to inhibitors of cholinesterase. J. pharm. Sci. **53**, 995—1007 (Part 1) and 1143—1150 (Part 2) (1964).
ELLMAN,G.L., COURTNEY,K.D., ANDRES,V., FEATHERSTONE,R.M.: A new and rapid colorimetric determination of acetylcholinesterase activity. Biochem. Pharmacol. **7**, 88—95 (1961).
ELMQVIST,D., HOFMANN,W., KUGELBERG,J., QUASTEL,D.M.J.: An electrophysiological investigation of neuromuscular transmission in myasthenia gravis. J. Physiol. (Lond.) **174**, 417—434 (1964).
ELMQVIST,D., QUASTEL,D.M.J.: A quantitative study of end-plate potentials in isolated human muscle. J. Physiol. (Lond.) **178**, 505—529 (1965).
ENANDER,I.: Experiments with methyl-fluorophosphorylcholine-inhibited cholinesterase. Acta chem. scand. **12**, 780—781 (1958).
ENGEL,A.G., SANTA,T.: Histometric analysis of the ultrastructure of the neuromuscular junction in myasthenia gravis and in the myasthenic syndrome. Ann. N.Y. Acad. Sci. **183**, 46—63 (1971).
ERANKÖ,O., TERÄVÄINEN,H.: Distribution of esterases in the myoneural junction of the striated muscle of the rat. J. Histochem. Cytochem. **15**, 399—403 (1967).
ERDMANN,W.D., LENDLE,L.: Vergiftungen mit esteraseblockierenden Insecticiden aus der Gruppe der organischen Phosphorsäureester (E 605 und Verwandte). In: HEILMEYER,L., SCHOEN,R., GLANZMANN,E., DE RUDDER,B. (Eds.): Ergeb. inn. Med. Kinderheilk., Bd. 10, pp.103—184. Berlin-Göttingen-Heidelberg: Springer 1958.
FAMBROUGH,D.M., HARTZELL,H.C.: Acetylcholine receptors: Number and distribution at neuromuscular junctions in rat diaphragm. Science **176**, 189—191 (1972).
FATT,P., KATZ,B.: An analysis of the endplate potential recorded with an intracellular electrode. J. Physiol. (Lond.) **115**, 320—370 (1951).
FATT,P., KATZ,B.: Spontaneous subthreshold activity at motor nerve endings. J. Physiol. (Lond.) **117**, 109—128 (1952).
FENG,T.P.: Studies on the neuromuscular junction. VI. Potentiation by eserine of response to single indirect stimulus in amphibian nerve-muscle preparations. Chin. J. Physiol. **12**, 51—58 (1937).
FENG,T.P.: Studies on the neuromuscular junction. XVIII. The local potentials around N-M junctions induced by single and multiple volleys. Chin. J. Physiol. **15**, 367—404 (1940).

Feng, T. P.: The local activity around the skeletal N-M junctions produced by nerve impulses. Biol. Symp. **3**, 121—152 (1941).

Feng, T. P., Li, T. H.: Studies on the neuromuscular junction. XXIII. A new aspect of the phenomena of eserine potentiation and post-tetanic facilitation in mammalian muscle. Chin. J. Physiol. **16**, 37—56 (1941).

Fischer, G.: Inhibierung und Restitution der Azetylcholinesterase an der motorischen Endplatte im Zwerchfell der Ratte nach Intoxikation mit Soman. Histochemie **16**, 144—149 (1968).

Fischer, G.: Die Acetylcholinesterase an der motorischen Endplatte des Rattenzwerchfells nach Intoxikation mit Paraoxon und Soman bei Applikation von Oximen. Experientia (Basel) **26**, 402—403 (1970).

Fleisher, J. H., Corrigan, J. P., Howard, J. W.: Potentiation of the response of frog rectus muscle to acetylcholine by isopropyl methyl phosphonofluoridate and its modification by pyridine-2-aldoxime methiodide. Brit. J. Pharmacol. **13**, 291—295 (1958).

Fleisher, J. H., Hansa, J., Killos, P. J., Harrison, C. S.: Effects of 1,1'-trimethylene bis(4-formyl-pyridinium bromide dioxime (TMB-4) on cholinesterase activity and neuromuscular block following poisoning with sarin and DFP. J. Pharmacol. exp. Ther. **130**, 461—468 (1960).

Fleisher, J. H., Moen, T. H., Ellington, N. R.: Effects of 2-PAM and TMB-4 on neuromuscular transmission. J. Pharmacol. exp. Ther. **149**, 311—319 (1965).

Foldes, F. T., Glaser, G. H.: Diagnostic tests in myasthenia gravis: an overview. Ann. N.Y. Acad. Sci. **183**, 275—286 (1971).

Fredriksson, T., Tibbling, G.: Reversal of effects on the rat nerve-diaphragm preparation produced by methylfluorophosphorylcholines. Biochem. Pharmacol. **2**, 63—67 (1959).

Funke, A., Bagot, J., Depierre, F.: Anticholinestérasiques. I. Synthèse de diphénoxyalcanes porteurs d'une ou deux fonctions phenoliques librés. C.R. Acad. Sci. (Paris) **239**, 329—331 (1954).

Gage, J. C.: A cholinesterase inhibitor derived from 0,0-diethyl 0-p-nitrophenyl thiophosphate in vivo. Biochem. J. **54**, 426—430 (1953).

Galindo, A.: Prejunctional effect of curare; its relative importance. J. Neurophysiol. **34**, 289—301 (1971).

Glaser, G. H.: Crisis, precrisis and drug resistance in myasthenia gravis. Ann. N.Y. Acad. Sci. **135**, 335—345 (1966).

Goyer, R. G.: The effects of P-2-AM on the release of acetylcholine from the isolated diaphragm of the rat. J. Pharm. Pharmacol. **22**, 42—45 (1970).

Grob, D.: Therapy of myasthenia gravis. In: Koelle, G. B. (Ed.): Handbuch der experimentellen Pharmakologie, Ergänzungswerk XV. Cholinesterases and Anticholinesterase Agents, pp. 989—1027. Berlin-Göttingen-Heidelberg: Springer 1963.

Grob, D.: Spontaneous end-plate activity in normal subjects and in patients with myasthenia gravis. Ann. N.Y. Acad. Sci. **183**, 248—269 (1971).

Grob, D., Johns, R. J.: Use of oximes in the treatment of intoxication by anticholinesterase compounds in patients with myasthenia gravis. Amer. J. Med. **24**, 512—518 (1958a).

Grob, D., Johns, R. J.: Treatment of anticholinesterase intoxication in normal subjects and myasthenia patients with oximes. J. Amer. med. Ass. **166**, 1855—1858 (1958b).

Grob, D., Johns, R. J., Harvey, Mc G.: Studies in neuromuscular function. Johns Hopk. Hosp. Bull. **99**, 115—238 (1956).

Groblewski, G. E., McNamara, B. P., Wills, J. H.: Stimulation of denervated muscle by DFP and related compounds. J. Pharmacol. exp. Ther. **118**, 116—122 (1956).

Häggqvist, G.: Cholinesterases and innervation of skeletal muscle. Acta physiol. scand. **48**, 63—70 (1960).

Hall, Z. W., Kelly, R. B.: Enzymatic detachment of endplate acetylcholinesterase from muscle. Nature (Lond.) New Biol. **232**, 62—63 (1971).

Hawkins, R. D., Gunter, J. M.: Studies on cholinesterase. 5. The selective inhibition of pseudo-cholinesterase in vivo. Biochem. J. **40**, 192—197 (1946).

Hayes, W. J., Jr.: Toxicity of pesticides to man, risks from present levels. Proc. roy. Soc. B **167**, 101—127 (1967).

Heath, D. F.: Organophosphorus poisons. Oxford: Pergamon Press 1961.

Heffron, P. F.: Actions of the selective inhibitor of cholinesterase tetramonoisopropyl pyrophosphortetramide on the rat phrenic nerve-diaphragm preparation. Brit. J. Pharmacol. **46**, 714—724 (1972).

HEILBRONN, E.: *In vitro* reactivation and "ageing" of tabun-inhibited blood cholinesterases. Studies with N-methylpyridinium-2-aldoxime methane sulphonate and N,N'-trimethylene *bis*(-pyridinium-4-aldoxime) dibromide. Biochem. Pharmacol. **12**, 25—36 (1963).

HEILBRONN, E.: Structure and reactions of DFP sensitive enzymes. E. HEILBRONN (Ed.): Stockholm: Research Institute of National Defence 1967.

HOBBIGER, F.: The action of carbamic esters and tetraethylpyrophosphate on normal and curarized frog rectus muscle. Brit. J. Pharmacol. **5**, 37—48 (1950).

HOBBIGER, F.: Inhibition of cholinesterase by irreversible inhibitors *in vitro* and *in vivo*. Brit. J. Pharmacol. **6**, 21—30 (1951).

HOBBIGER, F.: The mechanisms of anticurare action of certain neostigmine analogues. Brit. J. Pharmacol. **7**, 223—236 (1952).

HOBBIGER, F.: Chemical reactivation of phosphorylated human and bovine true cholinesterases. Brit. J. Pharmacol. **11**, 295—303 (1956).

HOBBIGER, F.: Protection against the lethal effects of organophosphates by pyridine-2-aldoxime methiodide. Brit. J. Pharmacol. **12**, 438—446 (1957).

HOBBIGER, F.: Reactivation of phosphorylated acetylcholinesterase. In: KOELLE, G. B. (Ed.): Handbuch der experimentellen Pharmakologie, Ergänzungswerk XV. Cholinesterases and Anticholinesterase Agents, pp. 921—988. Berlin-Göttingen-Heidelberg: Springer 1968.

HOBBIGER, F.: Anticholinesterases. In: LAURENCE, D. R., BACHARACH, A. L. (Eds.): Evaluation of Drug Activities Pharmacometrics, Part 2, pp. 459—489. London: Academic Press 1964.

HOBBIGER, F.: Anticholinesterases. In: ROBSON, T. M., STACEY, R. S. (Eds.): Recent Advances in Pharmacology, 4th Ed., pp. 291—310. London: J. & A. Churchill 1968.

HOBBIGER, F.: Chemotherapy in pesticide poisoning. In: KAHN, M. A., HAUFE, W. O. (Eds.): Toxicology, Biodegradation and Efficacy of Livestock Pesticides, pp. 252—281. Amsterdam: Swets & Zeitlinger 1972.

HOBBIGER, F., PECK, A. W.: Hydrolysis of suxamethonium by different types of plasma. Brit. J. Pharmacol. **37**, 258—271 (1969).

HOBBIGER, F., PECK, A. W.: The relationship between the level of cholinesterase in plasma and the action of suxamethonium in animals. Brit. J. Pharmacol. **40**, 775—789 (1970).

HOBBIGER, F., PITMAN, M., SADLER, P. W.: Reactivation of phosphorylated acetocholinesterases by pyridinium aldoximes and related compounds. Biochem. J. **75**, 363—372 (1960).

HOBBIGER, F., SADLER, P. W.: Protection against lethal organophosphate poisoning by quaternary pyridine aldoximes. Brit. J. Pharmacol. **14**, 192—201 (1959).

HOBBIGER, F., VOJVODIĆ, V.: The reactivating and antidotal actions of N,N'-trimethylene-*bis*(pyridinium-4-aldoxime) (TMB-4) and N,N'-oxydimethylene*bis*(pyridinium-4-aldoxime) (Toxogonin), with particular reference to their effect on phosphorylated acetylcholinesterase in the brain. Biochem. Pharmacol. **15**, 1677—1690 (1966).

HODGE, H. C., MAYNARD, E. A., HURWITZ, L., DISTEFANO, V., DOWNS, W. L., JONES, C. K., BLANCHET, H. J., JR.: Studies of the toxicity and enzyme kinetics of ethyl-p-nitrophenyl thionobenzene phosphonate (EPN). J. Pharmacol. exp. Ther. **122**, 29—39 (1954).

HOLMES, R., ROBINS, E. L.: The reversal by oximes of neuromuscular block produced by anticholinesterases. Brit. J. Pharmacol. **10**, 490—495 (1955).

HOLMSTEDT, B.: Synthesis and pharmacology of dimethylamidoethoxy-phosphoryl cyanide (Tabun) together with a description of some allied anticholinesterase compounds containing the N-P bond. Acta. physiol. scand. **25**, Suppl. **90**, 1—120 (1951).

HOLMSTEDT, B.: A modification of the thiocholine method for the determination of cholinesterase. I. Biochemical evaluation of selective inhibitors. Acta physiol. scand. **40**, 322—330. II. Histochemical application. Acta physiol. scand. **40**, 331—337 (1957).

HOLMSTEDT, B.: Pharmacology of organophosphorus cholinesterase inhibitors. Pharmacol. Rev. **11**, 567—688 (1959).

HOLMSTEDT, B.: Structure-activity relationships of the organophosphorus anticholinesterase agents. In: KOELLE, G. B. (Ed.): Handbuch der experimentellen Pharmakologie, Ergänzungswerk XV, pp. 428—485. Berlin-Göttingen-Heidelberg: Springer 1963.

HOLMSTEDT, B.: The ordeal bean of old calabar: the pageant of *physostigma venenosum* in medicine. In: SWAIN, T. (Ed.): Plants in the development of modern medicine, pp. 303—360. Cambridge: Harvard University Press 1972.

HOPPE, J. O., FUNNELL, J. E., LAPE, H.: The effects of structural variation in the quaternary nitrogen centers of benzoquinonium chloride upon neuromuscular blocking activity. J. Pharmacol. exp. Ther. **115**, 106—119 (1955).

HUBBARD, J. I.: The effect of calcium and magnesium on the spontaneous release of transmitters from mammalian nerve endings. J. Physiol. (Lond.) **159**, 507—517 (1961).

HUBBARD, J. I.: Mechanism of transmitter release. In: BUTLER, J. A. V., NOBLE, D. (Eds.): Progress in Biophysics and Molecular Biology. Oxford: Pergamon Press 1970.

HUBBARD, J. I., LLINÁS, R., QUASTEL, D. M.: In: DAVSON, H., GREENFIELD, A. D. M., WHITTAM, R., BRINDLEY, G. S. (Eds.): Monographs of the Physiological Society. Number 19. Electrophysiological analysis of synaptic transmission. London: Edward Arnold Ltd. 1969a.

HUBBARD, J. I., SCHMIDT, R. F.: Stimulation of motor nerve terminals. Nature (Lond.) **191**, 1103—1104 (1961).

HUBBARD, J. I., SCHMIDT, R. F., YOKOTA, T.: The effect of acetylcholine upon mammalian motor nerve terminals. J. Physiol. (Lond.) **181**, 810—829 (1965).

HUBBARD, J. I., WILLIS, W. D.: The effects of depolarisation of motor nerve terminals upon the release of transmitter by nerve impulses. J. Physiol. (Lond.) **194**, 381—405 (1968).

HUBBARD, J. I., WILSON, D. F.: Neuromuscular transmission in a mammalian preparation in the absence of blocking drugs and the effect of D-tubocurarine. J. Physiol. (Lond.) **228**, 307—325 (1973).

HUBBARD, J. I., WILSON, D. F., MIYAMOTO, M.: Reduction of transmitter release by D-tubocurarine. Nature (Lond.) **223**, 531—533 (1969b).

HUNT, C. C.: The effect of di-isopropyl fluorophosphate on neuromuscular transmission. J. Pharmacol. exp. Ther. **91**, 77—83 (1947).

HUNT, C. C., RIKER, W. F., JR.: The effect of chronic poisoning with di-isopropyl fluorophosphate on neuromuscular function in the cat. J. Pharmacol. exp. Ther. **91**, 298—305 (1947).

HUTTER, O. F.: Post-tetanic restoration of neuromuscular transmission blocked by D-tubocurarine. J. Physiol. (Lond.) **118**, 216—227 (1952).

JACOB, J., PECOT-DECHAVASSINE, M.: Hydrolyse enzymatique de la propionylcholine, de l'acétylthiocholine et de la butyrylthiocholine par le rectus de grenouille. Experientia (Basel) **14**, 330 (1958).

JOHNS, R. J., McQUILLEN, M. P.: Syndroms simulating myasthenia gravis: asthenia with anticholinesterase tolerance. Ann. N.Y. Acad. Sci. **135**, 385—397 (1966).

KALOW, W., GENEST, K.: A method for the detection of atypical forms of human serum cholinesterase. Determination of dibucaine numbers. Canad. J. Biochem. **35**, 339—346 (1957).

KALOW, W., GUNN, D. R.: The relations between dose of succinylcholine and duration of apnea in man. J. Pharmacol. exp. Ther. **120**, 203—214 (1957).

KALOW, W., STARON, N.: On distribution and inheritance of atypical forms of human serum cholinesterase, as indicated by dibucaine numbers. Canad. J. Biochem. **35**, 1305—1320 (1957).

KARCZMAR, A. G.: Antagonism between a *bis*-quaternary oxamide, WIN 8078, and depolarizing and competitive blocking drugs. J. Pharmacol. exp. Ther. **119**, 39—47 (1957).

KARCZMAR, A. G.: Neuromuscular pharmacology. Ann. Rev. Pharmacol. **7**, 241—276 (1967).

KATZ, B.: Nerve, muscle and synapse. New York: McGraw-Hill Inc. 1966.

KATZ, B.: The release of neural transmitter substances. Springfield/Ill.: Charles C. Thomas 1969.

KATZ, B., THESLEFF, S.: The interaction between edrophonium (Tensilon) and acetylcholine at the motor end-plate. Brit. J. Pharmacol. **12**, 260—264 (1957).

KELEMEN, M. H., VOLLE, R. L.: Plasma cholinesterase activity and neuromuscular paralysis by succinylcholine. Arch. int. Pharmacodyn. **159**, 477—483 (1966).

KEWITZ, H.: A specific antidote against lethal alkyl phosphate intoxication. III. Repair of chemical lesion. Arch. Biochem. **66**, 263—270 (1957).

KEWITZ, H., WILSON, I. B., NACHMANSOHN, D.: A specific antidote against lethal alkyl phosphate intoxication. II. Antidotal properties. Arch. Biochem. **64**, 456—465 (1956).

KOELLE, G. B.: Histochemical demonstration of reversible anticholinesterase action at selective cellular sites *in vivo*. J. Pharmacol. exp. Ther. **120**, 488—503 (1957).

KOELLE, G. B.: Handbuch der experimentellen Pharmakologie, Ergänzungswerk, XV. In: KOELLE, G. B. (Ed.): Cholinesterases and anticholinesterase agents. Berlin-Göttingen-Heidelberg: Springer 1963a.

KOELLE, G. B.: Cytological distributions and physiological functions of cholinesterase. In: KOELLE, G. B. (Ed.): Handbuch der experimentellen Pharmakologie, Ergänzungswerk, XV, pp. 187—298, Cholinesterases and Anticholinesterase Agents. Berlin-Göttingen-Heidelberg: Springer 1963 b.

KOELLE, G. B.: Current concepts of synaptic structure and function. Ann. N.Y. Acad. Sci. **183**, 5—25 (1971).

KOELLE, G. B., DAVIS, R., DEVLIN, M.: Acetyl disulfide, $(CH_3COS)_2$, and *bis*-(thioacetoxy) aurate (I) complex, $Au(CH_3COS)_2$, histochemical substrates of unusual properties with acetylcholinesterase. J. Histochem. Cytochem. **16**, 754—764 (1968).

KOELLE, G. B., DAVIS, R., GROMADZKI, C. G.: Electron microscopic localisation of cholinesterases by means of gold salts. Ann. N.Y. Acad. Sci. **144**, 613—625 (1967).

KOELLE, G. B., FRIEDENWALD, J. S.: A histochemical method for localizing cholinesterase activity. Proc. Soc. exp. Biol. (N.Y.) **70**, 617—622 (1949).

KOELLE, G. B., GILMAN, A.: Anticholinesterase drugs. Pharmacol. Rev. **1**, 166—216 (1949).

KOELLE, G. B., STEINER, E. C.: The cerebral distributions of a tertiary and a quaternary anticholinesterase agent following intravenous and intraventricular injection. J. Pharmacol. exp. Ther. **118**, 420—434 (1956).

KORDAS, M.: A study of the end-plate potential in sodium deficient solution. J. Physiol. (Lond.) **198**, 81—90 (1968).

KOSTER, R.: Synergisms and antagonisms between physostigmine and di-isopropyl fluorophosphate in cats. J. Pharmacol. exp. Ther. **88**, 39—46 (1946).

KRAUPP, O., STUMPF, CH., HERZFELD, E., PILLAT, B.: Pharmakologische Eigenschaften einiger langwirksamer Cholinesterase-Hemmkörper aus der Reihe der Polymethylen-*Bis*-(Carbaminoyl-m-Trimethylammoniumphenole). Arch. int. Pharmacodyn. **102**, 281—303 (1955).

KRNJEVIĆ, K., MILEDI, R.: Failure of neuromuscular propagation in rats. J. Physiol. (Lond.) **140**, 440—461 (1958).

KRNJEVIĆ, K., MITCHELL, J. F.: The release of acetylcholine in the isolated rat diaphragm. J. Physiol. (Lond.) **155**, 246—262 (1961).

KUBA, K., TOMITA, T.: Effect of prostigmine on the time course of the end-plate potential in the rat diaphragm. J. Physiol. (Lond.) **213**, 533—544 (1971).

KUFFLER, S. W.: Incomplete neuromuscular transmission in twitch system of frog's skeletal muscles. Fed. Proc. **11**, 87 (1952).

KUFFLER, S. W., VAUGHAN WILLIAMS, E. M.: Small nerve junctional potentials. The distribution of small motor nerves to frog skeletal muscle, and the membrane characteristics of the fibres they innervate. J. Physiol. (Lond.) **121**, 289—317 (1953 a).

KUFFLER, S. W., VAUGHAN WILLIAMS, E. M.: Properties of the slow skeletal muscle fibres of the frog. J. Physiol. (Lond.) **121**, 318—340 (1953 b).

KUPERMAN, A. S., GILL, E. W., RIKER, W. F., JR.: The relationship between cholinesterase inhibition and drug induced facilitation of mammalian neuromuscular transmission. J. Pharmacol. exp. Ther. **132**, 65—73 (1961).

KUPERMAN, A. S., OKAMOTO, M.: The relationship between anti-curare activity and time course of the end-plate potential; a structure-activity approach. Brit. J. Pharmacol. **23**, 575—591 (1964).

KUPFER, C., KOELLE, G. B.: A histochemical study of cholinesterase during the formation of the motor end-plate of the albino rat. Journal of Experimental Zoology **116**, 397—413 (1951).

LAMBERT, E. H., ELMQVIST, D.: Quantal components of end-plate potentials in the myasthenic syndrome. Ann. N.Y. Acad. Sci. **183**, 183—199 (1971).

LANCASTER, R.: Inhibition of acetylcholinesterase in the brain and diaphragm of rats by a tertiary organophosphorus anticholinesterase and its quaternary analogue; *in vivo* and *in vitro* studies. J. Neurochem. **19**, 2587—2597 (1972).

LANCASTER, R.: Relationships between *in vivo* and *in vitro* inhibition of acetylcholinesterase (AChE) and impairment of neuromuscular transmission in the rat phrenic-nerve diaphragm by a tertiary anticholinesterase and its quaternary analogue. Biochem. Pharmacol. **22**, 1875—1881 (1973).

LANDS, A. M., HOPPE, J. O., ARNOLD, A., KIRCHNER, F. K.: An investigation of the structure-activity correlations within a series of ambenonium analogs. J. Pharmacol. exp. Ther. **123**, 121—127 (1958).

Liley,A. W.: An investigation of spontaneous activity at the neuromuscular junction of the rat. J. Physiol. (Lond.) **132**, 650—656 (1956a).

Liley,A. W.: The effects of presynaptic polarization on the spontaneous activity at the mammalian neuromuscular junction. J. Physiol. (Lond.) **134**, 427—443 (1956b).

Lilleheil,G., Naess,K.: A presynaptic effect of D-tubocurarine in the neuromuscular junction. Acta physiol. scand. **52**, 120—136 (1961).

Litwiller,R. W.: Succinylcholine hydrolysis: a review. Anaesthesiology **31**, 356—360 (1969).

Lloyd,D. P. C.: Stimulation of peripheral nerve terminations by active muscle. J. Neurophysiol. **5**, 153—165 (1942).

Long,J. P.: Structure-activity relationships of the reversible anticholinesterase agents. In: Koelle,G. B. (Ed.): Handbuch der experimentellen Pharmakologie, Ergänzungswerk, XV, pp. 374—427. Cholinesterases and Anticholinesterase Agents. Berlin-Göttingen-Heidelberg: Springer 1963.

Lowndes,H., Johnson,D. D.: The effect of lidocaine on twitch potentiation and repetitive neural activity produced by soman and neostigmine. Canad. Physiol. Pharmac. **49**, 464—468 (1971).

Maanen,F. F. van: Effectiveness of anticurarizing agents at different frequencies of stimulation. Fed. Proc. **11**, 398—399 (1952).

Machne,X., Unna,R. W.: Actions on the central nervous system. In: Koelle,G. B. (Ed.): Handbuch der experimentellen Pharmakologie, Ergänzungswerk, XV, pp. 679—700. Cholinesterases and Anticholinesterase Agents. Berlin-Göttingen-Heidelberg: Springer 1963.

MacFarlane,D. W., Pelikán,E. W., Unna,K. R.: Evaluation of curarizing drugs in man. V. Antagonism to curarizing effects of D-tubocurarine by neostigmine, m-hydroxy phenyltrimethylammonium and m-hydroxy phenylethyldimethylammonium. J. Pharmacol. exp. Ther. **100**, 382—392 (1950).

MacIntosh,F. C.: Biological estimation of acetylcholine. In: Gerard,R. W. (Ed.): Methods in medical research, Vol. 3, pp. 78—92. Chicago: The Year Book Publ. 1950.

MacLagan,J.: A comparison of the responses of the tenuissimus muscle to neuromuscular blocking drugs *in vivo* and *in vitro*. Brit. J. Pharmacol. **18**, 204—216 (1962).

Marney,A., Nachmansohn,D.: Choline esterase in voluntary muscle. J. Physiol. (Lond.) **92**, 37—47 (1938).

Martin,A. R.: A further study of the statistical composition of the end-plate potential. J. Physiol. (Lond.) **130**, 114—122 (1955).

Martin,A. R.: Quantal nature of synaptic transmission. Physiol. Rev. **46**, 51—66 (1966).

Masland,R. L., Wigton,R. S.: Nerve activity accompanying fasciculation produced by prostigmin. J. Neurophysiol. **3**, 269—275 (1940).

McIsaac,R. J., Koelle,G. B.: Comparison of the effects of inhibition of external, internal, and total acetylcholinesterase upon ganglionic transmission. J. Pharmacol. exp. Ther. **126**, 9—20 (1959).

McPhillips,J. J.: Altered sensitivity to drugs following repeated injections of a cholinesterase inhibitor to rats. Toxicol. appl. Pharmacol. **14**, 67—73 (1969).

McPhillips,J. J., Coon,J. M.: Adaptation to octamethyl pyrophosphoramide in rats. Toxicol. appl. Pharmacol. **8**, 66—76 (1966).

Meer,C. van der, Meeter,E.: The mechanism of action of anticholinesterases. II. The effect of di*iso*propylfluorophosphonate (DFP) on the isolated rat phrenic nerve-diaphragm preparation. A. Irreversible effects. Acta physiol. pharmacol. neerl. **4**, 454—471 (1956).

Meer,C. van der, Wolthuis,O. L.: The effect of oximes on isolated organs intoxicated with organophosphorus anticholinesterases. Biochem. Pharmacol. **14**, 1299—1312 (1965).

Meeter,E.: The relation between end-plate depolarization and the repetitive response elicited in the isolated rat phrenic nerve-diaphragm preparation by DFP. J. Physiol. (Lond.) **144**, 38—51 (1958).

Miledi,R., Potter,L. T.: Acetylcholine receptors in muscle fibres. Nature (Lond.) **233**, 599—603 (1971).

Mittag,T. W., Ehrenpreis,S., Hehir,R. M.: Functional acetylcholinesterase of rat diaphragm muscle. Biochem. Pharmacol. **20**, 2263—2273 (1971).

Modell,W., Krop,S., Hitchcock,P., Riker,W. F., Jr.: General systemic actions of di*iso*propyl fluorophosphate (DFP) in cats. J. Pharmacol. exp. Ther. **87**, 400—413 (1946).

MOUNTER, L. A.: Metabolism of organophosphorus anticholinesterases. In: KOELLE, G. B. (Ed.): Handbuch der experimentellen Pharmakologie, Ergänzungswerk, XV, pp. 486—504. Cholinesterases and Anticholinesterase Agents. Berlin-Göttingen-Heidelberg: Springer 1963.

NAMBA, T., GROB, D.: Cholinesterase activity of the motor endplate in isolated muscle membrane, J. Neurochem. **15**, 1445—1454 (1968).

NASTUK, W. L., ALEXANDER, J. T.: The action of 3-hydroxyphenyldimethylethylammonium (Tensilon) on neuromuscular transmission in the frog. J. Pharmacol. exp. Ther. **111**, 302—328 (1954).

NEITLICH, H. W.: Increased plasma cholinesterase activity and succinylcholine resistance: a genetic variant. J. clin. Invest. **45**, 380—387 (1966).

O'BRIEN, R. D.: Toxic phosphorus esters. New York: Academic Press 1960.

O'BRIEN, R. D.: The reaction of carbamates with acetylcholinesterase. In: HEILBRONN, E. (Ed.): Structure and reactions of DFP sensitive enzymes, pp. 113—123. Stockholm: Research Institute of National Defence 1967.

OGSTON, A. G.: Removal of acetylcholine from a limited volume by diffusion. J. Physiol. (Lond.) **128**, 222—223 (1955).

OSSERMAN, K. E., GENKINS, G.: Critical reappraisal of the use of edrophonium (tensilon) chloride tests in myasthenia gravis and significance of clinical classification. Ann. N.Y. Acad. Sci. **135**, 312—326 (1966).

OSSERMAN, K. E., KAPLAN, L. I.: Studies in myasthenia gravis. Use of edrophonium chloride (tensilon) in differentiating myasthenic from cholinergic weakness. Arch. Neurol. Psychiat. (Chic.) **70**, 385—392 (1953).

PAL, J.: Physostigmin, ein Gegengift des Curare. Zbl. Physiol. **14**, 255—258 (1900).

PARKES, M. W., SACRA, P.: Protection against the toxicity of cholinesterase inhibitors by acetylcholine antagonists. Brit. J. Pharmacol. **9**, 299—305 (1954).

PECK, A. W.: Relative importance of the enzymic hydrolysis of suxamethonium in plasma and tissues: studies on rhesus monkeys. Brit. J. Pharmacol. **45**, 64—70 (1972).

POLAK, R. L., MEEUWS, M. M.: The influence of atropine on the release and uptake of acetylcholine by the isolated cerebral cortex of the rat. Biochem. Pharmacol. **15**, 989—992 (1966).

POTTER, L. T.: Synthesis, storage and release of [^{14}C] acetylcholine in isolated rat diaphragm muscles. J. Physiol. (Lond.) **206**, 145—166 (1970).

PREUSSER, H. J.: Die Ultrastruktur der motorischen Endplatte im Zwerchfell der Ratte und Veränderungen nach Inhibierung der Acetylcholinesterase. Z. Zellforsch. **80**, 436—457 (1967).

QUINBY, G. E., DOORNINK, G. M.: Tetraethyl pyrophosphate poisoning following airplane dusting. J. Amer. med. Ass. **191**, 1—6 (1965).

RANDALL, L. O.: Anticurare action of phenolic quaternary ammonium salts. J. Pharmacol. exp. Ther. **100**, 83—93 (1950).

RANDALL, L. O., LEHMANN, G.: Pharmacological properties of some neostigmine analogs. J. Pharmacol. exp. Ther. **99**, 16—32 (1950).

RANDIĆ, M., STRAUGHAN, D. W.: Antidromic activity in the rat phrenic nerve-diaphragm preparation. J. Physiol. (Lond.) **173**, 130—148 (1964).

RAVENTOS, J.: The effects of arterial injections of drugs on the frog's gastrocnemius. J. Physiol. (Lond.) **90**, 8 P—9 P (1937).

REINER, E., ALDRIDGE, W. N.: Effect of pH on inhibition and spontaneous reactivation of acetylcholinesterase treated with esters of phosphorus acids and of carbamic acids. Biochem. J. **105**, 171—179 (1967).

REMEN, L.: Zur Pathogenese und Therapie der Myasthenia gravis pseudo paralytica. Dtsch. Z. Nervenheilk. **128**, 66—78 (1932).

RIDER, J. A., ELLINWOOD, L. E., COON, J. M.: Production of tolerance in the rat to octamethyl pyrophosphoramide (OMPA). Proc. Soc. exp. Biol. (N.Y.) **81**, 455—459 (1952).

RIKER, W. F., JR.: Actions of acetylcholine on mammalian motor nerve terminals. J. Pharmacol. exp. Ther. **152**, 397—416 (1966).

RIKER, W. F., JR., OKAMOTO, M.: Pharmacology of motor nerve terminals. Ann. Rev. Pharmacol. **9**, 173—208 (1969).

RIKER, W. F., JR., ROBERTS, J., STANDAERT, F. G., FUJIMORI, H.: The motor nerve terminal as the primary focus for drug-induced facilitation of neuromuscular transmission. J. Pharmacol. exp. Ther. **121**, 286—312 (1957).

RIKER, W. F., JR., WERNER, G., ROBERTS, J., KUPERMAN, A.: Pharmacologic evidence for the existence of a presynaptic event in neuromuscular transmission. J. Pharmacol. exp. Ther. **125**, 150—158 (1959a).

RIKER, W. F., JR., WERNER, G., ROBERTS, J., KUPERMAN, A.: The presynaptic element in neuromuscular transmission. Ann. N.Y. Acad. Sci. **81**, 328—344 (1959b).

RIKER, W. F., JR., WESCOE, W. C.: The direct action of prostigmine on skeletal muscle; its relationship to the choline esters. J. Pharmacol. exp. Ther. **88**, 58—66 (1946).

RIKER, W. F., JR., WESCOE, W. C., BROTHERS, M. J.: Studies on the interrelationships of certain cholinergic compounds. II. The effects of 3-acetoxy phenyltrimethylammonium methylsulphate on neuromuscular transmission. J. Pharmacol. exp. Ther. **97**, 208—221 (1949).

ROBERTS, D. V., THESLEFF, S.: Acetylcholine release from motor-nerve endings in rats treated with neostigmine. Europ. J. Pharmacol. **6**, 281—285 (1969).

ROBERTS, D. V., WILSON, A.: The toxicity of pesticides to man. In: KHAN, M. A., HAUFE, W. O. (Eds.): Toxicology, Biodegradation and Efficacy of Livestock Pesticides, pp. 182—201. Amsterdam: Swets & Zeitlinger 1972.

ROTHBERGER, J. C.: Über die gegenseitigen Beziehungen zwischen Curare und Physostigmin. Pflügers Arch. ges. Physiol. **87**, 117—169 (1901).

SALPETER, M. M.: Electron microscope radioautography as a quantitative tool in enzyme cytochemistry. I. The distribution of acetylcholinesterase at motor endplates of a vertebrate twitch muscle. J. Cell Biol. **32**, 379—389 (1967).

SALPETER, M. M.: Electron microscope radioautography as a quantitative tool in enzyme cytochemistry. II. The distribution of DFP-reactive sites at motor endplates of a vertebrate twitch muscle. J. Cell Biol. **42**, 122—134 (1969).

SCHAUMANN, W.: Über den Einfluß von Atropin auf die zentrale Hemmung der Atmung durch Anticholinesterasen. Naunyn-Schmiedebergs Arch. exp. Path. Pharmak. **236**, 415—420 (1959).

SCHAUMANN, W.: Beziehungen zwischen den peripheren und zentralen Wirkungen von Cholinesterase-Hemmern und der Inaktivierung der Cholinesterase. Naunyn-Schmiedebergs Arch. exp. Path. Pharmak. **239**, 96—113 (1960).

SCHAUMANN, W., JOB, C.: Differential effects of a quaternary cholinesterase inhibitor, phospholine, and its tertiary analogue, compound 217-AO, on central control of respiration and on neuromuscular transmission. The antagonism by 217-AO of the respiratory arrest caused by morphine. J. Pharmacol. exp. Ther. **123**, 114—120 (1958).

SCHUBERTH, J., SUNDWALL, A.: Effects of some drugs on the uptake of acetylcholine in cortex slices of mouse brain. J. Neurochem. **14**, 807—812 (1967).

SMITH, C. M., COHEN, H. L., PELIKAN, E. W., UNNA, K. R.: Mode of action of antagonists to curare. J. Pharmacol. exp. Ther. **105**, 391—399 (1952).

STANDAERT, F. G.: Effect of pH on twitch facilitating potency of 3-hydroxyphenyltriethylammonium ion. Proc. Soc. exp. Biol. (N.Y.) **102**, 138—139 (1959).

STANDAERT, F. G.: Post tetanic repetitive activity in cat soleus nerve. Its origin, cause and mechanism of generation. J. gen. Physiol. **47**, 53—70 (1963).

STANDAERT, F. G.: The mechanism of post tetanic potentiation in cat soleus and gastrocnemius muscles. J. gen. Physiol. **47**, 987—1001 (1964).

STEDMAN, E.: XCIV. Studies on the relationship between chemical constitution and physiologic action. Part I. Position isomerism in relation to the miotic activity of some synthetic urethanes. Biochem. J. **20**, 719—734 (1926).

STEDMAN, E., BARGER, G.: Physostigmine. (Eserine); part III. J. chem. Soc. **127**, 247—258 (1925).

THESLEFF, S.: Acetylcholine utilization in myasthenia gravis. Ann. N.Y. Acad. Sci. **135**, 195—208 (1966).

THESLEFF, S., QUASTEL, D. M. J.: Neuromuscular pharmacology. Ann. Rev. Pharmacol. **5**, 263—284 (1965).

TIEGS, O. W.: Innervation of voluntary muscle. Physiol. Rev. **33**, 90—144 (1953).

TOIVONEN, T., OHELA, K., KAIPAINEU, W. J.: Parathion poisoning in Finland. Lancet **1**, 168 (1965).

VANDEKAR, M., HEATH, D. F.: The reactivation of cholinesterase after inhibition in vivo by some dimethyl phosphate esters. Biochem. J. **67**, 202—208 (1957).

WALKER, M. B.: Treatment of myasthenia gravis with physostigmine. Lancet **1934 I**, 1200—1201.

WALKER, M. B.: Case showing the effect of prostigmine on myasthenia gravis. Proc. roy. Soc. Med. **28**, 759—761 (1935).

WALTHER, H.: Zur Abhängigkeit der Wirkung von Neostigmin, Nivalin und Paraoxon von der Reizfrequenz. Acta biol. med. germ. **22**, 767—778 (1969).

WASER, P. G., RELLER, J.: Bestimmung der Zahl aktiver Zentren der Acetylcholinesterase in motorischen Endplatten. Experientia (Basel) **21**, 402—403 (1965).

WERNER, G.: Neuromuscular facilitation and antidromic discharges in motor nerves: their relation to activity in motor nerve terminals. J. Neurophysiol. **23**, 171—187 (1960a).

WERNER, G.: Generation of antidromic activity in motor nerves. J. Neurophysiol. **23**, 453—461 (1960b).

WERNER, G.: Antidromic activity in motor nerves and its relation to a generator event in nerve terminals. J. Neurophysiol. **24**, 401—416 (1961).

WERNER, G., KUPERMAN, A. S.: Actions on the neuromuscular junction. In: KOELLE, G. B. (Ed.): Handbuch der experimentellen Pharmakologie, Ergänzungswerk, XV, pp. 570—678. Cholinesterases and Anticholinesterase Agents. Berlin-Göttingen-Heidelberg: Springer 1963.

WESCOE, W. C., RIKER, W. F., JR.: The pharmacology of anti-curare agents. Ann. N.Y. Acad. Sci. **54**, 438—455 (1951).

WESCOE, W. C., RIKER, W. F., JR., BROTHERS, M. J.: Studies on the interrelationship of certain cholinergic compounds. I. The pharmacology of 3-acetoxy phenyltrimethylammonium methylsulphate. J. Pharmacol. exp. Ther. **97**, 190—207 (1949).

WESTERBERG, M. R., MAGEE, K. R., SHIDEMAN, F. E.: Effect of 3-hydroxyphenyldimethylethylammonium chloride (Tensilon) in myasthenia gravis. Univ. Mich. med. Bull. **17**, 311—316 (1951).

WHITE, A. C., STEDMAN, E.: On the physostigmine-like action of certain synthetic urethanes. J. Pharmacol. exp. Ther. **41**, 259—288 (1931).

WHITTAKER, V. P.: The application of subcellular fractionation techniques to the study of brain function. Progr. Biophys. **15**, 39—96 (1965).

WHITTAKER, V. P.: Origin and function of synaptic vesicles. Ann N.Y. Acad. Sci. **183**, 21—32 (1966).

WHITTAKER, V. P., WIJESUNDERA, S.: The hydrolysis of succinyldicholine by cholinesterase. Biochem. J. **51**, 475—479 (1952).

WILLS, J. H.: Pharmacological antagonists of the anticholinesterase agents. In: KOELLE, G. B. (Ed.): Handbuch der experimentellen Pharmakologie, Ergänzungswerk, XV, pp. 883—920. Cholinesterases and Anticholinesterase Agents. Berlin-Göttingen-Heidelberg: Springer 1963.

WILLS, J. H., KUNKEL, A. M., O'LEARY, J. F., OIKEMUS, A. H.: Effect of 2-PAM on neuromuscular blockade induced by certain chemicals. Proc. Soc. exp. Biol. (N.Y.) **101**, 196—197 (1959).

WILSON, I. B.: The interaction of tensilon and neostigmine with acetylcholinesterase. Arch. int. Pharmacodyn. **104**, 204—213 (1955).

WILSON, I. B., HARRISON, M. A., GINSBURG, S.: Carbamylderivatives of acetylcholinesterase. J. biol. Chem. **236**, 1498—1500 (1961).

WILSON, I. B., QUAN, C.: Acetylcholinesterase studies on molecular complimentariness. Arch. Biochem. **73**, 131—143 (1958).

WISLICKI, L.: Differences in the effect of oximes on striated muscle and respiratory centre. Arch. int. Pharmacodyn. **129**, 1—17 (1960).

WOLFE, H. R., DURHAM, W. F., ARMSTRONG, J. F.: Exposure of workers to pesticides. Arch. environm. Hlth **14**, 622—633 (1967).

WRIGHT, D. L., PLUMMER, D. T.: Multiple forms of acetylcholinesterase from human erythrocytes. Biochem. J. **133**, 521—527 (1973).

CHAPTER 5A

The Clinician Looks at Neuromuscular Blocking Drugs

R. D. DRIPPS

A. Introduction

Use of neuromuscular blocking drugs by physicians is alleged to have begun more than 160 years ago when WILLIAM SOULE and Sir BENJAMIN COLLINS BRODIE recommended "curare" for the treatment of tetanus and hydrophobia in 1812. Scattered reports of its administration for chorea, epilepsy, tetanus and strychnine poisoning appeared in the French medical literature of the 1850's. In the twentieth century, WEST in 1932, and BURMAN six years later wrote of management of spastic states with "curare". The introduction of pentamethylenetetrazol (Metrazol) and electric shock for the therapy of mental depression was accompanied by the disturbing occurrence of fractures and dislocations resulting from the massive contraction of skeletal muscles. It was natural to attempt to minimize this undesirable muscular reaction through the use of a neuromuscular blocking drug. Such a goal apparently led A. E. BENNETT to seek supplies of crude South American curare from RICHARD GILL in the late 1930's and to urge the manufacturing chemists, E. R. SQUIBB and SONS, to purify the crude material (see BENNETT, 1968). This, despite the fact that in England, HAROLD KING had isolated D-tubocurarine from so-called tube curare in 1935.

BENNETT became deeply involved in mental health institutional work during the course of which he observed that pelvic examination of disturbed female psychotic patients was made easier after the relaxation provided by curare. With great foresight he suggested to Dr. LEWIS H. WRIGHT of Squibb and Sons that the substance might be valuable for the production of muscular relaxation during general anaesthesia. Wright in turn discussed the matter with HAROLD R. GRIFFITH, an anaesthesiologist in Montreal. It was GRIFFITH, so far as I know, who in 1942, first described in a two and a half page report the apparent value of adding curare to cyclopropane "occasionally, as a means of providing the surgeon with excellent relaxation at critical times during certain operations". A mere twenty-five patients were included in the initial publication. Since 1942 thousands of papers have been published about neuromuscular blocking drugs and millions of individuals have been given one or more of these substances.

What are the reasons for the popularity of this class of compounds, what price has been paid for their use and what is their future?

From the clinical introduction of general anaesthesia in the mid-nineteenth century until three decades into the twentieth century, progress in the field was slow. Nitrous oxide, chloroform (for a time) and ether were the chief drugs used. Cyclopropane, used first by clinicians in the 1930's, provided certain advantages, but the introduction of short-acting barbiturates such as thiopentone and within a few years, the advent of muscle relaxants revolutionized the practice of general anaesthesia.

This is clearly revealed in remarks made by ECKENHOFF in 1959 for a Symposium on Muscle Relaxants. He wrote, "The introduction of muscle relaxants into clinical anaesthesiology has been one of the most significant advances made in the specialty". Because of these drugs, concepts of anaesthesia have changed so that in many areas today's anaesthetic techniques bear little resemblance to those of a short generation ago. Most anaesthesiologists who have begun practice in the past decade have little comprehension of the anaesthetic routine prior to the advent of the muscle relaxants. Then a rapid, smooth induction of anaesthesia and the maintenance of a steady state adequate for the surgical procedure was a work of art, accomplished regularly by relatively few. This ability was obtained only after years of diligent practice. No longer is this true. Unconsciousness can now be produced rapidly by the intravenous injection of barbiturates, and profound muscular relaxation is provided shortly thereafter.

B. General Anaesthesia before Neuromuscular Blocking Drugs

Muscular relaxation of varying degrees is needed in many surgical procedures. In abdominal surgery while approaching the duodenum during gastric resection for example, profound relaxation is expected, indeed, often required by the surgeon. When performing a pelvic examination prior to intra-abdominal gynaecological procedures, a lesser, but nonetheless, definite degree of relaxation is useful. Relaxation of the jaw muscles assists intubation of the trachea and the reduction of a dislocated shoulder can be facilitated by the use of a muscle relaxant. Prior to the introduction of neuromuscular blocking drugs, all of this was achieved by varying depths of inhalational anaesthesia. Diethylether, or ether as it is commonly known, was the drug most frequently used to produce conditions requested by the surgeon. Before respiratory acidosis secondary to inadequate ventilation was recognized as a sequel of general anaesthesia, ether was thought to permit rather marked muscular relaxation while spontaneous breathing was supposedly maintained by several reflex and direct forces driving the respiratory centre.

We now know that respiration was often not optimal, but it sufficed for at least two reasons; first, the tendency of surgeons to operate upon generally healthy persons and avoid those desperately ill, and secondly the fact that man can withstand considerable insult before succumbing. Penalties were paid, of course. In addition to respiratory inadequacy, hypotension occurred during anaesthesia in approximately direct relationship with its depth. Post-operative complications such as nausea, vomiting, drenching perspiration and metabolic acidosis also bore an almost linear relationship with the depth of anaesthesia. Understandably recovery from anaesthesia was often slow. It is humbling to recall that patients survive in spite of rather than because of the health professions on occasion.

With the advent of cyclopropane in the 1930's, anaesthetists came to recognize that abdominal muscular activity could only be reduced with safety and a state of quiet produced within the peritoneal cavity if respiration was controlled by intermittent manual compression of the breathing bag of the anaesthetic machine. The actual lessening of muscular tension did not appear as great as that achieved with ether, but this was difficult to measure. Most agreed, at least, that if spontaneous breathing was permitted during the administration of cyclopropane, particularly if opioids were given for premedication, both inadequate muscular relaxation and inadequate respiration would result. Cyclopropane also appeared to have the advantage of causing less hypotension than ether, largely due to the mobilization of adrenaline in the dog and of noradrenaline in man. The value of cyclopropane was diminished in some people's eyes, however, by the observation that abnormalities of ventricular rhythm were more likely with deeper planes of anaesthesia.

Certain surgeons and anaesthetists, albeit not a large number, discouraged by the problems of general anaesthesia, resorted to spinal anaesthesia, which could provide marked flaccidity in those muscles whose nerve supply was interrupted by the local anaesthetic. The technique, however, never achieved world-wide popularity for intra-abdominal operations, although it was espoused by a few clinics in the United States. The occurrence during surgery of hypotension, often made worse by hypovolaemia, the distress caused to the patient by remaining awake while the abdominal cavity was being explored, the post-anaesthetic development of headache attributable to lumbar puncture and an unreasonable fear by clinicians of permanent neurologic sequelae, all contributed to the unpopularity of the technique.

This was the situation when the paper of GRIFFITH and JOHNSON appeared in 1942 with its limited, almost hesitant suggestions.

C. Clinical Influence of Neuromuscular Blocking Drugs

Probably the greatest contribution of neuromuscular blocking drugs is in surgery, where the desired degree of muscular relaxation can be achieved without administering a dangerously high concentration of a general anaesthetic. Hypotension during surgery is reduced and the comfort of the patient is increased post-operatively since the deeper the anaesthesia the more troublesome is the hangover represented by such sequelae as nausea, vomiting, headache, perspiration and fluid loss. There is an analogy between the consequences of a considerable uptake of anaesthetic and those of excessive intake of alcohol.

The use of neuromuscular blocking drugs during surgery, however, deprives the anaesthetist of many signs traditionally relied upon to determine the depth of anaesthesia. Ocular movement, change in respiratory tidal volume, tightness of the jaw, and the ability to phonate, swallow, move or close the glottis are lost completely or in part in the general paralysis produced by neuromuscular blocking drugs. Fortunately, certain subtle signs indicate response to pain. These arise largely from the autonomic nervous system and include increase in arterial pressure and the development of tachycardia, pupillary dilation, salivation and sweating. In addition, emergence from anaesthesia and the loss of satisfactory muscle relaxation are often heralded by wrinkling of the brow, pursing of the lips and the appearance of other fine muscle movements. Finally, attempts at spontaneous respiration, the occurrence of bronchospasm, weak coughing and other changes in thoracic compliance can be sensed by the anaesthetist as an altered response to manual compression of the breathing bag.

As might have been predicted, the depth of anaesthesia can be so minimal in the presence of profound muscle paralysis that awareness of surroundings remains and recollection is evident. Surprisingly this has not proved common, nor when it does occur does it seem to disturb the patient, who often recalls incidents during his operation without apparent detrimental psychological reaction. This has not yet been satisfactorily explained, for a direct central nervous system action of the neuromuscular blocking drugs seems minimal. In this connection, one thinks of the lassitude and general feeling of ease which attends voluntary reduction in skeletal muscle tone, as though afferent impulses from muscles serve to maintain increased "activity" or alertness of the central nervous system.

Muscular relaxation produced by neuromuscular blocking drugs almost at once became a substitute for adequately conducted general anaesthesia (CULLEN, 1944). Anaesthetists no longer thought it necessary to learn how to use general anaesthetics to prevent and treat laryngospasm, provide relaxation prior to intubation of the trachea, or to facilitate intra-abdominal operations. "Curare" was relied upon to mask one's inaptitude. Intravenous administration of the blocking drug frequently took the place of mastery of the art of general, primarily inhalational anaesthesia. Perhaps the yearning on the part of critics of this aspect of the neuromuscular blocking drugs for the skills which they had had to develop slowly and painfully reflected the belief that things had become too easy. However there was a good deal of truth in the allegation that short cuts were being accepted and fundamentals neglected.

Prior to the use of relaxants, it was almost taken for granted that patients would be breathing spontaneously at the end of an operation. The chief exception to this was when one administered cyclopropane using controlled respiration. With the advent of the neuromuscular blocking drugs, and particularly as the doses administered increased, inadequate breathing or apnoea became more frequent. There seemed to be national differences here, with British anaesthetists, perhaps because they relied upon reversing tubocurarine action with neostigmine more often than did their U.S. counterparts, reporting respiratory problems less often. Indeed, almost a decade passed before reversal became an accepted part of anaesthetic management when tubocurarine was used in the United States. Thus, inadequate respiration postoperatively after tubocurarine tended to be reported initially more frequently in the U.S.A.

After the depolarizing drug decamethonium was introduced by PATON and ZAIMIS in 1948, the incidence of prolonged post-anaesthetic apnoea in certain series was alarming (DRIPPS, 1953). Pharmacologists were concerned about the wisdom of using depolarizing drugs in man, fearing that in some instances permanent or long-term depolarization might occur. Time has shown this concern to be unjustified, particularly since the use of the short-acting suxamethonium is now widespread. However, while long lasting depolarization did not appear to be a problem, concern was felt about prolonged post-operative respiratory inadequacy following the administration of suxamethonium by continuous intravenous infusion, as dozens of papers attested.

Means of showing whether the action of blocking drugs was continuing into the post-operative period were required. If the patient was sufficiently conscious, grip strength and head raising offered crude indices. For the unconscious individual, one had to await the development of techniques for measuring inspiratory force (BEN-DIXEN et al., 1959) and estimating transmission across the neuromuscular junction. The latter was greatly aided by the introduction of relatively inexpensive battery-powered stimulators such as the Block-Aid Monitor. Supramaximal single shocks and tetanic stimuli of varying frequencies could be delivered through intact skin or subcutaneously over peripheral nerves. One either observed or actually recorded the degree of response to each type of stimulus, noting the degree of block after single shocks and whether tetanus was sustained and post-tetanic facilitation developed following tetanic stimuli. Stimulators were used for a number of years before it was recognized that deterioration of the battery was accompanied by a change in tetanic frequency. In addition there was not always adequate voltage to deliver supramaximal stimuli.

Additional contributions were made to the patient's welfare when fear of arterial puncture in man was lessened, better pH electrodes developed and the CO_2 electrode introduced (SEVERINGHAUS and BRADLEY, 1958). These permitted the measurement of arterial pH and pCO_2, both important in the assessment of respiration and acid-base balance.

Deaths in patients who had received tubocurarine began to be discussed in the late 1940's. In a number of cases the cause was obscure and one could not be sure of the reason why death occurred. This led to the belief, expressed most forcefully by BEECHER and TODD (1954), that tubocurarine possessed an inherent toxicity which no amount of skill in usage could overcome. Surgeons hearing such opinions and failing to understand that the data were not convincing, often over-reacted and in some U.S. clinics the use of tubocurarine was forbidden. The Beecher-Todd contention provoked a good deal of controversy.

What was needed was a scientific, controlled, carefully planned prospective study. There were several obstacles to this. The incidence of fatality was so low that to show a statistically significant difference between operations performed in the presence or absence of tubocurarine required a huge volume of cases. It was also difficult to establish cause and effect and eliminate coincidence in an individual instance because of the large number of almost uncontrollable variables. Animal models were unsatisfactory, due to species differences and to variations in the quality of post-operative care of the animal.

One interesting prospective study was made in 693 patients undergoing upper abdominal operations; approximately half of these were managed with ether and no blocking drug and the remainder with thiopentone, nitrous oxide and suxamethonium (BUNKER et al., 1959). The series was too small for one to be confident that failure to show a difference in mortality contradicted the concept of inherent toxicity proposed by BEECHER and TODD. There were, however, significantly different complications following the two types of anaesthetic management. Ether anaesthesia for upper abdominal procedures offered an increased risk of hypotension in the elderly and women. Light general anaesthesia with suxamethonium for relaxation appeared to involve, in addition to the dangers of hypoventilation during and after operation, an increased incidence of atelectasis. Although inconclusive, the paper laid the ground-work for the more detailed and sophisticated analyses of the 1960's and 70's.

Perhaps the chief obstacle to the early development of reliable data was the fact that clinical investigation had been slow to develop in most countries. The American

Society for Clinical Investigation had relatively few members in the early 1940's, almost none of whom were anaesthetists. Although in much of the British Empire physicians had been entrusted with the administration of anaesthetics instead of technicians, for the most part these clinicans were untrained in the fundamentals of research. Scientific journals related to anaesthesia were virtually non-existent before 1940. The speciality itself was a belated arrival on the medical scene.

As the result of all of this, early papers on curare often reflected clinical impressions or relied upon unsound statistical analyses. Nonetheless, the use of neuromuscular blocking drugs steadily increased as anaesthetists almost instinctively judged their advantages to outweigh any possibilities of harm.

In 1959, I wrote: "the future of the neuromuscular blockers in anesthesia seems assured. It is reasonable to hope that the price for this use will soon be determined. My opinion is that it will almost certainly be sufficiently low to warrant their present widespread use." I see no reason to change this belief 15 years later, but shall attempt to indicate some aspect of the "price" as we understand it today.

With the widespread acceptance of neuromuscular blocking drugs basic and clinical investigation increased rapidly, and the number of drugs available for study became larger (see Chapter 4A and B and Chapter 5B). The quality of studies also improved as technology became more sophisticated and knowledge of fundamental aspects of cell function grew. Today there is a good deal of information about the two broad groups of blocking drugs, non-depolarizing or competitive inhibitors and depolarizing drugs. As knowledge increases, it is likely that it will become less acceptable to describe the substances in these terms, but the classification is still used by many clinicians. Scientific information will be presented by other contributors to this volume. I shall comment primarily upon the clinical importance of some of the more recent findings.

Experience soon suggested and studies confirmed a variety of clinical conditions in which the action of neuromuscular blocking drugs differed from that seen in normal patients. These included the age of the patient, electrolyte abnormalities, change in body temperature, the presence of certain diseases and the concomitant use of other drugs. While the mechanisms involved have not yet been fully explained, much has been learned. In most instances, sensitivity or increased response is observed. Less commonly, resistance seems evident. Nor is the direction of change always the same under a given condition if one uses a depolarizing blocking drug as compared to a competitive neuromuscular blocking drug. Dr. S.E. SMITH (Chapter 5B) will describe the present state of pharmacological knowledge in man of a number of these factors. I shall refer to a few considerations in order to indicate the degree of care required of an anaesthetist attempting to provide optimal patient protection.

The list of entities given above indicates many of the common sense approaches used. Neonates, for example, appear to be very sensitive to those competitive neuromuscular blocking drugs which have been studied, particularly tubocurarine. Sometimes they appear sensitive to suxamethonium also, possibly because of a fall in muscle temperature. Under clinical conditions hypothermia is likely to occur during operation on these little youngsters unless efforts are made to maintain body temperature and temperature is constantly monitored. Since reduction in body temperature depresses respiration *per se* as well as increasing the blocking action of suxamethonium, interpretation of clinical reports is not easy unless a complete description is offered. Nonetheless the influence of temperature upon the action of the neuromuscular blocking drugs is real (see also Chapter 4A).

The anaesthetist should try to elicit a history of muscular weakness from his patient, which might indicate latent myasthenia gravis or the myasthenic syndrome (also called neuromyopathy) associated with such malignancies as oat-cell carcinoma of the bronchus. In myasthenia gravis sensitivity to competitive neuromuscular blocking drugs can occur, while a certain resistance to depolarizing drugs has been noted. In the myasthenic syndrome sensitivity to both groups of muscle relaxants has been reported. A history of drug intake is also important. Some antibiotics, such as colistin, streptomycin, kanamycin and neomycin, interfere with neuromuscular transmission. Other drug interactions may also be relevant.

Laboratory investigations are important, particularly potassium plasma levels. A decrease in extracellular in relation to the intracellular potassium level, a not uncommon clinical finding, potentiates competitive and antagonizes depolarizing neuromuscular blocking drugs. Respiratory and metabolic acidosis produce a picture resembling partial curarization owing to central nervous system depression.

Probably the most common undesirable consequence of neuromuscular blocking drugs is prolonged post-operative apnoea. As CHURCHILL-DAVIDSON and WISE (1960) observed, the onset of spontaneous respiratory activity after a period of controlled respiration is not entirely dependent upon the disappearance of the effect of neuromuscular blockade. Depression of the respiratory centre can be caused by premedication, use of opioids during anaesthesia, and the presence of anaesthetic drugs. Reduction in body temperature can also contribute to respiratory depression. The carbon dioxide level of the blood must not fall too far. The respiratory centre often seems to require afferent stimuli before rhythmic activity is resumed. The stimulus may be provided by movement of an endotracheal tube, deflation of its balloon, or a painful stimulus of some kind.

Nonetheless there is an obvious relationship between the use of neuromuscular blocking drugs and inadequacy of breathing after operation. Overdosage contributes. With suxamethonium a reduction in plasma pseudocholinesterase levels, which may be hereditary, or the result of inanition or hepatic disease increases the drug's effect. Abnormal reactions may also be associated with electrolyte imbalance, drug interaction and diseases other than hepatic.

D. Three Possibly Fatal Reactions to Suxamethonium

1. One reaction to suxamethonium with potentially fatal consequences seems now quite clear, namely, the sudden release of potassium when the blocking drug is given to patients suffering from severe soft tissue trauma, burns, spinal cord injury, tetanus and perhaps uraemia. The mechanism will be outlined in Chapter 4A by ZAIMIS and HEAD and Chapter 5B by S. E. SMITH. Suffice it to say that caution must be exercised or the use of the drug avoided in such cases. It should be recognized that some time must elapse after trauma before an injured individual reacts to suxamethonium with a potentially dangerous liberation of potassium. Prompt recognition of the untoward effects of excess potassium on the heart together with closed-chest or open cardiac massage, will usually permit recovery as one washes the potassium out of the my-

ocardium. The phenomenon thus poses a relatively brief threat and can often, although not always, be reversed.

2. The relationship between suxamethonium and the development of malignant hyperthermia is somewhat less clear. This catastrophe is rare, but ultimately it can be prevented only when its aetiology has been more firmly established. At the moment, because of hereditary factors, one should be careful when administering general anaesthesia and suxamethonium to individuals with a personal or more likely a family history of unexplained high fever developing during anaesthesia. Unfortunately, this is not an easy history to elicit. An anaesthetist seeing such a response should inform patient and family of the potential dangers so that subsequent anaesthetists can be forewarned.

3. Injections of suxamethonium repeated within two to five minutes of one another may be followed by marked bradycardia, particularly in the young age group. Cardiac arrest has been reported although cause-effect has not been convincingly demonstrated. The response, which is prevented by atropine, should be in the mind of the clinician when a second dose of the blocking drug is considered necessary soon after the first, as for example, after failure to intubate the trachea.

E. Less Serious Reactions to Suxamethonium

Muscular pain and stiffness may follow the administration of suxamethonium. A variety of causes have been suggested, though none proven. This phenomenon, while occasionally annoying, obviously offers no threat to life.

Suxamethonium may initiate a rise in intra-ocular tension. Some ophthalmologic surgeons are more concerned about this than others, believing that the increased tension, brief though it is, may compromise the results of certain intra-ocular operations. We have not found this a difficult problem from the practical standpoint.

F. Personal Technique

Having grown up in the pre-relaxant era, I claim a certain justification as an elder citizen, for offering personal observations on clinical use of the neuromuscular blocking drugs. I tend to use moderately large doses of suxamethonium (80 to 100 mg) to assist with tracheal intubation. I believe it preferable not to rely on nitrous oxide as the sole general anaesthetic during maintenance. Perhaps increased amounts of narcotic drugs for premedication, or during maintenance of anaesthesia prevent patient awareness, but this is easily achieved by small amounts of one of the newer volatile liquid anaesthetics such as halothane or enflurane, and this is the approach I favour. If hepatic damage unrelated to dose is eventually attributed to halothane and a greater incidence proven after multiple exposures to this drug, then my position over halothane at least is incorrect.

Because of the considerable individual variation in response to tubocurarine (PELIKAN et al., 1953; KATZ, 1967), I prefer a test dose of 5 mg given intravenously. This procedure is easily performed, can suggest sensitivity, and if properly conducted causes no inconvenience to the patient. A test dose of suxamethonium does not seem worthwhile to me, particularly if one is going to give only a single injection. Since complete blockade of the neuromuscular junction is not essential, the use of a nerve stimulator and monitor seems reasonable. Laziness, I suspect, has worked against the common application of the technique.

I favour the reversal of the effects of competitive neuromuscular blocking drugs almost regardless of the total dose and the time of the last injection. Since the onset of action of atropine (given in order to prevent the muscarinic effects of neostigmine) is more rapid than that of neostigmine, I use a mixture of the two drugs as a matter of convenience. Finally, I am willing to administer the reversal mixture while the patient is apnoeic rather than await the return of some degree of spontaneous breathing. Multiple techniques for the administration of neuromuscular blocking drugs are in use. I record mine to assist readers in interpreting any clinical bias of which I may be unaware.

G. Conclusions

In the first edition of Goodman and Gilman's *The Pharmacological Basis of Therapeutics*, published in 1941, the statement was made that "curare is an important pharmacological tool for laboratory investigations, but as yet it has no well-established therapeutic uses".

Considerable progress has been made since then in the use of neuromuscular blocking drugs. Their clinical usefulness is firmly established and their cost/benefit ratio is favourable in my judgment.

But there remains a long way to go. We need increased knowledge in three areas: the mechanism(s) of action of neuromuscular blocking drugs, the mechanism(s) involved in the reversal of this action, and the mechanism(s) involved when blocking drugs interact with other drugs and when such drugs are given in disease states. Almost certainly this knowledge will not come from clinicians, although they may suggest clues. Answers must await the results of basic research, a cornerstone of advance in therapeutics.

References

BEECHER, H. K., TODD, D. P.: Study of deaths associated with anesthesia and surgery. Ann. Surg. **140**, 2—35 (1954).

BENDIXEN, H. H., SURTEES, A. D., OYAMA, T., BUNKER, J. P.: Postoperative disturbances in ventilation following use of muscle relaxants in anesthesia. Anesthesiology **20**, 121—122 (1959).

BENNETT, A. E.: The history of the introduction of curare into medicine. Curr. Res. Anesth. **47**, 484—492 (1968).

BUNKER, J. P., BENDIXEN, H. H., SYKES, M. K., TODD, D. P., SURTEES, A. D.: A comparison of ether anesthesia with thiopental-nitrous oxide-succinylcholine for upper abdominal surgery. Anesthesiology **20**, 745—752 (1959).

BURMAN, M. S.: Curare therapy for the release of muscle spasm and rigidity in spastic paralysis and dystonia musculorum deformans. J. Bone Jt Surg. **20**, 754—756 (1938).

CHURCHILL-DAVIDSON, H. C., WISE, R. P.: Prevention, diagnosis and treatment of prolonged apnoea. Brit. J. Anaesth. **32**, 384—387 (1960).

CULLEN, S. C.: Clinical and laboratory observations on the use of curare during inhalation anesthesia. Anesthesiology **5**, 166—173 (1944).

DRIPPS, R. D.: Abnormal respiratory responses to various "curare" drugs during surgical anesthesia: Incidence, etiology and treatment. Ann. Surg. **137**, 145—155 (1953).

DRIPPS, R. D.: The role of muscle relaxants in anesthesia deaths. Anesthesiology **4**, 542—545 (1959).

ECKENHOFF, J. E.: A symposium on muscle relaxants. Introduction. Anesthesiology **4**, 407—408 (1959).

GRIFFITH, H. R., JOHNSON, G. E.: The use of curare in general anesthesia. Anesthesiology **3**, 418—420 (1942).

KATZ, R. L.: Neuromuscular effects of D-Tubocurarine, Edrophonium and Neostigmine in man. Anesthesiology **28**, 327—336 (1967).

KING, H.: Curare alkaloids, l. tubocurarine. J. chem. Soc. **59**, 1381—1383 (1935).

PATON, W. D. M., ZAIMIS, E. J.: Clinical potentialities of certain bisquaternary salts causing neuromuscular and ganglionic block. Nature (Lond.) **162**, 810 (1948).

PELIKAN, E. W., TETHER, J. E., UNNA, K. R.: Sensitivity of myasthenia gravis patients to Tubocurarine and Decamethonium. Neurology (Minneap.) **3**, 284—296 (1953).

SEVERINGHAUS, J. W., BRADLEY, A. F.: Electrodes for Blood PO_2 and PCO_2 Determination. J. Appl. Physiol. **13**, 515—520 (1958).

WEST, R.: Curare in man. Proc. roy. Soc. Med. **25**, 1107—1116 (1932).

Neuromuscular Blocking Drugs in Man

S. E. SMITH

A. Introduction

The action of neuromuscular blocking drugs in man has been subject to widespread observation and experimentation ever since their introduction into clinical practice just over thirty years ago. Many of the reports in the extensive literature on the subject are concerned with experience in the use of these drugs in anaesthesia and provide assistance to the practising clinician. In many instances, however, their contribution to our understanding of the pharmacology of neuromuscular blockade is slight. The same is unfortunately also true of some of the research in this field, for much experimental work has been done in the past under conditions which were inadequately controlled, making interpretation of the findings difficult and occasionally invalid. In what follows, therefore, this chapter concentrates largely on results obtained in man by quantitative measurement and attempts to clarify conflicting data which appear in published experiments by special reference to the many pitfalls to research in this field.

The simplistic view of course exists that the clinician's requirements are satisfied by relatively simple investigations in which drug actions are studied under the conditions in which they are normally used. Yet such studies provide clinical impressions which are sometimes false or even misleading. The author has expressed the opinion elsewhere that there is at present a greater need for improved methods for using our existing therapeutic armamentarium than there is for the introduction of new drugs (SMITH and RAWLINS, 1973). Such improvement can follow only the most careful scientific evaluation of drug action. This chapter strikes such an attitude in an attempt to apply the strictest standards in assessing a complex and difficult subject.

B. Measurement of Drug Action

I. Voluntary Muscle Contractions

The methods and conditions used in the measurement of drug-induced neuromuscular blockade are almost as numerous as the investigators engaged in such studies. Early work, reviewed by MUSHIN and MAPLESON (1957), concentrated largely on the influence of drugs on the strength of voluntary muscle contractions, mainly because of the lack of direct methods for the measurement of events at the neuromuscular junction. Other studies dealt with the effects of the drugs on respiration, either spontaneous or forced, probably in the belief long fostered by anaesthetists, and

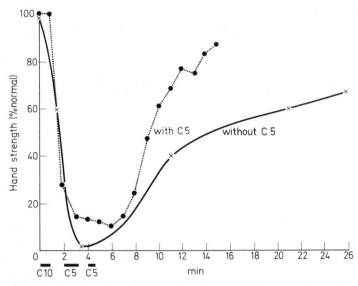

Fig. 1. Effect of decamethonium 3 mg (C 10) on hand strength in a conscious volunteer. Subsequent injection of pentamethonium 30 mg (C 5) causes more rapid recovery of grip strength. (Organe et al., 1949)

referred to by Dripps in his contribution to this volume, that muscle paralysis could be obtained in the anaesthetised patient without impairment of respiration. This belief was as misguided as it was dangerous and one can but regret that measurements of respiratory tidal or minute volume in anaesthetised subjects were ever used as indicators of neuromuscular blockade (Artusio et al., 1951; Zaimis, 1959; Foldes et al., 1963) without artificial ventilation to correct hypoxia and hypercarbia.

A number of authors have used grip strength in conscious volunteers to measure the degree of muscle paralysis produced by neuromuscular blocking drugs. The method was pioneered by Organe et al. (1949) who demonstrated the action of decamethonium and its partial antagonism by pentamethonium (Fig. 1); and also by Mushin et al. (1949) who showed the effect of gallamine and its reversal by neostigmine. Subsequent work has resulted in some elegant dose-response curves for a number of competitive neuromuscular blocking drugs, which are illustrated in Fig. 2 (Bodman, 1952; Lund and Stovner, 1970). The antagonistic action of tetraethylammonium on tubocurarine has been demonstrated using the same technique (Stovner, 1958). In a series of papers, Unna and his colleagues (for references see Unna and Pelikan, 1951) demonstrated that doses of competitive neuromuscular blocking drugs can cause 95% impairment of grip strength while having only slight influence on vital capacity. By contrast the effect of decamethonium on respiration at comparable dose levels was much greater (Table 1). Subsequent studies with tubocurarine and decamethonium on head-lifting, hand grip as well as respiratory muscle power revealed effects which were in keeping with those described by Unna et al. (Johansen et al., 1964; Nielsen and Bennike, 1965; Jørgensen et al., 1966). Unna et al. interpreted their findings as indicating that competitive blocking drugs show selec-

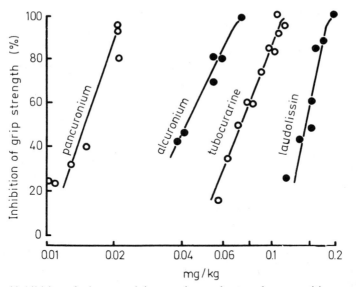

Fig. 2. Maximal inhibition of grip strength in conscious volunteers by competitive neuromuscular blocking drugs. (Data from BODMAN, 1952; LUND and STOVNER, 1970)

Table 1. Effect of neuromuscular blocking drugs on vital capacity in conscious volunteers. In each case the dose is that which reduces grip strength by 95%. (Data from UNNA et al., 1950)

Drug	n	Mean dose (± S.D.) μg/kg	Mean (± S.D.) % reduction in vital capacity
Tubocurarine	28	135 ± 11	31 ± 16
Dimethyltubocurarine	17	57 ± 3	16 ± 12
Gallamine	19	693 ± 46	20 ± 12
Decamethonium	30	32 ± 6	61 ± 2

tivity for limb muscles. Such a conclusion has been criticised (PATON and ZAIMIS, 1950) on the grounds that adrenaline secretion, which is probably considerable in experiments on conscious volunteers, increases the paralysing effects of decamethonium on respiratory muscles so that the actions of depolarising and competitive drugs are not necessarily dissimilar.

The findings in conscious volunteers are therefore not really applicable to subjects under anaesthesia and it is evident that, particularly if respiratory embarrassment is present (POULSEN and HOUGS, 1957), experiments on conscious volunteers do not necessarily provide useful indications of the intensity of action of these drugs in anaesthetised patients. Substance is given to this by the observations of THESLEFF (1952) who showed that in anaesthetised subjects suxamethonium also had much more effect on limb than on respiratory muscles.

In conscious subjects, muscle paralysis produced by competitive neuromuscular blocking drugs is exaggerated, as would be expected, by frequent exercise (FOLDES et

al., 1961) and is more apparent with continuous than intermittent exertion (MOL-
BECH and JOHANSEN, 1969). The latter observation is consistent with the theory that
such drugs influence slow muscle fibres more than fast ones.

II. Direct Measurement of Neuromuscular Transmission in Man

1. General Aspects

The magnitude of drug-induced neuromuscular block is now almost universally
assessed by direct measurements. In the interests of ready accessibility, most measurements are made using the small muscles of the hand, stimulated through their
motor nerves at the wrist or the elbow or in the forearm. The commonest practice is
to stimulate the ulnar nerve and record the response of the adductor pollicis or the
muscles of the hypothenar eminence. Methods suitable for the study of neuromuscular transmission in leg muscles have also been described (CANNARD and ZAIMIS,
1959; ZAIMIS, 1969). Reference to these is made later.

The response of muscle groups to nerve stimulation can be measured in two
ways; first, by recording integrated action potentials of a group of muscle fibres, and
secondly by measuring the muscle tension developed during contraction. It is important to recognise that action potentials and mechanical measurements are not necessarily comparable because they do not measure the same thing. The integrated
action potential provides a measure of the electrical activity in a limited number of
muscle fibres, while the tension measures the contractile response of the whole
muscle. For this reason, the results of electromyographic and mechanical recordings
must be expected to show discrepancies (KATZ, 1973). Failure to appreciate this
point has led to controversy, particularly in the interpretation of quantitative aspects
of blockade.

The introduction of direct measurements has enabled the principal features and
the qualitative aspects of neuromuscular blockade produced by depolarising and
competitive neuromuscular blocking drugs to be recorded readily. It is apparent,
however, that great care is required in the application of these techniques before
reliable and reproducible results can be obtained, particularly if accurate quantitation is required. Some of the possible sources of error are considered below. In
discussing these errors emphasis is placed on the details involved and the suggestion
is made that workers in this field use uniform conditions so that results from different
research centres may be compared meaningfully. To the same end, it is further
suggested that a universal system of descriptive terminology be adopted.

A number of assumptions are also made and conclusions reached which are
derived from animal studies and not from clinical pharmacological investigations at
all. For further details the reader is referred to Chapter 4 A and B.

2. Electrical Stimulation of Motor Nerves and Stimulus Schedules

A motor nerve can be stimulated in man through needle or surface electrodes. The
electrical stimulus applied must be of suitable waveform, duration, intensity and
frequency. For two reasons the pulse duration should be as short as possible, usually
less than 0.2 msec. First, motor nerve fibres are preferentially stimulated under such
conditions (VEALE et al., 1973). Secondly, if the interval is greater than the least

refractory period of the muscle double stimulation or repetitive firing of the muscle fibres results. This is very likely to have occurred in the experiments described by DANN (1971) who used a stimulator providing square-wave pulses of 110 msec duration. Such an extraordinary technique can lead only to erroneous consequences.

The intensity of the stimulus should be such as to produce a maximal response. This can be achieved with certainty by a supramaximal pulse from a stimulator of fairly low output impedance.

The frequency of stimulation and the time relationships of tetanic and single stimuli are critical and must be defined. EPSTEIN and his colleagues (for references see EPSTEIN and EPSTEIN, 1973) apply single stimuli at 5 sec intervals (0.2 Hz) and tetanic stimuli of 30 Hz frequency and 5 sec duration at 5 min intervals. The first post-tetanic single stimulus always follows the last tetanic stimulus after exactly 5 sec. It is not imperative that all investigators should use identical schedules, but closer comparisons between published work would be possible if they did so. In many papers the time intervals, particularly the critical one before the first post-tetanic twitch, are not given and some published illustrations of responses belie the stipulated stimulus frequencies.

Before the administration of a neuromuscular blocking drug, the recordings obtained should be studied carefully to ensure that the responses of the muscle to nerve stimulation are normal. In the absence of a neuromuscular blocking drug the shape and size of action potentials resulting from repeated stimulation should not change with time. In particular this requires that only a light depth of anaesthesia is maintained, that the stimulus is truly supramaximal so that tetanic stimulation cannot lead to recruitment of extra muscle fibres and that there is no movement of the recording electrodes which could subsequently respond to more or different muscle fibres (ZAIMIS, 1969).

Repetitive Responses. In some individuals stimuli of a satisfactory short duration can produce what appear to be repetitive electrical responses of the muscle. EPSTEIN and JACKSON (1970a) by recording muscle contractions and action potentials of the adductor pollicis muscle found that repetitive activity occurred in about one third of their subjects following the application of single stimuli of 0.1 msec duration. Paired stimuli at about 1.2 msec separation suppressed the second response and the tension developed was reduced (Fig. 3). It is unlikely that this is the result of reflex activity, since the repetitive response follows within about 5 msec, whereas the transmission time for nerve impulses via the spinal cord would be approximately 20 msec, given a nerve conduction velocity of about 100 m/sec and synaptic delay of 1 msec.

Similar results have previously been obtained in the cat by BROWN and MATTHEWS (1960). After a thorough analysis of the underlying mechanism BROWN and MATTHEWS concluded that during synchronous nerve stimulation the summed action potentials of the muscle fibres were large enough to re-excite some of the motor nerve fibres. This ephaptically induced "back response" of the nerve fibres (LLOYD, 1942) in turn can re-excite some of the muscle fibres giving rise to a large muscle contraction. As in the human experiments, a second stimulus timed to arrive during the refractory period of the muscle abolishes the back response and reduces the height of the synchronous muscle "twitch" (see Chapter 4 B for a fuller discussion).

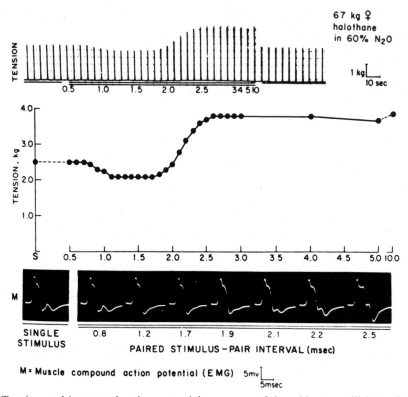

Fig. 3. Tension and integrated action potential responses of the adductor pollicis to single and paired electrical stimulation of the ulnar nerve in an anaesthetised patient. Repetitive muscle firing induced by the single stimulus was suppressed by paired stimulation at 1.2 and 1.7 msec separation. (EPSTEIN and JACKSON, 1970a)

In experimental studies it is preferable to use only individuals who show single responses to twitch stimulation. Such individuals can be identified only by electromyographic recording.

As nerve trunks contain both motor and sensory fibres, repetitive responses are also to be expected if H-reflex activity is set up by centripetal impulses travelling in the sensory fibres of the stimulated nerve trunk. Again, this can only be excluded by careful inspection of the electromyogram. If activity is seen approximately 20 msec after the initial response it is probably reflex in origin. It cannot be detected from the measurement of muscle contractions because of their long duration. Such reflex activity is less likely to occur if stimuli of very short duration (0.1 msec or less) are used, because under such conditions motor nerve fibres are preferentially stimulated, as mentioned above, and sensory stimulation is reduced to a minimum. It is unlikely to occur in experiments on the upper limb because H-reflex activity there is usually absent or only slight. In experiments on the lower limb, however, where H-reflex activity is strong, it is to be expected.

In the presence of reflex activity, as with the repetitive responses mentioned above, the tension developed by the muscle fibres in response to a single stimulus is increased. This has important implications. First, drugs with central depressant actions (e.g. anaesthetics, benzodiazepines and phenothiazines) must be expected to reduce reflex responses and diminish the mechanical tension developed, even though they have no direct action at the neuromuscular junction. Secondly, because of this effect and because these same drugs potentiate competitive neuromuscular blocking drugs the overall result may be exaggerated.

3. Electromyographic Recording

A satisfactory method for measuring the response of muscle fibres to nerve stimulation is to record the evoked action potentials. Either needle electrodes or surface electrodes can be used though they will not necessarily yield identical results. It is theoretically possible that deep and superficial muscle fibres might not behave identically, particularly under conditions involving temperature or blood flow changes in the limb. It is always essential to ensure that the electrodes cannot move, particularly following tetanic stimulation, so that activity of the same group of muscle fibres is recorded throughout the experimental procedure. This means that the muscle being tested must contract isometrically, since any shortening of the muscle inevitably alters the compound action potential picked up by the electrodes. A test should be carried out before neuromuscular blocking drugs are administered to ensure that the physiological response can be recorded satisfactorily. Reference has already been made to the unsatisfactory nature of records which can result from a movement of the recording electrodes. A recording system for continuous evoked electromyography is described by EPSTEIN et al. (1973).

4. Recording of Muscle Contractions

Early experimental work in this field relied on the use of mechanical lever systems designed to record near-isometric muscle contractions (MAPLESON and MUSHIN, 1955a). They have been used for measuring the actions of gallamine (MAPLESON and MUSHIN, 1955b), dipyrandium (MUSHIN and MAPLESON, 1964) and ingeniously adapted to provide automatic feed-back control of muscle relaxation produced by a slow intravenous infusion of suxamethonium (MCSHERRY et al., 1956). The obvious limitations of such mechanical devices have now largely been overcome with the advent of force displacement transducers, applied as a rule to measure thumb adduction. A caliper with incorporated transducers suitable for recording contractions of leg muscles has also been described (CANNARD and ZAIMIS, 1959).

Mechanical recording of muscle tension presents several difficulties which can be overcome with care. First, the force transducer must have sufficient capacity to record the highest tension likely to be developed by the muscle or muscles. Surprisingly, the adductor pollicis muscle may produce up to 9 kg tension during tetanic stimulation. Secondly, the direction of movement of the transducer must be aligned with the direction of the pull exerted by the contracting muscle. Thirdly, the resting tension should be measured and kept constant.

Other techniques for recording the strength of muscle contractions are available, such as devices for recording intramuscular pressure through indwelling needles (KAUFMAN, 1965) and various pneumatic devices for recording grip strength (NEMA-

ZIE and KITZ, 1967; SHANKS and HARRISON, 1973). Such techniques provide only indirect measurements of muscle tension and they are not suitable for quantitative studies.

5. Experimental Conditions

It is desirable that studies of neuromuscular blocking drugs during surgery in anaesthetised patients should be carried out under specifically designed conditions. Ill-suited conditions have profound quantitative and qualitative influences on the assessment of the action of these drugs (as discussed later) and it is not surprising that, even in the hands of the same experimenter, the response of different patients to neuromuscular blocking drugs administered in defined dosages should vary over a wide range (Fig. 4). To achieve reliable and reproducible results it is essential that pertinent influences such as environmental and muscle temperature and the nature of anaesthetic and other drugs administered should be controlled and described when the results are published.

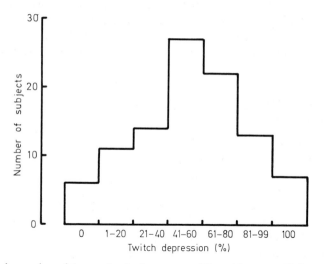

Fig. 4. Maximal depression of the mechanical response of the adductor pollicis to twitch stimulation of the ulnar nerve by tubocurarine 0.1 mg/kg in 100 anaesthetised patients. Mean depression = 53%. (From KATZ, 1967)

6. Definition of Terms

It is now appropriate and necessary to define in some detail the terminology to be used.

Post-Tetanic Potentiation. The increase in twitch tension which occurs physiologically in normal muscle following tetanic stimulation (BOTELHO and CANDER, 1953). During this post-tetanic potentiation of the twitch the muscle action potential remains unchanged; this indicates that the effect is due to a change in the contractile properties of the muscle (for further discussion see Chapter 4 A).

Tetanic Fade. The inability of the muscle to sustain a contraction in response to tetanic stimulation. In the absence of drugs fade can occur: a) in fatigued muscle; b) when the muscle is stimulated at rates above the physiological range; or c) when the duration of tetanic stimulation is unduly long. By contrast, fade occurs readily in the presence of competitive blocking drugs, as well as with drugs or factors which interfere with the synthesis or release of acetylcholine.

Post-Tetanic „Decurarisation". An increase in the compound muscle action potential and muscle tension in response to single stimuli following tetanic stimulation during partial competitive neuromuscular block. The increase in the size of the muscle action potential indicates that a greater number of muscle fibres are firing. It is seen only under conditions in which blockade can be overcome by increased transmitter availability.

Many anaesthetists use the term post-tetanic potentiation for both phenomena— the physiological increase in muscle contraction in the absence of a neuromuscular blocking drug following a tetanus with unaltered action potentials and for the decurarisation induced by a tetanus which is accompanied by an increase in tension and in the size of the action potential. Other authors prefer the term "post-tetanic facilitation" for both phenomena. As the mechanism underlying these increases in muscle contraction are fundamentally different it is important to use terms which distinguish clearly between them.

III. Quantitation of Neuromuscular Blockade and Assessment of Residual Blockade

The assessment of the degree of neuromuscular blockade during the course of experimental work presents few problems. In the presence of competitive or depolarising drugs it can be derived from measurements of either integrated action potentials or mechanical responses and conveniently expressed as the percentage twitch depression. Quantitation of neuromuscular blockade at the end of an operation when residual paralysis is suspected is, however, difficult if no control measurements were made prior to administration of the drug. Under the influence of depolarising blocking drugs it is impossible, but with competitive agents it can be achieved if single stimuli are replaced by faster rates of stimulation.

In subjects under steady state anaesthesia with 1% halothane in 60% nitrous oxide, EPSTEIN and EPSTEIN (1973) measured simultaneously twitch tension and muscle action potentials during partial paralysis by tubocurarine. They showed that fade, and post-tetanic decurarisation are found at all levels of blockade (Figs. 5 and 6) and concluded that either of these parameters can be used as reliable indicators of residual curarisation. Their findings, however, showed that at levels of blockade below about 50% twitch depression fade and post-tetanic decurarisation were detectable only from electromyographic recordings. They therefore proposed that for practical purposes tension responses are unlikely to be of value in the detection of residual curarisation of low degree.

An alternative technique, developed by ALI et al. (1971), allows residual paralysis to be assessed from twitch responses using a train of four nerve stimuli. In their experiments the ulnar nerve of the patient was stimulated and the resultant muscle

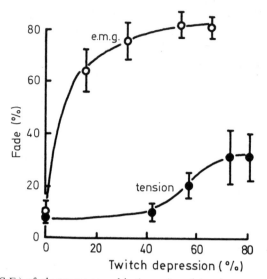

Fig. 5. Fade (mean ± S.E.) of electromyographic (e.m.g.) and tension responses of the adductor pollicis to tetanic stimulation of the ulnar nerve in anaesthetised subjects following administration of tubocurarine 0.1 mg/kg. The results are related to the degree of twitch depression present at various stages of recovery. See text for definitions. (Data from EPSTEIN and EPSTEIN, 1973)

activity assessed either mechanically (force of thumb adduction) or by recording compound action potentials from the belly of the first dorsal interosseus muscle of the hand. At 10 sec intervals trains of four stimuli, at a frequency of 2 to 24 Hz, were applied and the results quantified using three ratios: the height of the first twitch response of the train of four, after the relaxant had been given, was compared with the control response [ratio (a)]; the height of the second twitch response of the train of four was compared with the height of the first response [ratio (b)], and the height of the fourth response of the train of four to the first response [ratio (c)]. It was found that there was a good correlation between ratio (a) and ratios (b) and (c). ALI et al. considered this satisfactory since the first ratio involves a direct comparison between partially curarised and control responses, whereas the last two are obtained without the necessity of a control response having been first elicited.

Recordings of muscle tension were found satisfactory also by WAUD and WAUD (1972). They consider, however, that the response to tetanic stimulation at 100 Hz provides a considerably more sensitive indication of receptor block than either the twitch response or the fade in a train of four twitches. GISSEN and KATZ (1969) are of the same opinion and advise tetanic stimulation at several fixed frequencies. Finally, KATZ (1973) concludes that where possible both electrical and mechanical responses to nerve stimulation should be studied.

C. Pharmacokinetics of Neuromuscular Blocking Drugs

I. Distribution and Elimination

Neuromuscular blocking drugs, being quaternary ammonium compounds, are fully ionised at physiological pH and are consequently highly water soluble but largely

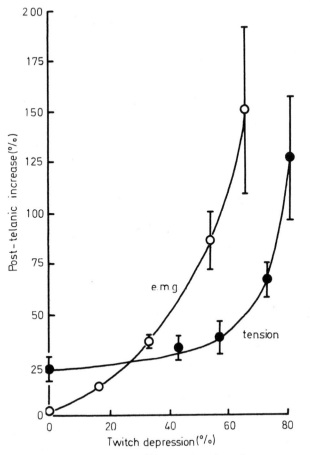

Fig. 6. Post-tetanic increases in electromyographic (e.m.g.) and tension responses of the adductor pollicis to single stimuli (ulnar nerve) in anaesthetised subjects following administration of tubocurarine 0.1 mg/kg. The results are related to the degree of twitch depression present at various stages of recovery. See text for definitions. (Data from EPSTEIN and EPSTEIN, 1973)

lipid insoluble. Their ability to cross cell membranes throughout the body is therefore slight and as a group they do not escape the extracellular space when injected into the circulation, nor are they significantly absorbed from the gastrointestinal tract. Indeed one could speculate that were this not so curare would never have been put to practical use as an arrow poison and these drugs might not be known today.

The distribution and fate of tubocurarine in man has been the subject of fairly extensive investigation. However, until recently the methods available for the estimation of tubocurarine in body fluids were not very sensitive. Bioassay (MAHFOUZ, 1949) and spectrophotometric techniques in particular (KALOW, 1953; ELERT and COHEN, 1962) could only detect microgram quantities of the drug, and the spectrofluorimetric method (COHEN, 1963) was only marginally more sensitive. For this reason plasma concentrations of tubocurarine could be measured only for two to three hours after the administration of the drug. However, the recent introduction of

a radioimmunoassay method (HOROWITZ and SPECTOR, 1973) has provided the necessary sensitivity to enable nanogram quantities to be measured.

Following intravenous administration, the concentration of tubocurarine in
plasma falls rapidly over the first 15 min or so. Early work by MAHFOUZ (1949)
indicated that during this period the concentration of the drug declined with a half-
life of a few minutes and that the distribution volume corresponded closely to the
plasma volume. At this stage, therefore, the drug appeared to be redistributed in the
body. Thereafter the rate of disappearance of tubocurarine was slow. KALOW (1959),
reviewing the findings of several authors, showed that over the next few hours
tubocurarine concentrations declined approximately exponentially with a half-life of
about 40 to 60 min and an apparent distribution volume of some 14% of body
weight. The bi-exponential decline in plasma tubocurarine concentration was confirmed by COHEN et al. (1965); it is illustrated in Fig. 7. These data yield half-lives for
the two processes of 6 and 52 min respectively and an equilibrium distribution
volume of 16.7% of body weight, confirming KALOW's earlier findings. Distribution
volumes within the range 14 to 16.7% are less than that of the extracellular space
(approximately 22% of body weight) and indicate that the drug is sequestered in
plasma, presumably by binding to plasma proteins. The data are consistent with
binding to the extent of about 30 to 45%.

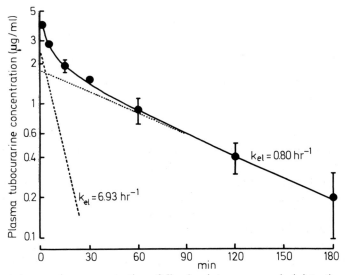

Fig. 7. Plasma tubocurarine concentrations following intravenous administration of 0.3 mg/kg.
The approximate values for the distributional (k_d) and elimination (k_{el}) constants are calculated
as 6.93 hrs^{-1} $(t_{1/2}=6$ min) and 0.80 hrs^{-1} $(t_{1/2}=52$ min) respectively and are indicated by interrupted lines. (Data from COHEN et al., 1965)

The time course of disappearance of the drug from the plasma following intravenous administration was therefore consistent with a two-compartment system, as
suggested earlier by KALOW (1953) on the basis of urinary excretion data. However,
recent measurements of plasma concentrations of tubocurarine, using the more sensitive radioimmunoassay method, indicate that the decline is probably multi-expo-

nential. HOROWITZ and SPECTOR (1973) reported that over long periods of time the drug disappears even more slowly than previously supposed; 24 hrs after the administration of 0.3 mg/kg, a dose similar to that used by COHEN et al. (1965), plasma concentrations in the range of 25 to 83 ng/ml were still detectable. One possible explanation for this finding is that binding to tissue ligands slows down the long-term elimination of the drug. Such ligands cannot yet be identified, however, and there is no evidence to indicate whether binding is mostly to end-plate receptors or to non-specific sites. Thus it appears that kinetic analysis requires a more complex model than that of the two compartment system. More recently, GIBALDI et al. (1972a) have fitted data obtained in man to a tri-exponential decay curve, using a three compartment model (see below).

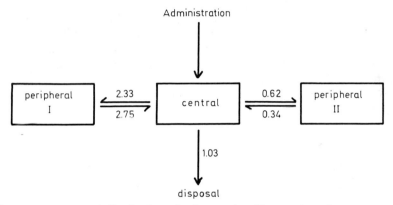

Fig. 8. Three-compartmental distribution of tubocurarine. The numbers denote rate constants (hr^{-1}). (GIBALDI et al., 1972a)

In subjects with normal renal function, the disappearance of tubocurarine from plasma is too rapid to be due solely to removal by glomerular filtration. The data shown in Fig. 7 yield a value for clearance in the second exponential phase of 150 ml/ min for a 70 kg subject, whereas clearance by glomerular filtration, assuming 30 to 45% binding of the drug to plasma protein, should be about half that value, within the range 65 to 85 ml/min. This confirms that tubocurarine is only partly eliminated by the kidney, a fact which has indeed been known for some years. MAHFOUZ (1949) and KALOW (1953) found only 30 to 40% of the administered dose in the urine of anaesthetised patients, and KALOW (1953) predicted from this that the duration of action of the drug would not be greatly influenced by renal failure. This has been confirmed by recent theoretical studies with computer models (GIBALDI et al., 1972b) and by clinical experience (CHURCHILL-DAVIDSON et al., 1967). On the basis of animal experiments it seems probable that the proportion of the drug not excreted by the kidney, both in normal subjects and patients with renal failure, is largely removed by biliary excretion (COHEN et al., 1967). Some metabolic degradation has also been claimed (MARSH, 1952) but is not definitely established (COHEN et al., 1967).

The other neuromuscular blocking drugs differ in their metabolic fate in the body. Unlike tubocurarine, gallamine is believed to be totally excreted by the kidney,

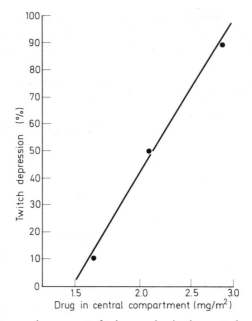

Fig. 9. Relationship between the amount of tubocurarine in the central compartment, calculated from elimination kinetics (see Fig. 8) and the mean degree of neuromuscular blockade in anaesthetised subjects. (GIBALDI et al., 1972a)

though no direct measurements appear to have been made in man. In renal failure the action of galamine is greatly prolonged (MONTGOMERY and BENNETT-JONES, 1956; FELDMAN and LEVI, 1963; CHURCHILL-DAVIDSON et al., 1967). Suxamethonium is rapidly hydrolysed by the cholinesterase enzymes in the plasma and at the end-plate region, whereas decamethonium is excreted unchanged (ZAIMIS, 1950). The elimination of pancuronium has been studied recently by AGOSTON et al. (1973). Their findings indicate that the drug is eliminated predominantly by the kidney although in the small group of subjects studied an average of 11% of the dose given was recovered in the bile. Analysis of the data shows that during the period immediately following its administration pancuronium leaves the plasma with a half-life of 6 to 7 min, a value which is close to that obtained with tubocurarine. During the period from two to four hours after administration, for which the data are complete, plasma concentrations decline with a mean half-life of 138 min, i.e. substantially more slowly than is the case with tubocurarine. The equilibrium distribution volume of approximately 36% of body weight is greater than that of the extracellular fluid, suggesting that the drug is sequestered in the tissues. The calculated plasma clearance value of 114 ml/min is consistent with elimination by renal glomerular filtration.

Perhaps the most interesting contributions to the field of pharmacokinetics have been the attempts to relate the duration of neuromuscular blockade produced by tubocurarine to its disposition in the body. By the intravenous administration of loading doses of tubocurarine to anaesthetised patients, followed by slow infusions at various rates, RYAN (1964) was able to deduce from the size of the blockade that the half-life of elimination of the drug was about 45 min, a value which accords roughly with the actual measurements of plasma concentrations already discussed. Furthermore, he observed that the time taken for the neuromuscular block to reach a steady level (approximately 13 min) was similar to that predicted from the pharmacokinetic data. The relationship between the disposition of tubocurarine and the time-course of its pharmacological action has been further explored most elegantly by GIBALDI et al. (1972a) using a three-compartment model (Fig. 8). They have calculated the concentration of the drug in the central compartment, which presumably corresponds fairly closely to the plasma concentration, and shown that this correlates well with the degree of the neuromuscular blockade measured in the experiments of WALTS and DILLON (1968a, b) (Fig. 9). This close correlation is perhaps surprising in view of the binding of the drug to plasma proteins. The three-compartment model also predicts remarkably accurately the observed relationship between the dose of tubocurarine and the duration of the neuromuscular blockade (Fig. 10) and the pattern of drug elimination described by KALOW (1953). From

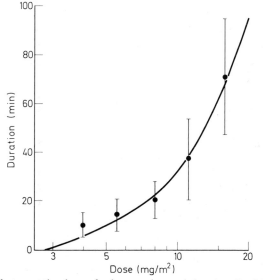

Fig. 10. Relationship between the dose of tubocurarine and the mean ($\pm$ S.D.) duration of neuromuscular blockade to 90% recovery in anaesthetised patients. The curve is the relationship predicted from elimination kinetics (see Fig. 8). (GIBALDI et al., 1972a)

theoretical considerations LEVY (1964) suggests that the pharmacological effect of tubocurarine should decline arithmetically rather than exponentially. This is because the magnitude of the effect is directly related to the logarithm of the concentration over a substantial range and also because the logarithm of the concentration declines approximately linearly with time. Evidence to support this concept is illustrated in Fig. 11 (LEVY, 1964); it is based on measurements made by BELLVILLE et al. (1964).

In the case of suxamethonium, because the drug is so rapidly hydrolysed a single compartment model is appropriate to describe the pharmacokinetic data (LEVY,

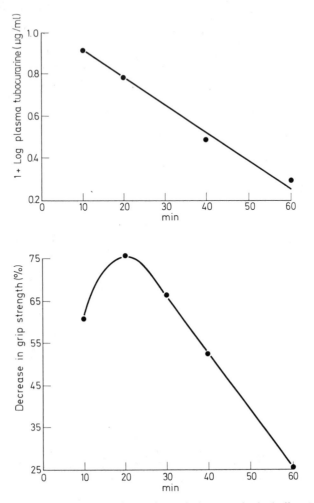

Fig. 11. Decline in plasma concentration (log scale) and pharmacological effect (reduction of grip strength: arithmetic scale) of tubocurarine with time following its intramuscular administration. (LEVY, 1964)

1967, 1970). Suxamethonium is first hydrolysed rapidly to succinylmonocholine and choline (WHITTAKER and WIJESUNDERA, 1952). Succinylmonocholine is then slowly hydrolysed in man to choline and succinic acid (FOLDES, 1953; FOLDES and TSUJI, 1953; LEHMANN and SILK, 1953; FRASER, 1954). Succinylmonocholine is much less potent pharmacologically than is suxamethonium. Using the measurements of neuromuscular blockade obtained by WALTS and DILLON (1967, 1969a), LEVY has calculated that the effect of the drug declines arithmetically with time at a rate which is independent of dosage (Fig. 12). As predicted by the model, the product of the duration and the rate of decline of the pharmacological effect is remarkably constant from one individual to another despite wide differences between them in the rate of drug elimination.

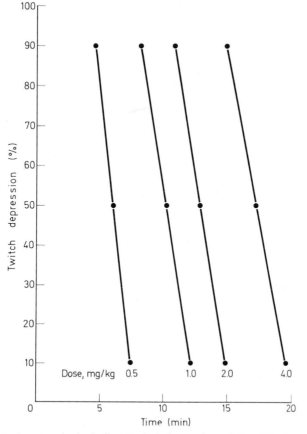

Fig. 12. Decline in pharmacological effect (twitch depression of the adductor pollicis) with time following administration of suxamethonium 0.5 to 4 mg/kg intravenously. The rate of decay of the pharmacological effect is independent of dosage. (LEVY, 1967)

The pharmacokinetic approach can therefore be used to predict the duration of the effect obtained by different dosage regimes and to assess the likely influence of renal failure and of other factors on the duration of action of both competitive and depolarising neuromuscular blocking drugs.

II. Plasma Protein Binding

Equilibrium dialysis experiments *in vitro* show that tubocurarine can be bound to both albumin and globulin. ALADJEMOFF et al. (1958) found in 10 patients that tubocurarine was bound more to globulin than to albumin. In contrast, in two patients who had previously shown marked resistance to tubocurarine during anaesthesia most of the drug was found to be attached to albumin. The results suggest that the clinical response to tubocurarine might be greatly influenced by the plasma protein pattern of the individual patient. It is noteworthy, for example, that resistance to the

Table 2. Correlations between dose requirements of neuromuscular blocking drugs in anaesthesia and plasma protein concentrations

Drug	Albumin	Globulins			
		α_1	α_2	β	γ
Tubocurarine	−0.27	0.28	0.23	0.11	0.48[c]
Dimethyltubocurarine	0.12	−0.24	−0.16	−0.26	0.02
Toxiferine	−0.46[c]	0.28	0.11	0.08	0.18
Alcuronium	0.62[c]	−0.40[b]	−0.16	0.13	−0.22
Pancuronium	−0.17	0	−0.06	−0.13	−0.13
Gallamine	0.34[a]	−0.33[a]	−0.23	−0.02	−0.18

See text for details.

[a] $P < 0.05$. — [b] $P < 0.01$. — [c] $p < 0.001$ (Stovner et al., 1971 a, b, 1972).

action of the drug occurs in liver disease when albumin: globulin ratios are often reversed (Dundee and Gray, 1953).

In some recent studies attempts have been made to relate individual dose requirements of several neuromuscular blocking drugs to the concentration of each fraction of plasma protein present (Stovner et al., 1971a, b, 1972). Hand-grip responses to ulnar nerve stimulation with short trains of stimuli at 2 Hz were used to determine the effective dose of the blocking drug. Following an initial loading dose, further doses were administered as dictated by the degree of blockade. Each drug was investigated in 50 patients who were anaesthetised with nitrous oxide and oxygen and who were also given diazepam. The total dose of each neuromuscular blocking drug, given during a 90 min period, was calculated in mg/m^2 body surface area and related to the plasma protein values determined on another occasion. Equilibrium dialysis, however, to determine the degree of binding was not performed. The regression coefficients obtained are summarised in Table 2 and show a correlation between tubocurarine requirement and the gamma globulin fraction; on the other hand gallamine and alcuronium requirements correlated with the albumin fraction. The results with tubocurarine are in agreement with the results obtained by Baraka and Gabali (1968).

These findings, though of considerable interest, are difficult to interpret because of a number of complicating factors. On a theoretical basis, if a drug is protein bound to an appreciable extent the concentration in free solution is correspondingly reduced. Consequently greater doses are needed to produce a neuromuscular block. At the same time, increased binding holds the drug in the circulation, thus reducing its volume of distribution. If the drug is eliminated from the plasma by glomerular filtration, increased binding would automatically reduce its elimination, thereby diminishing dose requirement over a long period. On the other hand, the same factors would increase its availability for elimination by metabolism or by biliary or renal excretion (Evans et al., 1973). The relationship between protein binding and dose requirement in studies of this type is therefore exceedingly complex, particularly if, as in the case of tubocurarine and pancuronium, more than one route of elimination may be involved.

The situation is further complicated by the fact that a low albumin and high gamma globulin level may coexist in certain patients, particularly in those suffering from cirrhosis of the liver, when a positive correlation between a drug-dose requirement and the level of one particular protein would automatically be associated with a negative correlation for the other protein. This particular difficulty could be overcome to some extent by multiple regression analysis but more effectively by the direct measurement of protein binding of the drug in the individual patient using equilibrium dialysis. The interpretation derived from the indirect measurements of STOVNER et al., should therefore be viewed with caution.

Hypersensitivity reactions to neuromuscular blocking drugs have been reported occasionally, suggesting that they are capable of provoking antibody formation in man. Indeed, drugs which are readily bound to plasma proteins can act as haptenes and cause antibody formation. In the case of tubocurarine, use has been made of this property to develop a radioimmunoassay technique (HOROWITZ and SPECTOR, 1973). Allergic types of reaction have also occurred during the clinical use of gallamine (LOPERT, 1955; WALMSLEY, 1959) and alcuronium (CHAN and YEUNG, 1972). However, whether these drugs can be implicated directly is open to doubt. First, the patients concerned have inevitably received a number of other drugs, any one of which may be the causative agent. This point is particularly important in that these patients often show multiple drug allergies. Secondly, the reactions produced are indistinguishable from those to be expected on the basis of simple histamine release by the drugs themselves (discussed later). True allergy to this group of drugs is therefore doubtful.

III. The Placental and Blood-Brain Barriers

Low concentrations of tubocurarine, about one twentieth to one tenth of those present in maternal plasma, (COHEN, 1962) and of dimethyltubocurarine (KIVALO and SAARIKOSKI, 1972) have been detected in foetal plasma within 10 to 15 min of administering the drug to the mother. SPEIRS and SIM (1972) reported that pancuronium could be found in foetal urine, suggesting placental transfer of this compound also. However, in the case of pancuronium interpretation of the results is in doubt as the authors used for their test a substance (methylorange) which reacts non-specifically with a variety of amines including nicotine and pethidine which are known to cross the placenta and reach the foetus. Suxamethonium has been found to be detectable in foetal plasma only when exceptionally large single doses of the drug were given to the mother (MOYA and KVISSELGARD, 1961; KVISSELGARD and MOYA, 1961). Under such circumstances histamine liberated by the drug may well have increased the permeability of the endometrial capillaries, thereby aiding transfer of the drug.

The importance of placental transport of neuromuscular blocking drugs in anaesthesia during Caesarian section is discussed by MOYA and SMITH (1965). It is well recognised, however, that infants born to mothers in such circumstances rarely if ever show evidence of neuromuscular blockade; failure to breathe is almost always due to other factors.

Tubocurarine and gallamine have also been recovered from the cerebrospinal fluid in man, though the concentrations involved are so small as to be of little significance

(Devasankaraiah et al., 1973; Haranath et al., 1973). A remarkable account of the subjective experience of a conscious volunteer under the influence of tubocurarine was presented by Smith et al. (1947). This indicates that even a large dose of the drug, reported as $2\frac{1}{2}$ times that needed for respiratory paralysis, does not influence sensation nor the pattern of the electroencephalogram (EEG). It has also been shown that gallamine does not produce EEG changes (Jones et al., 1956) in patients anaesthetised with ether. The ability of tubocurarine to prolong breath-holding capacity in the presence of gross increases in P_{CO_2} is probably determined peripherally rather than centrally (Campbell et al., 1969).

D. Action of Neuromuscular Blocking Drugs at the Neuromuscular Junction

I. General Characteristics

In a series of papers, Churchill-Davidson and his colleagues have described and illustrated compound action potentials obtained using surface electrodes over, or needle electrodes within, the hypothenar muscles in response to ulnar nerve stimulation under various conditions (Churchill-Davidson and Richardson, 1952a; Churchill-Davidson and Christie, 1959; Christie et al., 1959; Churchill-Davidson et al., 1960; Churchill-Davidson and Wise, 1963). The authors showed that in man a clear distinction could be made between depolarisation and competitive blockade on the basis of electromyographic responses.

It is well known that in animals, under partial blockade with depolarising neuromuscular blocking drugs, repeated stimulation, even at tetanic rates, does not further reduce either the action potential or the height of muscle contraction. When the tetanic stimulation ceases, both twitch tension and action potential remain unaltered. The same pattern has been described in man as illustrated in Fig. 13, taken from Churchill-Davidson et al. (1960). It is to be assumed that under such conditions the recorded muscle potentials are those of muscle fibres which are unaffected by the drug and that the affected fibres are inoperative because their endplates are depolarised. The electromyographic findings are consistent with these assumptions in that alterations of transmitter availability within reasonable limits would not influence either group of fibres. Unaffected fibres function normally; affected fibres cannot do so at all.

Partial blockade induced by drugs competing with acetylcholine shows quite different characteristics. During repeated and especially during tetanic stimulation, the height of both compound muscle action potential and muscle contraction declines. In competitive block, a dynamic equilibrium exists between the blocking drug and acetylcholine, and molecules of both rapidly combine with, and dissociate from, the end-plate receptors.

In the absence of any drug, during tetanic stimulation of the nerve, the amount of acetylcholine released in response to each nerve impulse rapidly diminishes. However, because of the safety factor in the amount of acetylcholine released under normal conditions (Paton and Waud, 1967), no fall in tension occurs during the tetanus unless the period of stimulation is excessively long or the rate of stimulation is outside the physiological range. During block by competition the proportion of

A Depolarisation blockade

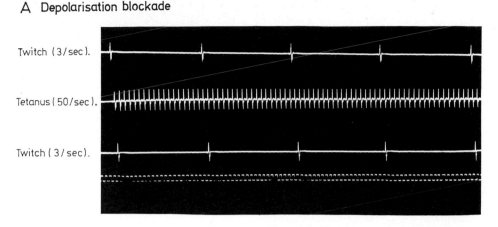

Twitch (3/sec).

Tetanus (50/sec).

Twitch (3/sec).

B Competitive blockade

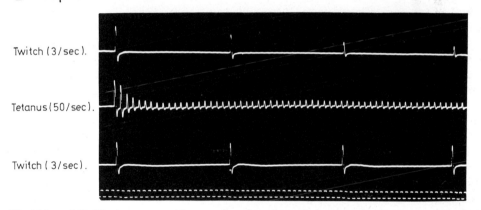

Twitch (3/sec).

Tetanus (50/sec).

Twitch (3/sec).

Fig. 13 A and B. Electromyographic recording from hypothenar muscles in response to ulnar nerve stimulation in anaesthetised subjects. (A) during blockade caused by a depolarising drug and (B) during competitive blockade. In (B), tetanic stimulation causes fade of the response. (CHURCHILL-DAVIDSON et al., 1960)

free receptors diminishes and therefore the threshold of the end-plate to acetylcholine is raised and the safety factor is reduced. Consequently the waning acetylcholine output during a tetanus is immediately reflected in the muscle's inability to sustain a tetanic contraction (Fig. 13). On returning to single stimuli both twitch and muscle potential increase for a short period of time. This well known post-tetanic decurarisation occurs because of recruitment of muscle fibres which had been paralysed before the tetanus and which now recover as a result of temporary accumulation of acetylcholine in the end-plate area, due to the rapid frequency of stimulation. Such an interpretation is consistent with the fact that competitive blockade is overcome by anticholinesterase drugs which appear to work by preventing the enzymatic hydrolysis of acetylcholine (see Chapter 4 B).

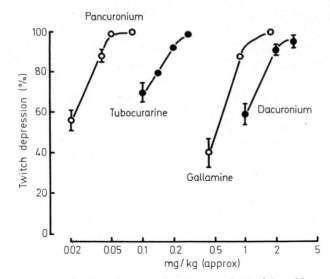

Fig. 14. Reduction of indirectly elicited contractions (mean ± S.E.) of the adductor pollicis muscle in anaesthetised subjects following administration of competitive neuromuscular blocking drugs. Doses of tubocurarine and gallamine are approximate only, and have been calculated from the original data where they were expressed in terms of body surface area. (Data from FOLDES et al., 1971; KATZ, 1971a, b; KATZ et al., 1969; NORMAN and KATZ, 1971; NORMAN et al., 1970; WALTS et al., 1967; WALTS and DILLON, 1968a)

Table 3. Equiactive doses and relative potencies of competitive neuromuscular blocking drugs in man, derived from data illustrated in Fig. 2 and 14

Drug	dose producing 70% impairment of response (mg/kg)	Relative potency
a) *Grip strength in conscious volunteers*		
Tubocurarine	0.089	1
Pancuronium	0.017	5.3
Alcuronium	0.052	1.7
Laudolissin	0.162	0.58
b) *Thumb adduction in response to ulnar nerve stimulation in anaesthetised subjects*		
Tubocurarine	0.100	1
Pancuronium	0.027	3.7
Gallamine	0.69	0.14
Dacuronium	1.27	0.08

KATZ and his colleagues (KATZ et al., 1963; KATZ et al., 1965; KATZ, 1966; KARIS et al., 1966; KATZ, 1967; KATZ and GISSEN, 1967; KATZ et al., 1968; GISSEN and KATZ, 1969; NORMAN et al., 1970; KATZ, 1971a, b; NORMAN and KATZ, 1971), MILLER and his colleagues (MILLER et al., 1968; MILLER et al., 1971a; MILLER and WAY, 1971; MILLER et al., 1971b and 1972), WALTS and DILLON (1967, 1968a, b,

1969a, b; WALTS et al., 1967) and other authors (FELDMAN and TYRELL, 1970b; FOLDES et al., 1971), have obtained similar results by recording muscle contractions only. Reference to many of these papers is made elsewhere in this chapter. Depression of the tension response of the adductor pollicis in anaesthetized subjects following administration of competitive drugs at various dose levels is illustrated in Fig. 14. Equiactive doses have been derived and are recorded in Table 3. The potencies of tubocurarine and pancuronium closely support the figures derived from studies of grip strength in conscious volunteers.

As anticipated from basic pharmacological observations in animals and from clinical impressions, neuromuscular blockade produced by suxamethonium is antagonised by prior administration of a small dose of tubocurarine (SCHUH et al., 1974).

Neuromuscular Refractory Period. EPSTEIN and his colleagues (EPSTEIN et al., 1969; EPSTEIN and JACKSON, 1973) recorded electromyograms and tension simultaneously from the adductor pollicis muscle in response to stimulation of the ulnar nerve with pairs of identical stimuli. They used this method to measure the "average refractory period" which they defined as "that pair interval which determines that tension which is the average of the tension evoked by a single stimulus and the maximum tension that can be evoked with a paired stimulus". Under normal conditions this average refractory period was found to range between 1.7 and 2.2 msec, but decreased slightly (by 0.35 msec) in the presence of either tubocurarine or gallamine in doses which were so small that they had no effect on muscle tension. After decamethonium, suxamethonium or an anticholinesterase drug the opposite effect was obtained, an increase of the average refractory period between 0.50 and 0.83 msec (EPSTEIN and JACKSON, 1973).

This indirect method of measuring refractory period has been used satisfactorily in the unanaesthetised man. However, it might be expected to give misleading results in any condition where there is repetitive firing, or where there is a change in the excitability of the post-synaptic membrane or in the presence of any change in muscle contractility. Consequently the interpretation of the results obtained by EPSTEIN and his colleagues remains unclear at present.

II. Influence of Anaesthetics

In clinical practice, the degree of muscle relaxation produced by competitive neuromuscular blocking drugs is greatly influenced by the anaesthetic agent and by the depth of anaesthesia present. Thus small doses of gallamine (e.g. 20 mg) which in conscious subjects produce no discernible blockade at all may lead to total respiratory paralysis in subjects anaesthetised to the third stage with diethylether. Such effects arise largely because the anaesthetic produces central nervous depression of somatic reflexes which in turn reduces transmitter liberation from the motor nerve terminals. Although no measurements of such changes have been recorded in man, it seems highly likely that this effect accounts both for the muscle relaxation produced by the anaesthetic and for much of its capacity to potentiate the competitive blocking drugs.

Anaesthetic agents do, however, also influence the neuromuscular junction directly. Experiments with animal preparations indicate that diethylether and haloth-

ane exert both prejunctional and postjunctional depressant actions (Karis et al.,
1967) and in man diethylether, fluroxene, halothane, methoxyflurane (Epstein and
Jackson, 1970b) and forane (Miller et al., 1971a) produce dose-dependent prolongation of the end-plate refractory period. One effect of this prolongation is to reduce
both the electromyographic and mechanical responses to high frequency nerve stimulation (Cohen et al., 1970). It is important to recognise here that there is an
approximately two-fold variability in the refractory period of different muscle fibres,
at least in the thenar eminence, which means that at high frequency stimulation some
muscle fibres must inevitably appear to be more affected than others. It can be
predicted, for example, from the observations of Epstein and Jackson (1970a),
illustrated in Fig. 15, that nerve stimulation at 300 Hz would produce a fade of
tension response due to blockade by fluroxene of about one third of the end-plates.
Blockade of this type is revealed only by very high stimulus frequencies and not at

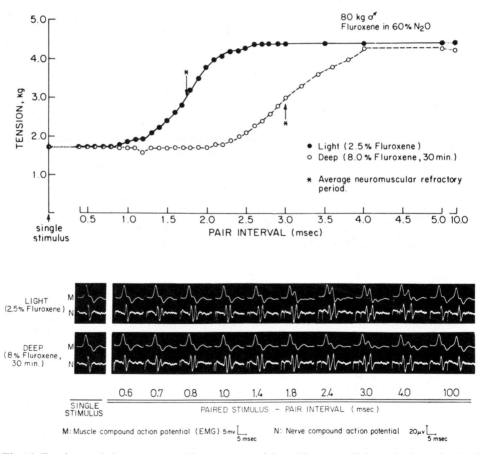

Fig. 15. Tension and electromyographic responses of the adductor pollicis to single and paired
stimulation of the ulnar nerve in an anaesthetised patient under fluroxene 2.5% (●) and fluroxene 8.0% (○). Deepening anaesthesia increased the average neuromuscular refractory period
from 1.75 to 3.00 msec. (From Epstein and Jackson, 1970b)

those occurring physiologically or those advocated for testing neuromuscular blockade. Such changes cannot therefore account for the potentiation of competitive
neuromuscular blocking drugs revealed by responses to twitch stimulation at about
0.3 Hz (KATZ, 1966; KATZ and GISSEN, 1967; HEISTERKAMP et al., 1969; KATZ,
1971 b; MILLER et al., 1971 a, b, 1972) nor necessarily to that at higher rates (BARAKA,
1968).

The origin of this phenomenon cannot be deduced from the human studies but
seems likely to be a consequence of the inhibition of end-plate depolarisation. Recent
work on isolated tissues by WAUD et al. (1973) indicates that halothane potentiates
tubocurarine and pancuronium but it does not influence the affinities of these drugs
for the receptors. Its action may therefore be exerted on the mechanisms which link
receptor activation to the contractile response. It is to be expected that anaesthetic
agents would potentiate only competitive neuromuscular blocking drugs and antagonise the depolarising agents. The former is well established but the latter is less
certain. The experiments of BARAKA (1968) suggest that 2% halothane does not
influence the action of suxamethonium. The situation is, however, complicated by
the fact that this and most other anaesthetics cause widespread increases in peripheral blood flow which would increase the availability of any neuromuscular blocking drug to the end-plate region during its first circulation after intravenous administration. Such an interpretation is consistent with the observations of MILLER et al.
(1971 b) which indicate that even suxamethonium is potentiated by the halogenated
ether forane.

Cyclopropane has been reported to produce increased contractility of isolated
human intercostal muscle at very high concentrations (SABAWALA and DILLON, 1958,
1961), though the origin and relevance of this action is obscure.

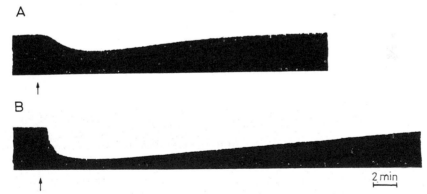

Fig. 16A and B. Depression of the tension response of the adductor pollicis to twitch stimulation
of the ulnar nerve (3 msec duration, 0.3 Hz) by tubocurarine 0.1 mg/kg in an anaesthetised
patient, tested on two occasions. (A) under N$_2$O, oxygen and pethidine; (B) under N$_2$O, oxygen
and halothane 1% (3 weeks later). Tubocurarine had a greater and more prolonged effect in the
presence of halothane. (KATZ and GISSEN, 1967)

It is clear that the recorded degree of blockade produced by competitive neuromuscular blocking drugs is highly dependent on the nature and the concentration of
the anaesthetic agent used. The effect of halothane is illustrated in Fig. 16. The

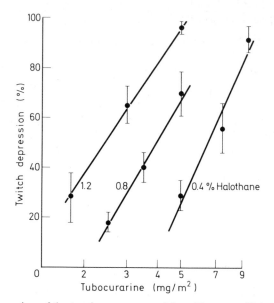

Fig. 17. Maximal depression of the tension response of the adductor pollicis to twitch stimulation of the ulnar nerve (0.1 msec duration, 0.3 Hz) by tubocurarine in patients anaesthetised with N_2O (70%), oxygen and different concentrations of halothane. Each point represents mean depression ($\pm$ S.E.) for 3 patients. Tubocurarine was potentiated by increasing concentrations of halothane. (Miller et al., 1972)

depencence is demonstrated most elegantly by the work of Miller et al. (1972) who showed that the doses of tubocurarine and pancuronium required to produce 50% twitch depression of the adductor pollicis to nerve stimulation are negatively and linearly related to the inhaled concentrations of the anaesthetic agents halothane and forane (Fig. 17). More recent studies indicate that enflurane and isoflurane exert even greater protentiating effects (Fogdall and Miller, 1975). Such observations indicate that clinical data on drug-induced neuromuscular blockade are meaningless unless the nature and intensity of anaesthesia are stated. It is pertinent here to record the frequent assertion that neuromuscular blocking drugs exert greater effects on North Americans than on patients in the United Kingdom. In their studies of this observation, Katz et al. (1969) showed that tubocurarine and suxamethonium had approximately twice as much effect on patients in New York as on those in London, a difference which might well have been a consequence of variations in anaesthetic technique.

It has been suggested that diazepam potentiated gallamine, possibly by a prejunctional action (Feldman and Crawley, 1970). The experimental design used, however, was such that the apparent potentiation almost certainly resulted from carry-over effect of the previous (test) dose of the blocking drug which had been administered only 80 to 120 min earlier. Subsequent studies by other authors failed to reveal potentiation, and experiments in dogs showed that the slight delay in recovery from competitive blocking drugs produced by diazepam could be produced equally well by its solvent (Dretschen et al., 1971).

III. Muscle Temperature and Blood Flow

Neuromuscular transmission is influenced by muscle temperature. Studies of ZAIMIS et al. (1958) and CANNARD and ZAIMIS (1959) on the response of leg muscles, and those of FELDMAN (1973) on hand muscles, have shown that cooling reduces peak twitch tension in response to nerve stimulation but prolongs its duration, slowing recovery. Cooling also greatly modifies the action of neuromuscular blocking drugs, the effect of depolarising agents being increased in magnitude and duration and that of tubocurarine being reduced (Fig. 18; CANNARD and ZAIMIS, 1959). On rewarming the muscle these effects are reversed. These observations are in agreement with results obtained from animal experiments and from studies of drug action in isolated preparations (see Chapter 4 A and B).

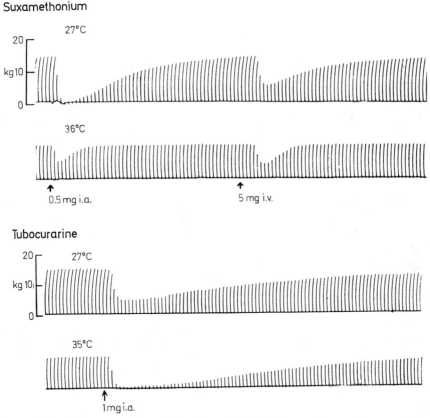

Fig. 18. Mechanical contractions of the right and left tibialis anterior muscles to twitch stimulation applied to their motor points (0.1 Hz) in anaesthetised patients. The muscles of one limb were cooled to the temperature indicated. At the lower temperature suxamethonium had a greater, but tubocurarine a smaller, effect. i.a.—intra-arterial injection; i.v.—intravenous injection. (CANNARD and ZAIMIS, 1959)

Such findings have obvious clinical relevance in that body temperature, and in particular limb temperature, may fall markedly during anaesthesia, or may be reduced deliberately, and rewarming occurs after the operation is over. WOLLMAN and CANNARD (1960) have shown that both core and muscle temperature fall under general anaesthesia particularly during thoracic operations. In one case, the authors found that the deltoid muscle had cooled to 27.4° C. Further information on temperature changes in various muscle groups during operation is urgently needed. In particular, it would be valuable to know what happens to the temperature of the thenar and hypothenar muscles of the hand, responses of which are almost universally used for assessing degrees of neuromuscular blockade. A number of questions spring to mind. Is there any temperature difference between the surface muscle fibres, the activity of which is predominantly recorded by surface electrodes, and the deeper muscle fibres which are relatively more involved in the contractile response? Such a difference might help to explain some of the discrepancies found by authors using different techniques of measurement, especially in experiments in which anaesthetic agents producing marked vascular changes were used. What is the effect on blood flow, and hence temperature, of the initiation and cessation of tetanic stimulation? FELDMAN and TYRRELL (1970a) found that frequent tetanic stimulation caused the effect of tubocurarine to wear off more rapidly. Was this due to an alteration in blood flow and was it influenced by temperature change? Do leg temperatures fall less than hand temperatures because the limb mass is so much greater, and could this influence the production of what anaesthetists recognise as dual block? It is worth noting in this respect that the majority of experiments done by ZAIMIS (1969) to test the possible existence of dual block in man were done on leg muscles, whereas those of all other authors are done on the hand. These questions need to be answered.

It is difficult to assess what effect blood flow changes would have *per se* on neuromuscular blockade because the techniques available at present are relatively crude and distinguish poorly between total flow and flow through particular capillary beds. It is suggested elsewhere that blood flow during the period immediately following injection of a neuromuscular blocking drug could be critical in determining how much of the drug reaches the end-plate, particularly with a drug like suxamethonium which disappears from the circulation at a very fast rate. Inspection of the upper record shown in Fig. 18 reveals that potentiation of suxamethonium by cooling is much more obvious after intra-arterial than after intravenous administration of the drug. Such a finding is consistent with the view that cooling reduces blood flow to the area concerned, as a result of which the proportion of the intravenous dose available to the cooled limb is smaller than that to the warm limb. By contrast, following intra-arterial administration the full dose enters the muscle independently of flow and direct potentiation of the drug by cold is seen without interference. It is also reasonable to suppose that an increase in flow would increase drug wash-out from the tissue and thus shorten the drugs duration of action. Such could easily explain the findings of FELDMAN and TYRRELL (1970a) discussed above. It would also explain why the effect of decamethonium is reduced by local anaesthesia of the motor nerve above the point of stimulation (CHURCHILL-DAVIDSON and RICHARDSON, 1952a) because such anaesthesia inevitably removes sympathetic tone in the area of study. It could also explain the apparent antagonism of decamethonium by pentamethonium shown by ORGANE et al. (1949) and illustrated in Fig. 1. In the absence of the pertinent measurements, however, such suppositions are merely conjectural.

IV. Carbon Dioxide and Plasma pH

In clinical anaesthesia the degree of muscle relaxation and respiratory depression, produced by anaesthetic agents or neuromuscular blocking drugs, is influenced by the degree of ventilation of the patient. Early reports suggested that hyperventilation increased the relaxation produced by tubocurarine or thiopentone (DUNDEE, 1952). Severe degrees of acidosis, however, can have the same result (BROOKS and FELDMAN, 1962). Reports of such effects are usually anecdotal and the cause remains uncertain. Some are likely to be the result of a reduction in reflex muscle activity due to central depression caused by the change in P_{CO_2}. It is well known that passive hyperventilation reduces activity in the abdominal muscles in the absence of a neuromuscular blocking drug (KATZ and WOLF, 1964). Changes in blood flow or plasma calcium and pharmacokinetic adjustments involving alterations in drug binding to plasma proteins and of drug concentrations in plasma water may also be involved. Furthermore, changes in pH may directly influence events at the neuromuscular junction and alter the response to the drug present at its site of action. From the data presently available one can only speculate on the relative importance of these different influences.

Measurements of neuromuscular transmission from electromyographic and tension responses of hand muscles show clearly that hyperventilation to a plasma P_{CO_2} of 19 or 22 mmHg and pH of 7.5 reduces blockade by tubocurarine (BARAKA, 1964; BRIDENBAUGH et al., 1966). Inhalation of carbon dioxide to give a plasma P_{CO_2} of 73 mmHg and pH of 7.2 has the opposite effect. Such effects could result from changes in drug distribution. BARAKA (1964) measured plasma concentrations of tubocurarine and found that in alkalosis the plasma concentration was reduced while in acidosis the plasma concentration was raised, but the changes produced were slight and probably insufficient to account for the alterations in drug action.

Animal experiments indicate that when ventilation changes alter neuromuscular transmission it is the pH rather than the P_{CO_2} which is the important factor (KALOW, 1954). Such changes in pH may influence the potency of tubocurarine via an effect on the ionisation of the molecule which would in turn alter its binding to plasma proteins and possibly affect its binding to the end-plate receptors. (See Chapter 4 C for further discussion of this point.)

Although gallamine is also a competitive neuromuscular blocking drug, it is affected by pH changes in the opposite direction to tubocurarine. Hyperventilation appears to increase gallamine blockade to a substantial degree (BRIDENBAUGH et al., 1966; WALTS et al., 1967). Ionization changes cannot be involved in the case of gallamine, and the mechanism underlying this effect is unknown (See Chapter 4 C). Suxamethonium blockade is reputed to be increased during acidosis (BARAKA, 1967). Pancuronium is apparently unaffected (DANN, 1971), but the methods used in this assessment are questionable because of the excessive duration (110 msec) of the stimuli applied to the nerve.

A great deal of additional information has been obtained from animal experiments as discussed in Chapter 4 C, and the conclusion which can be drawn for both animals and man is that the effect of alkalosis and acidosis on tubocurarine blockade is well documented while their effect on other neuromuscular blocking drugs is either unknown or obscure.

V. Dual Block

There is widespread acceptance by anaesthetists that in clinical practice the characteristics of neuromuscular blockade produced by depolarising blocking drugs change with time, particularly if the drugs have been used in high dosage or over a long period. The term used most frequently to describe the altered response is "Dual Block", though it is also known as "Phase II" and "Desensitisation Block", both of which terms were derived from studies on isolated nerve-muscle preparations (JENDEN et al., 1951; THESLEFF, 1955). For further discussion of the phenomenon the reader is referred to Chapter 4 A. The term dual block was first coined by ZAIMIS (1952) to describe the biphasic reaction of the monkey, dog and hare to the administration of decamethonium and the analogous reaction of birds to tridecamethonium. The term is used here because, of the three, it is the one most closely (though not exactly) appropriate and most frequently used by anaesthetists to describe the clinical syndrome encountered.

Considerable controversy exists over the frequency of occurrence of dual block, the readiness with which it can be produced, and the mechanism by which it occurs. The very existence of the phenomenon has been disputed. It must be admitted that much heat has gone out of the argument now that practising anaesthetists have learned to avoid using large doses of depolarising agents so that the syndrome is no longer frequently seen. Dual block is not observed in most studies on conscious volunteers but only in anaesthetised patients given large or repeated drug doses, usually over a period of 2 to 3 hrs. The restricted occurrence is probably critical as will be revealed from the discussion that follows.

The following findings are taken as indications of dual block in practice:

A Poorly Sustained Response to Repeated Nerve Stimulation. Substanial fade of electromyographic (CHURCHILL-DAVIDSON et al., 1960; DE JONG and FREUND, 1967) and tension (KATZ et al., 1963; CRUL et al., 1966; DE JONG and FREUND, 1967) responses to ulnar nerve stimulation at twitch and tetanic rates of stimulation is found. This is obviously unlike the response usually observed in the early stages after administration of suxamethonium or decamethonium (CHURCHILL-DAVIDSON and CHRISTIE, 1959).

Post-Tetanic Decurarisation. Increased electromyographic (CHURCHILL-DAVIDSON et al., 1960; DE JONG and FREUND, 1967) and tension (KATZ et al., 1963; CRUL et al., 1966; DE JONG and FREUND, 1967) responses are elicited by twitch stimulation following a short period of tetanic stimulation. Again, this is unlike the usual response to administration of depolarising blocking drugs.

Additive Effect of Competitive Neuromuscular Blocking Drugs. The administration of gallamine further increases the blockade, as judged by respiratory traces (BRENNAN, 1956).

Reversal of Blockade by Anticholinesterases. Edrophonium nd neostigmine reverse the blockade, as judged by the clinical degree of relaxation (RUDDELL, 1952; BRENNAN, 1956; BULLOUGH, 1957) and by electromyographic and tension responses

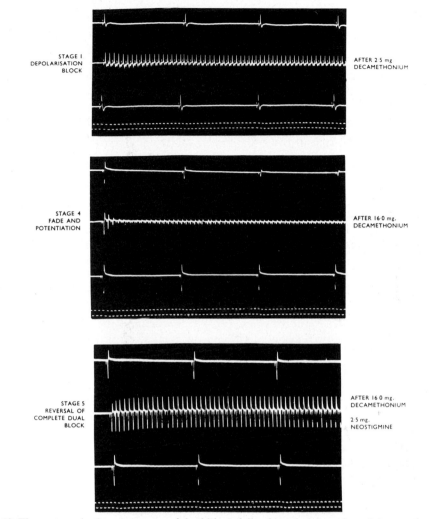

Fig. 19. Three stages in the occurrence of dual block following administration of decamethonium to anaesthetised subjects. Electromyographic response of hypothenar muscles to twitch and tetanic stimulation of the ulnar nerve. (CHURCHILL-DAVIDSON et al., 1960)

to nerve stimulation (CHURCHILL-DAVIDSON et al., 1960; KATZ et al., 1963; FREUND, 1969).

An electromyographic record of some of these findings is illustrated in Fig. 19. Coincident with the development of these signs of dual block progressive tachyphylaxis to the drugs occurs so that the second and subsequent doses produce fewer or no muscle fasciculations (HARRISON, 1965) and less neuromuscular blockade (POULSEN and HOUGS, 1958; PAYNE and HOLMDAHL, 1959; KATZ and RYAN, 1969). The responses are similar to those produced by decamethonium in myasthenic subjects and neonates, and reminiscent of the response of the tibialis anterior muscle in the monkey (ZAIMIS, 1953).

These alterations in response do not necessarily occur simultaneously and are not all apparent in every case. On the basis of electromyographic studies, CHURCHILL-DAVIDSON et al. (1960) have described five stages in the development of dual block, according to the extent to which the above signs have appeared. Such a classification implies a uniformity in the condition which is denied by a number of studies. At one extreme the observations of ZAIMIS (1969) suggested that such changes did not occur at all, even with repeated drug administration over several hours. At the other, DE JONG and FREUND (1967) observed changes which they interpreted as dual block in every subject to whom suxamethonium was administered.

The interpretation of these findings is rendered difficult by the multiplicity of techniques used by different authors. Consideration is given here to the possible origins of the changes observed.

The first is that the responses attributed to dual block originate from muscle fibres which have already recovered from the effects of the drug and which therefore respond like normal fibres. Minor degrees of fade in both electromyographic and tension responses to nerve stimulation might be seen in some subjects (EPSTEIN and EPSTEIN, 1973) but these are unlikely to be as great as those usually recorded in this situation. Post-tetanic potentiation of the mechanical response can be expected because it is physiological (BOTELHO and CANDER, 1953) and could increase tension by as much as 40% (EPSTEIN and EPSTEIN, 1973). It is worth noting that this figure is as great as that reported by KATZ et al. (1963) from responses of the adductor pollicis. Electrical responses should, however, remain unchanged and this is clearly not so at least under the conditions employed by CHURCHILL-DAVIDSON et al. (1960). Administration of anticholinesterases should increase both electrical and mechanical responses because under their influence the muscle action potential is converted into a brief asynchronous tetanus due to repetitive firing of the muscle fibres (HARVEY et al., 1941; ZAIMIS, 1969). The fact that anticholinesterases reverse the block cannot therefore be taken as incontrovertible evidence of dual block.

Secondly, attention should be given to the possible influence of the anaesthetic. It is clear that dual block is most readily observed when neuromuscular blocking drugs, and by implication anaesthetics, have been given over a long period. This being so, the anaesthetic agent will have reached its highest levels and its influence on the neuromuscular junction will be maximal. Prejunctional inhibition of acetylcholine release and post-junctional inhibition of end-plate depolarisation (KARIS et al., 1967) are known to occur. These actions will produce blockade of a competitive type, the features of which will be fade on tetanic stimulation, post-tetanic decurarisation, tachyphylaxis to depolarising agents and summation with (or potentiation by) competitive neuromuscular blocking drugs and reversibility by anticholinesterases. All these effects are observed in dual block. Their intensity depends on the nature and partial pressure of the anaesthetic used, the greatest effect occurring with deep anaesthesia with drugs such as diethylether or forane.

Thirdly, large doses of depolarising drugs could cause impairment of prejunctional function and reduce transmitter release, an action resembling that of hemicholinium. Although there is no direct evidence for this in man, observations on the cat whose neuromuscular junction responds similarly to most agents indicate that prejunctional failure can occur with quite moderate doses of suxamethonium (STAN-

DAERT and ADAMS, 1965). Such impairment might contribute to the fade, facilitation and response to anticholinesterases observed in the clinical situation, particularly in the presence of anaesthetics.

Fourthly, there is the possibility that the response of the receptors to the depolarising agent actually changes with time, either because of continuous loss of potassium from the end-plate, as suggested by PATON (1956), or entry of sodium or of the depolarising agent itself. While such changes undoubtedly occur, there is at the moment no direct evidence that they alter the response of the end-plate in the manner observed or assumed.

It is impossible to estimate the extent to which any of these influences are involved in producing the clinical picture of dual block. The relative importance of the factors discussed may vary from case to case. It seems reasonable to assume that the clinical condition could arise largely or exclusively as a consequence of the effects of anaesthesia without essential change in the mode of action of the drug or of the nature of the receptor, as proposed by ZAIMIS (1969). If this is the case, the terminology used is inappropriate. On the other hand, it is conceivable that receptor changes do occur; at the moment there is no evidence of this.

In order to clarify this situation, FELDMAN and TYRRELL (1970a) have investigated the action of decamethonium and other neuromuscular blocking drugs using a technique of retrograde intravenous administration of the drug (TORDA and KLONYMUS, 1966) which involves temporary occlusion of the circulation to the limb under examination. After release of the tourniquet, tension responses of the adductor pollicis recovered substantially more rapidly after administration of decamethonium than after gallamine or tubocurarine. On the assumption that the concentration of the blocking drug in the extracellular fluid in the region of the end-plate drops to zero when the tourniquet is released and normal circulation is reestablished, the authors have concluded that competitive neuromuscular blocking drugs bind much more tightly to the receptors than do depolarising drugs. Though the conclusion is probably correct, the conditions employed make its derivation from the data obtained unjustified. In the first place, the drug concentration at its site of action is unknown. The assumption that this concentration drops to zero upon release of the tourniquet is fundamentally untenable, delayed diffusion and recirculation both tending to keep the drug within the critical area. Furthermore, the conditions are complicated by the unknown degrees of hypoxia and hypercarbia produced by the circulatory obstruction which would exaggerate responses to competitive neuromuscular blocking drugs. The authors have attempted to demonstrate that recovery from decamethonium blockade is slowed after prolonged contact suggesting the existence of a stable drug-receptor complex akin to that produced by tubocurarine. Unfortunately the critical tracing does not reveal slowed so much as delayed recovery, which is not what would be expected on the basis of increased stability of the drug-receptor complex. The matter therefore remains open.

VI. Responses of Newborn Infants

The responses of neonates to the administration of neuromuscular blocking drugs differs somewhat from that of adult subjects. By comparison, they are highly sensitive to the action of competitive neuromuscular blocking drugs, particularly during the first 10 days of life (BUSH and STEAD, 1962), and resistant to that of depolarisers. This was first recorded by STEAD (1955) using a respiratory excursion tambour which of course provides only an indirect index of neuromuscular function. Similarly, related studies by LIM et al. (1964), using measurements of exhaled CO_2 concentrations and suggesting great sensitivity to blocking drugs of all types, cannot be interpreted accurately in terms of events at the neuromuscular junction. More precise observations indicate, however, that the differences in sensitivity are determined at the neuromuscular junction as shown by electromyographic recordings (CHURCHILL-DAVIDSON and WISE, 1963; NIGHTINGALE et al., 1966) and muscle tension changes (WALTS and DILLON, 1969a) in response to ulnar nerve stimulation.

These observations cannot be explained on the basis of differences in extracellular fluid volume which, in terms of body weight, is greater in neonates than in adults. Such differences would make neonates resistant to all types of blocking drugs. In his original paper, STEAD (1955) pointed out that the response of the neonate resembles that of the myasthenic in that he too is relatively supersensitive to competitive, but resistant to depolarising blocking drugs. Electromyographic studies of the action of decamethonium in the neonate have confirmed these observations (CHURCHILL-DAVIDSON and WISE, 1963) and have also revealed some qualitative resemblance.

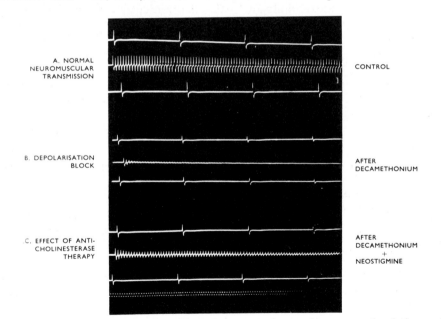

Fig. 20. Electromyographic response of hypothenar muscles to ulnar nerve stimulation and the influence of decamethonium in a newborn infant under anaesthesia. Neuromuscular blockade by decamethonium shows marked fade on repeated stimulation and partial reversal by neostigmine. (CHURCHILL-DAVIDSON and WISE, 1963)

They indicate, as shown in Fig. 20, that the response to tetanic stimulation at 30 Hz is poorly sustained and that blockade may be overcome with anticholinesterase drugs. Taken together with observations that depolarising blocking drugs do not produce fasciculations in young children, it is apparent that their action shows some of the features of competitive blockade and of dual block as seen in adults. STEAD (1955) himself blamed immaturity of the end-plate, though this merely records rather than explains the phenomenon.

Resistance of neonates to suxamethonium might also be due to other factors. Recent studies by COOK and FISCHER (1975) are consistent with the idea that resistance is due largely to differences in distribution and of elimination rate, rather than to intrinsic resistance of the neuromuscular junction itself.

These findings have only slight practical significance for anaesthesia of newborn children. In theory the dose of a depolarising drug should be somewhat larger and that of a competitive drug smaller if dosage is to be judged on the basis of body weight. The differences are, however, slight and consequently little practical adjustment is needed.

VII. Antibiotic Administration

It is well known that the instillation of aminoglycoside antibiotics into the peritoneal cavity during anaesthesia carried risk of respiratory arrest. Neomycin, for example, has been reported to have such an effect in patients anaesthetised with diethylether (PRIDGEN, 1956; PITTINGER et al., 1958) and streptomycin-induced weakness has been observed even in unanaesthetised subjects (LODER and WALKER, 1959). The effect is of greater consequence in the presence of competitive blocking drugs which appear to be potentiated (EMERY, 1963).

Neuromuscular blockade by aminoglycosides is only partially reversible by neostigmine, which indicates that these drugs do not exert typical curare-like actions on cholinergic receptors. Animal studies (BRAZIL and CORRADO, 1957) indicate that the blockade is at least partly prejunctional in origin and may be caused by ionic interference with transmitter release (GALINDO, 1972), perhaps as a result of chelation of calcium at this site. In clinical practice the blockade may be exacerbated by hypocalcaemia following blood transfusion (EMERY, 1963) and can be partially reversed by intravenous calcium chloride, as can the blockade produced by large doses of magnesium sulphate (GHONEIM and LONG, 1970).

VIII. Suxamethonium and Muscle Pain

Complaints of post-operative aches, pains or stiffness affecting the trunk and upper parts of the limbs are not uncommon in anaesthetic practice. It was pointed out by CHURCHILL-DAVIDSON (1954) that many patients complain of such symptoms following suxamethonium administration, particularly if they have been mobilised soon after the surgical operation concerned. He reported complaints from 21 of 36 outpatients who were sent home within hours of surgery but only from 5 of 36 inpatients who were confined to bed for a day or two. This observation has since been confirmed by FOSTER (1960) and many other authors. Women appear to be more susceptible than men (HEGARTY, 1956) and there is a strong association between the incidence of pain and lack of muscular fitness. NEWNAM and LOUDON (1966) found that 45% of subjects who were unaccustomed to exercise (some were partly disabled) complained of pain, while only 6% of subjects who were accustomed to strenuous exercise were affected. The authors likened this affect of suxamethonium to that of taking unaccustomed exercise and drew attention to an interesting observation that patients given the drug repeatedly for electroconvulsive therapy rarely complain of pain or stiffness. The overall incidence of pain following suxamethonium administration is exceedingly variable, presumably in part because of differences in training but also because such data depend very much on how the complaints are elicited, whether spontaneously or by direct questioning. In their review of over 2000 cases, DOTTORI et al. (1965) quote incidences ranging from 0.2 to 89%.

When suxamethonium has been administered during anaesthesia, post-operative levels of serum creatine phosphokinase are markedly elevated (TAMMISTO and AIRAKSINEN, 1966; INNES and STRØMME, 1973). INNES and STRØMME found a ninefold mean increase in the enzyme among a group of 26 children given halothane and suxamethonium but no change among 13 children who were given halothane alone. This finding and the occasional precipitation of myoglobinuria in susceptible individuals (BENNIKE and JARNUM, 1964; MCLAREN, 1968) indicate that suxamethonium pain is probably due to muscle damage caused by drug-induced fasciculations. In confirmation of this, an association is reported between pain and the occurrence of particularly high frequency discharge rates of muscle action potentials during the period of fasciculation (COLLIER, 1975). No direct correlation between pain and the visible intensity of such fasciculations has been found (NEWNAM and LOUDON, 1966), but this is hardly surprising considering the subjective nature of the observations.

The incidence of pain is reduced by the prior administration of small doses of competitive neuromuscular blocking drugs (FOSTER, 1960; GLAUBER, 1966; CULLEN, 1971) and of thiopentone (CRAIG, 1964). Such treatment reduces fasciculations in clinical practice and presumably reduces muscle damage for this reason.

IX. Suxamethonium and Plasma Cholinesterase

Early clinical experience with suxamethonium revealed that in the vast majority of patients the drug caused muscle relaxation and respiratory paralysis of very short duration, doses of 0.1 to 0.3 mg/kg causing muscle relaxation for only 1 or 2 min. By measuring the time taken for respiratory movements to re-appear after the injection of suxamethonium, BOURNE et al. (1952), however, showed that the duration of the response varied greatly between individuals (Fig. 21). They also reported that 6 patients who showed a prolonged response had abnormally low levels of plasma cholinesterase. A similar finding was reported by EVANS et al. (1952). Subsequent studies of the duration of apnoea together with measurements of serum cholinesterase activity (HODGES and HARKNESS, 1954; FOLDES et al., 1956) confirmed that variations in the latter determine the duration of action of the drug. The relationship was explored in more detail by KALOW and GUNN (1957) who recorded the duration of apnoea in 51 psychiatric patients given various doses of suxamethonium on different occasions, prior to electroconvulsive therapy. The duration of apnoea produced by suxamethonium could be correlated with the esterase activity, age and body weight. However, the correlation with the enzyme activity ($r = -0.75$) was preponderant and tended to obscure the role of body weight.

Administration of a concentrated preparation of the enzyme appears to shorten the duration of action of suxamethonium both in patients with deficient enzyme

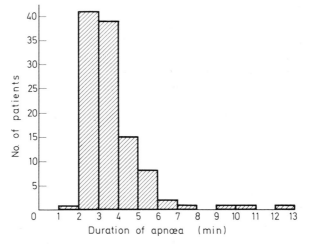

Fig. 21. Duration of apnoea in 110 anaesthetised patients following the administration of suxamethonium 1.1 mg/kg. (BOURNE et al., 1952)

(EVANS et al., 1953; CALVERT et al., 1954) and in those with normal enzyme levels (BORDERS et al., 1955). These observations should be accepted with caution, however, for they were the result of repeated administration of suxamethonium (given both before and after the enzyme preparation), a procedure which may in itself cause tachyphylaxis.

In normal healthy adults plasma cholinesterase activity varies over a fairly wide range (CALLAWAY et al., 1951). Where the enzyme concerned is of the usual type (see below) much of this variability is inherited and is determined by polygenic influences. WETSTONE et al. (1965) carried out a twin study and a parent-offspring study, and have shown from the degreee of resemblance between relatives that the value for heritability is approximately 66%. In view of the relationship discussed above between suxamethonium apnoea and cholinesterase levels, it can be concluded that the duration of action of the drug is largely genetically determined.

Neonates and infants under 6 months of age have low enzyme levels (ZSIGMOND and DOWNS, 1971) and may therefore be assumed to hydrolyse the drug relatively slowly. Abnormally low levels of cholinesterase are also found in malnutrition (McCANCE et al., 1948; WATERLOW, 1950), in liver disease, severe cardiac failure and uraemia (McARDLE, 1940), in hypothyroidism (THOMPSON and WHITTAKER, 1965), in severe illness associated with blood dyscrasias (SCUDAMORE et al., 1951) and following exposure to organophosphate insecticides (BARNES and DAVIES, 1951) or eyedrops (PANTUCK, 1966). The relevance of these findings to the anaesthetist are discussed in reviews by WIELHORSKI et al. (1962) and ROBERTSON (1966). Hyperthyroid patients have a somewhat higher plasma concentration of cholinesterase (ANTOPOL et al., 1937). A simple test-paper method suitable for screening cholinesterase levels in such patients has been described (CHURCHILL-DAVIDSON and GRIFFITHS, 1961).

The action of suxamethonium in patients with low, though qualitatively normal, cholinesterase activity is somewhat prolonged, though the effect of the drug usually wears off within 20 to 30 min unless the enzyme concentration is grossly reduced to about 10% of normal. Even patients with advanced secondary carcinomatosis, cirrhosis and cachexia often show responses to suxamethonium of almost normal duration (HUNTER, 1966).

The administration of drugs which inhibit plasma cholinesterase increases and prolongs the action of suxamethonium. This effect has been deliberately used during anaesthesia in order to prolong the muscle paralysis caused by suxamethonium. The drugs which have been used are tacrine (tetrahydroaminacrine) (GORDH and WÅHLIN, 1961; McCAUL and ROBINSON, 1962; KARIS et al., 1966); hexafluorenium (KATZ et al., 1965); N,N-bis-(B-piperidinoethyl)-gluteramide (HAMPTON et al., 1955); propanidid (MONKS and NORMAN, 1972; TORDA et al., 1972); and procaine (FOLDES et al., 1953; USUBIAGA et al., 1967). Drugs such as edrophonium, neostigmine and pyridostigmine have also been deliberately administered because of their well known anticholinesterase activity at the neuromuscular junction.

Severe prolongation of apnoea following the administration of suxamethonium is a well-recognised, though fortunately fairly rare, clinical occurrence. Failure to breathe under such circumstances can of course be due to many factors apart from prolonged neuromuscular blockade. Shortly after the appearance of the first reports of prolonged apnoea, DURRANS (1952) wrote: "... prolonged apnoea after administration of thiopentone together with a relaxant is many times more likely to have been caused by the thiopentone than by the relaxant." This timely warning was elaborated by FORBAT et al. (1953), who pointed out that apnoea can result from central respiratory depression caused by drugs used in premedication, by general anaesthetics themselves and by acidosis or hyperventilation. It is therefore imperative to view all such cases critically before concluding that the apnoea is due to prolongation of the action of suxamethonium at the neuromuscular junction. The assessment of such reports from the literature is further complicated by the fact that minor degrees of prolongation, e.g. 20 min, are regarded as being normal by some authors but not so by others. The interpretation of reports in this field is therefore difficult.

While minor degrees of prolongation of the action of suxamethonium are undoubtedly quite common, apnoea lasting more than 1 hr is rare. Genuine prolonged neuromuscular blockade, detected by testing neuromuscular transmission, immediately suggests that the individual concerned may lack the usual form of plasma cholinesterase having instead either an atypical variant form of the enzyme which is incapable of hydrolysing the drug or no enzyme at all. KALOW and GENEST (1957) showed that one variant form, now recognised to be that most often implicated in prolonged apnoea, could be readily distinguished from the usual enzyme by its resistance to inhibition *in vitro* by the local anaesthetic drug cinchocaine (dibucaine). The dibucaine number (DN) is defined as the percentage inhibition of enzyme activity produced by dibucaine 10^{-5} mol/l, using benzoylcholine 5×10^{-5} mol/l as substrate. KALOW's work indicated that inheritance of the atypical form of the enzyme is consistent with the existence of two autosomal allelic genes without dominance, each gene causing the formation of one type of enzyme. The distribution of dibucaine numbers in 135 members of 7 families was trimodal as shown in Fig. 22 (KALOW and STARON, 1957).

The usual enzyme, produced by the gene denoted E_1^u, and the atypical enzyme produced by the gene E_1^a, differ in several respects. The atypical form has less affinity

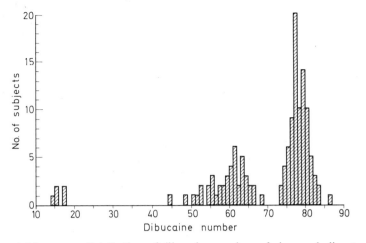

Fig. 22. Trimodal frequency distribution of dibucaine numbers of plasma cholinesterase among 135 members of 7 unrelated families. (KALOW and STARON, 1957)

for the substrate (GARRY, 1971), which is why atypical homozygotes $(E_1^a E_1^a)$ can be shown to have less cholinesterase activity in conventional test measurements. It is hardly surprising that early genetic observations in this field were interpreted as indicating inheritance of a low concentration of normal enzyme, rather than the presence of an atypical form of the enzyme (FORBAT et al., 1953; LEHMANN and SIMMONS, 1958). The atypical form of the enzyme is relatively resistant to inhibition by suxamethonium *in vitro* (STOVNER, 1955; KING and GRIFFIN, 1973), a finding consistent with the inability of the atypical enzyme to hydrolyse suxamethonium *in vivo* (KALOW, 1959). Indeed, one would expect the "suxamethonium number" to provide a good indication of the duration of apnoea *in vivo*. Recent kinetic studies show that the atypical enzyme has lesser affinity for the drug's thiol analogue succi-nyldithiocholine (HERSH et al., 1974). Certain physical characteristics, a lower temperature coefficient (KING and DIXON, 1969), different behaviour on chromatography and gel electrophoresis (LIDDELL et al., 1962a) and failure of activation by critical concentrations of chloride, also distinguish it from the usual enzyme. The latter has been used as the basis of a quick and simple population screening test (SWIFT and LA DU, 1966).

Since the discovery of the atypical enzyme, family and population studies have revealed other variant forms. One variant, resistant to inhibition by fluoride (HARRIS and WHITTAKER, 1961; LIDDELL et al., 1963), is produced by a gene on the same locus, denoted E_1^f. This enzyme hydrolyses suxamethonium at a rate intermediate between that of the usual and the atypical enzymes, and there is moderate prolongation of the drug's action in homozygotes $(E_1^f E_1^f)$. The enzyme shows only slight resistance to inhibition by suxamethonium *in vitro* (KING and GRIFFIN, 1973).

Rare individuals have been found with no plasma cholinesterase whatsoever (LIDDELL et al., 1962b; HART and MITCHELL, 1962). They occur with a frequency of only 1 per 100000 in the population and are believed to be homozygotes for a silent gene (E_1^s) situated at the same locus (SIMPSON and KALOW, 1964). Their response to

Table 4. Inherited variants of human plasma cholinesterase

Genotype	Incidence	Relative activity (benzoyl-choline)	Average dibucaine number	Average fluoride number	Average suxa-methonium number	Prolongation of suxa-methonium response
$E_1^u E_1^u$	0.94	1.00	80	61	90	–
$E_1^u E_1^a$	0.04	0.75	62	48	68	±
$E_1^u E_1^f$	0.004	0.85	74	52	84	±
$E_1^u E_1^s$	0.006	0.60	80	61	90	±
$E_1^a E_1^a$	0.0004	0.45	22	23	18	+ +
$E_1^a E_1^f$	0.00003	0.60	50	30	48	+
$E_1^a E_1^s$	0.0001	0.25	22	23	18	+ +
$E_1^f E_1^f$	0.000003	–	66	34	75	+
$E_1^f E_1^s$	0.000005	–	66	34	75	+
$E_1^s E_1^s$	0.00001	0	–	–	–	+ + +

(HARRIS, 1964; KALOW, 1964; KING and GRIFFIN, 1973; LEHMANN and LIDDELL, 1969)

suxamethonium is grossly prolonged to several hours (HART and MITCHELL, 1962). It is interesting to speculate on the likely mode, and speed, of elimination of the drug in such individuals. If suxamethonium is distributed evenly throughout the extracellular fluid (approximately 22% of body weight), normal glomerular filtration should eliminate the drug with a half-life of about 1 hr. The actual elimination may be accelerated somewhat by the drug's slight liability to spontaneous hydrolysis at physiological pH. Such observations are roughly consistent with the reported duration of apnoea (approximately 4 hrs).

Further phenotypes are suggested by tests with a variety of enzyme inhibitors, n-butanol (WHITTAKER, 1968a), chloride (WHITTAKER, 1968b, c) and urea (HANEL and MOGENSEN, 1971), though the full significance of these findings is as yet unclear.

The enzyme variants discussed so far arise from genes at a single locus E_1. A total of ten genotypes have been identified and their approximate frequencies in the population assessed. These frequencies are shown in Table 4, together with data for enzyme activity, for dibucaine, fluoride and suxamethonium members, and for the usual responses to suxamethonium *in vivo*. Frequencies of the various genotypes may vary slightly between different populations (KALOW, 1964), but many of them are so rare that accurate assessment of their frequencies is subject to considerable error. An unexpectedly high occurrence of atypical homozygotes has been found among Canadian mental hospital patients (KALOW and GUNN, 1959) and among leprosy patients in India (THOMAS and JOB, 1972). The validity of the latter observations is, however, suspect, as the phenotype frequencies reported do not fit the distribution to be expected on the basis of the HARDY-WEINBERG equilibrium (SMITH, 1972) and may therefore be an artifact.

Genotype studies of patients showing prolonged responses to suxamethonium do not always reveal recognisable enzyme abnormalities. Some relevant findings are summarised in Table 5. In each of these studies, approximately one third of the patients were of the common genotype $E_1^u E_1^u$. It is of course possible that central

Table 5. Cholinesterase genotypes of 437 cases of suxamethonium apnoea

Genotype	SIMPSON and KALOW (1966)	THOMPSON and WHITTAKER (1966)	LEHMANN and LIDDELL (1969)	WHITTAKER and VICKERS (1970)	BAULD et al. (1974)	all	%	Relative risk of suxamethonium apnoea[a]
$E_1^u E_1^u$	39	25	62	21	24	171	39	1
$E_1^u E_1^a$	11	10	12	1	10	44	10	7
$E_1^u E_1^f$	1	6	1	3	—	11	3	
$E_1^u E_1^s$	—	—	—	—	—	0	0	
$E_1^a E_1^a$	50	30	69	24	8	181	41	3000
$E_1^a E_1^f$	2	7	5	4	4	22	5	3700
$E_1^a E_1^s$	—	—	1	—	—	1	< 1	
$E_1^f E_1^f$	—	—	2	—	—	2	< 1	
$E_1^f E_1^s$	—	—	1	—	—	1	< 1	
$E_1^s E_1^s$	1	—	2	—	1	4	1	
	104	78	155	53	47	437		

[a] The relative risk of suxamethonium apnoea in four genotypes is calculated by reference to the genotype frequency indicated in Table 4.

nervous system depression may have led to prolonged apnoea in these patients, but in each study such a cause was thought to have been excluded. It is possible that some of the individuals may have been homozygotes for an enzyme of a particular chloride sensitivity recently implicated in similar circumstances (WHITTAKER, 1968 b). Further work in this field is clearly needed. In all threee studies, prolongation is reported among $E_1^u E_1^a$ and $E_1^u E_1^f$ heterozygotes, who should have possessed sufficient normal enzyme to hydrolyse the drug in a short time. Again, chloride inhibition studies are needed. On a theoretical basis, the risk of a prolonged response for any genotype can be calculated from the knowledge of the relative frequencies of occurrence and genotype distribution in the population. Such estimates are, however, subject to considerable error because of the rarity of some of the genotypes and because of variable reporting of incidents of prolonged drug effect. Values for relative risks in four of the genotypes (for which adequate numbers are available) are indicated in Table 5.

Cholinesterase variants determined by variations in genes at a second locus, E_2, have been detected by means of gel electrophoresis. However, the separation of isoenzymes in this manner has revealed little of importance about the action of suxamethonium. For further discussion the reader is referred to review articles by KALOW, 1964; LEHMANN and LIDDELL, 1969; LAMOTTA and WORONICK, 1971. One series of observations is pertinent, however. This concerns a family described by NEITLICH (1966), members of which show a high degree of resistance to the action of suxamethonium due to the presence of an abnormally active form of the enzyme. The gene, denoted $E_{\text{Cynthiana}}$, is probably a variant of the E_2^+ gene present in about 10% of the population, the enzyme for which can be separated as a fifth band (C_5) on electrophoresis. The C_5 variant is responsible for most instances of added cholinesterase activity, but in no other cases has actual suxamethonium resistance been reported.

X. Myopathy

Both the quantitative and qualitative responses to neuromuscular blocking drugs differ (from the normal) in patients suffering from various muscle diseases. These differences are discussed here in relation to the anatomical and physiological abnormalities known to be present in the diseases concerned and brief mention is made, where appropriate, of current theories about the aetiology of the conditions. For further details, however, the reader is advised to consult more specialised sources.

It is important to remember in anaesthetic practice that the action of drugs in patients suffering from disorders of voluntary muscles will vary, depending on the stage which the disease has reached and the treatment that the patient has received. Furthermore, if the disease has progressed more in some parts of the body than in others, as is often the case, it is inevitable that drug actions should show regional variation. This has important implications if tests of neuromuscular transmission and muscle function are applied in that such tests may not provide accurate indications of function in all parts of the body. The practical use of drugs during anaesthesia in patients suffering from various myopathies is reviewed by WISE (1963).

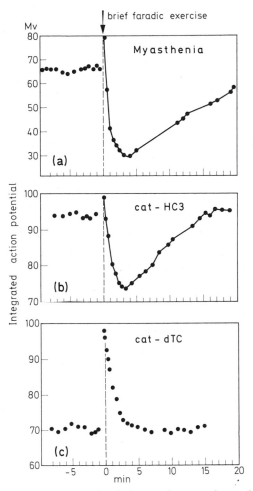

Fig. 23a—c. Influence of tetanic nerve stimulation on integrated muscle action potentials induced by twitch stimulation: (a) Conscious patient with myasthenia gravis. (b) Anesthetised cat under the influence of hemicholinium HC3. (c) Anesthetised cat under the influence of tubocurarine. (DESMEDT, 1958)

Myasthenia Gravis. Since the original description of the disease by BUZZARD in 1900 the functional and structural abnormalities involved in myasthenia gravis have been the subject of many investigations. For details, the reader is referred to extensive symposia on the subject (OSSERMAN, 1966; FIELDS, 1971).

It is currently thought that the disease is of autoimmune origin, an idea first proposed by SIMPSON (1960), and that antibodies are produced against end-plate receptors (LENNON and CARNEGIE, 1971). The proliferation of the motor nerve endings and the multiple innervation of end-plates (BICKERSTAFF and WOOLF, 1960; MACDERMOT, 1960) which follow may be compensatory (BROWNELL et al., 1972). Substance is given to this hypothesis by the recent indentification of a serum factor present in myasthenics which disappears following thymectomy (BACH et al., 1972), a procedure long known to benefit some of these patients. A further factor has now been found which inhibits α-bungarotoxin binding both by neuromuscular junctions of normal human subjects and by sarcolemmal membrane prepartions obtained from muscle biopsy specimens of patients with motor neurone disease (BENDER et al., 1975). In many cases the condition is greatly improved by the administration of prednisone (JENKINS, 1972) and it is likely that immunosuppressant therapy will be used widely in the future to supplement, or even supplant, the use of anticholinesterases which have been the mainstay of treatment for 40 years (WALKER, 1934).

The electromyographic response of myasthenic muscle to repeated stimulation of its motor nerve shows progressive impairment (HARVEY and MASLAND, 1941; JOHNS et al., 1955). Such changes resemble those seen in the normal subject under the influence of tubocurarine. Responses of the myasthenic muscle following tetanic stimulation are, however, somewhat different. DESMEDT (1958) showed that though there is a brief increase in post-tetanic response as found in partially curarised normal individuals or animals, the response of the myasthenic muscle is subsequently impaired for a long period (Fig. 23). DESMEDT pointet out that this sequence of events resembles that in the cat following administration of hemicholinium (HC3), an inhibitor of acetylcholine synthesis in the nerve ending (see Chapter 2). This suggests that transmitter availability is reduced in maysthenia, a finding which is in keeping with microelectrode studies of intercostal muscle which have shown that both the frequency (DALHBÄCK et al., 1961) as well as the magnitude (ELMQVIST et al., 1964) of m.e.p.p.s are much less than in normal muscle. Whether this indicates a primary disorder of the nerve endings or of the end-plate region is not clear.

The response of the myasthenic muscle to neuromuscular blocking drugs is consistent with the observation already made. There is a great increase in sensitivity to the action of competitive drugs and resistance to the action of the depolarising drugs. Increased sensitivity to tubocurarine was introduced as a diagnostic test of the disease by BENNETT and CASH (1943a and b) and that to gallamine by DUNDEE (1951). The degree of sensitivity appears to differ greatly between individuals, as would be expected, but can be 5 to 40 times greater than that in the normal subject (BENNETT and CASH, 1943b; PELIKAN et al., 1953). DUNDEE and GRAY (1951) showed that the response of myasthenic muscle to tubocurarine can decline following thymectomy, as judged by the respiratory response to a small test dose of the drug.

Resistance to the action of decamethonium was revealed by the studies of CHURCHILL-DAVIDSON and RICHARDSON (1952b, 1953), which showed that doses capable of producing substantial impairment of electromyographic responses in normal subjects induced little or no change in myasthenics (Fig. 24).

It would be expected that myasthenic muscle would be resistant to intra-arterially administered acetylcholine as it is to decamethonium. In fact the evidence is controversial (WILSON and STONER, 1947; BUCHTAL and ENGBAEK, 1948), possibly because many of the patients had been chronically treated with anticholinesterase drugs. Even when the treatment is discontinued for the test, the plasma or tissue cholinesterases may be partly inhibited, thus boosting the response to acetylcholine. Prolonged treatment with anticholinesterases can lead to a myasthenic crisis (ROWLAND et al., 1955), presumably due to depolarisation blockade produced by accumu-

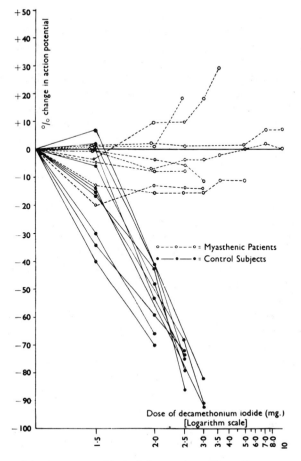

Fig. 24. Impairment of electromyographic twitch response of hypothenar muscles to ulnar nerve stimulation by decamethonium in normal and myasthenic conscious subjects. Myasthenics show resistance to the action of the drug. (CHURCHILL-DAVIDSON and RICHARDSON, 1952 b)

lating acetylcholine. This condition has been shown to resolve in time providing anticholinesterase therapy is withdrawn, tubocurarine administered and artificial respiration performed (CHURCHILL-DAVIDSON and RICHARDSON, 1957).

Ocular Myopathy. Increased sensitivity to tubocurarine has also been reported in ocular myopathy (ROSS, 1963). The response to decamethonium, however, is normal (ROSS, 1964) and anticholinesterase therapy is not beneficial (JACOB and VARKEY, 1966). This rare but interesting condition seems unlikely to be a local manifestation of myasthenia gravis since the drug responses differ. The unique multiple innervation of some of the extra-ocular muscle fibres (DIETERT, 1965), however, raises the possibility that the two conditions might involve different types of end-plate. Clearly, further study is warranted.

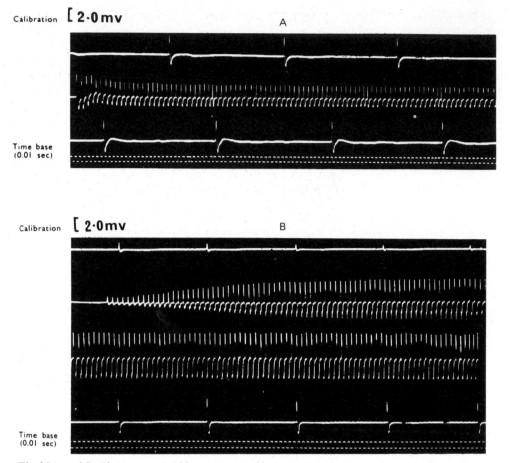

Fig. 25A and B. Electromyographic responses of hypothenar muscles to ulnar nerve stimulation in conscious subjects. (A) Myasthenia gravis. (B) Myasthenic syndrome. (WISE, 1962)

Myasthenic Syndrome. The generalised muscle weakness found in some patients with oat-cell carcinoma of the bronchus, referred to as the myasthenic syndrome (EATON and LAMBERT, 1957), is of unknown origin. It is associated with undue fatiguability and in anaesthetic practice respiratory arrest may be produced by small doses both of competitive and depolarising neuromuscular blocking drugs (ANDERSON et al., 1953).

Detailed electromyographic studies by WISE (1962) have revealed fundamental differences between myasthenia gravis and the myasthenic syndrome. Some of the results are illustrated in Fig. 25. In myasthenia gravis, twitch stimulation produces a response of reasonable magnitude but there is fade on tetanic stimulation and some post-tetanic restoration may occur. In the myasthenic syndrome, on the other hand, the initial response is of very low voltage but on tetanic stimulation there is a progressive increase in successive responses which, after a few seconds, reach normal size. Post-tetanic responses remain large for a few seconds but subsequently they decline and later on there is post-tetanic exhaustion. The studies made by WISE are in agreement with the earlier studies of ANDERSON et al. (1953) and indicate undue sensitivity to both competitive and depolarising neuromuscular blocking drugs.

It is clear that transmission failure in the myasthenic syndrome is different from that in myasthenia gravis and it is interesting to speculate on its possible aetiology. The increase in size of the compound action potential during tetanic stimulation indicates increasing release of transmitter from the nerve endings, and suggests that the primary fault lies in failure of release. The finding is somewhat analogous to that produced by excess magnesium or by botulinum toxin in animals (MASLAND and GAMMON, 1949). It is tempting to suggest that the myasthenic syndrome is produced by a circulating substance, secreted by the tumour, which impairs acetylcholine release. Further investigation is needed.

Myotonia. In a number of the rarer myopathies the administration of suxamethonium induces a prolonged contraction of muscle fibres instead of the usual flaccid paralysis. This has been shown to be common in cases of Dystrophia myotonica and Myotonia congenita (ÖRNDAHL, 1962) but it also occurs in Amyotrophic lateral sclerosis and as a local response in patients with unilateral brachial plexus nerve lesions a contracture occurs in the affected arm (ÖRNDAHL and STERNBERG, 1962; BRIM, 1973). Many cases have been reviewed by THIEL (1967). The exact reason for these responses is unclear.

Malignant Hyperpyrexia. This is a rare but potentially fatal complication of general anaesthesia which occurs both in patients known to have myopathy and also in occasional individuals who show no signs of myopathy. Some cases appear to be hereditary in origin while others are not. The condition can be precipitated by administration of suxamethonium (CODY, 1968), but in many cases anaesthesia alone, particularly with halothane, appears to be responsible. As soon as the triggering drug has been administered widespread muscle rigidity occurs and there is a considerable increase in heat production by muscle which may cause fatal hyperpyrexia unless the heat can be dissipated by deliberate cooling techniques. Inevitably there is progressive muscle damage with consequent high serum levels of creatine phosphokinase, phosphate and potassium, and severe acidosis occurs.

It is inappropriate here to discuss in detail the aetiology of malignant hyperpyrexia, which is complex and varies between cases. For details of its occurrence, discussion of its aetiology and of the structural and biochemical abnormalities involved the reader is referred to recent publications (FURNISS, 1971; ELLIS et al., 1972; RELTON et al., 1973; KYEI-MENSAH et al., 1973; ELLIS et al., 1973; BRADLEY et al., 1973; PENNINGTON and WORSFOLD, 1973), and to two detailed pharmacological and biochemical studies of muscle biopsy material from affected individuals (BRITT et al., 1973; MOULDS and DENBOROUGH, 1974). These latter studies have revealed three consistent abnormalities. First, the muscle fibres show microscopic peculiarities of various sorts and unusually large variability in fibre diameter. Secondly, isolated fibres *in vitro* respond to suxamethonium, halothane and caffeine with a sustained contracture although very high concentrations of the drugs are required. Thirdly, the sarcoplasmic reticulum shows impaired ability to bind calcium, particularly in the presence of halothane. It seems likely that this latter is the primary abnormality and that failure of calcium binding results in high myoplasmic calcium concentrations which then trigger the chemical and contractile responses found. The relatives of patients who have developed hyperpyrexia (BRITT et al., 1969) often show evidence of myopathy and may have raised serum levels of muscle enzymes (DENBOROUGH et al., 1970). Such individuals should not be given general anaesthetics if this can possibly be avoided.

Muscle fibres of susceptible individuals, stimulated to contract with halothane or caffeine *in vitro*, are relaxed by high concentrations of procaine (MOULDS and DENBOROUGH, 1972). Preliminary reports indicate that administration of this drug in large doses, together with bicarbonate to correct acidosis, may alleviate the condition in some instances (HÖIVIK and STOVNER, 1975). Whether this results from a specific action on the muscle or from increased heat loss induced by cutaneous vasodilatation is not clear at present.

E. Other Actions of Neuromuscular Blocking Drugs

I. Histamine Release

In animals many neuromuscular blocking drugs release histamine from its binding sites (see the review by PATON, 1957, for full discussion). Evidence that the same drugs can release histamine in man comes from three sources. First, tubocurarine produces cutaneous vasodilatation and wheals when injected intradermally or intra-arterially (COMROE and DRIPPS, 1946; GROB et al., 1947; MONGAR and WHELAN, 1953). Secondly, these cutaneous effects are reduced by prior treatment of the subjects with anti-histamines such as pyribenzamine (GROB et al., 1947) and mepyramine (SMITH, 1957). Thirdly, in the human arm intra-arterial administration of tubocurarine in large doses (10 to 50 mg) causes a rise in plasma histamine content (up to 190 ng/ml) in the venous blood draining the area (MONGAR and WHELAN, 1953). In concentrations which produce equivalent neuromuscular block dimethyltubocurarine, gallamine, laudexium, suxamethonium and decamethonium may produce cutaneous vasodilatation and wheals but they are much less potent than tubocurarine in this respect (COLLIER and MACAULEY, 1952; SNIPER, 1953; SMITH, 1957).

There seems no doubt, therefore, that these drugs can release histamine under certain experimental conditions. Evidence that they do so in clinical practice, however, is largely circumstantial. Intravenous administration of tubocurarine, the most potent histamine-releaser, may produce cutaneous flushing (McDOWALL and CLARKE, 1969) but wheals rarely occur, except occasionally at the site of injection (SMITH, 1957). Inconsistent changes in plasma histamine concentration have been reported (WESTGATE and VAN BERGEN, 1962). Increases in airway resistance, interpreted as indicating bronchoconstriction in response to liberated histamine, occasionally occur following the administration of tubocurarine to anaesthetised patients (LANDMESSER et al., 1952; WESTGATE et al., 1962; GERBERSHAGEN and BERGMAN, 1967). The changes produced are slight and in most instances of short duration. Reports of patients developing long-lasting respiratory obstructive changes, such as one of the cases described by WESTGATE et al. (1962), suggest the presence of mucous plugs in the bronchi.

Transient hypotension following the clinical administration of tubocurarine is common (THOMAS, 1957) and may be due to histamine release, ganglion blockade and/or a reduction in venous return to the heart due to muscle paralysis or to intermittent positive pressure ventilation of the subjects; it may also be due to one of the other drugs administered during anaesthesia. Very severe hypotensive responses have been described, sometimes with widespread erythema and an increase in haematocrit (SALEM et al., 1968), changes which are highly suggestive of histamine release occurring in particularly susceptible subjects. Gallamine (KENNEDY and FARMAN, 1968) and alcuronium (TAMMISTO and WELLING, 1969; COLEMAN et al., 1972) can also produce hypotension, presumably for the same reason. Unfortunately there has been no controlled study of the effect of antihistamine agents on the hypotension produced by neuromuscular blocking drugs.

As far as histamine release is concerned, the reports on pancuronium are conflicting. In man, there are two case reports of severe bronchoconstriction (BUCKLAND and AVERY, 1973; HEATH, 1973). In animals, however, pancuronium does not cause histamine release (BUCKETT et al., 1968). On the other hand, there is good agreement on the effect of pancuronium on blood pressure. Hypotension does not occur in animals or man, and the administration of pancuronium is usually followed by a small rise in blood pressure (LOH, 1970; KELMAN and KENNEDY, 1971; COLEMAN et al., 1972).

A considerable discrepancy appears to exist between the concentration of neuromuscular blocking drugs which can produce histamine release on intradermal testing and that which is likely to be found in the plasma when the drugs are administered clinically by intravenous injection. PATON (1959) has pointed out that when drugs are rapidly injected intravenously a slug or bolus effect may occur because mixing of the drug solution with the whole blood volume is slow and may take about 5 circulation times to complete (FLEXNER et al., 1948). A concentration of the drug in the plasma sufficiently large to release histamine may therefore exist transiently during the first circulation or so. The marked variation which appears to exist between individuals is possibly determined not only by the susceptibility of the individual but also by the rate at which the drugs are injected.

II. Cardiovascular Actions

This section is concerned with the direct influence of neuromuscular blocking drugs on the cardiovascular system. Transient hypotension, with or without reflex tachycardia, is a common sequel to the administration of tubocurarine and other drugs. Although this effect may be in part a consequence of histamine release, animal studies indicate that these agents can also cause ganglion blockade, sometimes preceded by transient ganglion stimulation. Whether this occurs in man is not certain. Pancuronium is unique among the competitive neuromuscular blocking drugs in causing an increase in systemic blood pressure, tachycardia and a fall in central venous pressure, and these effects might be the result of ganglionic stimulation (KELMAN and KENNEDY, 1971; COLEMAN et al., 1972; NIGHTINGALE and BUSH, 1973).

Gallamine is known to cause tachycardia in anaesthetised patients, and the suggestion has been made that this effect is due to its atropine-like action. It is almost impossible to accept some of the evidence for this assertion, however, because of the number of drugs administered concurrently to the subjects under investigation. This is well illustrated by the type of experiment reported by KENNEDY and FARMAN (1968) who gave to all their subjects papaveretum, hyoscine, thiopentone, nitrous oxide, trichloroethylene and tubocurarine before the test-doses of gallamine.

In a study of dose-response relationships in a group of 48 anaesthetised subjects, EISELE et al. (1971) observed that heart rates of about 100/min were obtained with single intravenous doses of 100 mg of gallamine and that above this dose no further increases in heart rate occurred. In each subject, however, atropine produced a further increase in rate to about 125/min. It is therefore apparent that vagal blockade by gallamine is always submaximal. The reason for this is obscure.

In the absence of atropine premedication, suxamethonium causes bradycardia, sometimes associated with a variety of transient arrhythmias (LEIGH et al., 1957; CRAYTHORNE et al., 1960b; LUPPRIAN and CHURCHILL-DAVIDSON, 1960). This appears to occur quite frequently in children, but in both adults and children the effect is particularly associated with repeated administration of the drug. Much discussion has focussed on the origin of this effect which is usually explained as an acetylcholine-like action exerted directly on the heart. Early work by WILLIAMS et al. (1961) indicated that bradycardia was likely to occur only if repeated doses were given within a critical time interval of 2 to 5 min, a finding which is inconsistent with simple summation of responses. The authors also reported that the administration of thiopentone and diethylether would prevent the response. Subsequent work has shown that the bradycardia can also be prevented by competitive neuromuscular blocking agents such as tubocurarine, alcuronium and pancuronium (MATTHIAS et al., 1970), by hexafluorenium (SCHOENSTADT and WHITCHER, 1963) and by ganglion blockade with trimetaphan (WILLIAMS et al., 1961). MATTHIAS et al. (1970) suggested that the bradycardia is brought about by reflex activity, possibly initiated by stimulation of vagal afferents in the carotid body. The critical timing of suxamethonium doses and the inhibitory effect of competitive blocking drugs, however, indicate that other factors are also involved. The most likely explanation is that the second dose of suxamethonium exerts a greater effect on the heart because of the hyperkalaemia induced by the first dose (see next Section) which reaches its maximum about 2 to 3 min after the injection of suxamethonium. It is pertinent to comment that in the experiments described by MATTHIAS et al. the competitive blocking agents were administered before, rather than after, the first dose of suxamethonium; information on the effect of reversing the order of the two types of drugs would strengthen the suggestion. Unfortunately an early attempt to test the hypothesis that potassium was involved (WILLIAMS et al., 1961) did not help greatly because it failed to demonstrate consistent changes in serum potassium. Suxamethonium produces other effects on peripheral blood vessels (HALLDIN et al., 1959; GRAF et al., 1963) and on the uterus (FELTON and GODDARD, 1966), which are almost certainly muscarinic in origin.

III. Suxamethonium and Hyperkalaemia

Depolarisation of the end-plate followed by muscle contraction results in the efflux of intracellular potassium ions into the extracellular space. In man, as in animals, the magnitude of this efflux is sufficient for potassium to enter the venous blood, thus causing detectable increases in plasma potassium concentrations. GROB et al. (1957) were able to demonstrate small but consistent increases of about 0.25 mmol/l in

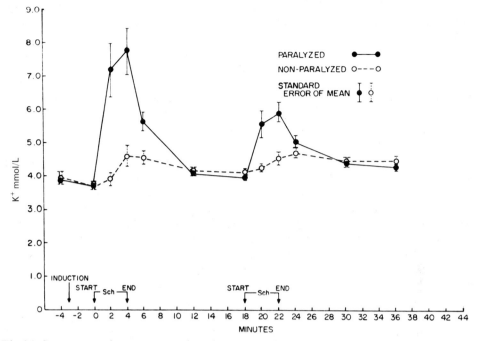

Fig. 26. Serum potassium concentrations in venous blood from paralysed and non-paralysed limbs of previously injured patients following administration of suxamethonium 1 mg/kg under anaesthesia. Points represent mean concentrations ($\pm$S.E.) for 7 patients. (TOBEY et al., 1972)

plasma obtained from venous blood draining the arm following contractions of the thenar muscles induced by electrical stimulation of the ulnar nerve. Depolarisation produced by suxamethonium has a similar, though usually somewhat larger, effect. Increases of 0.4 to 0.6 mmol/l have been reported (PATON, 1959; MAZZE et al., 1969; WEINTRAUB et al., 1969) but it is unusual for plasma potassium concentrations (normally 3.8 to 5.0 mmol/l) to rise above 5 to 5.5 mmol/l. This level is insufficient to cause untoward cardiac effects. Predictably, the hyperkalaemic response to suxamethonium is antagonised by prior administration of tubocurarine which reduces or abolishes the depolarisation produced by suxamethonium (WEINTRAUB et al., 1969).

Interest in suxamethonium-induced hyperkalaemia has increased in recent years following reports of cardiac arrest after the administration of the drug to patients with neurological injuries or with severe burns. THOMAS (1969), for example, described a neurologically injured patient in whom suxamethonium raised the plasma potassium concentration to 7.2 mmol/l, with associated electrocardiographic changes (T-wave peaking) and subsequent ventricular tachycardia. A higher figure has been reported in a hemiplegic subject (COOPERMAN et al., 1970) and in one paraplegic patient, with severe spinal cord injuries, the extraordinary level of 13.6 mmol/l was recorded (TOBEY, 1970). BIRCH et al. (1969) have reviewed a number of similar cases involving various degrees of hyperkalaemia occurring at different times after injury. Predictably, in patients with unilateral injury, suxamethonium causes hyperkalaemia on the affected side only (TOBEY et al., 1972). Twenty-three anaesthetised patients

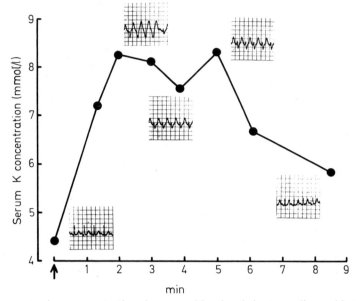

Fig. 27. Serum potassium concentrations in venous blood and electrocardiographic tracings from an anaesthetised patient 45 days after severe burn injury at intervals following administration of suxamethonium 60 mg. (TOLMIE et al., 1967)

with peripheral nerve injuries and muscle paralysis were studied. Three venous catheters were inserted percutaneously: one for sampling blood draining a limb with atrophied muscles, a second for sampling blood from a normal limb, and a third elsewhere for the administration of drugs. After suxamethonium (1 mg/kg infused intravenously at a constant rate during a 4 min period), the concentration of potassium in the venous blood draining the paralysed limbs was much greater than that in the blood draining the nonparalysed ones. Figure 26 shows these results. Electrocardiographic changes suggestive of hyperkalaemia have been found also in a paralysed patient following the administration of suxamethonium a few months after an attack of poliomyelitis (author's observation). A common feature of all the epidoses of hyperkalaemia described is that several weeks had elapsed between the time of injury and the adverse response to suxamethonium. During the early stages after the injury suxamethonium was administered uneventfully (MAZZE et al., 1969). It is therefore likely that the increased potassium loss from the muscles is related to the increased area of muscle membrane which is depolarised by the drug during the period of denervation supersensitivity (see Chapter 4 A). The more extensive the denervation, the greater the hyperkalaemic response to suxamethonium. It is not surprising, therefore, that most cases of cardiac arrest have involved extensive neurological involvement of the lower, rather than the upper, limbs because of the large mass of muscle tissue involved.

It has long been recognised that suxamethonium is liable to produce cardiac arrest in severly burned patients. BUSH et al. (1962), reviewing a number of such reported incidents, suggested that cardiac arrest was the result of enhanced vagal activity, though why this should occur particularly in the burned subject was not clear. It was later suggested (BUSH, 1964; BELIN and KARLEEN, 1966) that the effect of suxamethonium might be increased in these subjects by loss of plasma cholinesterase, by hypovolaemia and by metabolic acidosis secondary to the injury. Though such factors may contribute to the risk of cardiac arrest, it is apparent that the main one is hyperkalaemia. TOLMIE et al. (1967) have shown most elegantly (Fig. 27) the coincidence of electrocardiographic changes with alterations in serum potassium following suxamethonium administration to a severely burned patient. Similar observations have been made by SCHANER et al. (1969), who have found that severe hyperkalaemia does not occur until between 25 and 60 days have elapsed since the injury. It seems likely therefore that denervation supersensitivity is again involved, and that the muscle loss of potassium is not merely a consequence of leakage through muscle membranes injured at the time of the burn. The exact cause of the change is not clear, however, and most of these cases lack definite evidence of denervation changes.

Hyperkalaemic responses have also been found in patients with encephalitis (COWGILL et al., 1974), with tetanus and with uraemia (ROTH and WÜTHRICH, 1969).

IV. Ocular Actions

In some individuals the clinical administration of suxamethonium causes a rise in intra-ocular pressure lasting for a few minutes. Consequently, there is a risk of vitreous body expulsion or retinal damage or both in patients undergoing open ocular surgery for cataract, glaucoma or penetrating injury. The original observations in this field were made by HOFMANN and HOLZER (1953) soon after the introduction of the drug into clinical use. These authors were careful to point out that in ocular surgery failure of proper respiratory control might exacerbate the condition because both hypoxia and hypercarbia are capable of inducing an increase in intra-ocular pressure. In practice, therefore, it is hardly surprising that the studies in this field, using both tonometric and manometric recording techniques, have revealed wide differences between individuals (LINCOFF et al., 1955; CRAYTHORNE et al., 1960a; ROBERTSON and GIBSON, 1968). Such variability could arise, at least in part, from differences in the extent to which the subjects were ventilated, prior to, or during, the action of suxamethonium. LINCOFF et al. (1955), for example, in their study of 73 patients found rises in intra-ocular pressure of 20 mmHg or more in 7 subjects but of less than 10 mm Hg in 43, while ROBERTSON and GIBSON (1968) found no change at all in 7 of their 30 subjects. Decamethonium has been found to induce similar pressure increases (MAIER and CLARK, 1965) while tubocurarine causes a reduction in intra-ocular pressure (HOFMANN and HOLZER, 1953).

Suxamethonium and decamethonium are thought to increase intra-ocular pressure because of their effect on the extra-ocular muscles. HOFMANN and HOLZER (1953) observed that suxamethonium caused fixed divergence of the eyes and DILLON et al. (1957) have demonstrated that isolated preparations of human external ocular muscle respond to the drug with sustained contraction (contracture). An external ocular muscle, when detached from its insertion on the eye in the course of operation for strabismus, will undergo contracture for several minutes, producing

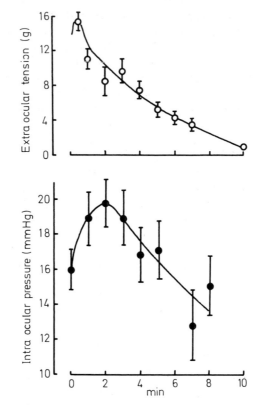

Fig. 28. Extra-ocular muscle tension (g) and intra-ocular pressure (mm Hg) (mean±S.E.) of an-aesthetised patients following administration of suxamethonium. (Data from Kaufman, 1967)

tension of up to 24 g (Fig. 28; Kaufman, 1967). Clearly this is quite sufficient to raise the intra-ocular pressure by the amounts which have been recorded, and it is appar-ently also sufficient to cause measurable degrees of enophthalmos (Björk et al., 1957). Electromyographic recordings *in vivo* by means of needle electrodes inserted in the external rectus muscle have shown almost complete absence of electrical activity (Björk et al., 1957); this again is characteristic of muscle contracture (see Chapter 4 A).

A sustained contraction in response to depolarising drugs is characteristic of muscle fibres which are multiply innervated, and indeed electron microscopic and histochemical studies demonstrate that these muscles do contain a percentage of fibres with multiple innervation (Dietert, 1965; and present volume, Chapter 1). In this respect ocular muscle is unique. Perhaps the variation in response to suxame-thonium *in vivo* may therefore depend on the proportion of multiply innervated fibres.

Prior administration of competitive neuromuscular blocking drugs antagonises the rise in intra-ocular pressure caused by suxamethonium (Miller et al., 1968), as does an increase in the depth of anaesthesia (Craythorne et al., 1960a). Hexafluorenium also prevents the response (SOBEL, 1962; KATZ et al., 1968) presumably because of its weak competitive blocking action at the neuromuscular junction.

All the evidence quoted indicates that the rise in intraocular pressure which follows the administration of depolarising drugs is due to their action on the extra-ocular muscles. In support of this, LINCOFF et al. (1955) quote one set of observations in which an intial dose of suxamethonium raised the intra-ocular pressure by 11 mm Hg but subsequent larger doses, given after cutting all the external muscles from their insertions prior to enucleation of the eye, caused intra-ocular pressure rises of 2 to 4 mm Hg only. Nonetheless it is often suggested that other effects like systemic hypertension, transient stimulation of cervical sympathetic ganglia and contraction of intra-ocular muscle, may play a part in the response. The brief time-course of events makes these hypotheses untenable, because vascular changes could affect intra-ocular pressure only by altering secretion or filtration of the aqueous humor, a process which would take much too long to influence pressure within the few minutes involved. Furthermore, contraction of the intraocular muscles in re-sponse to a muscarinic action of suxamethonium would lower pressure by opening the irido-corneal angle and increasing drainage of aqueous humor. It therefore seems unlikely that such factors are of any great importance.

References

AGOSTON, S., VERMEER, G. A., KERSTEN, U. W., MEIJER, D. K. F.: The fate of pancuronium bromide in man. Acta anaesth. scand. **17**, 267—275 (1973).

ALADJEMOFF, L., DIKSTEIN, S., SHAFRIR, E.: The binding of *d*-tubocurarine chloride to plasma proteins. J. Pharmacol. exp. Ther. **123**, 43—47 (1958).

ALI, H. H., UTTING, J. E., GRAY, T. C.: Quantitative assessment of residual antidepolarizing block (Part I). Brit. J. Anaesth. **43**, 473—477 (1971).

ANDERSON, H. J., CHURCHILL-DAVIDSON, H. C., RICHARDSON, A. T.: Bronchial neoplasm with myasthenia. Prolonged apnoea after administration of succinylcholine. Lancet **1953 II**, 1291—1293.

ANTOPOL, W., TUCHMAN, L., SCHIFRIN, A.: Choline-esterase activity of human sera, with special reference to hyperthyroidism. Proc. Soc. exp. Biol. (N.Y.) **36**, 46—50 (1937).

ARTUSIO, J. F., MARBURY, B. E., CREWS, M. A.: A quantitative study of *d*-tubocurarine, tri-(diethyl-aminoethoxy)1,2,3 benzene (Flaxedil) and a series of tri-methyl and dimethylethyl-ammonium compounds in anesthetized man. Ann. N.Y. Acad. Sci. **54**, 512—527 (1951).

BACH, J.-F., DARDENNE, M., PAPIERNIK, M., BAROIS, A., LEVASSEUR, P., LE BRIGAND, H.: Evidence for a serum-factor secreted by the human thymus. Lancet **1972 II**, 1056—1058.

BARAKA, A.: The influence of carbon dioxide on the neuromuscular block caused by tubocurarine chloride in the human subject. Brit. J. Anaesth. **36**, 272—278 (1964).

BARAKA, A.: Effect of carbon dioxide on gallamine and suxamethonium block in man. Brit. J. Anaesth. **39**, 786—788 (1967).

BARAKA, A.: Effect of halothane on tubocurarine and suxamethonium block in man. Brit. J. Anaesth. **40**, 602—606 (1968).

BARAKA, A., GABALI, F.: Correlation between tubocurarine requirements and plasma protein pattern. Brit. J. Anaesth. **40**, 89—93 (1968).

BARNES, J. M., DAVIES, D. R.: Blood cholinesterase levels in workers exposed to organo-phospho-rus insecticides. Brit. med. J. **1951 II**, 816—819.

BAULD, H. W., GIBSON, P. F., JEBSON, P. T., BROWN, S. S.: Aetiology of prolonged apnoea after suxamethonium. Brit. J. Anaesth. **46**, 273—281 (1974).

BELIN, R. P., KARLEEN, C. I.: Cardiac arrest in the burned patient following succinyldicholine administration. Anesthesiology **27**, 516—518 (1966).

BELLVILLE, J. W., COHEN, E. N., HAMILTON, J.: The interaction of morphine and d-tubocurarine on respiration and grip strength in man. Clin. Pharmacol. Ther. **5**, 35—43 (1964).

BENDER, A. N., RINGEL, S. P., ENGEL, W. K., DANIELS, M. P., VOGEL, Z.: Myasthenia gravis: a serum factor blocking acetylcholine receptors of the human neuromuscular junction. Lancet **1975 I**, 607—609.

BENNETT, A. E., CASH, P. T.: Myasthenia gravis and curare sensitivity. Dis. nerv. Syst. **4**, 299—301 (1943 a).

BENNETT, A. E., CASH, P. T.: Myasthenia gravis—curare sensitivity; a new diagnostic test and approach to causation. Arch. Neurol. Psychiat. (Chic.) **49**, 537—547 (1943 b).

BENNIKE, K.-A., JARNUM, S.: Myoglobinuria with acute renal failure possibly induced by suxamethonium. Brit. J. Anaesth. **36**, 730—736 (1964).

BICKERSTAFF, E. R., WOOLF, A. L.: The intramuscular nerve endings in myasthenia gravis. Brain **83**, 10—23 (1960).

BIRCH, A. A., MITCHELL, G. D., PLAYFORD, G. A., LANG, C. A.: Changes in serum potassium response to succinylcholine following trauma. J. Amer. med. Ass. **210**, 490—493 (1969).

BJÖRK, Å., HALLDIN, M., WAHLIN, Å.: Enophthalmos elicited by succinylcholine. Some observations on the effect of succinylcholine and noradrenaline on the intraorbital muscles studied in man and experimental animals. Acta anaesth. scand. **1**, 41—53 (1957).

BODMAN, R. I.: Evaluation of two synthetic curarizing agents in conscious volunteers. Brit. J. Pharmacol. **7**, 409—416 (1952).

BORDERS, R. W., STEPHEN, C. R., NOWILL, W. K., MARTIN, R.: The interrelationship of succinylcholine and the blood cholinesterases during anesthesia. Anesthesiology **16**, 401—422 (1955).

BOTELHO, S. Y., CANDER, L.: Post-tetanic potentiation before and during ischemia in intact human skeletal muscle. J. appl. Physiol. **6**, 221—228 (1953).

BOURNE, J. G., COLLIER, H. O. J., SOMERS, G. F.: Succinylcholine (succinoylcholine). Muscle relaxant of short duration. Lancet **1952 I**, 1225—1229.

BRADLEY, W. G., WARD, M., MURCHISON, D., HALL, L., WOOLF, N.: Clinical, electrophysiological and pathological studies on malignant hyperpyrexia. Proc. roy. Soc. Med. **66**, 67—68 (1973).

BRAZIL, O. V., CORRADO, A. P.: The curariform action of streptomycin. J. Pharmacol. exp. Ther. **120**, 452—459 (1957).

BRENNAN, H. J.: Dual action of suxamethonium chloride. Brit. J. Anaesth. **28**, 159—168 (1956).

BRIDENBAUGH, P. O., CHURCHILL-DAVIDSON, H. C., CHURCHER, M. D.: Effects of carbon dioxide on actions of d-tubocurarine and gallamine. Curr. Res. Anesth. **45**, 804—809 (1966).

BRIM, V. D.: Denervation supersensitivity: the response to depolarizing muscle relaxants. Brit. J. Anaesth. **45**, 222—226 (1973).

BRITT, B. A., KALOW, W., GORDON, A., HUMPHREY, J. G., REWCASTLE, N. B.: Malignant hyperthermia: an investigation of five patients. Canad. Anaesth. Soc. J. **20**, 431—467 (1973).

BRITT, B. A., LOCHER, W. G., KALOW, W.: Hereditary aspects of malignant hyperthermia. Canad. Anaesth. Soc. J. **16**, 89—98 (1969).

BROOKS, D. K., FELDMAN, S. A.: Metabolic acidosis. A new approach to "neostigmine resistant curarisation". Anaesthesia **17**, 161—169 (1962).

BROWN, M. C., MATTHEWS, P. B. C.: The effect on a muscle twitch of the back-response of its motor nerve fibres. J. Physiol. (Lond.) **150**, 332—346 (1960).

BROWNELL, B., OPPENHEIMER, D. R., SPALDING, J. M. K.: Neurogenic muscle atrophy in myasthenia gravis. J. Neurol. Neurosurg. Psychiat. **35**, 311—322 (1972).

BUCHTAL, F., ENGBAEK, L.: On the neuromuscular transmission in normal and myasthenic subjects. Acta Psychiat. (Kbh.) **23**, 3—11 (1948).

BUCKETT, W. R., MARJORIBANKSE, C. E. B., MARWICK, F. A., MORTON, M. B.: The pharmacology of pancuronium bromide (ORG.NA 97) a new potent steroidal neuromuscular blocking agent. Brit. J. Pharmacol. **32**, 671—682 (1968).

BUCKLAND, R. W., AVERY, A. F.: Histamine release following pancuronium: a case report. Brit. J. Anaesth. **45**, 518—521 (1973).

BULLOUGH, J.: Suxamethonium paralysis reversed by edrophonium. Lancet **1957 II**, 804.

BUSH, G. H.: The use of muscle relaxants in burnt children. Anaesthesia **19**, 231—238 (1964).

BUSH, G. H., GRAHAM, H. A. P., LITTLEWOOD, A. H. M., SCOTT, L. B.: Danger of suxamethonium and endotracheal intubation in anaesthesia for burns. Brit. med. J. **1962 II**, 1081—1085.

BUSH, G. H., STEAD, A. L.: The use of D-tubocurarine in neonatal anaesthesia. Brit. J. Anaesth. **34**, 721—728 (1962).

BUZZARD, T.: Myasthenia gravis pseudo-paralytica. Brit. med. J. **1900 I**, 493—496.

CALLAWAY, S., DAVIES, D. R., RUTLAND, J. P.: Blood cholinesterase levels and range of personal variation in a healthy adult population. Brit. med. J. **1951 II**, 812—816.

CALVERT, J., LEHMANN, H., SILK, E., SLACK, W. K.: Prolonged apnoea after suxamethonium. A case study of pseudocholinesterase. Lancet **1954 II**, 354—356.

CAMPBELL, E. J. M., GODFREY, S., CLARK, T. J. H., FREEDMAN, S., NORMAN, J.: The effect of muscular paralysis induced by tubocurarine on the duration and sensation of breath-holding during hypercapnia. Clin. Sci. **36**, 323—328 (1969).

CANNARD, T. H., ZAIMIS, E.: The effect of lowered muscle temperature on the action of neuromuscular blocking drugs in man. J. Physiol. (Lond.) **149**, 112—119 (1959).

CHAN, C. S., YEUNG, M. L.: Anaphylactic reaction to alcuronium. Brit. J. Anaesth. **44**, 103—105 (1972).

CHRISTIE, T. H., WISE, R. P., CHURCHILL-DAVIDSON, H. C.: Hexamethylene 1—6 biscarbaminoylcholine bromide, a new synthetic muscle relaxant. Lancet **1959 II**, 648—650.

CHURCHILL-DAVIDSON, H. C.: Suxamethonium (succinylcholine) chloride and muscle pains. Brit. med. J. **1954 I**, 74—75.

CHURCHILL-DAVIDSON, H. C., CHRISTIE, T. H.: The diagnosis of neuromuscular block in man. Brit. J. Anaesth. **31**, 290—301 (1959).

CHURCHILL-DAVIDSON, H. C., CHRISTIE, T. H., WISE, R. P.: Dual neuromuscular block in man. Anesthesiology **21**, 144—149 (1960).

CHURCHILL-DAVIDSON, H. C., GRIFFITHS, W. J.: Simple test-paper method for the clinical determination of plasma pseudocholinesterase. Brit. med. J. **1961 II**, 994—995.

CHURCHILL-DAVIDSON, H. C., RICHARDSON, A. T.: Decamethonium iodide (C 10): some observations on its action using electromyography. Proc. roy. Soc. Med. **45**, 179—185 (1952a).

CHURCHILL-DAVIDSON, H. C., RICHARDSON, A. T.: The action of decamethonium iodide (C 10) in myasthenia gravis. J. Neurol. Neurosurg. Psychiat. **15**, 129—133 (1952b).

CHURCHILL-DAVIDSON, H. C., RICHARDSON, A. T.: Neuromuscular transmission in myasthenia gravis. J. Physiol. (Lond.) **122**, 252—263 (1953).

CHURCHILL-DAVIDSON, H. C., RICHARDSON, A. T.: Myasthenic crisis. Therapeutic use of *d*-tubocurarine. Lancet **1957 I**, 1221—1224.

CHURCHILL-DAVIDSON, H. C., WAY, W. L., DE JONG, R. H.: The muscle relaxants and renal excretion. Anesthesiology **28**, 540—546 (1967).

CHURCHILL-DAVIDSON, H. C., WISE, R. P.: Neuromuscular transmission in the newborn infant. Anesthesiology **24**, 271—278 (1963).

CODY, J. R.: Muscle rigidity following administration of succinylcholine. Anesthesiology **29**, 159—162 (1968).

COHEN, E. N.: Thiopental-curare-nitrous oxide anesthesia for Cesarian section 1950—1960. Curr. Res. Anesth. **41**, 122—127 (1962).

COHEN, E. N.: Fluorescent analysis of *d*-tubocurarine hydrochloride. J. Lab. clin. Med. **61**, 338—345 (1963).

COHEN, E. N., BREWER, H. W., SMITH, D.: The metabolism and elimination of *d*-tubocurarine — H^3. Anesthesiology **28**, 309—317 (1967).

COHEN, E. N., CORBASCIO, A., FLEISCHLI, G.: The distribution and fate of *d*-tubocurarine. J. Pharmacol. exp. Ther. **147**, 120—129 (1965).

COHEN, P. J., HEISTERKAMP, D. V., SKOVSTED, P.: The effect of general anaesthetics on the response to tetanic stimulus in man. Brit. J. Anaesth. **42**, 543—547 (1970).

COLEMAN, A. J., DOWNING, J. W., LEARY, W. P., MOYES, D. G., STYLES, M.: The immediate cardiovascular effects of pancuronium, alcuronium and tubocurarine in man. Anaesthesia **27**, 415—422 (1972).

COLLIER, C.: Suxamethonium pains and fasciculations. Proc. roy. Soc. Med. **68**, 105—108 (1975).

COLLIER, H. O. J., MACAULEY, B.: The pharmacological properties of "Laudolissin"—a long-acting curarizing agent. Brit. J. Pharmacol. **7**, 398—408 (1952).

COMROE, J. H., DRIPPS, R. D.: The histamine-like action of curare and tubocurarine injected intracutaneously and intra-arterially in man. Anesthesiology **7**, 260—262 (1946).

COOK, D. R., FISCHER, C. G.: Neuromuscular blocking effects of succinylcholine in infants and children. Anesthesiology **42**, 662—665 (1975).

COOPERMAN, L. H., STROBEL, G. E., KENNELL, E. M.: Massive hyperkalaemia after administration of succinylcholine. Anesthesiology **32**, 161—164 (1970).

COWGILL, D. B., MOSTELLO, L. A., SHAPIRO, H. M.: Encephalitis and a hyperkalaemic response to succinylcholine. Anesthesiology **40**, 409—411 (1974).

CRAIG, H. J. L.: The protective effect of thiopentone against muscular pain and stiffness which follows the use of suxamethonium chloride. Brit. J. Anaesth. **36**, 612—619 (1964).

CRAYTHORNE, N. W. B., ROTTENSTEIN, H. S., DRIPPS, R. D.: The effect of succinylcholine on intra-ocular pressure in adults, infants and children during general anesthesia. Anesthesiology **21**, 59—63 (1960a).

CRAYTHORNE, N. W. B., TURNDORF, H., DRIPPS, R. D.: Changes in pulse rate and rhythm associated with the use of succinylcholine in anesthetized children. Anesthesiology **21**, 465—470 (1960b).

CRUL, J. F., LONG, G. L., BRUNNER, E. A., COOLEN, J. M. W.: The changing pattern of neuromuscular blockade caused by succinylcholine in man. Anesthesiology **27**, 729—735 (1966).

CULLEN, D. J.: The effect of pretreatment with nondepolarizing muscle relaxants on the neuromuscular blocking action of succinylcholine. Anesthesiology **35**, 572—578 (1971).

DAHLBÄCK, O., ELMQVIST, D., JOHNS, T. R., RADNER, S., THESLEFF, S.: An electrophysiologic study of the neuromuscular junction in myasthenia gravis. J. Physiol. (Lond.) **156**, 336—343 (1961).

DANN, W. L.: The effect of different levels of ventilation on the action of pancuronium in man. Brit. J. Anaesth. **43**, 959—962 (1971).

DE JONG, R. H., FREUND, F. G.: Characteristics of the neuromuscular block with succinylcholine and decamethonium in man. Anesthesiology **28**, 583—591 (1967).

DENBOROUGH, M. A., EBELING, P., KING, J. O., ZAPF, P.: Myopathy and malignant hyperpyrexia. Lancet **1970 I**, 1138—1140.

DESMEDT, J. E.: Myasthenic-like features of neuromuscular transmission after administration of an inhibitor of acetylcholine synthesis. Nature (Lond.) **182**, 1673—1674 (1958).

DEVASANKARAIAH, G., HARANATH, P. S. R. K., KRISHNAMURTY, A.: Passage of intravenously administered tubocurarine into the liquor space in man and dog. Brit. J. Pharmacol. **47**, 787—798 (1973).

DIETERT, S. E.: The demonstration of different types of muscle fibres in human extraocular muscle by electron microscopy and cholinesterase staining. Invest. Ophthal. **4**, 51—63 (1965).

DILLON, J. B., SABAWALA, P., TAYLOR, D. B., GUNTER, R.: Action of succinylcholine on extraocular muscles and intraocular pressure. Anesthesiology **18**, 44—49 (1957).

DOTTORI, O., LÖF, B. A., YGGE, H.: Muscle pains after suxamethonium. Acta anaesth. scand. **9**, 247—256 (1965).

DRETSCHEN, K., GHONEIM, M. M., LONG, J. P.: The interaction of diazepam with myoneural blocking agents. Anesthesiology **34**, 463—468 (1971).

DUNDEE, J. W.: Gallamine in the diagnosis of myasthenia gravis. Brit. J. Anaesth. **23**, 39—41 (1951).

DUNDEE, J. W.: Influence of controlled respiration on dosage of thiopentone and *d*-tubocurarine chloride required for abdominal surgery. Brit. med. J. **1952 II**, 893—896.

DUNDEE, J. W., GRAY, T. C.: Variations in response to relaxant drugs. Lancet **1951 II**, 1015—1018.

DUNDEE, J. W., GRAY, T. C.: Resistance to *d*-tubocurarine chloride in the presence of liver damage. Lancet **1953 II**, 16—17.

DURRANS, S. F.: Prolonged apnoea. Lancet **1952 II**, 539.

EATON, L. M., LAMBERT, E. H.: Electromyography and electrical stimulation of nerves in diseases of motor unit. Observations on myasthenic syndrome associated with malignant tumours. J. Amer. med. Ass. **163**, 1117—1124 (1957).

EISELE, J. H., MARTA, J. A., DAVIS, H. S.: Quantitative aspects of the chronotropic and neuromuscular effects of gallamine in anesthetized man. Anesthesiology **35**, 630—633 (1971).

ELERT, S., COHEN, E. N.: A microspectrophotometric method for the analysis of minute concentrations of *d*-tubocurarine in plasma. Amer. J. med. Technol. **28**, 125—134 (1962).

ELLIS, F. R., KEANEY, N. P., HARRIMAN, D. G. F.: Histopathological and neuropharmacological aspects of malignant hyperpyrexia. Proc. roy. Soc. Med. **66**, 66—67 (1973).

ELLIS, F. R., KEANEY, N. P., HARRIMAN, D. G. F., SUMNER, D. W., KYEI-MENSAH, K., TYRRELL, J. H., HARGREAVES, J. B., PARIKH, R. K., MULROONEY, P. L.: Screening for malignant hyperpyrexia. Brit. med. J. **1972 III**, 559—561.

ELMQVIST, D., HOFMANN, W. W., KUGELBERG, J., QUASTEL, D. M. J.: An electrophysiological investigation of neuromuscular transmission in myasthenia gravis. J. Physiol. (Lond.) **174**, 417—434 (1964).

EMERY, E. R. J.: Neuromuscular blocking properties of antibiotics as a cause of post-operative apnoea. Anaesthesia **18**, 57—65 (1963).

EPSTEIN, R. A., EPSTEIN, R. M.: The electromyogram and the mechanical response of indirectly stimulated muscle in anesthetized man following curarization. Anesthesiology **38**, 212—223 (1973).

EPSTEIN, R. A., JACKSON, S. H.: Repetitive muscle depolarization from single indirect stimulation in anesthetized man. J. appl. Physiol. **28**, 407—410 (1970a).

EPSTEIN, R. A., JACKSON, S. H.: The effect of depth of anesthesia on the neuromuscular refractory period of anesthetized man. Anesthesiology **32**, 494—499 (1970b).

EPSTEIN, R. A., JACKSON, S. H.: The effect of deplarizing relaxants on the neuromuscular refractory period in anesthetized man. Anesthesiology **38**, 166—172 (1973).

EPSTEIN, R. A., JACKSON, S. H., WYTE, S. R.: The effects of nondepolarizing relaxants on the neuromuscular refractory period in anesthetized man. Anesthesiology **31**, 69—77 (1969).

EPSTEIN, R. M., EPSTEIN, R. A., LEE, A. S. J.: A recording system for continuous evoked electromyography. Anesthesiology **38**, 287—289 (1973).

EVANS, F. T., GRAY, P. W. S., LEHMANN, H., SILK, E.: Sensitivity to succinylcholine in relation to serum-cholinesterase. Lancet **1952 I**, 1229—1230.

EVANS, F. T., GRAY, P. W. S., LEHMANN, H., SILK, E.: Effect of pseudo-cholinesterase level on action of succinylcholine in man. Brit. med. J. **1953 I**, 136—138.

EVANS, G. H., NIES, A. S., SHAND, D. G.: The disposition of propranolol. III. Decreased half-life and volume of distribution as a result of plasma binding in man, monkey, dog and rat. J. Pharmacol. exp. Ther. **186**, 114—122 (1973).

FELDMAN, S. A.: Muscle relaxants. London: W. B. Saunders 1973.

FELDMAN, S. A., CRAWLEY, B. E.: Interaction of diazepam with the muscle-relaxant drugs. Brit. med. J. **1970 II**, 336—338.

FELDMAN, S. A., LEVI, J. A.: Prolonged paresis following gallamine. Brit. J. Anaesth. **35**, 804—806 (1963).

FELDMAN, S. A., TYRRELL, M. F.: A new theory of the termination of action of the muscle relaxants. Proc. roy. Soc. Med. **63**, 692—695 (1970a).

FELDMAN, S. A., TYRRELL, M. F.: A new steroid muscle relaxant. Dacuronium-NB. 68 (Organon). Anaesthesia **25**, 349—355 (1970b).

FELTON, D. J. C., GODDARD, B. A.: The effect of suxamethonium chloride on uterine activity. Lancet **1966 I**, 852—854.

FIELDS, W. S. (Ed.): Myasthenia gravis, Symposium. Ann. N.Y. Acad. Sci. **183**, 1—386 (1971).

FLEXNER, L. B., COWIE, D. B., VOSBURGH, G. J.: Studies on capillary permeability with tracer substances. Cold Spr. Harb. Symp. quant. Biol. **13**, 88—97 (1948).

FOGDALL, R. P., MILLER, R. D.: Neuromuscular effects of enflurane, alone and combined with d-tubocurarine, pancuronium and succinylcholine in man. Anesthesiology **42**, 173—178 (1975).

FOLDES, F. F.: Succinylmonocholine: its enzymatic hydrolysis and neuromuscular activity. Proc. Soc. exp. Biol. (N.Y.) **83**, 187 (1953).

FOLDES, F. F., BROWN, I. M., LUNN, J. N., MOORE, J., DUNCALF, D.: The neuromuscular effects of diallylnortoxiferine in anesthetized subjects. Curr. Res. Anesth. **42**, 177—187 (1963).

FOLDES, F. F., KLONYMUS, D. H., MAISEL, W., SCIAMMAS, F., PAN, T.: Studies of pancuronium in conscious and anesthetized man. Anesthesiology **35**, 496—503 (1971).

FOLDES, F. F., MCNALL, P. G., DAVIS, D. L., ELLIS, C. H., WNUCK, A. L.: Substrate competition between procaine and succinylcholine diiodide for plasma cholinesterase. Science **117**, 383—386 (1953).

FOLDES, F. F., MONTE, A. P., BRUNN, H. M., WOLFSON, B.: The influence of exercise on neuromuscular activity of relaxant drugs. Canad. Anaesth. Soc. J. **8**, 118—127 (1961).

Foldes, F. F., Swerdlow, M., Lipschitz, E., van Hees, G. R., Shanor, S. P.: Comparison of the respiratory effects of suxamethonium and suxethonium in man. Anesthesiology 17, 559—568 (1956).

Foldes, F. F., Tsuji, F. J.: Enzymatic hydrolysis and neuromuscular activity of succinylmono-choline iodide. Fed. Proc. 12, 321 (1953).

Forbat, A., Lehmann, H., Silk, E.: Prolonged apnoea following injection of succinyldicholine. Lancet 1953 II, 1067—1068.

Foster, C. A.: Muscle pains that follow administration of suxamethonium. Brit. med. J. 1960 II, 24—25.

Fraser, P. T.: Hydrolysis of succinylcholine salts. Brit. J. Pharmacol. 9, 429 (1954).

Freund, F. G.: Tachyphylaxis to decamethonium and reversibility of the block by anticholines-terase drugs. Anesthesiology 30, 7—11 (1969).

Furniss, P.: The etiology of malignant hyperpyrexia. Proc. roy. Soc. Med. 64, 216—220 (1971).

Galindo, A.: The role of prejunctional effects in myoneural transmission. Anesthesiology 36, 598—608 (1972).

Garry, P. J.: Serum cholinesterase variants: examination of several differential inhibitors, salts and buffers used to measure enzyme activity. Clin. Chem. 17, 183—191 (1971).

Gerbershagen, H. U., Bergman, N. A.: The effect of d-tubocurarine on respiratory resistance in anesthetized man. Anesthesiology 28, 981—984 (1967).

Ghoneim, M. M., Long, L. P.: The interaction between magnesium and other neuromuscular blocking agents. Anesthesiology 32, 23—27 (1970).

Gibaldi, M., Levy, G., Hayton, W.: Kinetics of the elimination and neuromuscular blocking effect of d-tubocurarine in man. Anesthesiology 36, 213—218 (1972 a).

Gibaldi, M., Levy, G., Hayton, W.: Tubocurarine and renal failure. Brit. J. Anaesth. 44, 163—165 (1972 b).

Gissen, A. J., Katz, R. L.: Twitch, tetanus and post-tetanic potentiation as indices of nerve-mus-cle block in man. Anesthesiology 30, 481—487 (1969).

Glauber, D.: The incidence and severity of muscle pains after suxamethonium when preceded by gallamine. Brit. J. Anaesth. 38, 541—544 (1966).

Gordh, T., Wåhlin, Å.: Potentiation of the neuromuscular effect of succinylcholine by tetrahy-dro-amino-acridine. Acta anaesth. scand. 5, 55—61 (1961).

Graf, K., Ström, G., Wåhlin, Å.: Circulatory effects of succinylcholine in man. Acta anaesth. scand. 7 (suppl. 14), 1—48 (1963).

Grob, D., Lilienthal, J. L., Harvey, A. M.: On certain vascular effects of curare in man: the "histamine" reaction. Bull. Johns Hopk. Hosp. 80, 299—322 (1947).

Grob, D., Liljestrand, Å., Johns, R. J.: Potassium movement in normal subjects. Effect on mus-cle function. Amer. J. Med. 23, 340—355 (1957).

Halldin, M., Wåhlin, Å., Koch, T.: Observations of the conjunctival vessels under the influence of succinylcholine with intravenous anaesthesia. Acta anaesth. scand. 3, 163—171 (1959).

Hampton, L. J., Little, D. M., Rodabaugh, S. G., Chaffee, W. R.: Studies concerning the prolon-gation of activity of succinylcholine. Anesthesiology 16, 67—72 (1955).

Hanel, H. K., Mogensen, J. V.: Urea inhibition of human pseudocholinesterase. Brit. J. Anaesth. 43, 51—53 (1971).

Haranath, P. S. R. K., Krishnamurty, A., Rao, L. N., Seshagirirao, K.: Passage of gallamine from blood into the liquor space in man and in dog. Brit. J. Pharmacol. 48, 640—645 (1973).

Harris, H.: The genetics of serum cholinesterase "deficiency" in relation to suxamethonium apnoea. Proc. roy. Soc. Med. 57, 503—506 (1964).

Harris, H., Whittaker, M.: Differential inhibition of human serum cholinesterase with fluoride: recognition of two new phenotypes. Nature (Lond.) 191, 496—498 (1961).

Harrison, G. A.: The incidence of visible muscular fasciculations following a second dose of suxamethonium chloride. Brit. J. Anaesth. 37, 129—132 (1965).

Hart, S. M., Mitchell, J. V.: Suxamethonium in the absence of pseudocholinesterase. A case report. Brit. J. Anaesth. 34, 207—209 (1962).

Harvey, A. M., Lilienthal, J. L., Talbot, S. A.: On the effects of the intra-arterial injection of acetylcholine and prostigmine in normal man. Bull. Johns Hopk. Hosp. 69, 529—546 (1941).

HARVEY,A. M., MASLAND,R. L.: The electromyogram in myasthenia gravis. Bull. Johns Hopk. Hosp. **69**, 1—13 (1941).
HEATH,M. L.: Bronchospasm in an asthmatic patient following pancuronium. Anaesthesia **28**, 437—440 (1973).
HEGARTY,P.: Postoperative muscle pains. Brit. J. Anaesth. **28**, 209—212 (1956).
HEISTERKAMP,D. V., SKOVSTED,P., COHEN,P.J.: The effects of small incremental doses of d-tubocurarine on neuromuscular transmission in anesthetized man. Anesthesiology **30**, 500—505 (1969).
HERSH,L. B., RAJ,P. P., OHLWEILER,D.: Kinetics of succinyldithiocholine hydrolysis by serum cholinesterase: comparison to dibucaine and succinylcholine numbers. J. Pharmacol. exp. Ther. **189**, 544—549 (1974).
HODGES,R.J. H., HARKNESS;J.: Suxamethonium sensitivity in health and disease. A clinical evaluation of pseudocholinesterase levels. Brit. med. J. **1954**II, 18—22.
HOFMANN,H., HOLZER,H.: Die Wirkung von Muskelrelaxantien auf den intraokularen Druck. Klin. Mbl. Augenheilk. **123**, 1—15 (1953).
HÖIVIK,B., STOVNER,J.: Procaine and malignant hyperthermia. Lancet **1975 II**, 185.
HOROWITZ,P. E., SPECTOR,S.: Determination of serum d-tubocurarine concentration by radioimmunoassay. J. Pharmacol. exp. Ther. **185**, 94—100 (1973).
HUNTER,A.R.: Prolongation of the action of suxamethonium. A clinical investigation. Anaesthesia **21**, 337—345 (1966).
INNES,R. K. R., STRØMME,J. H.: Rise in serum creatine phosphokinase associated with agents used in anaesthesia. Brit. J. Anaesth. **45**, 185—190 (1973).
JACOB,J.C., VARKEY,G. P.: Curare sensitivity in ocular myopathy. Canad. Anaesth. Soc. J. **13**, 449—452 (1966).
JENDEN,D.J., KAMIJO,K., TAYLOR,D.B.: The action of decamethonium (C 10) on the isolated rabbit lumbrical muscle. J. Pharmacol. exp. Ther. **103**, 348—349 (1951).
JENKINS,R. B.: Treatment of myasthenia gravis with prednisone. Lancet **1972**I, 765—767.
JOHANSEN,S. H., JØRGENSEN,M., MOLBECH,S.: Effect of tubocurarine on respiratory muscle power in man. J. appl. Physiol. **19**, 990—994 (1964).
JOHNS,R.J., GROB,D., HARVEY,A. M.: Electromyographic changes in myasthenia gravis. Amer. J. Med. **19**, 679—683 (1955).
JONES,C.S., MEYEROVITZ,L. S., SWEENEY,G.D.: The effect of curarizing doses of gallamine triethiodide (Flaxedil) on the electroencephalogram in man. Curr. Res. Anesth. **35**, 425—428 (1956).
JØRGENSEN,M., MOLBECH,S., JOHANSEN,S. H.: Effect of decamethonium on head lift, hand grip and respiratory muscle power in man. J. appl. Physiol. **21**, 509—512 (1966).
KALOW,W.: Urinary excretion of d-tubocurarine in man. J. Pharmacol. exp. Ther. **109**, 74—82 (1953).
KALOW,W.: The influence of pH on the ionization and biological activity of d-tubocurarine. J. Pharmacol. exp. Ther. **110**, 433—442 (1954).
KALOW,W.: The distribution, destruction and elimination of muscle relaxants. Anesthesiology **20**, 505—518 (1959).
KALOW,W.: Pharmacogenetics and anesthesia. Anesthesiology **25**, 377—387 (1964).
KALOW,W., GENEST,K.: A method for the detection of atypical forms of human serum cholinesterase. Determination of dibucaine numbers. Canad. J. Biochem. **35**, 339—346 (1957).
KALOW,W., GUNN,D. R.: The relation between dose of succinylcholine and duration of apnoea in man. J. Pharmacol. exp. Ther. **120**, 203—214 (1957).
KALOW,W., GUNN,D. R.: Some statistical data on atypical cholinesterase of human serum. Ann. human Genet. **23**, 239—250 (1959).
KALOW,W., STARON,N.: On distribution and inheritance of atypical forms of human serum cholinesterase, as indicated by dibucaine numbers. Canad. J. Biochem. **35**, 1305—1317 (1957).
KARIS,J. H., GISSEN,A.J., NASTUK,W.L.: The effect of volatile anesthetic agents on neuromuscular transmission. Anesthesiology **28**, 128—133 (1967).
KARIS,J. H., NASTUK,W. L., KATZ,R. L.: The action of tacrine on neuromuscular transmission: a comparison with hexafluorenium. Brit. J. Anaesth. **38**, 762—774 (1966).
KATZ,R. L.: Neuromuscular effects of diethyl ether and its interaction with succinylcholine and d-tubocurarine. Anesthesiology **27**, 52—63 (1966).

KATZ, R. L.: Neuromuscular effects of d-tubocurarine, edrophonium and neostigmine in man. Anesthesiology **28**, 327—336 (1967).

KATZ, R. L.: Clinical neuromuscular pharmacology of pancuronium. Anesthesiology **34**, 550—556 (1971 a).

KATZ, R. L.: Modification of the action of pancuronium by succinylcholine and halothane. Anesthesiology **35**, 602—606 (1971 b).

KATZ, R. L.: Electromyographic and mechanical effects of suxamethonium and tubocurarine on twitch, tetanic and post-tetanic responses. Brit. J. Anaesth. **45**, 849—859 (1973).

KATZ, R. L., EAKINS, K. E., LORD, C. O.: The effects of hexafluorenium in preventing the increase in intraocular pressure produced by succinylcholine. Anesthesiology **29**, 70—78 (1968).

KATZ, R. L., GISSEN, A. J.: Neuromuscular and electromyographic effects of halothane and its interaction with d-tubocurarine in man. Anesthesiology **28**, 564—567 (1967).

KATZ, R. L., GISSEN, A. J., KARIS, J. H.: The effects of hexafluorenium and edrophonium on the neuromuscular blocking actions of succinylcholine, decamethonium, Imbretil and d-tubocurarine. Anesthesiology **26**, 154—161 (1965).

KATZ, R. L., NORMAN, J., SEED, R. F., CONRAD, L.: A comparison of the effect of suxamethonium and tubocurarine in patients in London and New York. Brit. J. Anaesth. **41**, 1041—1047 (1969).

KATZ, R. L., RYAN, J. F.: The neuromuscular effects of suxamethonium in man. Brit. J. Anaesth. **41**, 381—390 (1969).

KATZ, R. L., WOLF, C. E.: Neuromuscular and electromyographic studies in man: effects of hyperventilation, carbon dioxide inhalation and d-tubocurarine. Anesthesiology **25**, 781—787 (1964).

KATZ, R. L., WOLF, C. E., PAPPER, E. M.: The nondepolarizing neuromuscular blocking action of succinylcholine in man. Anesthesiology **24**, 784—789 (1963).

KAUFMAN, L.: Measurement of intramuscular pressure. J. Physiol. (Lond.) **179**, 1 P (1965).

KAUFMAN, L.: General anaesthesia in ophthalmology. Proc. roy. Soc. Med. **60**, 1275—1280 (1967).

KELMAN, G. R., KENNEDY, B. R.: Cardiovascular effects of pancuronium in man. Brit. J. Anaesth. **43**, 335—338 (1971).

KENNEDY, B. R., FARMAN, J. V.: Cardiovascular effects of gallamine triethiodide in man. Brit. J. Anaesth. **40**, 773—780 (1968).

KING, J., DIXON, R. I.: A further factor contributing to inherited suxamethonium sensitivity. Brit. J. Anaesth. **41**, 1023—1028 (1969).

KING, J., GRIFFIN, D.: Differentiation of serum cholinesterase variants by succinyldicholine inhibition. Brit. J. Anaesth. **45**, 450—454 (1973).

KIVALO, I., SAARIKOSKI, S.: Placental transmission and foetal uptake of ^{14}C-dimethyltubocurarine. Brit. J. Anaesth. **44**, 557—561 (1972).

KVISSELGAARD, N., MOYA, F.: Investigation of placental thresholds to succinylcholine. Anesthesiology **22**, 7—10 (1961).

KYEI-MENSAH, K., TYRRELL, J. H., SUMNER, D. W.: Clinical genetic aspects of malignant hyperpyrexia. Proc. roy. Soc. Med. **66**, 63—66 (1973).

LaMOTTA, R. V., WORONICK, C. L.: Molecular heterogeneity of human serum cholinesterase. Clin. Chem. **17**, 135—144 (1971).

LANDMESSER, C. M., CONVERSE, J. G., HARMEL, M. H.: Quantitative evaluation of the bronchoconstrictor action of curare in the anesthetized patient: a preliminary report. Anesthesiology **13**, 275—280 (1952).

LEHMANN, H., LIDDELL, J.: Human cholinesterase (pseudocholinesterase): genetic variants and their recognition. Brit. J. Anaesth. **41**, 235—244 (1969).

LEHMANN, H., SILK, E.: Succinylmonocholine. Brit. med. J. **1953 I**, 767.

LEHMANN, H., SIMMONS, P. H.: Sensitivity to suxamethonium. Apnoea in two brothers. Lancet **1958 II**, 981—982.

LEIGH, M. D., McCOY, D. D., BELTON, M. K., LEWIS, G. B.: Bradycardia following intravenous administration of succinylcholine chloride to infants and children. Anesthesiology **18**, 698—702 (1957).

LENNON, V. A., CARNEGIE, P. R.: Immunopharmacological disease: a break in tolerance to receptor sites. Lancet **1971 I**, 630—633.

LEVY, G.: Relationship between rate of elimination of tubocurarine and rate of decline of its pharmacological activity. Brit. J. Anaesth. **36**, 694—695 (1964).

LEVY, G.: Kinetics of pharmacological activity of succinylcholine in man. J. pharm. Sci. **56**, 1687—1688 (1967).

LEVY, G.: Pharmacokinetics of succinylcholine in newborns. Anesthesiology **32**, 551—552 (1970).

LIDDELL, J., LEHMANN, H., DAVIES, D.: Harris and Whittaker's pseudocholinesterase variant with increased resistance to fluoride. A study of four families and the identification of the homozygote. Acta genet. (Basel) **13**, 95—108 (1963).

LIDDELL, J., LEHMANN, H., DAVIES, D., SHARIH, A.: Physical separation of pseudocholinesterase variants in human serum. Lancet **1962 a I**, 463—464.

LIDDELL, J., LEHMANN, H., SILK, E.: A "silent" pseudocholinesterase gene. Nature (Lond.) **193**, 561—562 (1962 b).

LIM, H. S., DAVENPORT, H. T., ROBSON, J. G.: The response of infants and children to muscle relaxants. Anesthesiology **25**, 161—168 (1964).

LINCOFF, H. A., ELLIS, C. H., DEVOE, A. G., DEBEER, E. J., IMPASTATO, D. J., BERG, S., ORKIN, L., MAGDA, H.: The effect of succinylcholine on intraocular pressure. Amer. J. Ophthal. **40**, 501—510 (1955).

LLOYD, D. P. C.: Stimulation of peripheral nerve terminations by active muscle. J. Neurophysiol. **5**, 153—165 (1942).

LODER, R. E., WALKER, G. F.: Neuromuscular-blocking action of streptomycin. Lancet **1959 I**, 812—813.

LOH, L.: The cardiovascular effects of pancuronium bromide. Anaesthesia **25**, 356—363 (1970).

LOPERT, H.: Allergic reaction to gallamine triethiodide. Anaesthesia **10**, 76—77 (1955).

LUND, I., STOVNER, J.: Dose-response curves for tubocurarine, alcuronium and pancuronium. Acta anaesth. scand., Suppl. **37**, 238—242 (1970).

LUPPRIAN, K. G., CHURCHILL-DAVIDSON, H. C.: Effect of suxamethonium on cardiac rhythm. Brit. med. J. **1960 II**, 1774—1777.

MAHFOUZ, M.: The fate of tubocurarine in the body. Brit. J. Pharmacol. **4**, 295—303 (1949).

MAIER, E. S., CLARK, R. B.: Effect of decamethonium on intraocular pressure in man. Curr. Res. Anesth. **44**, 753—757 (1965).

MAPLESON, W. W., MUSHIN, W. W.: Relaxant action in man. An experimental study. I. Method. Anaesthesia **10**, 265—278 (1955 a).

MAPLESON, W. W., MUSHIN, W. W.: Relaxant action in man. An experimental study. II. Results with intravenous gallamine triethiodide. Anaesthesia **10**, 379—390 (1955 b).

MARSH, D. F.: The distribution, metabolism and excretion of d-tubocurarine chloride and related compounds in man and other animals. J. Pharmacol. exp. Ther. **105**, 299—316 (1952).

MASLAND, R. L., GAMMON, G. D.: The effect of botulinus toxin on the electromyogram. J. Pharmac. exp. Ther. **97**, 499—506 (1949).

MATTHIAS, J. A., EVANS-PROSSER, C. D. G., CHURCHILL-DAVIDSON, H. C.: The role of the non-depolarizing drugs in the prevention of suxamethonium bradycardia. Brit. J. Anaesth. **42**, 609—613 (1970).

MAZZE, R. I., ESCUE, H. M., HOUSTON, J. B.: Hyperkalaemia and cardiovascular collapse following administration of succinylcholine to the traumatized patient. Anesthesiology **31**, 540—547 (1969).

MCARDLE, B.: The serum choline esterase in jaundice and diseases of the liver. Quart. J. Med. **9**, 107—127 (1940).

MCCANCE, R. A., WIDDOWSON, E. M., HUTCHINSON, A. O.: Effect of undernutrition and alterations in diet on the choline esterase activity of serum. Nature (Lond.) **161**, 56—57 (1948).

MCCAUL, K., ROBINSON, G. D.: Suxamethonium "extension" by tetrahydroaminacrine. Brit. J. Anaesth. **34**, 536—542 (1962).

MACDERMOT, V.: The changes in the motor end-plate in myasthenia gravis. Brain **83**, 24—36 (1960).

MCDOWALL, S. A., CLARKE, R. S. J.: A clinical comparison of pancuronium and tubocurarine. Anaesthesia **24**, 581—590 (1969).

MCLAREN, C. A. B.: Myoglobinuria following the use of suxamethonium chloride. A case report. Brit. J. Anaesth. **40**, 901—902 (1968).

MCSHERRY, R. T., GOODWIN, G. Y., HAMPTON, L. J.: The measurement and regulation of neuro-
muscular blockade in the anesthetized patient. Curr. Res. Anesth. **35**, 363—368 (1956).
MILLER, R. D., EGER, E. I., WAY, W. L., STEVENS, W. C., DOLAN, W. M.: Comparative neuromuscular effects of forane and halothane alone and in combination with *d*-tubocurarine in man.
Anesthesiology **35**, 38—42 (1971a).
MILLER, R. D., WAY, W. L.: The interaction between succinylcholine and subparalyzing doses of
d-tubocurarine and gallamine in man. Anesthesiology **35**, 567—571 (1971).
MILLER, R. D., WAY, W. L., DOLAN, W. M., STEVENS, W. C., EGER, E. I.: Comparative neuromuscular effects of pancuronium, gallamine, and succinylcholine during forane and halothane
anesthesia in man. Anesthesiology **35**, 509—514 (1971b).
MILLER, R. D., WAY, W. L., DOLAN, W. M., STEVENS, W. C., EGER, E. I.: The dependence of pancu-
ronium- and d-tubocurarine-induced neuromuscular blockades on alveolar concentrations
of halothane and forane. Anesthesiology **37**, 573—581 (1972).
MILLER, R. D., WAY, W. L., HICKEY, R. F.: Inhibition of succinylcholine-induced increased intra-
ocular pressure by non-depolarizing muscle relaxants. Anesthesiology **29**, 123—126 (1968).
MOLBECH, S., JOHANSEN, S. H.: Endurance time in static work during partial curarization. J. appl.
Physiol. **27**, 44—48 (1969).
MONGAR, J. L., WHELAN, R. F.: Histamine release by adrenaline and d-tubocurarine in the human
subject. J. Physiol. (Lond.) **120**, 146—154 (1953).
MONKS, P. S., NORMAN, J.: Prolongation of suxamethonium-induced paralysis by propanidid.
Brit. J. Anaesth. **44**, 1303—1305 (1972).
MONTGOMERY, J. B., BENNETT-JONES, N.: Gallamine triethiodide and renal disease. Lancet
1956 II, 1243—1244.
MOULDS, R. F. W., DENBOROUGH, M. A.: Procaine in malignant hyperpyrexia. Brit. med. J.
1972 IV, 526—528.
MOULDS, R. F. W., DENBOROUGH, M. A.: Biochemical basis of malignant hyperpyrexia. Brit. med.
J. **1974 II**, 241—244.
MOYA, F., KVISSELGAARD, N.: The placental transmission of succinylcholine. Anesthesiology **22**,
1—6 (1961).
MOYA, F., SMITH, B. E.: Uptake, distribution and placental transport of drugs and anesthetics.
Anesthesiology **26**, 465—476 (1965).
MUSHIN, W. W., MAPLESON, W. W.: The assessment of relaxation in man. Brit. J. Anaesth. **29**,
249—260 (1957).
MUSHIN, W. W., MAPLESON, W. W.: Relaxant action in man of dipyrandium chloride (M & B
9105A). Brit. J. Anaesth. **36**, 761—768 (1964).
MUSHIN, W. W., WIEN, R., MASON, D. F. J., LANGSTON, G. T.: Curare-like actions of tri-(diethyl-
aminoethoxy)-benzene triethyliodide. Lancet **1949 I**, 726—728.
NEITLICH, H. W.: Increased plasma cholinesterase activity and succinylcholine resistance: a genetic variant. J. clin. Invest. **45**, 380—387 (1966).
NEMAZIE, A. S., KITZ, R. J.: A quantitative technique for the evaluation of peripheral neuromuscular blockade in man. Anesthesiology **28**, 215—217 (1967).
NEWNAM, P. T. F., LOUDON, J. M.: Muscle pain following administration of suxamethonium: the
aetiological role of muscular fitness. Brit. J. Anaesth. **38**, 533—540 (1966).
NIELSEN, E., BENNIKE, K.-Å.: The head-lift test after administration of d-tubocurarine. Acta anaesth. scand. **9**, 13—20 (1965).
NIGHTINGALE, D. A., BUSH, G. H.: A clinical comparison between tubocurarine and pancuronium
in children. Brit. J. Anaesth. **45**, 63—70 (1973).
NIGHTINGALE, D. A., GLASS, A. G., BACHMAN, L.: Neuromuscular blockade by succinylcholine in
children. Anesthesiology **27**, 736—741 (1966).
NORMAN, J., KATZ, R. L.: Some effects of the steroidal muscle relaxant, dacuronium bromide, in
anaesthetized patients. Brit. J. Anaesth. **43**, 313—319 (1971).
NORMAN, J., KATZ, R. L., SEED, R. F.: The neuromuscular blocking action of pancuronium in man
during anaesthesia. Brit. J. Anaesth. **42**, 702—710 (1970).
ÖRNDAHL, G.: Myotonic human musculature: stimulation with depolarizing agents. II. A clin-
ico-pharmacological study. Acta med. scand. **172**, 753—765 (1962).
ÖRNDAHL, G., STERNBERG, K.: Myotonic human musculature: stimulation with depolarizing
agents. Acta med. scand. **172** (suppl. 389), 3—29 (1962).

ORGANE,G., PATON,W.D.M., ZAIMIS,E.J.: Preliminary trials of bistrimethylammonium decane and pentane diiodide (C 10 and C 5) in man. Lancet **1949 I**, 21—23.

OSSERMAN, K.E. (Ed.): Myasthenia gravis. Symposium. Ann. N.Y. Acad. Sci. **135**, 1—680 (1966).

PANTUCK, E.J.: Ecothiopate iodide eye drops and prolonged response to suxamethonium. Brit. J. Anaesth. **38**, 406—407 (1966).

PATON, W.D.M.: Mode of action of neuromuscular blocking agents. Brit. J. Anaesth. **28**, 470—480 (1956).

PATON, W.D.M.: Histamine release by compounds of simple chemical structure. Pharmacol. Rev. **9**, 269—328 (1957).

PATON, W.D.M.: The effects of muscle relaxants other than muscle relaxation. Anesthesiology **20**, 453—463 (1959).

PATON, W.D.M., WAUD,D.R.: The margin of safety of neuromuscular transmission. J. Physiol. (Lond.) **191**, 59—90 (1967).

PATON, W.D.M., ZAIMIS,E.J.: Actions and clinical assessment of drugs which produce neuromuscular block. Lancet **1950 II**, 568—570.

PAYNE,J.P., HOLMDAHL,M.H.SON: The effect of repeated doses of suxamethonium in man. Brit. J. Anaesth. **31**, 341—347 (1959).

PELIKAN, E.W., TETHER,J.E., UNNA, K.R.: Sensitivity of myasthenia gravis patients to tubocurarine and decamethonium. Neurology (Minneap.) **3**, 284—296 (1953).

PENNINGTON,R.J.T., WORSFOLD,M.: Biochemical studies on malignant hyperpyrexia. Proc. roy. Soc. Med. **66**, 69—70 (1973).

PITTINGER,C.B., LONG,J.P., MILLER,J.R.: The neuromuscular blocking action of neomycin. Curr. Res. Anesth. **37**, 276—282 (1958).

POULSEN,H., HOUGS,W.: The effect of some curarizing drugs in unanaesthetized man. I. Acta anaesth. scand. **1**, 15—39 (1957).

POULSEN,H., HOUGS,W.: The effect of some curarizing drugs in unanaesthetized man. II. Acta anaesth. scand. **2**, 107—115 (1958).

PRIDGEN,J.E.: Respiratory arrest thought to be due to intraperitoneal neomycin. Surgery **40**, 571—574 (1956).

RELTON,J.E.S., BRITT,B.A., STEWARD,D.J.: Malignant hyperpyrexia. Brit. J. Anaesth. **45**, 269—275 (1973).

ROBERTSON,G.S.: Serum cholinesterase deficiency. I. Disease and inheritance. Brit. J. Anaesth. **38**, 355—360 (1966).

ROBERTSON,G.S., GIBSON,P.F.: Suxamethonium and intraocular pressure. Anaesthesia **23**, 342—349 (1968).

ROSS,R.T.: Ocular myopathy sensitive to curare. Brain **86**, 67—74 (1963).

ROSS,R.T.: The effect of decamethonium on curare sensitive ocular myopathy. Neurology (Minneap.) **14**, 684—689 (1964).

ROTH,F., WÜTHRICH,H.: The clinical importance of hyperkalaemia following suxamethonium administration. Brit. J. Anaesth. **41**, 311—316 (1969).

ROWLAND,L.P., KORENGOLD,M.C., JAFFE,I.A., BERG,L., SHY,G.M.: Prostigmine-induced muscle weakness in myasthenia gravis patients. Neurology (Minneap.) **5**, 89—99 (1955).

RUDDELL,J.S.: Succinylcholine. Lancet **1952 II**, 341—342.

RYAN,A.R.: Tubocurarine administration based upon its disappearance and accumulation curves in anaesthetized man. Brit. J. Anaesth. **36**, 287—294 (1964).

SABAWALA,P.B., DILLON,J.B.: The positive inotropic action of cyclopropane on human intercostal muscle *in vitro*, and its modification by d-tubocurarine. Anesthesiology **19**, 473—477 (1958).

SABAWALA,P.B., DILLON,J.B.: The combined effect of cyclopropane and the depolarizers on isolated human muscle. Anesthesiology **22**, 564—568 (1961).

SALEM, M.R., KIM, Y., EL ETR,A.A.: Histamine release following intravenous injection of d-tubocurarine. Anesthesiology **29**, 380—382 (1968).

SCHANER,P.J., BROWN,R.L., KIRKSEY,T.D., GUNTHER,R.C., RITCHEY,C.R., GRONERT,G.A.: Succinylcholine-induced hyperkalaemia in burned patients. I. Curr. Res. Anesth. **48**, 764—770 (1969).

SCHOENSTADT,D.A., WHITCHER,C.E.: Observations on the mechanism of succinyldicholine-induced cardiac arrhythmias. Anesthesiology **24**, 358—362 (1963).

Schuh, F. T., Viguera, M. G., Terry, R. N.: The effect of a subthreshold dose of d-tubocurarine on the neuromuscular blocking action of succinylcholine in anesthetized man. Acta anaesth. scand. **18**, 71—78 (1974).

Scudamore, H. H., Vorhaus, L. J., Kark, R. M.: Observations on erythrocyte and plasma cholinesterase activity in dyscrasias of the blood. Blood **6**, 1260—1273 (1951).

Shanks, C. A., Harrison, G. A.: Mechanical measurement of neuromuscular blockade. A comparison between the force transducer and a simple muscle twitch monitor. Brit. J. Anaesth. **45**, 75—78 (1973).

Simpson, J. A.: Myasthenia gravis: a new hypothesis. Scot. med. J. **5**, 419—436 (1960).

Simpson, N. E., Kalow, W.: The "silent" gene for serum cholinesterase. Amer. J. hum. Genet. **16**, 180—188 (1964).

Simpson, N. E., Kalow, W.: Pharmacology and biological variation. Ann. N.Y. Acad. Sci. **134**, 864—872 (1966).

Smith, N. L.: Histamine release by suxamethonium. Anaesthesia **12**, 293—298 (1957).

Smith, S. E.: Atypical cholinesterase in leprosy. Brit. med. J. **1972III**, 827—828.

Smith, S. E., Rawlins, M. D.: Variability in human drug response. London: Butterworths 1973.

Smith, S. M., Brown, H. O., Toman, J. E. P., Goodman, L. S.: The lack of cerebral effects of d-tubocurarine. Anesthesiology **8**, 1—14 (1947).

Sniper, W.: The estimation and comparison of histamine release by muscle relaxants in man. Brit. J. Anaesth. **24**, 232—237 (1953).

Sobel, A. M.: Hexafluorenium, succinylcholine, and intraocular tension. Curr. Res. Anesth. **41**, 399—404 (1962).

Speirs, I., Sim, A. W.: The placental transfer of pancuronium bromide. Brit. J. Anaesth. **44**, 370—373 (1972).

Standaert, F. G., Adams, J. E.: The actions of succinylcholine on the mammalian motor nerve terminal. J. Pharmacol. exp. Ther. **149**, 113—123 (1965).

Stead, A. L.: The response of the newborn infant to muscle relaxants. Brit. J. Anaesth. **27**, 124—130 (1955).

Stovner, J.: Variation in the cholinesterase-inhibiting effect of succinylcholine. Scan. J. clin. lab. Invest. **7**, 197—200 (1955).

Stovner, J.: The anticurare activity of tetraethylammonium (T.E.A.) in man. Acta anaesth. scand. **2**, 165—168 (1958).

Stovner, J., Theodorsen, L., Bjelke, E.: Sensitivity to tubocurarine and alcuronium with special reference to plasma protein pattern. Brit. J. Anaesth. **43**, 385—391 (1971 a).

Stovner, J., Theodorsen, L., Bjelke, E.: Sensitivity to gallamine and pancuronium with special reference to serum proteins. Brit. J. Anaesth. **43**, 953—958 (1971 b).

Stovner, J., Theodorsen, L., Bjelke, E.: Sensitivity to dimethyltubocurarine and toxiferine with special reference to serum proteins. Brit. J. Anaesth. **44**, 374—380 (1972).

Swift, M. R., La Du, B. N.: A rapid screening test for atypical serum-cholinesterase. Lancet **1966 I**, 513—514.

Tammisto, T., Airaksinen, M.: Increase of creatine kinase activity in serum as sign of muscular injury caused by intermittently administered suxamethonium during halothane anaesthesia. Brit. J. Anaesth. **38**, 510—515 (1966).

Tammisto, T., Welling, I.: The effect of alcuronium and tubocurarine on blood pressure and heart rate: a clinical comparison. Brit. J. Anaesth. **41**, 317—322 (1969).

Thesleff, S.: An investigation of the muscle-relaxing action of succinyl-choline-iodide in man. Acta physiol. scand. **25**, 348—367 (1952).

Thesleff, S.: The mode of neuromuscular block caused by acetylcholine, nicotine, decamethonium and succinylcholine. Acta physiol. scand. **34**, 218—231 (1955).

Thiel, R. E.: The myotonic response to suxamethonium. Brit. J. Anaesth. **39**, 815—821 (1967).

Thomas, E. T.: The effect of d-tubocurarine chloride on the blood-pressure of anaesthetised patients. Lancet **1957II**, 772—773.

Thomas, E. T.: Circulatory collapse following succinylcholine: report of a case. Curr. Res. Anesth. **48**, 333—337 (1969).

Thomas, M., Job, C. K.: Serum atypical pseudocholinesterase and genetic factors in leprosy. Brit. med. J. **1972III**, 390—391.

THOMPSON, J. C., WHITTAKER, M.: Pseudocholinesterase activity in thyroid disease. J. clin. Path. **18**, 811—812 (1965).
THOMPSON, J. C., WHITTAKER, M.: A study of the pseudocholinesterase in 78 cases of apnoea following suxamethonium. Acta genet. (Basel) **16**, 209—222 (1966).
TOBEY, R. E.: Paraplegia, succinylcholine and cardiac arrest. Anesthesiology **32**, 359—364 (1970).
TOBEY, R. E., JACOBSEN, P. M., KAHLE, C. T., CLUBB, R. J., DEAN, M. A.: The serum potassium response to muscle relaxants in neural injury. Anesthesiology **37**, 332—337 (1972).
TOLMIE, J. D., JOYCE, T. H., MITCHELL, G. D.: Succinylcholine danger in the burned patient. Anesthesiology **28**, 467—470 (1967).
TORDA, T. A., BURKHART, J., TOH, W.: The interaction of propanidid with suxamethonium and decamethonium. Anaesthesia **27**, 159—164 (1972).
TORDA, T. A. G., KLONYMUS, D. H.: Regional neuromuscular block. Acta anaesth. scand. **10** (suppl. 24), 177—182 (1966).
UNNA, K. R., PELIKAN, E. W.: Evaluation of curarizing drugs in man. VI. Critique of experiments in unanesthetized subjects. Ann. N.Y. Acad. Sci. **54**, 480—490 (1951).
UNNA, K. R., PELIKAN, E. W., MacFARLANE, D. W., CAZORT, R. J., SADOVE, M. S., NELSON, J. T.: Evaluation of curarizing agents in man. J. Amer. med. Ass. **144**, 448—451 (1950).
USUBIAGA, J. E., WIKINSKI, J. A., MORALES, R. L., USUBIAGA, L. E. J.: Interaction of intravenously administered procaine, lidocaine and succinylcholine in anesthetized subjects. Curr. Res. Anesth. **46**, 39—45 (1967).
VEALE, J. L., REES, S., MARK, R. F.: Renshaw cell activity in normal and spastic man. In: DESMEDT, J. E. (Ed.): New developments in electromyography and clinical neurophysiology, pp. 523, Vol. 3. Basel: Karger 1973.
WALKER, M. B.: Treatment of myasthenia gravis with physostigmine. Lancet **1934 I**, 1200—1201.
WALMSLEY, D. A.: Sensitivity reaction to gallamine triethiodide. Lancet **1959 II**, 237—238.
WALTS, L. F., DILLON, J. B.: Clinical studies on succinylcholine chloride. Anesthesiology **28**, 372—376 (1967).
WALTS, L. F., DILLON, J. B.: Duration of action of d-tubocurarine and gallamine. Anesthesiology **29**, 499—504 (1968 a).
WALTS, L. F., DILLON, J. B.: D-tubocurarine cumulation studies. Curr. Res. Anesth. **47**, 696—700 (1968 b).
WALTS, L. F., DILLON, J. B.: The response of newborns to succinylcholine and d-tubocurarine. Anesthesiology **31**, 35—38 (1969 a).
WALTS, L. F., DILLON, J. B.: Clinical studies of the interaction between d-tubocurarine and succinylcholine. Anesthesiology **31**, 39—44 (1969 b).
WALTS, L. F., LEBOWITZ, M., DILLON, J. B.: The effects of ventilation on the action of tubocurarine and gallamine. Brit. J. Anaesth. **39**, 845—850 (1967).
WATERLOW, J.: Liver choline-esterase in malnourished infants. Lancet **1950 I**, 908—909.
WAUD, B. E., CHENG, M. C., WAUD, D. R.: Comparison of drug-receptor dissociation constants at the mammalian neuromuscular junction in the presence and absence of halothane. J. Pharmacol. exp. Ther. **187**, 40—46 (1973).
WAUD, B. E., WAUD, D. R.: The relation between the response to "train-of-four" stimulation and receptor occlusion during competitive neuromuscular block. Anesthesiology **37**, 413—416 (1972).
WEINTRAUB, H. D., HEISTERKAMP, D. V., COOPERMAN, L. H.: Changes in plasma potassium concentration after depolarizing blockers in anaesthetized man. Brit. J. Anaesth. **41**, 1048—1052 (1969).
WESTGATE, H. D., VAN BERGEN, F. H.: Changes in histamine blood levels following d-tubocurarine administration. Canad. Anaesth. Soc. J. **9**, 497—503 (1962).
WESTGATE, H. D.; GORDON, J. R., VAN BERGEN, F. H.: Changes in airway resistance following intravenously administered d-tubocurarine. Anesthesiology **23**, 65—73 (1962).
WETSTONE, H. J., HONEYMAN, M. S., McCOMB, R. B.: Genetic control of the quantitative activity of a serum enzyme in man. J. Amer. med. Ass. **192**, 1007—1009 (1965).
WHITTAKER, M.: Differential inhibition of human serum cholinesterase with n-butyl alcohol: recognition of new phenotypes. Acta genet. (Basel) **18**, 335—340 (1968 a).
WHITTAKER, M.: An additional pseudocholinesterase phenotype occurring in suxamethonium apnoea. Brit. J. Anaesth. **40**, 579—582 (1968 b).

WHITTAKER, M.: The pseudocholinesterase variants. Differentiation by means of sodium chloride. Acta genet. (Basel) 18, 556—562 (1968c).

WHITTAKER, M., VICKERS, M. D.: Initial experiences with the cholinesterase research unit. Brit. J. Anaesth. 42, 1016—1020 (1970).

WHITTAKER, V. P., WIJESUNDERA, S.: Hydrolysis of succinyldicholine by cholinesterase. Biochem. J. 52, 475—479 (1952).

WIELHORSKI, W. A., DUBEAU, M., RIOPEL, P.: Plasma cholinesterase studies in some pathological conditions in man. Canad. Anaesth. Soc. J. 3, 31—38 (1962).

WILLIAMS, C. H., DEUTSCH, S., LINDE, H. W., BULLOUGH, J. W., DRIPPS, R. D.: Effects of intravenously administered succinyldicholine on cardiac rate, rhythm, and arterial blood pressure in anesthetized man. Anesthesiology 22, 947—954 (1961).

WILSON, A., STONER, H. B.: The effect of the injection of acetylcholine into the brachial artery of normal subjects and patients with myasthenia gravis. Quart. J. Med. 16, 237—243 (1947).

WISE, R. P.: A myasthenic syndrome complicating bronchial carcinoma. Anaesthesia 17, 488—504 (1962).

WISE, R. P.: Muscle disorders and the relaxants. Brit. J. Anaesth. 35, 558—564 (1963).

WOLLMAN, H., CANNARD, T. H.: Skeletal muscle, esophageal and rectal temperatures in man during general anesthesia and operation. Anesthesiology 21, 476—481 (1960).

WYLIE, W. D., CHURCHILL-DAVIDSON, H. C.: A practice of anaesthesia, 3rd Edn. London: Lloyd-Luke 1973.

ZAIMIS, E.: The synthesis of methonium compounds, their isolation from urine, and their photometric determination. Brit. J. Pharmacol. 5, 424—430 (1950).

ZAIMIS, E.: Motor end-plate differences as a determining factor in the mode of action of neuromuscular blocking substances. Nature (Lond.) 170, 617 (1952).

ZAIMIS, E.: Motor end-plate differences as a determining factor in the mode of action of neuromuscular blocking substances. J. Physiol. (Lond.) 122, 238—251 (1953).

ZAIMIS, E.: Measurement of neuromuscular block. In: LAURENCE, D. R. (Ed.): Quantitative methods in human pharmacology and therapeutics. London: Pergamon Press 1959.

ZAIMIS, E.: General physiology and pharmacology of neuromuscular transmission. In: WALTON, J. (Ed.): Disorders of voluntary muscle, pp. 57-87. London: Churchill 1969.

ZAIMIS, E., CANNARD, T. H., PRICE, H. L.: Effects of lowered muscle temperature upon neuromuscular blockade in man. Science 128, 34—35 (1958).

ZSIGMOND, E. K., DOWNS, J. R.: Plasma cholinesterase activity in newborns and infants. Canad. Anaesth. Soc. J. 18, 278—285 (1971).

CHAPTER 5C

Twenty Years' Experience with Decamethonium

G. E. HALE ENDERBY

A. Introduction

The successful introduction of curare into anaesthesia by GRIFFITH and JOHNSON (1942) was a major advance in modern medicine which stimulated the search for other "curare-like" drugs. In 1948 BARLOW and ING, PATON and ZAIMIS synthesized and tested independently a number of compounds in which quaternary nitrogen atoms were separated by straight carbon chains of various lengths. In the two letters published by "Nature", BARLOW and ING, PATON and ZAIMIS described the curare-like action of these polymethylene *bis*-quaternary ammonium salts. Later that same year a report from PATON and ZAIMIS on the clinical potentialities of certain *bis*-quaternary salts causing neuromuscular and ganglionic block, namely decamethonium and hexamethonium, also appeared. Understandably tubocurarine was taken as the standard, the main difference between decamethonium and tubocurarine being then reported as a "sparing of respiration" by decamethonium in the monkey and cat. Indeed a "ratio of respiratory activity" was described, being the dose producing cessation of respiration in 50% of the animals divided by the dose which produced muscle weakness for 10 min. Other advantages claimed for decamethonium were that it had less ganglionic action than tubocurarine, caused less histamine release and could be synthesised easily. Although the action of decamethonium was not antagonised by neostigmine or eserine it was antagonised by pentamethonium. Quite rightly, PATON and ZAIMIS claimed that decamethonium "merits consideration as a substitute for tubocurarine". It is interesting to note that they also made the suggestion that hexamethonium might be useful in the treatment of hypertension.

B. First Clinical Reports

The first trials of decamethonium in man, reported by ORGANE et al. (1949), were based on their observations of its use in three volunteers at the Westminster Hospital, London. They noted that man was very sensitive to the drug, but commented on the relative sparing of respiration and the absence of antagonism by anticholinesterases. Pentamethonium was used as an antidote and they demonstrated falls of blood pressure with this drug on standing.

These general findings were confirmed by GROB et al. (1949) and during that same year a number of accounts on the use of decamethonium in clinical anaesthesia appeared in the literature, the first being that of ORGANE (1949) with an interim report on 150 cases. He considered 3 mg decamethonium to be equivalent to 15 mg tubocurarine, and to have a duration of action of 10 to 20 min. Other workers reported on the use of decamethonium in electroconvulsive therapy and general surgery, but its early release before the first interim report caused some adverse comments from THOMAS (1949) and HEWER et al. (1949), and caution was recommended in the use of pentamethonium as an antagonist. ARMSTRONG DAVISON (1950) reported on the use of hexamethonium as a reversal agent, stressing the need for caution due to falls in blood pressure.

An authoritative report by HARRIS and DRIPPS (1950) described the satisfactory use of decamethonium for muscle relaxation in 250 patients. The absence of bronchospasm, hypotension, local irritation and histamine reactions were noted, as were decamethonium's free miscibility with thiopentone, its stability and ease of manufacture. They used doses of 2 to 4 mg for abdominal operations with increments of 1 to 3 mg if necessary. The largest dose used was 20 mg over a five hour period. Prolonged apnoea was reported in four patients, one having been given 11 mg. As pentamethonium was not available for reversal, they commented with considerable insight that "as respiratory depression was the only complication, adequate ventilation with oxygen is the most satisfactory treatment for overdosage".

However, such clear thinking was not always the case. GRAY (1950), reporting "delayed intoxication" and absence of respiration with decamethonium, referred to one patient who after a total dose of 8 mg exhibited prolonged apnoea for four hours, was treated with pentamethonium, methylamphetamine and oxygen, but apparently no intermittent positive pressure ventilation, and (surprisingly) survived. SADOVE et al. (1950) reported a case of prolonged apnoea following a two hour abdominal operation during which doses of 2.3 mg, 2 mg and finally 4 mg of decamethonium were given over a period of 55 min. It was stated that "artificial respiration was required" following the last dose and it is therefore reasonable to doubt whether artificial respiration had been used before this. The need for ventilation was however becoming more widely understood and ROBERTS (1950) in reply to GRAY's article recommended the use of controlled ventilation as the only treatment for respiratory muscle paralysis. Even so it is clear from reports as late as that of SPENCER et al. (1955) that ventilation was still not being controlled adequately for they state that "following recovery of nearly normal respiratory exchange breathing was usually smooth and relaxation adequate for periods up to 30 minutes", and it is illuminating to find that they list "depression of respiration" as one of the properties of decamethonium.

During this period prolonged respiratory paralysis with decamethonium was reported by several workers and although errors of technique appear to have been responsible in some instances, this was not always so. There was also little doubt that the use of pentamethonium or hexamethonium as antagonists could lead to cardiovascular collapse. DRIPPS (1953) analysed 1335 cases in which decamethonium had been used and reported 6 with prolonged apnoea and 7 with respiratory depression, and again with considerable insight he questioned the anaesthetic techniques used, the physical status of the patients and the dose of decamethonium. These were often greater than 10 mg, and in one case as high as 21 mg. He did not find any statistical difference in the incidence of prolonged apnoea or respiratory depression between decamethonium and tubocurarine.

These early reports indicate that not only was decamethonium released prematurely, before adequate trials and reports had been completed, but that there was prevalent then the concept of "respiratory sparing" which led to the mistaken belief that abdominal relaxation could be obtained without interfering with spontaneous respiration. Although this may now seem to show an extraordinary lack of understanding, it is perhaps less surprising when one recalls the difficulties then experienced in relaxing abdominal muscles with the paucity of anaesthetic drugs (and skills) available. The use of controlled respiration with cyclopropane, which had been introduced in the 1930's by WALTERS, was only occasionally practised, and then usually in desperation and often with considerable apprehension. The introduction of a drug which on injection would cause effective relaxation of the abdominal muscles was indeed an enormous step forward whilst its concomitant effects on respiration were, perhaps understandably, not so critically observed. The early reports, and particularly those of prolonged apnoea, should therefore be considered with this in mind. Indeed HARRIS and DRIPPS (1950) commenting on the concept of "respiratory sparing" pointed out that HEWER et al. (1949) found that relaxation entailed respiratory paralysis, and that ORGANE (1949) suggested that it might be necessary to paralyse respiration in order to provide adequate relaxation for peritoneal closure. HARRIS and DRIPPS concluded that controlled ventilation was always necessary for profound relaxation.

The years 1949 to 1952 saw the introduction of other relaxants, among them gallamine (Flaxedil) which became popular after the first clinical trials published by MUSHIN et al. (1949). In this they described abdominal relaxation without respiratory paralysis as a main feature of the drug's action. PATON and ZAIMIS (1950) emphasized the difficulties in making comparisons between competitive and depolarizing neuromuscular blocking drugs and SCURR (1951) who reviewed all the relaxants then in use considered that the "respiratory sparing" claimed for all agents was over-emphasised. He stated that in his own experience there was no qualitative difference in relaxation between adequate doses of decamethonium, tubocurarine and gallamine, although he noted the relatively shorter action of decamethonium. He found the durations of action to be 15 to 20 min for decamethonium, 25 to 30 min for gallamine and 30 to 40 min for tubocurarine.

The difficulties encountered with large doses of decamethonium, the remarkable tachyphylaxis described by HUNTER (1950) and the lack of a trouble-free antidote, brought criticism, best summarised by a Lancet editorial (1950) in which it was stated "Much more experience will be needed before its place in anaesthesia can be fully assessed". However, favourable reports were also forthcoming and HUNTER concluded that it was (1) a valuable agent for short operations, and (2) also useful in obstetrics as it did not apparently cross the placenta. YOUNG (1949) had previously demonstrated the absence of placental transfer in guinea-pigs and rabbits.

The early clinical reports on decamethonium indicate that the difficulties encountered were mainly due to either prolonged apnoea or to the lack of a satisfactory antagonist (COLLIER, 1953). In the same year the report which DRIPPS published from the University of Pennsylvania appeared to substantiate these adverse criticisms, and it seems from the paucity of published work thereafter, that the clinical use of decamethonium was largely abandoned except by a few enthusiasts.

In 1958 Murray Lawson wrote a re-appraisal of decamethonium which coincided, ironically, with the decision of Burroughs Wellcome to cease marketing the drug in England. Murray Lawson concluded that decamethonium is a reliable relaxant with no side effects and that the drug's disadvantages, such as lack of a suitable antagonist and the danger of pentamethonium and hexamethonium as reversal agents, were over-emphasised. He added that decamethonium did not need an antidote, that by avoiding excessive doses one could prevent prolonged paralysis and that cardiovascular effects were rare. The maximum dose of decamethonium recommended by him was 10 mg, but rather surprisingly, he advised against its use for operations longer than 30 to 45 min. Murray Lawson considered it the relaxant of choice for Caesarian section, which opinion has been upheld recently by Leng (1970) who reported its use in 102 deliveries.

One of the last published reports was by Enderby (1959) based on a series of 4000 cases in which the advantages of decamethonium were described as freedom from histamine release and bronchospasm, ease of control of respiration with hyperventilation and the absence of muscle pains and tachycardia. In the writer's opinion large doses of decamethonium were not needed, as relaxation could be supplemented by small doses of short-acting depolarising agents.

The shortcomings of the drug were the need for experience in its use, the slow onset time for relaxation (3 to 5 min), the "threshold level" of its action, and the need for hyperventilation to produce optimal effects. Similarly, Fisk (1961), outlining its use in clinical anaesthesia analysed the published reports of difficulties and complications. His conclusions upheld those of Murray Lawson and of Enderby and like them he recommended restriction of the dose used and the addition of suxamethonium if required, pointing out the virtual freedom from other complications.

Thus in retrospect we find there are only 5 years (1949 to 1953) of importance in the clinical assessment of decamethonium. It was received, like all new agents, with relative enthusiasm, but it was released for general use too quickly, and in the next two years there were a number of reports, mostly good, but with some definite criticisms. These criticisms were almost entirely concerned with prolonged apnoea and the difficulties which arose from the use of pentamethonium or hexamethonium as antagonists. However, as the literature clearly indicates, there is little doubt that mismanagement was responsible for many of them, and indeed looking back now with our present knowledge of pulmonary physiology and gas exchange, it is perhaps surprising that such problems were not encountered more frequently. Nevertheless it is obvious that the many good qualities of decamethonium were soon ignored and that most workers concerned themselves with its peculiarities. It must be recalled too that during this time it was being compared clinically with tubocurarine and gallamine. The effects of both these competitive blocking drugs could be reversed with neostigmine (although there were a number of reported cases of apparent failure of reversal), and their popularity grew whilst that of decamethonium decreased for lack of a successful antagonist. The need for an antagonist seems to have been accepted then quite blindly by the majority of anaesthetists, apparently ignoring the use of controlled ventilation to treat apnoea. Prolonged apnoea appears to have been the rock on which the prospects of clinical acceptance of decamethonium foundered, and the report by Dripps (1953) had a particularly adverse effect on its use, even though the figures he gave were not statistically significant.

The recent neglect of decamethonium, in spite of its re-appraisal by MURRAY LAWSON (1958), FISK (1961), and ENDERBY (1959), may be attributed to the fact that the drug has not been marketed in England since 1958 and that the only intravenous preparation now available in this country comes at considerable expense from USA. It can, however, be made up easily and cheaply by most hospital pharmacists, using decamethonium powder (B.P.C., 1954).

In this context it is interesting to note that decamethonium is extensively used in experimental pharmacology, as numerous publications testify. Its popularity is largely due to its purity of action and the absence of side effects such as histamine release and cardiovascular changes. It seems pertinent to ask whether these advantages should not be claimed for man to a greater extent than is the case today.

C. Analysis of 32 000 Administrations of Decamethonium

This number of cases represents work done at the Queen Victoria Hospital, East Grinstead by a group of anaesthetists and my own work in other clinics and hospitals. Hospital records have enabled me to assess the total number of patients receiving decamethonium during 1953 to 1972 at 23 000. Of these, 8000 patients received decamethonium alone and 15 000 decamethonium in combination with other relaxants. My personal records of 9200 patients have enabled me to extract more detailed information concerning doses administered, the use of additional relaxants, and the instance of adverse reactions.

It is interesting to recall why decamethonium was given a clinical trial and why our Hospital Group has continued to use it ever since, over a period of more than 23 years. In the early years after the introduction of muscle relaxants, the spectre of prolonged irreversible apnoea hung heavily over all anaesthetists, and as a safeguard against the accidental administration of a large dose to an incipient myasthenic or other sensitive individual, a test dose was recommended. SELLICK (1950), CHURCHILL-DAVIDSON and RICHARDSON (1952) had reported on the resistance of myasthenics to decamethonium and this, together with the apparent reduction of the drug's neuromuscular blocking action by adrenaline (PATON and ZAIMIS, 1950), appeared to minimise the need for a test dose and indeed to bring into question the results obtained under what were usually stressful conditions. Decamethonium was, therefore, used freely from the start, and at that time we considered this a great advantage over the competitive neuromuscular blocking drugs. In retrospect one can also point out that its introduction coincided with the early work on induced hypotension, and the absence of any cardiovascular effects was keenly appreciated. Freedom from histamine release and brochospasm were at first considered mainly theoretical advantages, and although they have proved to be true, it cannot be claimed that at the start we deliberately used this drug because of them. They were a "bonus" which we accepted and for which we have always been grateful.

I. Surgical Experience

Our surgical experience covers the routine practice of what is a busy General Hospital but without thoracic or obstetric departments. My own records, as well as those

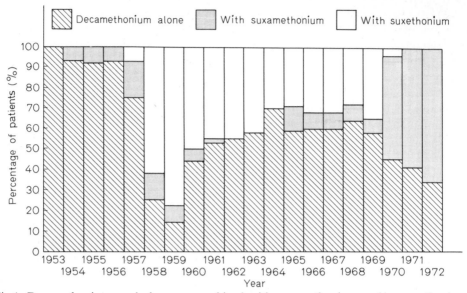

Fig. 1. Decamethonium used alone, or combined with suxamethonium and/or suxethonium, during the 20 year period 1953 to 1972

from the Queen Victoria Hospital, are very heavily weighted towards maxillo-facial and plastic surgical operations.

A sample analysis of operations in my personal records is as follows:

head and neck   71%
abdominal   11%
body wall   11%
extremities   7%

A similar analysis gives the following estimate of physical status based on the classification adopted by the American Society of Anaesthesiologists:

Physical status   1 : 78%
                   2 : 19%
                   3 : 2%
                   4 : 1%

The age of patients to whom decamethonium has been administered has ranged from 3 to 94 years.

II. Analysis

By 1953 decamethonium was our relaxant of choice. My records show that it was given to 98% of all patients receiving a relaxant in that year, and the figure has shown no significant change in subsequent years. For 20 years it has maintained a

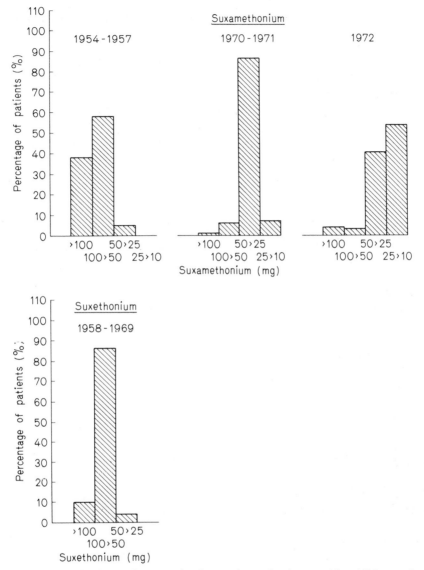

Fig. 2. The change in the doses of suxamethonium and suxethonium used in addition to decamethonium over the years 1954 to 1972

dominant and unchallenged position as the major relaxant, even though from 1954 onwards it has often been combined with suxamethonium or suxethonium. The yearly chart (Fig. 1) illustrates how frequent these combinations have been. As Fig. 2 shows during 1954 to 1957 it was combined mainly with suxamethonium, the dose of which was usually 50 to 100 mg, although doses in excess of 100 mg were also quite frequent. This was followed by a period of almost 12 years (1958 to 1969) during which suxethonium largely replaced suxamethonium, and with this drug too the

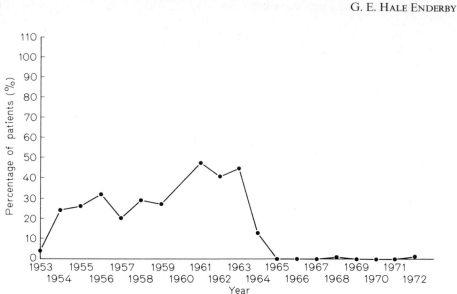

Fig. 3. Percentage of patients receiving 6 to 10 mg decamethonium over the period 1953 to 1972

dose was 50 to 100 mg in a high percentage of cases. By 1970 a return had been made to suxamethonium but during that year and the next the dose had fallen to 25 to 50 mg in 86% of cases while the figures for 1972 indicate that the dosage pattern has now fallen still further so that more than half of the patients now receive only 10 to 25 mg of suxamethonium.

At the same time there has been a gradual reduction in the average dose of decamethonium. During the period 1953 to 1956 doses in excess of 10 mg were relatively frequent, occurring in $2\frac{1}{2}$ to 11% of all administrations. In 1960 the proportion was 8%, but since that year amounts in excess of 10 mg have been very rare. In no case has a dose greater than 15 mg been given. It is also interesting to observe how the number of doses within the 6 to 10 mg range has changed. Figure 3 illustrates this and shows that there was at first a gradual increase, no doubt reflecting the simultaneous decrease in the numbers of patients receiving more than 10 mg, reaching a peak in 1961 to 1963 after which there was a striking reduction, so that since 1965 there have been very few cases indeed receiving more than 6 mg. The largest group each year has been that receiving 4 to 6 mg which since 1964 has comprised between 80% and 93% of all patients. The figures for dosages in 1972 are shown separately (Fig. 4) and from these it will be observed that 93% fall within the range of 4 to 6 mg, and that no patient received a dose in excess of 10 mg.

III. Methods of Administration

1. Early Techniques

In the years before the introduction of halothane a mixture of decamethonium and thiopentone was administered. Increments of such a mixture were often used to maintain anaesthesia, and given under controlled ventilation with nitrous oxide and

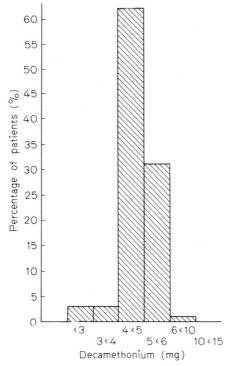

Fig. 4. Percentage of patients and dose of decamethonium (in mg) during 1972

oxygen. In recent years each drug has been administered separately and halothane added to the ventilatory gases.

It was apparent from the start that the full relaxant effects with decamethonium could only be achieved in association with respiratory control and hyperventilation. For many years this was attributed to increased carbon dioxide excretion and a reduced pCO_2. BRENNAN (1952) drew attention to the value of over-ventilation when using relaxants under nitrous oxide and oxygen anaesthesia, and PAYNE (1958) demonstrated the antagonism by carbon dioxide of the neuromuscular block with decamethonium, suxamethonium and gallamine in the cat. PATON and ZAIMIS (1950) pointed out that adrenaline increases the stimulant effect of decamethonium and lessens the maximum paralysis, the opposite occurring with tubocurarine. Understandably ENDERBY (1959) considered that there might be a direct relationship between the pCO_2 level during anaesthesia, catecholamine secretion and the duration and degree of relaxation. More recently NUNN (1972) has drawn attention to the importance of the intercostal muscle spindle reflex in respiratory control and the interruption of this mechanism is now considered to play a dominant role.

2. Present Techniques

Following the intravenous induction of anaesthesia, decamethonium is injected in a dose which is now remarkably constant at 4 to 6 mg although this is sometimes increased for heavily built and muscular patients and for upper-abdominal surgery. In children of 20 to 40 kg a dose of 2 to 3 mg is not excessive bearing in mind the need to exceed the "threshold level", for good relaxation. A small dose of suxamethonium (10 to 25 mg) is administered simultaneously in cases where it is considered necessary to hasten the onset of relaxation for intubation. Hyperventilation with end-tidal positive pressure (ETPP) using a mixture of nitrous oxide and oxygen together with halothane or another volatile anaesthetic agent is initiated after the relaxant has been injected and is maintained for the duration of the operation. This hyperventilation is usually performed by hand, with a minute volume of approximately 10 to 14 litres with the lungs constantly over-inflated throughout the respiratory cycle. With this technique good muscular relaxation, profound enough for upper abdominal surgery and most other surgical operations, is invariably achieved. With ventilatory control maintained in this manner, it becomes apparent that decamethonium is not a short-acting relaxant, for its effects can be extended to such a degree that it is difficult to know when its relaxant action has ceased. Respiratory paralysis passes imperceptibly into the apnoea of ventilatory control, and muscle tone usually remains minimal. The exact stage of the paralysis may be determined by encouraging natural respiration to resume by decreasing inflation pressures. If the depolarisation block has worn off, respiration will then recommence easily and naturally. Intermediate stages of partial respiratory paralysis do not often occur for the effect of decamethonium on respiration tends, surprisingly, to be an "all or nothing" one. Respiratory control can, of course, be practised effectively with other relaxants, but decamethonium has a smoothness and duration of action which is usually superior to most other agents.

The initial dose of decamethonium is now usually limited to a single one of approximately 4 to 6 mg in an average adult and it is expected that the initial profound relaxation will persist for 10 to 20 min, the exact duration depending on age, weight, sex and pulmonary compliance. During this period the neuromuscular block is complete and cannot be reversed by neostigmine, although an injection of pentamethonium or hexamethonium could be used to restore natural respiration if necessary. It can, however, be stated with great confidence that it is unnecessary to use these antagonists and indeed neither of them is now available for this purpose. The return of muscle tone and respiration postoperatively always ensure that the patient can be returned to bed in a satisfactory condition, and the antagonist is needed only on those rare occasions when an operation terminates suddenly or unexpectedly. Whenever it is known that operation time will be longer than 20 min, decamethonium can be used with complete confidence. It should not be employed for operations of shorter duration.

The initial profound relaxation with decamethonium cannot be repeated readily by further doses and it is important to stress that no attempt should be made to do so. In most operations this is not necessary provided respiratory control is maintained, but small incremental doses of 0.5 to 1.0 mg decamethonium with thiopentone were often used in the early years in order to maintain both anaesthesia and relaxation. This technique has now given way to ventilation with halothane, cyclopropane, or other inhalation agents, and there is seldom any need to administer additional decamethonium. However, if relaxation becomes inadequate, as may occur during surgery within the abdominal cavity (judged by the surgeon's assessment of abdominal muscle tone), 10 to 25 mg of suxamethonium may be given and repeated if necessary to maintain optimal conditions. It is an advantage to be able to use a depolarising relaxant in association with decamethonium without fear of a mixed block ensuing. If additional relaxation is required for closure of the peritoneum suxamethonium should always be used in preference to additional decamethonium whose action at this stage, while sometimes only partially effective, is nevertheless always too prolonged.

It is our experience that both young and old patients react favourably to decamethonium. In the young it often appears to have a more profound and prolonged action, which may be due either to the often unintentional higher dose/weight ratio used in smaller subjects or to the fact that easier ventilatory control often occurs in younger persons and facilitates relaxation. Patients in older age groups (40 plus) are usually less sensitive than the young, a full dose seldom having an action longer than 20 min. There is, therefore, no need to reduce the dose with increasing age, and 3 to 5 mg can be given with complete confidence even to patients over 90 years of age. Indeed a remarkable resistance to decamethonium has been observed on a few occasions in elderly patients and in one man of 80 years of age 15 mg of decamethonium produced only a short period of relaxation lasting less than 5 min.

It is important to realise that some experience is needed before the best results can be obtained from this drug. This is because there is a "threshold level" which must be exceeded before adequate paralysis is achieved. Practice is also needed in order to ventilate in the most effective manner. Adequate time must be allowed for full relaxation to occur, and a period of 3 to 5 min is necessary if laryngoscopy and intubation are to be performed with comfort. Dosage cannot be easily related to age or weight, and it is wise to be patient during induction and to ventilate for a few min before intubation is attempted.

IV. Complications

Prolonged apnoea, which undoubtedly was responsible for the majority of complications reported by earlier workers, and for many of the adverse criticisms of decamethonium, has been remarkably absent in this series. The 20 years covered by this analysis includes over 13000 cases where decamethonium was the only relaxant used, and in this large number *there were no cases of prolonged apnoea*. It appears reasonable to state therefore that prolonged neuromuscular block is extremely unlikely to occur *if the total dose of decamethonium has not exceeded 10 mg*. Consequently it is our practice to use this relaxant freely, within this admittedly rather arbitrary limit, with full confidence that prolonged neuromuscular blockade will not occur.

The only cases of prolonged apnoea which we have experienced are those of three patients, all of whom received a mixture of decamethonium with suxamethonium or suxethonium. They are described individually below.

(1) 1961. Male aged 71 years: Operation—Laparotomy for acute abdomen (appendix)
Physical status—4E—Chronic Bronchitis—Râles and Rhonchi. Emphysema and cough, but little sputum. BP 140/80 mm Hg. Large abdomen.

Premedication—Morphine 10 mg; atropine 0.6 mg.

Induction—Thiopentone 400 mg, decamethonium 4 mg with suxethonium 50 mg for intubation (oral tube cuffed). Controlled ventilation with nitrous oxide, oxygen and halothane. A total of 200 mg of suxethonium was used during operation, but more relaxation was needed for the closure of a difficult abdomen, and as no more suxethonium was available 25 mg of suxamethonium was given, following which there was a prolonged apnoea lasting for $1\frac{1}{2}$ hrs. (This appears to be a suxamethonium apnoea.) This man had been anaesthetised by me four months previously when there were no complications following induction with thiopentone 250 mg and maintenance under spontaneous respiration with nitrous oxide and halothane for a short operation to incise an abscess in the groin.

(2) 1962. Male aged 69 years: Operation—Laparotomy for intestinal obstruction.
Physical status—4E—Chronic Bronchitis. Emphysema. Large heart. Harsh systolic murmur. Ankle oedema.
BP 180/100 mm Hg. Giddy attacks. Vomiting blood-stained fluid.
Premedication—Levorphan 1.0 mg; atropine 0.6 mg.
Induction—Thiopentone 100 mg, oral intubation (cuffed tube) under suxamethonium 80 mg. Anaesthesia maintained by controlled ventilation with nitrous oxide, oxygen and ether, assisted by decamethonium 5 mg, and two subsequent doses of suxamethonium, 50 mg each. Total suxamethonium 180 mg. Spontaneous respiration returned after the initial suxamethonium and decamethonium, but after further doses of suxamethonium an irreversible apnoea occurred. There was no reponse to edrophonium (Tensilon) or nalorphine (Lethidrone). Ventilation was maintained but the patient died three days later. Post mortem examination revealed gross bowel obstruction was the cause of death. There was also marked pulmonary emphysema with oedema and lobar pneumonia, together with hypertensive cardiovascular disease. (This, therefore, appears to have been a suxamethonium apnoea, complicated by an unrelieved intestinal obstruction which was the cause of death.)

(3) 1963. Female aged 52 years: Operation—facial plastic (Rhytidectomy)
Physical status—1—Normotensive. Fit.
Premedication—Pethidine 100 mg; scopolamine 0.4 mg.
Induction—Thiopentone 400 mg. Oral intubation under decamethonium 4,5 mg, suxethonium 100 mg. Controlled ventilation thereafter for $1\frac{1}{2}$ hrs with controlled hypotension. Postoperative recovery was delayed, with a slow return of all motor power. Adequate spontaneous respiration resumed after two hours. Eight hours later the patient had recovered completely. Examination of her blood three days later revealed "fluoride number 21", characteristic of the homozygote for the atypical cholinesterase gene. The apnoea therefore was a classical "suxamethonium" apnoea.

During this same period my own records reveal two other cases of prolonged apnoea, one following gallamine (120 mg) and the other suxamethonium (50 mg). Both recovered satisfactorily after an hour of controlled ventilation.

One further case history is of interest. It concerns a man aged 64 who came to operation for an acute appendicitis. He was physically fit (Status 1), normotensive, but with a moderately high intake of alcohol. In view of the anticipated short duration of operation decamethonium was not used and small doses of suxamethonium were given in conjunction with nitrous oxide and halothane. The operation proved to be far more extensive than anticipated as a large neoplasm was found in the pelvis necessitating an extensive gut resection. Adequate relaxation became increasingly difficult to achieve with intermittent doses of suxamethonium, and after a total dose of 175 mg a change was made to decamethonium, a single three mg dose proving entirely satisfactory for the remainder of the operation (45 min). Spontaneous respiration returned uneventfully.

Histamine Release. There has been no obvious association between the administration of decamethonium and histamine release. Although this is said to occur with high doses of decamethonium (GOODMAN and GILMAN, 1970; SNIPER, 1952) it can be stated with confidence that it has not been observed with the doses commonly given in this series. Bronchospasm has been remarkably absent, and it is our practice to use decamethonium freely in all patients, including those who are asthmatic. Other signs of histamine release such as erythema, hypertension, excess salivation and bronchial secretion have likewise been absent.

V. Cardiovascular System and Decamethonium

Decamethonium has been used extensively in operations in which the technique of controlled hypotension by pharmacological blockade was used (ENDERBY, 1974). The lack of any obvious action on heart rate, blood vessels or autonomic ganglia makes it a very satisfactory agent for this purpose, and indeed makes it the relaxant of choice. In all cases, provided there was circulatory stability before anaesthesia was induced, decamethonium has not lowered blood pressure or precipitated cardiovascular collapse.

VI. Muscle Pains and Decamethonium

It can be stated with confidence that muscle pains similar to those following suxamethonium have not occurred with decamethonium. Muscle fasiculations have been seen occasionally but are so rare as to cause comment when observed. They have never been severe and are usually limited to slight facial and limb muscle twitching.

D. Assessment

This analysis of a very large number of cases makes possible an assessment of the qualities and usefulness of decamethonium as a relaxant in modern anaesthetic techniques. One factor of outstanding importance is immediately apparent—there has not been a single instance of prolonged apnoea when decamethonium has been used alone, and this gives it a unique position with regard to safety. In view of our extensive experience it seems reasonable to claim that a single dose not greater than 6 mg or a total not greater than 10 mg is extremely unlikely to cause prolonged neuromuscular blockade in any adult patient. In addition there has been a remarkable freedom from either cardiovascular or respiratory side-effects, so much so that the action of decamethonium appears, at least clinically, to be restricted to the neuromuscular junction.

It is apparent, however, that the drug has shortcomings. The initial profound relaxation cannot easily be repeated with subsequent doses, and this led many of the early workers into mistakes and difficulties in attempting to prolong its action. Furthermore, as mentioned previously, it may prove inadequate for intubation in certain circumstances. The combination of decamethonium with suxamethonium (or suxethonium), as these results indicate, has enabled us to circumvent these major deficiencies successfully. However it is wise to bear in mind that such problems are partly of our own making and can be largely avoided by patience and skill. Thus intubation can nearly always be performed successfully under decamethonium alone provided adequate time has been allowed for its full action to develop. This advice, if taken, would have made a very significant reduction in the use of additional relaxants in this series.

We have found that the manner in which ventilatory control is practised, e.g. by hyperventilation with end-tidal positive pressure determines the speed of return of spontaneous ventilation, and hence the possible need for further increments of the relaxant drug. Relaxation often remains adequate even though neuromuscular block has largely disappeared.

We can claim that decamethonium is still the relaxant of choice, even though there are occasions when the help of short-acting depolarising drugs is necessary. Only very small doses of suxamethonium are needed, and it is clear from these results that few complications have arisen from their use in this manner. These figures underline the need to restrict the total dose of decamethonium and to avoid large additional doses. Apart from the early years when incremental doses were given with thiopentone the vast majority of the work reported here has been with decamethonium as a single dose only.

Thus we have in decamethonium a unique drug which is used as a background for ventilatory control of the anaesthetised patient, achieving on its own very satisfactory relaxation for a limited period of time, but whose initial effects are not reproducible with subsequent doses without the possible danger of prolonged apnoea. It is however a drug which suits our anaesthetic techniques so perfectly that its peculiarities are soon forgiven while its virtues are easily taken for granted. It is a trusted and faithful servant, but as with most servants it has limitations which must be understood and accepted if it is to be retained within the anaesthetic household. It seems reasonable therefore to underline the claim made by ENDERBY (1959) that "it is probably these limitations which impose on this drug its peculiar characteristics and endow it with such a remarkable degree of safety".

References

ARMSTRONG DAVISON, M. H.: Pentamethonium iodide in anaesthesia. Lancet 1950, 1, 252—253.
BARLOW, R. B., ING, H. R.: Curare-like action of polymethylene bis-quaternary ammonium salts. Nature (Lond.) **161**, 718 (1948).
BRENNAN, H. J.: Nitrous oxide-oxygen analgesia in major surgery. Anaesthesia **7**, 27—33 (1952).
CHURCHILL-DAVIDSON, H. C., RICHARDSON, A. T.: Motor end-plate differences as a determining factor in the mode of action of neuromuscular blocking substances. Nature (Lond.) **170**, 617 (1952).

COLLIER, H. O. J.: Descendants of Decamethonium. Brit. J. Anaesth. **25**, 100—115 (1953).

DRIPPS, R. D.: Abnormal respiratory responses to various "curare" drugs during surgical anesthesia: incidence, etiology and treatment. Ann. Surg. **137**, 145—155 (1953).

ENDERBY, G. E. HALE: Muscle relaxation with decamethonium (C 10). Anaesthesia **14**, 138—143 (1959).

ENDERBY, G. E. HALE.: Pharmacological Blockade. Postgraduate Medical Journal 1974, 50, 553.

FISK, G. C.: Decamethonium in clinical anesthesia. Anaesthesia **16**, 89—94 (1961).

GOODMAN, L. S., GILMAN, A.: Pharmacological Basis of Therapeutics (4th Edn), p. 612. London: Collier-Macmillan 1970.

GRAY, A. J.: Decamethonium iodide as a muscle relaxant in abdominal surgery. Lancet **1950 I**, 253—255.

GRIFFITH, H. R., JOHNSON, G. E.: The use of curare in general anaesthesia. Anesthesiology **3**, 418—420 (1942).

GROB, D., HARVEY, A. McG., HOLADAY, D. A.: Some preliminary observations on the neuromuscular and ganglionic blocking action in man of *bis*-Trimethylammonium Decane and Pentane Diiodide. Bull. Johns Hopk. Hosp. **84**, 279—282 (1949).

HARRIS, L. C., DRIPPS, R. D.: The use of decamethonium bromide for the production of muscular relaxation. Anesthesiology **11**, 215—223 (1950).

HEWER, A. J. H., LUCAS, B. G. B., PRESCOTT, F., ROWBOTHAM, E. S.: Decamethonium iodide as a muscle relaxant in anaesthesia. Lancet **1949 I**, 817—819.

HUNTER, A. R.: Decamethonium and Hexamethonium—A Clinical and experimental study. Brit. J. Anaesth. **22**, 218—234 (1950).

LANCET Editorial: Substitutes for curare. **1950 I**, 1043—1044.

LENG, C. O.: Decamethonium in Anaesthesia for Caesarian Section. Singapore med. J. **11**, 173—175 (1970).

MURRAY LAWSON, J. I.: Decamethonium Iodide: A reappraisal. Brit. J. Anaesth. **30**, 240—244 (1958).

MUSHIN, W. W., WIEN, R., MASON, D. F. J., LANGSTON, G. T.: Curare-like actions ot Tri-(Diethylaminoethoxy)-Benzene Triethyliodide. Lancet **1949 I**, 726—728.

NUNN, J. F.: Applied Respiratory Physiology—With special reference to Anaesthesia, pp. 16—44. London: Butterworths 1969.

ORGANE, G. S. W., PATON, W. D. M., ZAIMIS, E. J.: Preliminary trial of *bis*-trimethylammonium decane and pentane di-iodide (C_{10} & C_5) in man. Lancet **1949 I**, 21—23.

PATON, W. D. M., ZAIMIS, E. J.: Curare-like action of polymethylene *bis*-quaternary ammonium salts. Nature (Lond.) **161**, 718—719 (1948).

PATON, W. D. M., ZAIMIS, E. J.: Clinical potentialities of certain *bis*-quaternary salts causing neuromuscular and ganglionic block Nature (Lond.) **162**, 810 (1948).

PATON, W. D. M., ZAIMIS, E. J.: Action and clinical assessment of drugs which produce neuromuscular block. Lancet **1950 II**, 568—570.

PAYNE, J. P.: The influence of carbon dioxide on the neuromuscular blocking activity of relaxant drugs in the cat. Brit. J. Anaesth. **30**, 206—216 (1958).

ROBERTS, T. B. L.: Decamethonium iodide. Lancet **1950 I**, 373.

SADOVE, M. S., MACFARLANE, D. W., PELIKAN, E. W.: Prolonged postanesthetic depression and apnea attributed to Decamethylene-*bis*(Trimethylammonium Bromide). J. Int. Coll. Surg. **13**, 745—747 (1950).

SELLICK, B. A.: Decamethonium iodide in Mayasthenia gravis. Lancet **1950 II**, 822—823.

SCURR, C. F.: A comparative review of the relaxants. Brit. J. Anaesth. **23**, 103—116 (1951).

SNIPER, W.: The estimation and comparison of histamine release by muscle relaxants in man. Brit. J. Anaesth. **24**, 232—237 (1952).

SPENCER, C. H., COAKLEY, C. S.: Clinical evaluation of syncurine (Decamethonium Bromide). A 2 yr. study. Anesthesiology **16**, 125—132 (1955).

THOMAS, K. B.: Decamethonium iodide in anaesthesia. (Correspondence) Lancet **1949 I**, 936.

YOUNG, I. M.: Abdominal relaxation with decamethonium iodide (C 10) during caesarean section. Lancet **1949 I**, 1052.

Author Index

Page numbers in *italics* refer to bibliography.

724

Zablocka-Esplin, B., Esplin,
D. W. 187, *228*
Zablocka-Esplin, B., see
McCandless, D. L.
124, 153, *217*
Zachar, J. 231, 340, *364*
Zacks, S. I. 25, *97*
Zacks, S. I., Blumberg, J. M.
449, 450, *486*
Zacks, S. I., Metzger, J. F.,
Smith, C. W., Blumberg, J. M.
74, *97*, 143, *228*
Zacks, S. I., see Kelly, A. M.
56, *92*
Zadunaisky, J. A., see Conway,
E. J. 378, *415*
Zaimis, E. 4, 9, 10, 11, 13, 14,
20, *21*, 261, 277, *364*, 366, 367,
368, 387, 388, 389, 390, 394,
395, 396, 398, 399, 402, *419*,
443, 453, 454, 458, *486*, 594,
596, 597, 606, 620, 622, 623,
624, 625, *660*
Zaimis, E., Cannard, T. H.,
Price, H. L. 619, *660*
Zaimis, E., Head 589
Zaimis, E., Metaxas, N.,
Havard, C. W. H.,
Campbell, E. D. R. 14, *21*
Zaimis, E., see Bennett, G. 11,
12, *18*
Zaimis, E., see Bigland, B. 14,
18, 400, 401, 402, *414*, 461,
462, 467, *475*

Zaimis, E., see Buttle, G. A. H.
396, *415*, 457, *476*
Zaimis, E., see Cannard, T. H.
4, 7, *18*, 400, 401, 402, *415*,
429, 430, 431, 461, *476*
Zaimis, E., see Child, K. G.
399, *415*
Zaimis, E., see Downman,
C. B. B. 382, *416*
Zaimis, E., see Jewell, P. A.
388, 394, 395, 404, 405, *417*,
460, *480*
Zaimis, E., see Maclagan, J.
429, *481*
Zaimis, E., see Organe, G. S. W.
594, 620, *657*, 661, 663, *675*
Zaimis, E., see Paton, W. D. M.
8, *20*, 365, 366, 368, *418*, 421,
443, 445, 453, 458, 460, 461,
470, *487*, 586, *592*, 595, *657*,
661, 663, 665, 669, *675*
Zaimis, E., see Perry, W. L. M.
385, 386, 396
Zaimis, E., see Vernikos-
Danellis, J. 14, *20*
Zander, E., see Weddell, G. 97
Zander, H. L., see Fellini, A. A.
468, *478*
Zapf, P., see Denborough, M. A.
640, *650*
Zar, M. A., see Paton, W. D. M.
101, 110, 111, 129, 133, 139,
141, 142, 144, 157, *219*
Zatman, L. J., see Burgen, A. S. V.
73, 74, *87*

Zeimal, E. V., see Michelson,
M. J. 3, *20*, 288, *358*, 365,
417, 465, *482*
Zeleńa, J., see Fex, S. 56, *90*
Zeleńa, J., see Jirmanova, I.
74, *92*
Zeleńa, J., see Lubińska, L.
256, *356*
Zeleńa, J., see Miledi, R. 256,
358, 459, *482*
Zengel, J. E., see Magleby, K. L.
336, *357*
Zenker, W., Anzenbacher, H.
27, *97*
Zenker, W., see Anzenbacher, H.
30, *86*
Zieher, L. M., see De Robertis,
E. 104, 120, 178, *201*
Zieher, L. M., see Rodriguez de
Lores Arnaiz, G. 116,
117, 172, *221*
Zierler, K. L., Rogus, E.,
Hazelwood, C. F. 231,
364
Zimmermann, H.,
Whittaker, V. P. 129, 151,
157, 164, 165, *228*
Zimmermann, M., see Braun, M.
336, *343*
Zsigmond, E. K., Downs, J. R.
629, *660*
Zucker, R. S. 313, 314, 315, *364*
Župančič, A. O., see Stalč, A.
259, *361*

Subject Index

(Compiled by the Editor with the collaboration of the individual contributors)

The following abbreviations are used, excepting as primary headings, throughout:

ACh: acetylcholine;
AChE: acetylcholinesterase;
anti-ChE: anticholinesterase;
ATP: adenosine triphosphate;
DFP: di*iso*propyl phosphorofluoridate;

e.p.p.:   end-plate potential;
m.e.p.p.: miniature end-plate potential;
n.m.:   neuromuscular;
TEPP: tetraethyl pyrophosphate

Handbook of Sensory Physiology

Editorial Board: H. Autrum, R. Jung, W. R. Loewenstein,
D. M. MacKay, H. L. Teuber

Vol. I:
Principles of Receptor Physiology
Edited by W. R. Loewenstein

This is an authoritative book dealing with basic chemical and physical
mechanisms on receptor action and with the question of how nerve
connections are made in sensory systems.

Vol. II:
Somatosensory System
Edited by A. Iggo

This book gives an integrated account of the function of the somatosensory
system from the initiation of impulses in specific cutaneous and joint
receptors to the receipt of information in the cerebral cortex of mammals,
including man.

Vol. III/1:
Enteroceptors
Edited by E. Neil

This book consists of essays on the functional characteristics of cardiovascular
mechanoreceptors, arterial chemoreceptors, receptors of the lungs and airways
and abdomino-pelvic visceral receptors with two final chapters on central
receptors concerned with thermoregulation and hunger and thirst.

Vol. III/2:
Muscle Receptors
Edited by C. C. Hunt

This volume describes the structure, function and sensory role of muscle
receptors with emphasis on vertebrate forms, especially mammalian.

Vol. III/3:
**Electroreceptors and Other Specialized
Receptors in Lower Vertebrates**
Edited by A. Fessard

This volume describes electroreceptors in fish with and without electric organs,
lateral-line organs in fish and amphibia, chemo- and pressoreceptor
organs of the pseudobranchial system in some fishes, and the infrared-sensitive
pit organs in some snakes.

Handbuch der experimentellen Pharmakologie/
Handbook of Experimental Pharmacology

Heffter-Heubner, New Series